METHODS IN MOLECULAR BIOLOGY

D1823477

Series Editor
John M. Walker
School of Life and Medical Sciences
University of Hertfordshire
Hatfield, Hertfordshire, UK

For further volumes:
http://www.springer.com/series/7651

For over 35 years, biological scientists have come to rely on the research protocols and methodologies in the critically acclaimed *Methods in Molecular Biology* series. The series was the first to introduce the step-by-step protocols approach that has become the standard in all biomedical protocol publishing. Each protocol is provided in readily-reproducible step-by-step fashion, opening with an introductory overview, a list of the materials and reagents needed to complete the experiment, and followed by a detailed procedure that is supported with a helpful notes section offering tips and tricks of the trade as well as troubleshooting advice. These hallmark features were introduced by series editor Dr. John Walker and constitute the key ingredient in each and every volume of the *Methods in Molecular Biology* series. Tested and trusted, comprehensive and reliable, all protocols from the series are indexed in PubMed.

Toxoplasma gondii

Methods and Protocols

Edited by

Christopher J. Tonkin

Division of Infectious Disease and Immune Defense, The Walter and Eliza Hall Institute of Medical Research, Melbourne, VIC, Australia

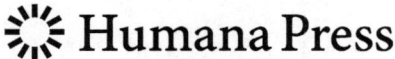 Humana Press

Editor
Christopher J. Tonkin
Division of Infectious Disease and
Immune Defense
The Walter and Eliza Hall Institute
of Medical Research
Melbourne, VIC, Australia

ISSN 1064-3745   ISSN 1940-6029   (electronic)
Methods in Molecular Biology
ISBN 978-1-4939-9859-3   ISBN 978-1-4939-9857-9   (eBook)
https://doi.org/10.1007/978-1-4939-9857-9

Preface

Welcome to the first *Methods in Molecular Biology* edition on *Toxoplasma gondii*. Chapters in this book have been commissioned by leaders in the field and have been designed to cover a diverse array of protocols currently being used by the *Toxoplasma* research community. I have been sure to include protocols that have been standard in the field for many years, as well as those that are pushing the boundaries of what is possible. This will hopefully mean that this volume will be useful for students or groups starting off in the field, as well as for those labs wanting to implement some of the latest techniques that have been developed by other groups.

I would like to take this opportunity to thank all the authors that have contributed to this volume; almost everyone that I approached was willing to contribute. Furthermore, it is a testament to the openness of our community that *Toxoplasma* research groups are so willing to share techniques that have taken years to develop and refine so that others may use these precious resources. It has been a pleasure to edit this volume, and I hope you all enjoy reading it. My wish is that this edition will help all those that want to "crack" some of the many mysteries that *Toxoplasma* still possesses.

Melbourne, Victoria, Australia   *Christopher J. Tonkin*

Contents

Contributors

CATALINA ALVAREZ • *Instituto Gulbenkian de Ciência, Oeiras, Portugal*

BEEJAN ASADY • *Center for Tropical and Emerging Global Diseases, University of Georgia, Athens, GA, USA*

LIAM M. ASHANDER • *College of Medicine and Public Health, Flinders University, Bedford Park, SA, Australia*

MARCO BIDDAU • *Wellcome Centre for Integrative Parasitology, University of Glasgow, Glasgow, UK*

JOHN C. BOOTHROYD • *Department of Microbiology and Immunology, Stanford University School of Medicine, Stanford, CA, USA*

JON P. BOYLE • *Department of Biological Sciences, Dietrich School of Arts and Sciences, University of Pittsburgh, Pittsburgh, PA, USA*

PETER J. BRADLEY • *Department of Microbiology, Immunology and Molecular Genetics, University of California, Los Angeles, CA, USA; Molecular Biology Institute, University of California, Los Angeles, CA, USA*

MALGORZATA BRONCEL • *The Francis Crick Institute, London, UK*

KEVIN M. BROWN • *Department of Microbiology and Immunology, University of Oklahoma Health Sciences Center, Oklahoma City, OK, USA; Department of Molecular Microbiology, Washington University School of Medicine, St. Louis, MO, USA*

CARLA M. CABRAL • *BIO5 Institute, University of Arizona, Tucson, AZ, USA*

ABIGAIL CALIXTO • *Center for Tropical and Emerging Global Diseases, University of Georgia, Athens, GA, USA*

ANA CLAUDIA CAMPOS • *Instituto Gulbenkian de Ciência, Oeiras, Portugal*

VERN B. CARRUTHERS • *Department of Microbiology and Immunology, University of Michigan Medical School, Ann Arbor, MI, USA*

BARBARA CLOUGH • *Host-Toxoplasma Interaction Laboratory, The Francis Crick Institute, London, UK*

SIMON A. COBBOLD • *Department of Biochemistry and Molecular Biology, Bio21 Institute of Molecular Science and Biotechnology, The University of Melbourne, Parkville, VIC, Australia*

MANLIO DI CRISTINA • *Department of Chemistry, Biology, and Biotechnology, University of Perugia, Perugia, Italy*

JITENDER P. DUBEY • *Agricultural Research Service, Animal Parasitic Diseases Laboratory, United States Department of Agriculture (USDA), Beltsville Agricultural Research Center, Beltsville, MD, USA*

DANIEL FISCH • *Host-Toxoplasma Interaction Laboratory, The Francis Crick Institute, London, UK*

EVA-MARIA FRICKEL • *Host-Toxoplasma Interaction Laboratory, The Francis Crick Institute, London, UK*

JOÃO M. FURTADO • *Faculdade de Medicina de Ribeirão Preto, Universidade de São Paulo, Ribeirão Preto, Brazil*

OMAR S. HARB • *Lynch Laboratories, Department of Biology, University of Pennsylvania, Philadelphia, PA, USA*

JONATHAN C. HOWARD • *Instituto Gulbenkian de Ciência, Oeiras, Portugal; Institute for Genetics, Cologne, Germany*

DAMIEN JACOT • *Department of Microbiology and Molecular Medicine, CMU, University of Geneva, Geneva, Switzerland*

ELIZABETH F. B. KING • *Department of Biochemistry and Molecular Biology, Bio21 Institute of Molecular Science and Biotechnology, The University of Melbourne, Parkville, VIC, Australia*

KIARAN KIRK • *Research School of Biology, Australian National University, Acton, ACT, Australia*

ANITA A. KOSHY • *BIO5 Institute, University of Arizona, Tucson, AZ, USA; Department of Immunobiology, University of Arizona, Tucson, AZ, USA; Department of Neurology, University of Arizona, Tucson, AZ, USA*

MARYSE LEBRUN • *UMR 5235 CNRS, Université de Montpellier, Montpellier, France*

ZHU-HONG LI • *Center for Tropical and Emerging Global Diseases, University of Georgia, Athens, GA, USA*

MELISSA B. LODOEN • *Department of Molecular Biology and Biochemistry, University of California, Irvine, Irvine, CA, USA; Institute for Immunology, University of California, Irvine, Irvine, CA, USA*

JOANA LOUREIRO • *Instituto Gulbenkian de Ciência, Oeiras, Portugal*

SEBASTIAN LOURIDO • *Whitehead Institute for Biomedical Research, Cambridge, MA, USA; Biology Department, Massachusetts Institute of Technology, Cambridge, MA, USA*

YUEFANG MA • *College of Medicine and Public Health, Flinders University, Bedford Park, SA, Australia*

JOSHUA MAYORAL • *Department of Pathology, Albert Einstein College of Medicine, Bronx, NY, USA*

MALCOLM J. MCCONVILLE • *Department of Biochemistry and Molecular Biology, Bio21 Institute of Molecular Science and Biotechnology, The University of Melbourne, Parkville, VIC, Australia*

JASON MERCER • *MRC-Laboratory for Molecular Cell Biology, University College London, London, UK*

EMILY F. MERRITT • *Department of Immunobiology, University of Arizona, Tucson, AZ, USA*

SILVIA N. J. MORENO • *Center for Tropical and Emerging Global Diseases, University of Georgia, Athens, GA, USA; Department of Cellular Biology, University of Georgia, Athens, GA, USA*

DEBANJAN MUKHOPADHYAY • *Department of Pathology, Microbiology and Immunology, School of Veterinary Medicine, University of California, Davis, Davis, CA, USA*

URS BENEDIKT MÜLLER • *Institute for Genetics, Cologne, Germany*

SANTHOSH M. NADIPURAM • *Department of Microbiology, Immunology and Molecular Genetics, University of California, Los Angeles, Los Angeles, CA, USA; Division of Pediatric Infectious Diseases, Department of Pediatrics, Cedars-Sinai Medical Center, Los Angeles, CA, USA*

JANA OVCIARIKOVA • *Wellcome Centre for Integrative Parasitology, University of Glasgow, Glasgow, UK*

GEORGIOS PAVLOU • *Institute for Advanced Biosciences (IAB), Team Membrane Dynamics of Parasite-Host Cell Interactions, CNRS UMR5309, INSERM U1209, Université Grenoble Alpes, Grenoble, France*

FEDERICA PIRO • *Department of Chemistry, Biology, and Biotechnology, University of Perugia, Perugia, Italy*

ESTHER RAJENDRAN • *Research School of Biology, Australian National University, Acton, ACT, Australia*

SHIMA RAYATPISHEH • *Department of Biological Chemistry and Institute of Genomics and Proteomics, University of California, Los Angeles, Los Angeles, CA, USA*

ELISE ROCHET • *College of Medicine and Public Health, Flinders University, Bedford Park, SA, Australia*

ANA LINA RODRIGUES • *Instituto Gulbenkian de Ciência, Oeiras, Portugal*

DAVID S. ROOS • *Lynch Laboratories, Department of Biology, University of Pennsylvania, Philadelphia, PA, USA*

JEROEN P. J. SAEIJ • *Department of Pathology, Microbiology and Immunology, School of Veterinary Medicine, University of California, Davis, Davis, CA, USA*

LILACH SHEINER • *Wellcome Centre for Integrative Parasitology, University of Glasgow, Glasgow, UK*

EMILY SHORTT • *Whitehead Institute for Biomedical Research, Cambridge, MA, USA*

L. DAVID SIBLEY • *Department of Molecular Microbiology, Washington University School of Medicine, St. Louis, MO, USA*

JUSTINE R. SMITH • *College of Medicine and Public Health, Flinders University, Bedford Park, SA, Australia*

SARAH L. SOKOL • *Department of Biological Sciences, Dietrich School of Arts and Sciences, University of Pittsburgh, Pittsburgh, PA, USA*

DOMINIQUE SOLDATI-FAVRE • *Department of Microbiology and Molecular Medicine, CMU, University of Geneva, Geneva, Switzerland*

CHUNLEI SU • *Department of Microbiology, University of Tennessee, Knoxville, TN, USA*

CATHERINE SUAREZ • *UMR 5235 CNRS, Université de Montpellier, Montpellier, France*

ISABELLE TARDIEUX • *Institute for Advanced Biosciences (IAB), Team Membrane Dynamics of Parasite-Host Cell Interactions, CNRS UMR5309, INSERM U1209, Université Grenoble Alpes, Grenoble, France*

CHRISTOPHER J. TONKIN • *Division of Infectious Disease and Immune Defense, The Walter and Eliza Hall Institute of Medical Research, Parkville, VIC, Australia*

MORITZ TREECK • *The Francis Crick Institute, London, UK*

ALESSANDRO D. UBOLDI • *Division of Infection and Immunity, The Walter and Eliza Hall Institute of Medical Research, Melbourne, VIC, Australia; Department of Medical Biology, The University of Melbourne, Parkville, Victoria, Australia*

GIEL G. VAN DOOREN • *Research School of Biology, Australian National University, Acton, ACT, Australia*

STEPHEN A. VELLA • *Center for Tropical and Emerging Global Diseases, University of Georgia, Athens, GA, USA*

QIULING WANG • *Department of Molecular Microbiology, Washington University School of Medicine, St. Louis, MO, USA*

LOUIS M. WEISS • *Department of Pathology, Albert Einstein College of Medicine, Bronx, NY, USA; Department of Medicine, Albert Einstein College of Medicine, Bronx, NY, USA*

JAMES A. WOHLSCHLEGEL • *Molecular Biology Institute, University of California, Los Angeles, CA, USA; Department of Biological Chemistry and Institute of Genomics and Proteomics, University of California, Los Angeles, CA, USA*

ZHEE SHEEN WONG • *Department of Biological Sciences, Dietrich School of Arts and Sciences, University of Pittsburgh, Pittsburgh, PA, USA*

ARTUR YAKIMOVICH • *MRC-Laboratory for Molecular Cell Biology, University College London, London, UK*

Chapter 1

What a Difference 30 Years Makes! A Perspective on Changes in Research Methodologies Used to Study *Toxoplasma gondii*

John C. Boothroyd

Abstract

Toxoplasma gondii is a remarkable species with a rich cell, developmental, and population biology. It is also sometimes responsible for serious disease in animals and humans and the stages responsible for such disease are relatively easy to study in vitro or in laboratory animal models. As a result of all this, *Toxoplasma* has become the subject of intense investigation over the last several decades, becoming a model organism for the study of the phylum of which it is a member, *Apicomplexa*. This has led to an ever-growing number of investigators applying an ever-expanding set of techniques to dissecting how *Toxoplasma* "ticks" and how it interacts with its many hosts. In this perspective piece I first wind back the clock 30 years and then trace the extraordinary pace of methodologies that have propelled the field forward to where we are today. In keeping with the theme of this collection, I focus almost exclusively on the parasite, rather than host side of the equation. I finish with a few thoughts about where the field might be headed—though if we have learned anything, the only sure prediction is that the pace of technological advance will surely continue to accelerate and the future will give us still undreamed of methods for taking apart (and then putting back together) this amazing organism with all its intricate biology. We have so far surely just scratched the surface.

Key words Development, Genetics, 'Omics, Host–pathogen interaction, Imaging, Biochemistry, Imaging

1 The State of Play in 1988

I was asked by the editors to provide some perspective on how the methodologies used for the study of *Toxoplasma* have changed over the years and where they might be headed in the future. Given that the median age of those reading this chapter is likely to be about 30, I have decided to start by winding back the clock to the year of your birth, 1988. Ronald Reagan was president of the USA, the Iron Curtain was a formidable barrier dividing Europe, and the BRIC nations (Brazil, Russia, India, and China) had yet to fully burst onto the world stage as economic powerhouses.

Christopher J. Tonkin (ed.), *Toxoplasma gondii: Methods and Protocols*, Methods in Molecular Biology, vol. 2071,
https://doi.org/10.1007/978-1-4939-9857-9_1, © Springer Science+Business Media, LLC, part of Springer Nature 2020

The small group of researchers studying *Toxoplasma gondii* back then knew that it was a fascinating beast with amazing biology and extraordinary cell biology to match. It had been known as an important infectious agent since its first description by Brazilian and Italian researchers 80 years earlier [1]. Its complete life cycle was known but even that knowledge was, remarkably, only 18 years old—the discovery of felines as the definitive host coming from the efforts of many researchers in just 1970 [2, 3]. Among the many implications of this discovery, it showed that *Toxoplasma* was a sexual organism, and thanks to the pioneering efforts of Pfefferkorn and colleagues, it was clear that standard Mendelian genetics could be used to study its haploid genome [4]. As of 1988, it was thought that that haploid genome consisted of about 89 Mbp [5]; this would turn out to be a bit high based on later DNA sequencing of the genome but impressively close for the methods then available. It was also known that the parasites had a curious, circular DNA of about 35 kbp with a very large inverted repeat [6]; with good reason, this was presumed to be mitochondrial DNA but within a decade even that conclusion would prove wrong in a most exciting way, as revealed below.

But perhaps the most powerful tool to be used in studying cell biology in the years leading up to 1988 was the electron microscope (EM) and this amazing instrument had been put to good use, with careful descriptions of the unique and remarkable ultrastructure for each of the *Toxoplasma* life cycle stages, ranging from the sexual cycle in the intestine of the cat (e.g., [7]) to the asexual stages (tachyzoites and bradyzoites) in multiple organs of the parasite's many intermediate hosts. The earliest EM studies, in the mid-1960s, had shown that asexual growth and division in the parasitophorous vacuole (PV) involves a remarkable process wherein two parasites develop within a mother cell, appropriately called endodyogeny [8]. These and earlier EM studies [9] had also revealed a remarkable mixture of membrane-limited organelles ranging from the trinity of dedicated and highly distinct secretory organelles—now called rhoptries, dense granules, and micronemes—to a collection of other distinct but somewhat mysterious structures; these included the spiraling conoid, the convoluted mitochondrion, the girdling inner membrane complex, and a mysterious organelle known by various names, (e.g., "Golgi adjunct" [10]), that was anterior to the nucleus and delimited by multiple membranes. As discussed below, the true identity of this unusual feature would take another three decades to resolve unambiguously.

Many researchers had begun to dissect the adaptive immune response, showing that infection elicited strong B- and T-cell responses and that in most instances this was capable of eliciting protective immunity to reinfection. Immunoblotting had identified a smattering of antigens, each named for its apparent molecular weight in SDS-PAGE (P22, P30, P43, etc.; [11–14]) and some of these were known to be specific to one or other of the different developmental stages [15]. Monoclonal antibodies were a major advance for all of cell biology and many were developed and used to define specific *Toxoplasma* proteins, including their location within the parasites or infected cell [16–18].

Even though in 1988 the molecular biology revolution was well advanced, a grand total of just three protein-coding genes from *Toxoplasma* had been cloned and sequenced (all published just that year, in fact; [19, 20]). Preliminary sequencing of the 18S rRNA had confirmed *Toxoplasma's* phylogenetic placement in the *Apicomplexa* [21]. But even this scant information was enough to show that, unlike the amazingly different gene expression that was being described in the 1980s for trypanosomes (RNA editing, trans-splicing, polycistronic transcription, etc.), the usual rules of eukaryotic gene expression—discrete promoters, abundant mRNA cis-splicing, etc.—were operating in *Toxoplasma*. Although a little disappointing to those of us who had been spoiled by the amazing and exciting differences in the *Kinetoplastida*, this relatively simple molecular biology would ultimately prove to be mostly good news as it would make some of the genetic manipulations to come much easier and let us focus on the intricate cell biology and host–parasite interaction.

At the time, very little was known about how *Toxoplasma* interacts with the host cells it infects, although it had been shown that the tachyzoite stage escapes one of the most potent ways of defending against an invader by avoiding fusion of the PV with the lysosome (unless the parasites had been opsonized and taken up by phagocytosis; [22]). Invasion was known to be an active process and a large number of experimentally tractable host cells had been described in the lab and in nature. The ability to grow the tachyzoites indefinitely in vitro, their ability to form plaques on host monolayers (a wonderfully easy way to assess gross phenotypic differences between strains and mutants, as any virologist will tell you), and the fact that mice are natural hosts, all made development of *Toxoplasma* into a model organism for the study of *Apicomplexa* extremely attractive. And this was the impetus that spurred the development of the many in vitro and in vivo methods to come.

By 1988, epidemiological data had shown that in women, so long as a first infection did not occur during pregnancy, disease was rare even though infection was almost unbelievably common; one oft-cited study from the time reported that in screening pregnant women in Paris, 71% of those of French origin were found to be seropositive [23]! That prevalence would decline in future decades but clearly we were dealing with an organism that was almost omnipresent and, given those staggering numbers, obviously not very pathogenic in the vast majority of at least adult infections. Tragically, though, 1983 was the year that toxoplasmic encephalitis was first reported as a devastating "opportunistic infection" (OI) of those afflicted with a frightening new disease known as AIDS [24–28]. This would prove a game changer for the field as it added to everyone's motivation and provided a sense of real urgency about needing to combat *Toxoplasma* infections. Commensurate with this, incremental funding to combat AIDS and its associated "OIs" began to flow and this would prove key to some of the collective efforts that were soon to be launched.

2   The Next 30 Years: An Explosion of Research, Methods, and Knowledge

Between 1988 and 2018, much was to change and the articles in this volume are all focused on the remarkable range of methods that are available to the field today. The focus in this volume and in this perspective piece is on the study of the parasite, rather than the host, but the same methods that have revolutionized our ability to dissect the parasite have proven no less powerful in dissecting the immune response that is in constant dialogue with the parasite. In the remainder of this article, I will trace some of the major advances that have unfolded on the parasite side since 1988 and then end with what I hope the next decade might bring—although if the history of science has taught us anything about predicting future directions in science, I am a fool for agreeing to do that!

2.1   Harnessing Development: Bradyzoites Yield to In Vitro Methods

Methods for in vitro culture of tachyzoites were fully mature by 1988 but studies of bradyzoites still required sacrificing infected animals. This changed in 1993 when the first in vitro methods for efficiently inducing tachyzoites to switch to bradyzoites were developed [29]. Subsequently, many further ways were found to induce this asexual switch, leading to the ability to select mutants and discover some of the pathways controlling asexual development [30–34]. As discussed further below, and despite much effort by many, however, the sexual stages that occur within the intestinal epithelium of felines have remained resistant to all attempts to drive their development in vitro.

2.2   Genetics: Forward/Reverse/Sideways

While by 1988, the Dartmouth group had shown that forward genetics (isolation of mutants with desired phenotypes) was eminently doable in *Toxoplasma* [35, 36], the full power of these approaches had to wait for the application of molecular biology methods to determine the exact identity of the mutations involved. The first step toward this goal was the development in the early 1990s of methods for introducing DNA into tachyzoites [37–39]. The selectable marker used in those early experiments, chloramphenicol acetyl transferase, was soon augmented with many additional selections ranging from other drug selections, like the elegant hypoxanthine/xanthine/guanine phosphoribosyltransferase that can be both positively and negatively selected [40]), to fusions with fluorescent proteins like GFP and the rainbow of related molecules [41]. All this made possible complementation methods for rescuing the mutants obtained from forward genetic screens and the first such approaches used cosmid libraries made of large pieces of wild type DNA [42]. But these methods were relatively laborious and the full power of forward genetics would have to wait another decade until the development of low-cost, "next-generation" sequencing methods that could provide a complete, reliable genome sequence and thus a rapid and efficient way to identify all the nucleotide changes in a mutant [43, 44].

The ability to introduce DNA into the parasites, including at a specific locus, also enabled "reverse genetics" approaches wherein a specifically mutated allele could be generated within a parasite, either as a point mutation, insertion or a deletion, and then the effect of that mutation on phenotype assessed [37]. This allowed the function of a great many genes and proteins to be dissected with great precision. Reverse genetics can quickly run into a "Catch-22," however, especially in haploid organisms like *Toxoplasma*, where mutants with disruptions in essential genes are hard to obtain since, by definition, they will ablate the ability of the parasites to grow. To overcome this limitation, much effort was put into the development of conditional expression systems whereby a gene can be turned on and off. In this way, the effect of even lethal mutations can be assessed. The first such system used the bacterial tetracycline (*tet*) operator/regulator system [45], but since then additional methods have been developed for turning on/off or up/down a gene's expression including, for example, the use of a dimerizable Cre-recombinase [46]. These have been further augmented by methods to regulate levels of the protein itself (rather than the mRNA) using mammal-derived FKBP degradation domains or "degrons" [47] and the plant-derived auxin-inducible degron or AID [48].

Forward genetics also suffers from this Catch-22 regarding essential genes and the first attempts to obtain such mutants involved selection for temperature-sensitive, "conditional" mutants [49]. These were tricky to generate and analyze, however, and such methods really only came of age with the advent of efficient complementation and/or next-generation sequencing that would reveal the identity of the mutation [50–54]. These led to the discovery of several processes that are crucial, even essential, to the parasite's survival inside a cell. Genes essential for survival in vivo but not for growth in vitro could be identified by an interesting twist on the use of conditional mutants called "signature-tagged mutagenesis." In this approach, insertional mutants are made that each carry a unique tag between common PCR primers, and the mutants that grow in vitro but do not persist in an animal are identified by virtue of the fact that their "signature tag" is present in the input population but missing from the output. This yielded several mutants with a defect in the ability to cause a productive infection [55].

The most recent and even more powerful approach to genome-wide screens for "essential" genes has come with adaptation of the game-changing CRISPR for efficiently targeting insertions to specific loci in *Toxoplasma* [56, 57]. Targeting all predicted genes of *Toxoplasma* followed by growth in culture and then asking which CRISPR tags are absent in the final population reveals which genes are necessary for fitness, defined here as growth in vitro. Doing this for the entire *Toxoplasma* genome has generated a "fitness score" for each of the ~8000 genes [58], an invaluable resource to the community. Further CRISPR screens will soon follow and will enable genes to be identified that are necessary for other conditions, including infection in animal models. In the meantime, the method has vastly accelerated and simplified the ability to target genes for "editing" (e.g., deletion or alteration), making reverse genetics even easier to perform on specific genes identified through other means.

What I will call "sideways" genetics also emerged in the 1990s; that is, the use of laboratory crosses (in cats) of naturally occurring variants/strains to create genetic maps and to map traits like virulence or other phenotypes that naturally vary between strains. Given the very wide host range and worldwide distribution of *Toxoplasma*, it is not too surprising that naturally occurring strains can vary enormously in everything from their antigenicity [15, 59] and lethality in lab mice [60] to how they interact with the host [61] and even whether they recruit host mitochondria to the parasitophorous vacuole [62]. But the necessary prerequisite to using crosses to identify the causal genes was to create a detailed genetic map by exploiting restriction-fragment-length-polymorphisms (RFLPs) to analyze F1 progeny from crosses performed between two strains in cats [63]. By way of historical footnote, I think it is fair to say that it was a mix of good fortune and the intuition of Elmer Pfefferkorn that the two strains used for that first cross were of different clonotypes as this work was done before the population biology studies had revealed the dominance of just three strains in most European and American labs' collections [64–66]; absent such intuition, this early cross could easily have been done using strains that were in fact clonally related (e.g., both Type II or Type I strains) and the progeny from such a cross would have been completely useless for genetic mapping (since the two parents would have essentially identical genomes and thus no mappable polymorphisms).

Once a genetic map was in hand, it became possible to map any naturally variable phenotype by returning to these same F1 progeny and looking for which loci cosegregated with the phenotype of interest. The extraordinary results to come from this "sideways" genetics are described further below.

2.3 Nascent Genomics/ Transcriptomics: Data, Data, Data ...

One of the most exciting discoveries to come early on from advances in DNA sequencing was the finding that the 35 kbp circular DNA mentioned above was not mitochondrial in origin but instead derived from an ancestral red algal plastid and that the mysterious multimembraned organelle anterior to the nucleus was its home [67, 68]!

Advances in DNA sequencing were exploding in the 1990s and these helped launch the 'omics revolution and "big data" science. Within the community of *Toxoplasma* researchers as well as some of the major funders (like NIH in the USA and Wellcome Trust in the UK), there was a recognition that making the most of these approaches would require a concerted effort and budgets that, as a rule, were not within sight for individual researchers. Partly sparked by the ongoing AIDS pandemic, and through meetings organized by major funders, there was a coalescence around the idea of making strategic efforts on specific, achievable "omics" goals. At each of these meetings, there was extensive dialogue about what was the intersection of the community's greatest need and cutting-edge methods to deliver on that need in a cost-effective way. I think it fair to say that the "Davids" (Roos and Sibley) were the major forces pushing for this approach and the first deliverable was a collection of "expressed sequence tags" (ESTs) from tachyzoites, which was a fancy way of saying a large number of random cDNA sequences [69]. These were initially generated from tachyzoite mRNA and even the first datasets proved enormously informative. Suddenly, the community could see the presence of extensive gene families encoding proteins unique to *Toxoplasma* and related *Apicomplexa*. These included the family encoding surface proteins defined by their homology to the first such gene to be cloned, *SAG1* [19], and hence termed SAG1-Related Sequences or SRSs [70]. Also revealed by this first glimpse into the *Toxoplasma* genome were genes encoding proteins related to the intriguing rhoptry protein kinases, the so-called ROP2 family [71, 72]. Later, and as discussed below, some of these ROP kinases would be found to serve as major, polymorphic virulence factors responsible for certain strain-specific differences in virulence seen in experimental mouse infections.

EST sequencing, while a powerful method that massively accelerated the discovery of many important genes, was limited by relative mRNA abundance; genes that were lowly expressed or perhaps not expressed at all in the tachyzoite stage that was used for these initial studies were not represented within these first EST datasets. With the development of yet further improvements and even lower costs of DNA sequencing, therefore, efforts turned to going for a complete genome! This was an ambitious and, for its time, expensive goal but the community again coalesced around the importance of such a resource and a concerted effort was made to sequence at least one "reference" strain. The choice for the first strain was ME49 because it was representative of the one of the most common clonotypes (Type II, which is responsible for the vast majority of infections in western Europe, at least [64–66]) and strains existed that were known to be "cat-competent"—that is, capable of completing the full life cycle of the parasites, including sexual development in cats. Later, a representative of the more commonly studied Type I lab strain RH was added to the list (GT1 was used in place of RH since it was clonally related to RH but did not suffer from RH's limitation of having been grown in tissue culture for decades with all the attendant genetic changes that might have been selected by such biologically artificial passage). More strains would soon follow, and probably because the sequence data were annotated and loaded onto a publically available website in almost "real time" (ToxoDB, *see* below), a formal publication describing the genome sequence only came out in 2016, when the number of sequenced strains had grown to 62 [73]! These sequences represent an extraordinarily rich resource for the entire community, one that is really only just beginning to be mined.

2.4 ToxoDB Is Born: A Place to Make Sense of All That 'Omics Data . . .

With these various large datasets came the need for a way to make the data accessible to all. In the spirit of other communities of scientists, such as those studying model systems like yeast and flies, this led to the creation of ToxoDB [74]. From its first inception to now, ToxoDB has grown exponentially and become a resource not only for storing the ever-growing types of 'omic datasets but also for interrogating the information in a way that allows researchers to discover new biological processes. Indeed, its popularity and utility served as a model for many other pathogens, resulting in its expansion into EuPathDB that now provides "one-stop shopping" for researchers studying most of the major eukaryotic pathogens ranging from fungi like *Cryptococcus* and *Aspergillus* to protists like *Plasmodium, Trypanosoma, Giardia,* and *Trichomonas.*

The importance of ToxoDB to researchers in and out of the field is hard to overstate. For example, the ability to go to one "page" and see all the information for a given gene/protein consolidated in a well-organized format means someone interested in that gene for whatever reason—for example, data from a CRISPR screen, a mutation in a forward-genetic screen or a "hit" in a proteomic analysis of a novel protein complex—can instantly know almost all there is to know about that gene. Similarly, someone doing an 'omics analysis of their own can download all the data from other 'omics efforts and look for intersections and commonalities that can reveal otherwise obscure connections, pathways, etc.

2.5 'Omics Efforts Expand: No Such Thing as Too Much Data!

While genome sequences are a key tool, at their simplest, they simply represent lists of genes. Except in cases of obvious homology, like evolutionarily conserved housekeeping genes and the *SRS* and *ROP2* gene families described above, such lists reveal little about function. To get to that, other 'omics datasets were needed. Among the 'omics efforts that proved most informative were gene expression (transcriptomics) studies that at first were based on hybridization of fluorescently tagged cDNAs from a given stage to spotted microarrays comprised of mechanically applied EST fragments [75, 76]. These first generation microarrays suffered from the same limitations as the EST libraries from which they were made, however: they were derived from only a subset of the most abundantly expressed genes and from only the most easily obtained developmental stages (tachyzoites and bradyzoites). These were soon superseded by use of the recently derived, complete genome sequence and Affymetrix's technology that allowed DNA synthesis on a "chip" [77]. Using mRNA from a range of developmental stages and different conditions, including using tachyzoites synchronized with respect to their progression through the cell cycle, these "Affy arrays" gave crucial clues to the function of many genes, including in developmental stages like oocysts emanating from cats [78] that, even today, remain technically challenging to study by other means.

Parallel to these studies of the parasite's gene expression, transcriptomic analysis of the infected host cells or tissue was occurring. This too started with spotted cDNA microarrays [79–81] but soon progressed to the far more sophisticated and powerful Affymetrix arrays. Today, next-generation sequencing has made possible extremely high-throughput RNASeq that yields millions of reads for each experimental condition and including data on both the parasite and host transcriptomes [82–86]. These studies have helped dissect the cross-talk between host and parasite in intricate detail, revealing many of the interactions described in the section that follows.

Another powerful 'omics dataset to be produced that helped make sense of all the genomic data was the use of high-throughput analysis of DNA fragments bound to histones carrying specific post-translational modifications indicative of an active or silenced locus. In addition to data on whether a gene was "on" or "off" in a given condition, these datasets also revealed important information about where genes begin and end [87–89].

As for other model organisms, the 'omics revolution also early on expanded to proteomic studies, including stage- and organelle-specific proteomes, that helped reveal the functions of some of the many discrete organelles that make *Toxoplasma* zoites such extraordinary beasts [90–92]. These include analysis of proteins secreted by free parasites [93] as well as proteins found in purified rhoptries [94], ultimately leading to the identification of key components of the invasion machinery (the so-called RONs because they derive from the rhoptry necks [95, 96]) and injected effectors dominated by the ROP2 family mentioned above [72]. Glycomic [97], lipidomic [98, 99], and metabolomic [100] studies are fast catching up as described in some of the chapters that follow. These promise to give us a much more complete picture of the totality of how these remarkable parasites operate as cells within cells.

Regulation of key functions is often controlled through phosphorylation, and *Toxoplasma* kinases that control processes such as invasion and egress have been described. Identification of these enzymes emerged from a mix of candidate gene approaches and genetics; and phosphoproteomics—an attempt to determine the complete set of all phosphorylation sites on all proteins—soon allowed at least a beginning determination of the targets and functions of these proteins [101–104]. This is one of many areas, however, where today we know only a tiny fraction of what remains to be discovered.

2.6 Small Molecules as Probes: "Chemical Genetics"

Although not a method that is easily deployed by your average biologist, the use of vast libraries of small molecules to interrogate function can produce unique results. Sometimes referred to as "chemical genetics" because, like its namesake, it makes no assumptions about what might be found and involves screening of large numbers of variants, this approach has yielded some important and intriguing targets. One of the first uses of this approach [105] eventually yielded the finding that myosin light chain is necessary for motility and invasion, as revealed by the activity of a small molecule that was found to be modifying, and thereby inactivating, the myosin component [106, 107]. In another screen, this time using molecules deliberately designed to covalently modify their target, it was relatively easy to move from showing activity against the parasite to identifying the target of the molecule [108]. This yielded an evolutionarily conserved but enigmatic protein, DJ-1, that proved to be key to calcium signaling in invasion and that might have been hard to discover by other means. As advances in chemistry are combined with yet further developments in robotics, the ability to explore molecular "space" and probe many of the most important functions of *Toxoplasma* seems likely to yield further insights. Perhaps most important, however, is the fact that this approach starts with a small, chemically synthesized molecule of known structure and this should vastly accelerate the process of translating a "basic research" finding into a therapeutically useful compound.

2.7 Interaction with the Host: Complexity Squared

Toxoplasma is an obligate intracellular infectious agent. Almost by definition, then, its life is intertwined with that of the many hosts it infects. Studying or thinking about it in isolation will miss much of the most intriguing biology that has attracted many of us the most to its study. This interaction with a host cell can be broken down into two general areas: the physical interaction that includes invasion into a host cell; and the biological interaction involving a molecular dialogue within the cell.

Mostly thanks to a mix of some of the 'omics methods mentioned above, along with some judicious use of methods like immunoprecipitation and mass spectrometry to identify protein complexes, we now know much more about how *Toxoplasma* zoites invade into a cell and it is a remarkable process. It likely begins with an initial interaction with the surface SRS proteins, soon followed by more intimate and higher affinity interactions between micronemal proteins shed onto the surface and proteins on the hosts cell surface [109]. Something that I do not think anyone anticipated in 1988 is the finding that these "host" surface proteins can include proteins that *Toxoplasma* zoites inject into the host cell [95, 110, 111]. This is a remarkable asset for an intracellular parasite, providing at least the possibility of expanding the host range since they bring their own receptor to the party.

As mentioned above, in 1988 we had only intuition to point to how intricate the interaction with the host might be, with actual data at the time largely indicating only that tachyzoites were relatively passive players expressing unsophisticated antigens that could be targeted by an intelligent and sophisticated immune response. But adopting the mindset that a tachyzoite or bradyzoite is really a giant virus, with the same opportunities and challenges of those simple entities, inevitably led to the suspicion that these parasites were likely much more active than passive in the host–parasite dialogue. And thanks to the combination of genetics and 'omics, on both the parasite and host sides, we now know that *Toxoplasma* zoites are phenomenally active participants in the conversation.

One of the first pieces of evidence to suggest this came with the observation that the rhoptry protein, ROP2, sat on the parasitophorous vacuole membrane, facing into the host cell cytosol [112], and that this was a likely property of other members of this extensive family [72]. An indication that the parasites might not be just muttering to their host cell but were engaged in full-on shouting came from the novel finding that another rhoptry protein, a protein phosphatase, no less, could cross the parasitophorous vacuole membrane (PVM) and transit across the host cell's cytosol, eventually reaching the host nucleus [113]! These results indicated that "effectors" as had been recently described in bacteria and as had long been known (but not called that) in viruses were in play here too. Soon, it was clear that many, perhaps all lumenal rhoptry proteins are injected into the host cell and that these interact with the host cell in many important ways. For example, it had long been known that there were major differences in the virulence of different strains, and genetic crosses described above proved a powerful way to map some of the genes responsible for those differences.

These crosses soon revealed that several polymorphic members of the ROP2-related ROPK family, ROP16, ROP17 and ROP18, are involved in a "molecular arms race" with the host immunity-related GTPases (IRGs) [114–120]. The IRGs are a key way that mice defend against intracellular infectious agents like *Toxoplasma*, attacking and destroying the PVM. Given that the IRGs are themselves a polymorphic family of ~20 genes in commonly studied mouse strains, it appears that there has been a long-lasting situation wherein mutations on one side are countered by mutations in the other and that there has been substantial evolutionary pressure on each leading to the expansion of both the IRG and ROP2 family genes, among others [121].

A recently developed tool that may help fill in the missing gaps about how *Toxoplasma* interacts with the host cell makes use of the powerful Cre-recombinase system and the many animals that have "floxed" (*flanked by lox* sites) genes. When Cre recombinase is fused to a rhoptry protein (toxofilin) that is injected into host cells [122], the Cre can excise the floxed segment in the host DNA removing or turning on (if the "floxed" portion is a stop signal) individual genes. When the host cells have "floxed stop" fluorescent reporters, this results in turn-on of the reporter allowing the injected host cell to be readily apparent [123]. Using this method allows even rare infected cells to stand out in infected tissue and, perhaps more interestingly, reveals the existence of uninfected-injected cells that have received the injected Cre but are not infected [124, 125]. What role such "uninfected-injected" cells play in the host–parasite interaction is not yet known but they could prove to be important players in both the acute and chronic stages of an infection.

For a few years, dense granules seemed to take a back seat to the rhoptries, at least in terms of dramatic impacts on the host cell; but that all changed with the discovery that these organelles too could be a source of potent "effectors" that could reach all the way to the host nucleus. Clever analysis of the 'omics datasets revealed proteins that were predicted to be secreted but that also had a classic nuclear-localization signal that hinted they might travel beyond the "usual" destination for such proteins—at least as far as was thought at the time—the parasitophorous vacuole. Indeed, when these were pursued using the methods highlighted here, two were found to be potent dense granule effectors that reach the host nucleus, GRA16 and GRA24 [126–128]. These have a profound effect on the host cell through interacting with key host signaling pathways. Their export is dependent on the aspartyl protease, ASP5 [129–131], and genetic screens for mutants unable to interfere with host c-*Myc* regulation (and hence dubbed Myr mutants) helped reveal the novel machinery used to translocate them across the PVM [132, 133]. It seems certain that the full complement of dense granule effectors performing key functions will prove to be substantial—TgIST, which interferes with STAT1-dependent transcription, has already been added to the list [134, 135] and more surely await discovery. Indeed, RNASeq experiments using cells infected with Myr1-mutants predicts the involvement of many effectors, both activators and suppressors, that are translocated by the Myr machinery [136].

2.8 Back to Basics: Leveraging Individual Proteins to Discover Key Complexes

Powerful as all those 'omics are, eventually one has to return to the individual gene or protein to dissect its exact function. A first question that is often posed as a start to understanding function is, "with what other proteins does my protein interact?" Immunoprecipitation of the protein in question (often epitope tagged for convenience) followed by mass spectrometry to identify the associating partners has become a "go-to" method for deducing such complexes. A few examples of key structures so revealed are the "glideosome" that mediates the gliding motility and invasion of tachyzoites [137–142] and the "moving junction" (MJ) complex that sits at the interface between the invading zoite and host plasma membrane during invasion [95, 110]. Interactions with host proteins have also been determined in this way, including with the rhoptry protein toxofilin [143], the GRA16 and GRA24 effectors mentioned above [126, 128] and the MJ components [144].

Development of proximity labeling (e.g., using a promiscuous biotin ligase, or "BioID") similarly has facilitated the discovery of one protein to identify nearby, potentially interacting partners. This has helped reveal a rich collection of proteins functioning in locations as diverse as the inner membrane complex [145, 146], the developing parasitophorous vacuole [147] and the apical conoid [148]. These systems of proximity labeling will no doubt have great utility in the future as they potentially have the capacity to identify interactions that occur in a narrow window of time or have a lower affinity.

2.9 Advances in Imaging: Could any Cell Be More Elegant and Beautiful?

Imaging methods have continued to advance and the resolution obtained has progressed commensurately. As just one example, helium-ion microscopy has revealed the parasites as they reside within the vacuole, including the startling detail of the intravacuolar network [149], and cryo-electron tomography is revealing subcellular structures with unprecedented resolution [150]. And while the 'omics revolution has given us long lists of genes, proteins, and other molecules, one of the most powerful ways to understand their functions is to know when and where those molecules are expressed. And for this, the field has made good use of major advances in imaging technology (e.g., light microscopy combined with immunofluorescence to localize proteins using antibodies generated to recombinant protein or, with the advent of the reverse genetics methods, antibodies to epitope tags like HA, Myc, and FLAG, and/or fusions to fluorescent proteins) [41]. Combined with improved imaging systems, such as confocal and superresolution light microscopy, and another time-honored workhorse, immunoelectron microscopy, the result has been an extraordinary "atlas" of *Toxoplasma* proteins in the context of an infected cell. As always, this work has been dominated by use of tachyzoites but glimpses into the other stages reveal additional elegant structures that are no less spectacular [151].

As exciting and impressive as the analysis of protein location within the parasite and infected host cell have been, the ability to see into the infected animal has revealed no less remarkable and unexpected findings. Two-photon microscopy, for example, has revealed how the parasites function and migrate within tissue, including the lymph node [152], brain [153] and intestine [154].

A more macroscopic view of how infections progress came with the development of bioluminescent methods for imaging the parasites in the entirety of an infected animal [155]. This so-called bioluminescent imaging built on studies first done with bacteria but exploiting the fact that firefly luciferase emits a wavelength of light (red) that travels remarkably well through tissue and even through thin bone like the cranium of mice. This method has helped monitor *Toxoplasma* infection in individual animals over a prolonged period, thereby improving the quality of the data obtained (time-course experiments can be done monitoring the same animal over days, weeks or even months) while simultaneously decreasing the number of animals that needed to be used, a clear win-win.

3   The Future: There Is NO Sign That Things Will Slow Down Anytime Soon ...

It is probably safe to say that back in 1988 no one could have predicted where we are today and so I worry that speculating on what the future might hold is a fool's errand. But there are some trends, and it is probably reasonable to at least speculate about a few methods that are already on the horizon and are likely to impact the field in ways every bit as powerfully as the advances described above. The chapters that follow will do this for the areas they each describe but I will offer a few of my own here.

One way in which trends are clear is the ever-increasing sensitivity of the methods available to the modern biologist. We can do much more with much less material, albeit at ever-increasing financial cost! Single-cell analyses are already here and these can provide powerful insights into gene expression in the individual parasite and host cell. Such can provide unprecedented information about variation that cannot be deduced from studies with populations of cells, for example, about how gene expression might differ throughout the cell cycle of the parasite as well as differences that might exist between individual parasites and host cells that are otherwise in nominally exactly the same state (e.g., in the same stage of the cell cycle).

Likewise, the ability to examine the function of individual molecules is a game-changer in providing atomic detail of the extraordinary molecular machines operating as *Toxoplasma* interacts with its host. This is especially true as these advances are paired with the further advances in imaging that now allow atomic resolution of complex biological structures through methods like cryo-electron tomography. It is hard to look at the apical end of a zoite and not be in awe of the phenomenal biological machine looking back at you. How this mix of cytoskeletal structures and multiple secretory organelles functions as it moves in and out with the conoid's protrusion will be rich pickings for cell biologists.

The speed and power of DNA sequencing continues to accelerate and the price continues to drop. This has the potential to make genetic studies even easier—we may soon be able to sequence complex populations and detect mutations in this complex mix making the identification of mutations responsible for important phenotypes even easier.

On top of all this, there can be little doubt that we are in an unusual time in biology where what seems to be limiting is not the ability to generate large amounts of interesting data but the ability to process it in a way that yields discrete and meaningful conclusions. When an RNASeq experiment can yield literally a billion unique datapoints (sequences) from both the parasite and the infected host, it is almost certain that far more information resides within these datasets than can be gleaned by the investigators harvesting the data in real time. Bioinformaticians are racing to devise yet faster and more powerful ways of analyzing ever-larger datasets and we live in a world where it is possible to make a good living as a researcher simply analyzing the data generated by others. One can, for example, ask which genes of *Toxoplasma* encode proteins that are (1) likely to be secreted because of a predicted signal peptide, (2) stage-specific, (3) highly variable between strains and thus under positive selection; (4) expressed at a stage of the cell cycle that indicates it is likely a component of a particular secretory organelle like the rhoptries, and (5) unique to *Toxoplasma* and its closest cousins. Add that all up and, voila, you almost certainly have "discovered" a collection of important effectors that are interacting with the infected host cell. And all from the comfort of your favorite reading chair (like the one I am writing this review in)!! Analyses such as this are completely dependent on complete and accurate databases like ToxoDB and the power and importance of this key resource will only grow with the mass of data it includes. The community of parasitologists owes a large debt to the continued leadership of Jessica Kissinger and David Roos in maintaining this truly extraordinary resource.

As parasitologists, we have both the challenge and the privilege of dealing with "complexity-squared"—the study of incredibly complex parasites interacting with equally complex hosts. This squaring of the problem makes taking a true "systems" approach correspondingly far more complex but such must clearly be the goal of anyone wanting to fully understand host–parasite interaction.

Integrating databases consisting of parasite and host 'omics data is an enormous bioinformatic challenge but one that we, as parasitologists, must embrace if we are to fully understand the dances we watch. ToxoDB has begun that process, but it is far from a simple task.

I will end with what might be considered the start of *Toxoplasma's* complex life cycle. Although many investigators have tried to reproduce the sexual (feline) part of the cycle in vitro, all efforts have so far failed to yield the desired oocysts. But there is clearly no "law of physics" that needs to be broken to accomplish this and the efforts of the field as a whole seem like they must eventually force the parasite to cede us this crucial tool. Being able to complete the entire life cycle in vitro would provide a huge saving in cost and convenience for those anxious to exploit genetic crosses for all their power of understanding the roles of various genes; but much more importantly, it would open up the amazing sexual development occurring in the cat intestine that remains largely mysterious, beyond the elegant but essentially descriptive work from electron and immunofluorescence microscopy and, most recently, RNASeq [156, 157]. This part of the parasite's developmental biology is probably even richer than the asexual tachyzoite and bradyzoite stages which seem relatively simple, at least when reduced to their essence: invade—divide—exit (or encyst and stay put). The sexual cycle involves far more complexity with radically different forms and development. One of my favorite conundrums is how a microgamete finds and fertilizes a macrogamete inside (we presume) an epithelial cell, not to mention how these gametes form and develop with such efficiency and with so little associated sequelae in the feline host. I used the word "shouting," above, when referring to the conversation that can occur between a tachyzoite and the infected host cell but perhaps "argument" would have been a better word to describe this interchange; at least during infections like those seen with a Type I strain where a raging cytokine storm inevitably kills a lab mouse within about 9–10 days. Within the cat intestine, the conversation may be much more nuanced, maybe more akin to an oft-repeated dialogue established long ago between simpatico life partners who happily accept and respect each other's independence, despite or perhaps because of years of cohabitation. Time, and a *lot* of exciting work yet to be done, will surely tell . . . .

References

1. Nicolle C, Manceaux L (1908) Sur une infection a corps de Leishman (ou organismes voisins) du gondi. C R Acad Sci III 146:207–209

2. Dubey JP, Miller NL, Frenkel JK (1970) *Toxoplasma gondii* life cycle in cats. J Am Vet Med Assoc 157(11):1767–1770

3. Witte HM, Piekarski G (1970) Oocyst excretion in experimentally infected cats depending on the *Toxoplasma* strain. Z Parasitenkd 33 (4):358–360

4. Pfefferkorn ER, Pfefferkorn LC (1980) *Toxoplasma gondii*: genetic recombination between drug resistant mutants. Exp Parasitol 50:305–316

5. Cornelissen AW, Overdulve JP, van der Ploeg M (1984) Determination of nuclear DNA of

five eucoccidian parasites, *Isospora* (*Toxoplasma*) *gondii*, Sarcocystis cruzi, Eimeria tenella, E. acervulina and Plasmodium berghei, with special reference to gamontogenesis and meiosis in *I.* (*T.*) *gondii*. Parasitology 88(Pt 3):531–553

6. Borst P, Overdulve JP, Weijers PJ, Fase-Fowler F, Van den Berg M (1984) DNA circles with cruciforms from Isospora (*Toxoplasma*) *gondii*. Biochim Biophys Acta 781 (1–2):100–111

7. Ferguson DJ, Hutchison WM, Dunachie JF, Siim JC (1974) Ultrastructural study of early stages of asexual multiplication and microgametogony of *Toxoplasma gondii* in the small intestine of the cat. Acta Pathol Microbiol Scand B: Microbiol Immunol 82 (2):167–181

8. Wildfuhr W (1966) Electron microscopic studies on the morphology and reproduction of *Toxoplasma gondii*. II. Observations on the reproduction of *Toxoplasma gondii* (endodyogeny). Zentralbl Bakteriol Orig 201 (1):110–130

9. Scholtyseck E, Piekarski G (1965) Electron microscopic studies on merozoites of Eimeria (Eimeria perforans and E. stidae) and *Toxoplasma gondii*. On the systematic position of *T. gondii*. Z Parasitenkd 26(2):91–115

10. Ogino N, Yoneda C (1966) The fine structure and mode of division of *Toxoplasma gondii*. Arch Ophthalmol 75(2):218–227

11. Handman E, Goding JW, Remington JS (1980) Detection and characterization of membrane antigens of *Toxoplasma gondii*. J Immunol 124(6):2578–2583

12. Johnson AM (1985) The antigenic structure of *Toxoplasma gondii*: a review. Pathology 17 (1):9–19

13. Kasper LH, Crabb JH, Pfefferkorn ER (1983) Purification of a major membrane protein of *Toxoplasma gondii* by immunoabsorption with a monoclonal antibody. J Immunol 130 (5):2407–2412

14. Couvreur G, Sadak A, Fortier B, Dubremetz JF (1988) Surface antigens of *Toxoplasma gondii*. Parasitology 97(Pt 1):1–10

15. Ware PL, Kasper LH (1987) Strain-specific antigens of *Toxoplasma gondii*. Infect Immun 55(3):778–783

16. Araujo FG, Handman E, Remington JS (1980) Use of monoclonal antibodies to detect antigens of *Toxoplasma gondii* in serum and other body fluids. Infect Immun 30(1):12–16

17. Sethi KK, Endo T, Brandis H (1980) Hybridomas secreting monoclonal antibody with specificity for *Toxoplasma gondii*. J Parasitol 66(2):192–196

18. Johnson AM, McNamara PJ, Neoh SH, McDonald PJ, Zola H (1981) Hybridomas secreting monoclonal antibody to *Toxoplasma gondii*. Aust J Exp Biol Med Sci 59 (Pt 3):303–306

19. Burg JL, Perelman D, Kasper LH, Ware PL, Boothroyd JC (1988) Molecular analysis of the gene encoding the major surface antigen of *Toxoplasma gondii*. J Immunol 141 (10):3584–3591

20. Nagel SD, Boothroyd JC (1988) The alpha- and beta-tubulins of *Toxoplasma gondii* are encoded by single copy genes containing multiple introns. Mol Biochem Parasitol 29 (2–3):261–273

21. Johnson AM, Murray PJ, Illana S, Baverstock PJ (1987) Rapid nucleotide sequence analysis of the small subunit ribosomal RNA of *Toxoplasma gondii*: evolutionary implications for the Apicomplexa. Mol Biochem Parasitol 25 (3):239–246

22. Sibley LD, Weidner E, Krahenbuhl JL (1985) Phagosome acidification blocked by intracellular *Toxoplasma gondii*. Nature 315 (6018):416–419

23. Jeannel D, Niel G, Costagliola D, Danis M, Traore BM, Gentilini M (1988) Epidemiology of toxoplasmosis among pregnant women in the Paris area. Int J Epidemiol 17 (3):595–602

24. Danziger A, Leibman AJ (1983) Cerebral toxoplasmosis in a patient with acquired immunodeficiency syndrome. Surg Neurol 20(4):332–334. PubMed PMID: 6623346

25. Dozier N, Ballentine R, Adams SC, Okafor KC (1983) Acquired immune deficiency syndrome and the management of associated opportunistic infections. Drug Intell Clin Pharm 17(11):798–807

26. Handler M, Ho V, Whelan M, Budzilovich G (1983) Intracerebral toxoplasmosis in patients with acquired immune deficiency syndrome. J Neurosurg 59(6):994–1001. PubMed PMID: 6631520

27. Horowitz SL, Bentson JR, Benson F, Davos I, Pressman B, Gottlieb MS (1983) CNS toxoplasmosis in acquired immunodeficiency syndrome. Arch Neurol 40(10):649–652

28. Moskowitz LB, Kory P, Chan JC, Haverkos HW, Conley FK, Hensley GT (1983) Unusual causes of death in Haitians residing in Miami. High prevalence of opportunistic infections. JAMA 250(9):1187–1191

29. Soete M, Fortier B, Camus D, Dubremetz JF (1993) *Toxoplasma gondii*: kinetics of

bradyzoite-tachyzoite interconversion in vitro. Exp Parasitol 76(3):259–264

30. Singh U, Brewer JL, Boothroyd JC (2002) Genetic analysis of tachyzoite to bradyzoite differentiation mutants in *Toxoplasma gondii* reveals a hierarchy of gene induction. Mol Microbiol 44(3):721–733. PubMed PMID: 11994153

31. Matrajt M, Donald RG, Singh U, Roos DS (2002) Identification and characterization of differentiation mutants in the protozoan parasite *Toxoplasma gondii*. Mol Microbiol 44(3):735–747. PubMed PMID: 11994154

32. Anderson MZ, Brewer J, Singh U, Boothroyd JC (2009) A pseudouridine synthase homologue is critical to cellular differentiation in *Toxoplasma gondii*. Eukaryot Cell 8(3):398–409. https://doi.org/10.1128/EC.00329-08. PubMed PMID: 19124578; PubMed Central PMCID: PMC2653242

33. Craver MP, Rooney PJ, Knoll LJ (2010) Isolation of *Toxoplasma gondii* development mutants identifies a potential proteophosphogylcan that enhances cyst wall formation. Mol Biochem Parasitol 169(2):120–123. https://doi.org/10.1016/j.molbiopara.2009.10.006. PubMed PMID: 19879901; PubMed Central PMCID: PMC2791180

34. Patil V, Lescault PJ, Lirussi D, Thompson AB, Matrajt M (2012) Disruption of the expression of a non-coding RNA significantly impairs cellular differentiation in *Toxoplasma gondii*. Int J Mol Sci 14(1):611–624. https://doi.org/10.3390/ijms14010611. PubMed PMID: 23275028; PubMed Central PMCID: PMC3565285

35. Kasper LH, Crabb JH, Pfefferkorn ER (1982) Isolation and characterization of a monoclonal antibody-resistant antigenic mutant of *Toxoplasma gondii*. J Immunol 129(4):1694–1699

36. Kasper LH, Pfefferkorn ER (1982) Hydroxyurea inhibition of growth and DNA synthesis in *Toxoplasma gondii*: characterization of a resistant mutant. Mol Biochem Parasitol 6(3):141–150

37. Kim K, Soldati D, Boothroyd JC (1993) Gene replacement in *Toxoplasma gondii* with chloramphenicol acetyltransferase as selectable marker. Science 262(5135):911–914

38. Soldati D, Boothroyd JC (1993) Transient transfection and expression in the obligate intracellular parasite *Toxoplasma gondii*. Science 260(5106):349–352

39. Donald RG, Roos DS (1993) Stable molecular transformation of *Toxoplasma gondii*: a selectable dihydrofolate reductase-thymidylate synthase marker based on drug- resistance mutations in malaria. Proc Natl Acad Sci U S A 90(24):11703–11707

40. Roos DS, Donald RG, Morrissette NS, Moulton AL (1994) Molecular tools for genetic dissection of the protozoan parasite *Toxoplasma gondii*. Methods Cell Biol 45:27–63

41. Striepen B, He CY, Matrajt M, Soldati D, Roos DS (1998) Expression, selection, and organellar targeting of the green fluorescent protein in *Toxoplasma gondii*. Mol Biochem Parasitol 92(2):325–338

42. Striepen B, White MW, Li C, Guerini MN, Malik SB, Logsdon JM Jr et al (2002) Genetic complementation in apicomplexan parasites. Proc Natl Acad Sci U S A 99(9):6304–6309. PubMed PMID: 11959921

43. Farrell A, Thirugnanam S, Lorestani A, Dvorin JD, Eidell KP, Ferguson DJ et al (2012) A DOC2 protein identified by mutational profiling is essential for apicomplexan parasite exocytosis. Science 335(6065):218–221. https://doi.org/10.1126/science.1210829. PubMed PMID: 22246776

44. Garrison E, Treeck M, Ehret E, Butz H, Garbuz T, Oswald BP et al (2012) A forward genetic screen reveals that calcium-dependent protein kinase 3 regulates egress in *Toxoplasma*. PLoS Pathog 8(11):e1003049. https://doi.org/10.1371/journal.ppat.1003049. PubMed PMID: 23209419; PubMed Central PMCID: PMC3510250

45. Meissner M, Brecht S, Bujard H, Soldati D (2001) Modulation of myosin a expression by a newly established tetracycline repressor-based inducible system in *Toxoplasma gondii*. Nucleic Acids Res 29(22):E115. PubMed PMID: 11713335

46. Andenmatten N, Egarter S, Jackson AJ, Jullien N, Herman JP, Meissner M (2013) Conditional genome engineering in *Toxoplasma gondii* uncovers alternative invasion mechanisms. Nat Methods 10(2):125–127. https://doi.org/10.1038/nmeth.2301. PubMed PMID: 23263690; PubMed Central PMCID: PMC3605914

47. Herm-Gotz A, Agop-Nersesian C, Munter S, Grimley JS, Wandless TJ, Frischknecht F et al (2007) Rapid control of protein level in the apicomplexan *Toxoplasma gondii*. Nat Methods 4(12):1003–1005. https://doi.org/10.1038/nmeth1134. PubMed PMID: 17994029; PubMed Central PMCID: PMC2601725

48. Brown KM, Long S, Sibley LD (2018) Conditional knockdown of proteins using Auxin-inducible Degron (AID) fusions in

Toxoplasma gondii. Bio Protoc 8(4). https://doi.org/10.21769/BioProtoc.2728. PubMed PMID: 29644255; PubMed Central PMCID: PMCPMC5890294

49. Pfefferkorn ER, Pfefferkorn LC (1976) *Toxoplasma gondii*: isolation and preliminary characterization of temperature-sensitive mutants. Exp Parasitol 39(3):365–376

50. Coleman BI, Gubbels MJ (2012) A genetic screen to isolate *Toxoplasma gondii* host-cell egress mutants. J Vis Exp 60. https://doi.org/10.3791/3807. PubMed PMID: 22349295

51. Chen CT, Gubbels MJ (2013) The *Toxoplasma gondii* centrosome is the platform for internal daughter budding as revealed by a Nek1 kinase mutant. J Cell Sci 126 (Pt 15):3344–3355. https://doi.org/10.1242/jcs.123364. PubMed PMID: 23729737; PubMed Central PMCID: PMC3730244

52. Suvorova ES, Croken M, Kratzer S, Ting LM, de Felipe MC, Balu B et al (2013) Discovery of a splicing regulator required for cell cycle progression. PLoS Genet 9(2):e1003305. https://doi.org/10.1371/journal.pgen.1003305. Epub 2013/02/26. PGENETICS-D-12-01651 [pii]. PubMed PMID: 23437009; PubMed Central PMCID: PMC3578776

53. Suvorova ES, Francia M, Striepen B, White MW (2015) A novel bipartite centrosome coordinates the apicomplexan cell cycle. PLoS Biol 13(3):e1002093. https://doi.org/10.1371/journal.pbio.1002093. PubMed PMID: 25734885; PubMed Central PMCID: PMCPMC4348508

54. Naumov A, Kratzer S, Ting LM, Kim K, Suvorova ES, White MW (2017) The *Toxoplasma* Centrocone houses cell cycle regulatory factors. MBio 8(4). https://doi.org/10.1128/mBio.00579-17. PubMed PMID: 28830940; PubMed Central PMCID: PMCPMC5565962

55. Knoll LJ, Furie GL, Boothroyd JC (2001) Adaptation of signature-tagged mutagenesis for *Toxoplasma gondii*: a negative screening strategy to isolate genes that are essential in restrictive growth conditions. Mol Biochem Parasitol 116(1):11–16. PubMed PMID: 11463461

56. Shen B, Brown KM, Lee TD, Sibley LD (2014) Efficient gene disruption in diverse strains of *Toxoplasma gondii* using CRISPR/CAS9. MBio 5(3):e01114–e01114. https://doi.org/10.1128/mBio.01114-14. PubMed PMID: 24825012; PubMed Central PMCID: PMC4030483

57. Sidik SM, Hackett CG, Tran F, Westwood NJ, Lourido S (2014) Efficient genome engineering of *Toxoplasma gondii* using CRISPR/Cas9. PLoS One 9(6):e100450. https://doi.org/10.1371/journal.pone.0100450. PubMed PMID: 24971596; PubMed Central PMCID: PMC4074098

58. Sidik SM, Hortua Triana MA, Paul AS, El Bakkouri M, Hackett CG, Tran F et al (2016) Using a genetically encoded sensor to identify inhibitors of *Toxoplasma gondii* Ca^{2+} signalling. J Biol Chem. https://doi.org/10.1074/jbc.M115.703546. PubMed PMID: 26933036

59. Windeck T, Gross U (1996) *Toxoplasma gondii* strain-specific transcript levels of SAG1 and their association with virulence. Parasitol Res 82(8):715–719

60. de Roever-Bonnet H (1969) Congenital *Toxoplasma* infections in mice and hamsters infected with avirulent and virulant strains. Trop Geogr Med 21(4):443–450

61. Suzuki Y, Yang Q, Remington JS (1995) Genetic resistance against acute toxoplasmosis depends on the strain of *Toxoplasma gondii*. J Parasitol 81(6):1032–1034

62. Pernas L, Adomako-Ankomah Y, Shastri AJ, Ewald SE, Treeck M, Boyle JP et al (2014) *Toxoplasma* effector MAF1 mediates recruitment of host mitochondria and impacts the host response. PLoS Biol 12(4):e1001845. https://doi.org/10.1371/journal.pbio.1001845. PubMed PMID: 24781109; PubMed Central PMCID: PMC4004538

63. Sibley LD, LeBlanc AJ, Pfefferkorn ER, Boothroyd JC (1992) Generation of a restriction fragment length polymorphism linkage map for *Toxoplasma gondii*. Genetics 132 (4):1003–1015

64. Sibley LD, Boothroyd JC (1992) Virulent strains of *Toxoplasma gondii* comprise a single clonal lineage. Nature 359(6390):82–85

65. Darde ML, Bouteille B, Pestre-Alexandre M (1992) Isoenzyme analysis of 35 *Toxoplasma gondii* isolates and the biological and epidemiological implications. J Parasitol 78 (5):786–794

66. Howe DK, Sibley LD (1995) *Toxoplasma gondii* comprises three clonal lineages: correlation of parasite genotype with human disease. J Infect Dis 172(6):1561–1566

67. Fichera ME, Roos DS (1997) A plastid organelle as a drug target in apicomplexan parasites. Nature 390(6658):407–409

68. McFadden GI, Reith ME, Munholland J, Lang-Unnasch N (1996) Plastid in human parasites [letter]. Nature 381(6582):482

69. Ajioka JW, Boothroyd JC, Brunk BP, Hehl A, Hillier L, Manger ID et al (1998) Gene discovery by EST sequencing in *Toxoplasma gondii* reveals sequences restricted to the Apicomplexa. Genome Res 8(1):18–28

70. Manger ID, Hehl AB, Boothroyd JC (1998) The surface of *Toxoplasma* tachyzoites is dominated by a family of glycosylphosphatidylinositol-anchored antigens related to SAG1. Infect Immun 66 (5):2237–2244

71. Herion P, Hernandez-Pando R, Dubremetz JF, Saavedra R (1993) Subcellular localization of the 54-kDa antigen of *Toxoplasma gondii*. J Parasitol 79(2):216–222

72. El Hajj H, Demey E, Poncet J, Lebrun M, Wu B, Galeotti N et al (2006) The ROP2 family of *Toxoplasma gondii* rhoptry proteins: proteomic and genomic characterization and molecular modeling. Proteomics 6 (21):5773–5784. PubMed PMID: 17022100

73. Lorenzi H, Khan A, Behnke MS, Namasivayam S, Swapna LS, Hadjithomas M et al (2016) Local admixture of amplified and diversified secreted pathogenesis determinants shapes mosaic *Toxoplasma gondii* genomes. Nat Commun 7:10147. https://doi.org/10.1038/ncomms10147. PubMed PMID: 26738725; PubMed Central PMCID: PMCPMC4729833

74. Kissinger JC, Gajria B, Li L, Paulsen IT, Roos DS (2003) ToxoDB: accessing the *Toxoplasma gondii* genome. Nucleic Acids Res 31 (1):234–236. PubMed PMID: 12519989

75. Cleary MD, Singh U, Blader IJ, Brewer JL, Boothroyd JC (2002) *Toxoplasma gondii* asexual development: identification of developmentally regulated genes and distinct patterns of gene expression. Eukaryot Cell 1 (3):329–340. PubMed PMID: 12455982

76. Su C, Hott C, Brownstein BH, Sibley LD (2004) Typing single-nucleotide polymorphisms in *Toxoplasma gondii* by allele-specific primer extension and microarray detection. Methods Mol Biol 270:249–262. PubMed PMID: 15153632

77. Bahl A, Davis PH, Behnke M, Dzierszinski F, Jagalur M, Chen F et al (2010) A novel multifunctional oligonucleotide microarray for *Toxoplasma gondii*. BMC Genomics 11:603. https://doi.org/10.1186/1471-2164-11-603. Epub 2010/10/27. doi: 1471-2164-11-603 [pii]. PubMed PMID: 20974003; PubMed Central PMCID: PMC3017859

78. Buchholz KR, Fritz HM, Chen X, Durbin-Johnson B, Rocke DM, Ferguson DJ et al (2011) Identification of tissue cyst wall components by transcriptome analysis of in vivo and in vitro *Toxoplasma gondii* bradyzoites. Eukaryot Cell 10(12):1637–1647. https://doi.org/10.1128/EC.05182-11. Epub 2011/10/25. doi: EC.05182-11 [pii]. PubMed PMID: 22021236; PubMed Central PMCID: PMC3232729

79. Blader IJ, Manger ID, Boothroyd JC (2001) Microarray analysis reveals previously unknown changes in *Toxoplasma gondii*-infected human cells. J Biol Chem 276 (26):24223–24231. PubMed PMID: 11294868

80. Chaussabel D, Semnani RT, McDowell MA, Sacks D, Sher A, Nutman TB (2003) Unique gene expression profiles of human macrophages and dendritic cells to phylogenetically distinct parasites. Blood 102(2):672–681. PubMed PMID: 12663451

81. Knight BC, Kissane S, Falciani F, Salmon M, Stanford MR, Wallace GR (2006) Expression analysis of immune response genes of Muller cells infected with *Toxoplasma gondii*. J Neuroimmunol 179(1–2):126–131. PubMed PMID: 16934877

82. Tuda J, Mongan AE, Tolba ME, Imada M, Yamagishi J, Xuan X et al (2011) Full-parasites: database of full-length cDNAs of apicomplexa parasites, 2010 update. Nucleic Acids Res 39(Database issue):D625–D631. https://doi.org/10.1093/nar/gkq1111. Epub 2010/11/06. doi: gkq1111. PubMed PMID: 21051343; PubMed Central PMCID: PMC3013703

83. Hassan MA, Melo MB, Haas B, Jensen KD, Saeij JP (2012) De novo reconstruction of the *Toxoplasma gondii* transcriptome improves on the current genome annotation and reveals alternatively spliced transcripts and putative long non-coding RNAs. BMC Genomics 13:696. https://doi.org/10.1186/1471-2164-13-696. Epub 2012/12/13. doi: 1471-2164-13-696. PubMed PMID: 23231500; PubMed Central PMCID: PMC3543268

84. Tanaka S, Nishimura M, Ihara F, Yamagishi J, Suzuki Y, Nishikawa Y (2013) Transcriptome analysis of mouse brain infected with *Toxoplasma gondii*. Infect Immun.. Epub 2013/07/17. https://doi.org/10.1128/IAI.00439-13. PubMed PMID: 23856619.

85. Pittman KJ, Aliota MT, Knoll LJ (2014) Dual transcriptional profiling of mice and *Toxoplasma gondii* during acute and chronic infection. BMC Genomics 15:806. https://doi.org/10.1186/1471-2164-15-806. PubMed PMID: 25240600; PubMed Central PMCID: PMC4177681

86. Swierzy IJ, Handel U, Kaever A, Jarek M, Scharfe M, Schluter D et al (2017) Divergent co-transcriptomes of different host cells infected with *Toxoplasma gondii* reveal cell type-specific host-parasite interactions. Sci Rep 7(1):7229. https://doi.org/10.1038/s41598-017-07838-w. PubMed PMID: 28775382; PubMed Central PMCID: PMCPMC5543063

87. Gissot M, Kelly KA, Ajioka JW, Greally JM, Kim K (2007) Epigenomic modifications predict active promoters and gene structure in *Toxoplasma gondii*. PLoS Pathog 3(6):e77. https://doi.org/10.1371/journal.ppat.0030077. Epub 2007/06/15. doi: 07-PLPA-RA-0114. PubMed PMID: 17559302; PubMed Central PMCID: PMC1891328

88. Sautel CF, Cannella D, Bastien O, Kieffer S, Aldebert D, Garin J et al (2007) SET8-mediated methylations of histone H4 lysine 20 mark silent heterochromatic domains in apicomplexan genomes. Mol Cell Biol 27 (16):5711–5724. https://doi.org/10.1128/MCB.00482-07. Epub 2007/06/15. doi: MCB.00482-07. PubMed PMID: 17562855; PubMed Central PMCID: PMC1952134

89. Bougdour A, Sautel CF, Cannella D, Braun L, Hakimi MA (2008) *Toxoplasma gondii* gene expression is under the control of regulatory pathways acting through chromatin structure. Parasite 15(3):206–210. Epub 2008/09/26 PubMed PMID: 18814682

90. Dlugonska H, Dytnerska K, Reichmann G, Stachelhaus S, Fischer HG (2001) Towards the *Toxoplasma gondii* proteome: position of 13 parasite excretory antigens on a standardized map of two-dimensionally separated tachyzoite proteins. Parasitol Res 87 (8):634–637. PubMed PMID: 11511000

91. Nischik N, Schade B, Dytnerska K, Dlugonska H, Reichmann G, Fischer HG (2001) Attenuation of mouse-virulent *Toxoplasma gondii* parasites is associated with a decrease in interleukin-12-inducing tachyzoite activity and reduced expression of actin, catalase and excretory proteins. Microbes Infect 3(9):689–699. PubMed PMID: 11489417

92. Cohen AM, Rumpel K, Coombs GH, Wastling JM (2002) Characterisation of global protein expression by two-dimensional electrophoresis and mass spectrometry: proteomics of *Toxoplasma gondii*. Int J Parasitol 32 (1):39–51. PubMed PMID: 11796121

93. Zhou XW, Kafsack BF, Cole RN, Beckett P, Shen RF, Carruthers VB (2005) The opportunistic pathogen *Toxoplasma gondii* deploys a diverse legion of invasion and survival proteins. J Biol Chem 280 (40):34233–34244. PubMed PMID: 16002397

94. Bradley PJ, Ward C, Cheng SJ, Alexander DL, Coller S, Coombs GH et al (2005) Proteomic analysis of rhoptry organelles reveals many novel constituents for host-parasite interactions in *Toxoplasma gondii*. J Biol Chem 280 (40):34245–34258. PubMed PMID: 16002398

95. Lebrun M, Michelin A, El Hajj H, Poncet J, Bradley PJ, Vial H et al (2005) The rhoptry neck protein RON4 re-localizes at the moving junction during *Toxoplasma gondii* invasion. Cell Microbiol 7(12):1823–1833. PubMed PMID: 16309467

96. Alexander DL, Arastu-Kapur S, Dubremetz JF, Boothroyd JC (2006) Plasmodium falciparum AMA1 binds a rhoptry neck protein homologous to TgRON4, a component of the moving junction in *Toxoplasma gondii*. Eukaryot Cell 5(7):1169–1173. PubMed PMID: 16835460

97. Fauquenoy S, Morelle W, Hovasse A, Bednarczyk A, Slomianny C, Schaeffer C et al (2008) Proteomics and glycomics analyses of N-glycosylated structures involved in *Toxoplasma gondii*--host cell interactions. Mol Cell Proteomics 7(5):891–910. https://doi.org/10.1074/mcp.M700391-MCP200. Epub 2008/01/12. PubMed PMID: 18187410

98. Welti R, Mui E, Sparks A, Wernimont S, Isaac G, Kirisits M et al (2007) Lipidomic analysis of *Toxoplasma gondii* reveals unusual polar lipids. Biochemistry 46 (48):13882–13890. https://doi.org/10.1021/bi7011993. Epub 2007/11/09. PubMed PMID: 17988103; PubMed Central PMCID: PMC2576749

99. Besteiro S, Bertrand-Michel J, Lebrun M, Vial H, Dubremetz JF (2008) Lipidomic analysis of *Toxoplasma gondii* tachyzoites rhoptries: further insights into the role of cholesterol. Biochem J 415(1):87–96. https://doi.org/10.1042/BJ20080795. Epub 2008/06/20. PubMed PMID: 18564055

100. Ramakrishnan S, Docampo MD, Macrae JI, Pujol FM, Brooks CF, van Dooren GG et al (2012) Apicoplast and endoplasmic reticulum cooperate in fatty acid biosynthesis in apicomplexan parasite *Toxoplasma gondii*. J Biol Chem 287(7):4957–4971. https://doi.org/10.1074/jbc.M111.310144. Epub 2011/

12/20. PubMed PMID: 22179608; PubMed Central PMCID: PMC3281623

101. Treeck M, Sanders JL, Elias JE, Boothroyd JC (2011) The Phosphoproteomes of plasmodium falciparum and *Toxoplasma gondii* reveal unusual adaptations within and beyond the Parasites' boundaries. Cell Host Microbe 10 (4):410–419. https://doi.org/10.1016/j. chom.2011.09.004. Epub 2011/10/25. doi: S1931-3128(11)00288-5 [pii]. PubMed PMID: 22018241

102. Treeck M, Sanders JL, Gaji RY, LaFavers KA, Child MA, Arrizabalaga G et al (2014) The calcium-dependent protein kinase 3 of *Toxoplasma* influences basal calcium levels and functions beyond egress as revealed by quantitative phosphoproteome analysis. PLoS Pathog 10(6):e1004197. https://doi.org/ 10.1371/journal.ppat.1004197. PubMed PMID: 24945436; PubMed Central PMCID: PMC4063958

103. Al-Bajalan MMM, Xia D, Armstrong S, Randle N, Wastling JM (2017) *Toxoplasma gondii* and Neospora caninum induce different host cell responses at proteome-wide phosphorylation events; a step forward for uncovering the biological differences between these closely related parasites. Parasitol Res 116(10):2707–2719. https://doi.org/10. 1007/s00436-017-5579-7. PubMed PMID: 28803361

104. He C, Chen AY, Wei HX, Feng XS, Peng HJ (2017) Phosphoproteome of *Toxoplasma gondii* infected host cells reveals specific cellular processes predominating in different phases of infection. Am J Trop Med Hyg 97 (1):236–244. https://doi.org/10.4269/ ajtmh.16-0901. PubMed PMID: 28719319; PubMed Central PMCID: PMCPMC5508905

105. Carey KL, Westwood NJ, Mitchison TJ, Ward GE (2004) A small-molecule approach to studying invasive mechanisms of *Toxoplasma gondii*. Proc Natl Acad Sci U S A 101 (19):7433–7438. PubMed PMID: 15123807

106. Heaslip AT, Leung JM, Carey KL, Catti F, Warshaw DM, Westwood NJ et al (2010) A small-molecule inhibitor of *T. gondii* motility induces the posttranslational modification of myosin light chain-1 and inhibits myosin motor activity. PLoS Pathog 6(1):e1000720. https://doi.org/10.1371/journal.ppat. 1000720. Epub 2010/01/20. PubMed PMID: 20084115; PubMed Central PMCID: PMC2800044

107. Leung JM, Tran F, Pathak RB, Poupart S, Heaslip AT, Ballif BA et al (2014) Identification of *T. gondii* myosin light chain-1 as a direct target of TachypleginA-2, a small-molecule inhibitor of parasite motility and invasion. PLoS One 9(6):e98056. https://doi.org/10.1371/journal.pone. 0098056. PubMed PMID: 24892871; PubMed Central PMCID: PMC4043638

108. Hall CI, Reese ML, Weerapana E, Child MA, Bowyer PW, Albrow VE et al (2011) Chemical genetic screen identifies *Toxoplasma* DJ-1 as a regulator of parasite secretion, attachment, and invasion. Proc Natl Acad Sci U S A 108(26):10568–10573. https://doi.org/ 10.1073/pnas.1105622108. Epub 2011/ 06/15. PubMed PMID: 21670272; PubMed Central PMCID: PMC3127939

109. Carruthers VG, Sibley LD (1997) Sequential protein secretion from three distinct organelles of *Toxoplasma gondii* accompanies invasion of human fibroblasts. Eur J Cell Biol 73:114–123

110. Alexander DL, Mital J, Ward GE, Bradley P, Boothroyd JC (2005) Identification of the moving junction complex of *Toxoplasma gondii*: a collaboration between distinct secretory organelles. PLoS Pathog 1(2):e17. PubMed PMID: 16244709

111. Tonkin ML, Roques M, Lamarque MH, Pugniere M, Douguet D, Crawford J et al (2011) Host cell invasion by apicomplexan parasites: insights from the co-structure of AMA1 with a RON2 peptide. Science 333 (6041):463–467. https://doi.org/10.1126/ science.1204988. Epub 2011/07/23. doi: 333/6041/463. PubMed PMID: 21778402

112. Sinai AP, Joiner KA (2001) The *Toxoplasma gondii* protein ROP2 mediates host organelle association with the parasitophorous vacuole membrane. J Cell Biol 154(1):95–108. PubMed PMID: 11448993

113. Gilbert LA, Ravindran S, Turetzky JM, Boothroyd JC, Bradley PJ (2007) *Toxoplasma gondii* targets a protein phosphatase 2C to the nuclei of infected host cells. Eukaryot Cell 6 (1):73–83. PubMed PMID: 17085638

114. Saeij JP, Boyle JP, Coller S, Taylor S, Sibley LD, Brooke-Powell ET et al (2006) Polymorphic secreted kinases are key virulence factors in toxoplasmosis. Science 314 (5806):1780–1783. https://doi.org/10. 1126/science.1133690. Epub 2006/12/ 16. doi: 314/5806/1780. PubMed PMID: 17170306; PubMed Central PMCID: PMC2646183

115. Taylor S, Barragan A, Su C, Fux B, Fentress SJ, Tang K et al (2006) A secreted serine-threonine kinase determines virulence in the eukaryotic pathogen *Toxoplasma gondii*.

Science 314(5806):1776–1780. PubMed PMID: 17170305

116. Saeij JP, Coller S, Boyle JP, Jerome ME, White MW, Boothroyd JC (2007) *Toxoplasma* co-opts host gene expression by injection of a polymorphic kinase homologue. Nature 445 (7125):324–327. PubMed PMID: 17183270

117. Khaminets A, Hunn JP, Konen-Waisman S, Zhao YO, Preukschat D, Coers J et al (2010) Coordinated loading of IRG resistance GTPases on to the *Toxoplasma gondii* parasitophorous vacuole. Cell Microbiol 12 (7):939–961. https://doi.org/10.1111/j. 1462-5822.2010.01443.x. Epub 2010/01/ 30. PubMed PMID: 20109161; PubMed Central PMCID: PMC2901525

118. Reese ML, Zeiner GM, Saeij JP, Boothroyd JC, Boyle JP (2011) Polymorphic family of injected pseudokinases is paramount in *Toxoplasma* virulence. Proc Natl Acad Sci U S A 108(23):9625–9630. https://doi.org/10. 1073/pnas.1015980108. Epub 2011/03/ 26. PubMed PMID: 21436047; PubMed Central PMCID: PMC3111280

119. Behnke MS, Fentress SJ, Mashayekhi M, Li LX, Taylor GA, Sibley LD (2012) The polymorphic pseudokinase ROP5 controls virulence in *Toxoplasma gondii* by regulating the active kinase ROP18. PLoS Pathog 8(11): e1002992. https://doi.org/10.1371/jour nal.ppat.1002992. Epub 2012/11/13. PPATHOGENS-D-12-01380 [pii]. PubMed PMID: 23144612; PubMed Central PMCID: PMC3493473

120. Niedelman W, Gold DA, Rosowski EE, Sprokholt JK, Lim D, Farid Arenas A et al (2012) The rhoptry proteins ROP18 and ROP5 mediate *Toxoplasma gondii* evasion of the murine, but not the human, interferon-gamma response. PLoS Pathog 8(6): e1002784. https://doi.org/10.1371/jour nal.ppat.1002784. Epub 2012/07/05. PPATHOGENS-D-11-02761 [pii]. PubMed PMID: 22761577; PubMed Central PMCID: PMC3386190

121. Gazzinelli RT, Mendonca-Neto R, Lilue J, Howard J, Sher A (2014) Innate resistance against *Toxoplasma gondii*: an evolutionary tale of mice, cats, and men. Cell Host Microbe 15(2):132–138. https://doi.org/ 10.1016/j.chom.2014.01.004. PubMed PMID: 24528860

122. Lodoen MB, Gerke C, Boothroyd JC (2010) A highly sensitive FRET-based approach reveals secretion of the actin-binding protein toxofilin during *Toxoplasma gondii* infection. Cell Microbiol 12(1):55–66. https://doi.

org/10.1111/j.1462-5822.2009.01378.x. Epub 2009/09/08. PubMed PMID: 19732057

123. Koshy AA, Fouts AE, Lodoen MB, Alkan O, Blau HM, Boothroyd JC (2010) *Toxoplasma* secreting Cre recombinase for analysis of host-parasite interactions. Nat Methods 7 (4):307–309. https://doi.org/10.1038/ nmeth.1438. Epub 2010/03/09. PubMed PMID: 20208532; PubMed Central PMCID: PMC2850821

124. Koshy AA, Dietrich HK, Christian DA, Melehani JH, Shastri AJ, Hunter CA et al (2012) *Toxoplasma* co-opts host cells it does not invade. PLoS Pathog 8(7):e1002825. https://doi.org/10.1371/journal.ppat. 1002825. Epub 2012/08/23. PPATHO-GENS-D-11-02798. PubMed PMID: 22910631; PubMed Central PMCID: PMC3406079

125. Christian DA, Koshy AA, Reuter MA, Betts MR, Boothroyd JC, Hunter CA (2014) Use of transgenic parasites and host reporters to dissect events that promote interleukin-12 production during toxoplasmosis. Infect Immun 82(10):4056–4067. https://doi. org/10.1128/IAI.01643-14. PubMed PMID: 25024368; PubMed Central PMCID: PMC4187868

126. Bougdour A, Durandau E, Brenier-Pinchart MP, Ortet P, Barakat M, Kieffer S et al (2013) Host cell subversion by *Toxoplasma* GRA16, an exported dense granule protein that targets the host cell nucleus and alters gene expression. Cell Host Microbe 13(4):489–500. https://doi.org/10.1016/j.chom.2013.03. 002. Epub 2013/04/23. doi: S1931-3128 (13)00112-1. PubMed PMID: 23601110

127. Braun L, Brenier-Pinchart MP, Yogavel M, Curt-Varesano A, Curt-Bertini RL, Hussain T et al (2013) A *Toxoplasma* dense granule protein, GRA24, modulates the early immune response to infection by promoting a direct and sustained host p38 MAPK activation. J Exp Med 210(10):2071–2086. https://doi. org/10.1084/jem.20130103. PubMed PMID: 24043761; PubMed Central PMCID: PMCPMC3782045

128. Bougdour A, Tardieux I, Hakimi MA (2014) *Toxoplasma* exports dense granule proteins beyond the vacuole to the host cell nucleus and rewires the host genome expression. Cell Microbiol 16(3):334–343. https://doi.org/ 10.1111/cmi.12255. PubMed PMID: 24373221

129. Coffey MJ, Sleebs BE, Uboldi AD, Garnham A, Franco M, Marino ND et al (2015) An aspartyl protease defines a novel

pathway for export of *Toxoplasma* proteins into the host cell. Elife 4. https://doi.org/10.7554/eLife.10809. PubMed PMID: 26576949; PubMed Central PMCID: PMCPMC4764566

130. Hammoudi PM, Jacot D, Mueller C, Di Cristina M, Dogga SK, Marq JB et al (2015) Fundamental Roles of the Golgi-associated *Toxoplasma* aspartyl protease, ASP5, at the Host-Parasite Interface. PLoS Pathog 11 (10):e1005211. https://doi.org/10.1371/journal.ppat.1005211. PubMed PMID: 26473595; PubMed Central PMCID: PMCPMC4608785

131. Curt-Varesano A, Braun L, Ranquet C, Hakimi MA, Bougdour A (2016) The aspartyl protease TgASP5 mediates the export of the *Toxoplasma* GRA16 and GRA24 effectors into host cells. Cell Microbiol 18 (2):151–167. https://doi.org/10.1111/cmi.12498. PubMed PMID: 26270241

132. Franco M, Panas MW, Marino ND, Lee MC, Buchholz KR, Kelly FD et al (2016) A novel secreted protein, MYR1, is central to *Toxoplasma's* manipulation of host cells. MBio 7 (1). https://doi.org/10.1128/mBio.02231-15. PubMed PMID: 26838724; PubMed Central PMCID: PMCPMC4742717

133. Marino ND, Panas MW, Franco M, Theisen TC, Naor A, Rastogi S et al (2018) Identification of a novel protein complex essential for effector translocation across the parasitophorous vacuole membrane of *Toxoplasma gondii*. PLoS Pathog 14(1):e1006828. https://doi.org/10.1371/journal.ppat.1006828. PubMed PMID: 29357375; PubMed Central PMCID: PMCPMC5794187

134. Gay G, Braun L, Brenier-Pinchart MP, Vollaire J, Josserand V, Bertini RL et al (2016) *Toxoplasma gondii* TgIST co-opts host chromatin repressors dampening STAT1-dependent gene regulation and IFN-gamma-mediated host defenses. J Exp Med 213(9):1779–1798. https://doi.org/10.1084/jem.20160340. PubMed PMID: 27503074; PubMed Central PMCID: PMCPMC4995087

135. Olias P, Etheridge RD, Zhang Y, Holtzman MJ, Sibley LD (2016) *Toxoplasma* effector recruits the Mi-2/NuRD complex to repress STAT1 transcription and block IFN-gamma-dependent gene expression. Cell Host Microbe 20(1):72–82. https://doi.org/10.1016/j.chom.2016.06.006. PubMed PMID: 27414498; PubMed Central PMCID: PMCPMC4947229

136. Naor A, Panas MW, Marino N, Coffey MJ, Tonkin CJ, Boothroyd JC (2018) MYR1-dependent effectors are the major drivers of a host cell's early response to *Toxoplasma*, including counteracting MYR1-independent effects. MBio 9(2). https://doi.org/10.1128/mBio.02401-17. PubMed PMID: 29615509; PubMed Central PMCID: PMCPMC5885026

137. Opitz C, Soldati D (2002) 'The glideosome': a dynamic complex powering gliding motion and host cell invasion by *Toxoplasma gondii*. Mol Microbiol 45(3):597–604. PubMed PMID: 12139608

138. Gaskins E, Gilk S, DeVore N, Mann T, Ward G, Beckers C (2004) Identification of the membrane receptor of a class XIV myosin in *Toxoplasma gondii*. J Cell Biol 165 (3):383–393. PubMed PMID: 15123738

139. Gilk SD, Gaskins E, Ward GE, Beckers CJ (2009) GAP45 phosphorylation controls assembly of the *Toxoplasma* myosin XIV complex. Eukaryot Cell 8(2):190–196. https://doi.org/10.1128/EC.00201-08. Epub 2008/12/03. PubMed PMID: 19047362; PubMed Central PMCID: PMC2643604

140. Bullen HE, Tonkin CJ, O'Donnell RA, Tham WH, Papenfuss AT, Gould S et al (2009) A novel family of Apicomplexan glideosome-associated proteins with an inner membrane-anchoring role. J Biol Chem 284 (37):25353–25363. https://doi.org/10.1074/jbc.M109.036772. Epub 2009/06/30. PubMed PMID: 19561073; PubMed Central PMCID: PMC2757237

141. Nebl T, Prieto JH, Kapp E, Smith BJ, Williams MJ, Yates JR 3rd et al (2011) Quantitative in vivo analyses reveal calcium-dependent phosphorylation sites and identifies a novel component of the *Toxoplasma* invasion motor complex. PLoS Pathog 7(9): e1002222. https://doi.org/10.1371/journal.ppat.1002222. Epub 2011/10/08. PPATHOGENS-D-10-00615 [pii]. PubMed PMID: 21980283; PubMed Central PMCID: PMC3182922

142. Williams MJ, Alonso H, Enciso M, Egarter S, Sheiner L, Meissner M et al (2015) Two essential light chains regulate the myoa lever arm to promote *Toxoplasma* gliding motility. MBio 6(5):e00845–e00815. https://doi.org/10.1128/mBio.00845-15. PubMed PMID: 26374117; PubMed Central PMCID: PMCPMC4600101

143. Jan G, Delorme V, David V, Revenu C, Rebollo A, Cayla X et al (2007) The toxofilin-actin-PP2C complex of *Toxoplasma*: identification of interacting domains. Biochem J 401(3):711–719. PubMed PMID: 17014426

144. Guerin A, Corrales RM, Parker ML, Lamarque MH, Jacot D, El Hajj H et al (2017)

Efficient invasion by *Toxoplasma* depends on the subversion of host protein networks. Nat Microbiol 2(10):1358–1366. https://doi.org/10.1038/s41564-017-0018-1. PubMed PMID: 28848228

145. Chen AL, Kim EW, Toh JY, Vashisht AA, Rashoff AQ, Van C et al (2015) Novel components of the *Toxoplasma* inner membrane complex revealed by BioID. MBio 6(1):e02357–e02314. https://doi.org/10.1128/mBio.02357-14. PubMed PMID: 25691595; PubMed Central PMCID: PMCPMC4337574

146. Chen AL, Moon AS, Bell HN, Huang AS, Vashisht AA, Toh JY et al (2017) Novel insights into the composition and function of the *Toxoplasma* IMC sutures. Cell Microbiol 19(4). https://doi.org/10.1111/cmi.12678. PubMed PMID: 27696623

147. Nadipuram SM, Kim EW, Vashisht AA, Lin AH, Bell HN, Coppens I et al (2016) In vivo biotinylation of the *Toxoplasma* parasitophorous vacuole reveals novel dense granule proteins important for parasite growth and pathogenesis. MBio 7(4). https://doi.org/10.1128/mBio.00808-16. PubMed PMID: 27486190; PubMed Central PMCID: PMCPMC4981711

148. Long S, Anthony B, Drewry LL, Sibley LD (2017) A conserved ankyrin repeat-containing protein regulates conoid stability, motility and cell invasion in *Toxoplasma gondii*. Nat Commun 8(1):2236. https://doi.org/10.1038/s41467-017-02341-2. PubMed PMID: 29269729; PubMed Central PMCID: PMCPMC5740107

149. de Souza W, Attias M (2015) New views of the *Toxoplasma gondii* parasitophorous vacuole as revealed by helium ion microscopy (HIM). J Struct Biol 191(1):76–85. https://doi.org/10.1016/j.jsb.2015.05.003. PubMed PMID: 26004092

150. Cyrklaff M, Kudryashev M, Leis A, Leonard K, Baumeister W, Menard R et al (2007) Cryoelectron tomography reveals periodic material at the inner side of subpellicular microtubules in apicomplexan parasites. J Exp Med 204(6):1281–1287. https://doi.org/10.1084/jem.20062405. Epub 2007/06/15. PubMed PMID: 17562819; PubMed Central PMCID: PMC2118598

151. Ferguson DJ, Brecht S, Soldati D (2000) The microneme protein MIC4, or an MIC4-like protein, is expressed within the macrogamete and associated with oocyst wall formation in *Toxoplasma gondii*. Int J Parasitol 30

(11):1203–1209. PubMed PMID: 11027789

152. Chtanova T, Schaeffer M, Han SJ, van Dooren GG, Nollmann M, Herzmark P et al (2008) Dynamics of neutrophil migration in lymph nodes during infection. Immunity 29(3):487–496. https://doi.org/10.1016/j.immuni.2008.07.012. Epub 2008/08/23. doi: S1074-7613(08)00364-6 [pii]. PubMed PMID: 18718768; PubMed Central PMCID: PMC2569002

153. Wilson EH, Harris TH, Mrass P, John B, Tait ED, Wu GF et al (2009) Behavior of parasite-specific effector CD8+ T cells in the brain and visualization of a kinesis-associated system of reticular fibers. Immunity 30(2):300–311. https://doi.org/10.1016/j.immuni.2008.12.013. Epub 2009/01/27. doi: S1074-7613(09)00060-0 [pii]. PubMed PMID: 19167248; PubMed Central PMCID: PMC2696229

154. Coombes JL, Charsar BA, Han SJ, Halkias J, Chan SW, Koshy AA et al (2013) Motile invaded neutrophils in the small intestine of *Toxoplasma gondii*-infected mice reveal a potential mechanism for parasite spread. Proc Natl Acad Sci U S A 110(21):E1913–E1922. https://doi.org/10.1073/pnas.1220272110. Epub 2013/05/08. PubMed PMID: 23650399; PubMed Central PMCID: PMC3666704

155. Saeij JP, Boyle JP, Grigg ME, Arrizabalaga G, Boothroyd JC (2005) Bioluminescence imaging of *Toxoplasma gondii* infection in living mice reveals dramatic differences between strains. Infect Immun 73(2):695–702. PubMed PMID: 15664907

156. Behnke MS, Zhang TP, Dubey JP, Sibley LD (2014) *Toxoplasma gondii* merozoite gene expression analysis with comparison to the life cycle discloses a unique expression state during enteric development. BMC Genomics 15:350. https://doi.org/10.1186/1471-2164-15-350. PubMed PMID: 24885521; PubMed Central PMCID: PMC4035076

157. Hehl AB, Basso WU, Lippuner C, Ramakrishnan C, Okoniewski M, Walker RA et al (2015) Asexual expansion of *Toxoplasma gondii* merozoites is distinct from tachyzoites and entails expression of non-overlapping gene families to attach, invade, and replicate within feline enterocytes. BMC Genomics 16:66. https://doi.org/10.1186/s12864-015-1225-x. PubMed PMID: 25757795; PubMed Central PMCID: PMCPMC4340605

Chapter 2

ToxoDB: Functional Genomics Resource for *Toxoplasma* and Related Organisms

Omar S. Harb and David S. Roos

Abstract

ToxoDB is a free online resource that provides access to genomic and functional genomic data. All data is made available through an intuitive queryable interface that enables scientists to build in silico experiments and develop testable hypothesis. The resource contains 32 fully sequenced and annotated genomes, with genomic sequence from multiple strains available for variant detection and copy number variation analysis. In addition to genomic sequence data, ToxoDB contains numerous functional genomic datasets including microarray, RNAseq, proteomics, ChIP-seq, and phenotypic data. In addition, results from a number of whole-genome analyses are incorporated including mapping to orthology clusters which allows users to leverage phylogenetic relationships in their analyses. Integration of primary data is made possible through a private galaxy interface and custom export tools that allow users to interrogate their own results in the context of all other data in the database.

Key words ToxoDB, EuPathDB, Apicomplexa, Genomics, Database, Bioinformatics

1 Introduction

ToxoDB (http://ToxoDB.org) is part of the Eukaryotic Pathogen Database (EuPathDB) bioinformatic resource center (BRC) which provides free online informatics support facilitating data access and analysis. Currently, there are four BRCs supported by the National Institutes of Allergy and Infectious Diseases (NIAID) with missions to enable bioinformatic access to bacterial (http://patrcibrc.org) [1], viral (http://vipr.org) [2], eukaryotic pathogens (http://EuPathDB.org) [3], and vectors of these pathogens (http://vectorbase.org) [4]. In addition to ToxoDB, EuPathDB includes the following resources: AmoebaDB, CryptoDB, GiardiaDB, MicrosporidiaDB, PlasmoDB, PiroplasmaDB, TriTrypDB, OrthoMCL, and HostDB. Recently, additional resources have been developed using the EuPathDB model and infrastructure to

On Behalf of the EuPathDB Team

Christopher J. Tonkin (ed.), *Toxoplasma gondii: Methods and Protocols*, Methods in Molecular Biology, vol. 2071, https://doi.org/10.1007/978-1-4939-9857-9_2, © Springer Science+Business Media, LLC, part of Springer Nature 2020

integrate clinical epidemiological data (http://clinepidb.org) and microbiome data (http://microbiomedb.org) [5].

Over the past two decades the idea of an online resource for *Toxoplasma* data evolved from a database for BLASTing sequences against *Toxoplasma* expressed sequence tag libraries (ESTs) to a fully integrated functional genomics resource [6, 7]. An explosion of "next generation" molecular techniques along with advances in computational power and the global reach of the Internet has made online resources such as ToxoDB not only feasible but also a necessary companion to laboratory research. Moreover, integration of multiple resources under the EuPathDB bioinformatic resource umbrella improves overall efficiency and distribution of recourses.

One feature of EuPathDB resources is that they adhere to some basic principles that have remained in place over the past 15 years. These include the following:

–   Reliable integration of annotation along with automated analysis such as predicted genes, proteins, motifs, structures, functions, and pathways for eukaryotic microbes, and their host species.

–   Incorporation of diverse data types including genomes; comparative genomics; polymorphisms and population genomics; field-clinical isolates and mutant strains (w/phenotypic metadata, including host–pathogen interactions); chromatin marks; transcriptomic, proteomic, and metabolomic data; interactomes; and subcellular localization/images.

–   Rapid access to both finished and draft datasets. Unfinished (and unpublished) data is increasingly important, as genomic-scale datasets are typically incomplete (or incompletely analyzed). Most EuPathDB datasets are now deposited and/or released prior to publication (but depositors always control release dates).

–   Development of tools that enable researchers to ask their own questions about the underlying data thus expediting discovery and translational science.

–   Providing a sustainable resource with universal access and extensive outreach to support researchers both through online and in-person support.

This chapter provides a description of the current data content of ToxoDB, information about some key ToxoDB tools and features and access to online guides for further self-learning. It is important to note that the fluid nature of databases will by design very quickly render this chapter out of date. A new version of ToxoDB, along with all EuPathDB resource, is released every 2 months. Readers are encouraged to consult the news section of ToxoDB on a regular basis: http://toxodb.org/news.

1.1   Data Content   ToxoDB aims to incorporate sufficient datasets and types to enable researchers to develop in silico hypothesis that can be tested on the bench. The following section lists the available data types and datasets available in ToxoDB. In addition, readers are encouraged to explore the searchable datasets section of ToxoDB: http://toxodb.org/toxo/app/search/dataset/AllDatasets/result.

1.1.1   Genomes   ToxoDB includes genome sequence data from 64 *Toxoplasma* strains and related organism including *Cyclospora cayetanensis, Cystoisospora suis, Neospora caninum, Hammondia hammondi, Sarcocystis neurona*, and *Eimeria* spp. Most of the genomes have been annotated. Table 1 lists all the genomes with information about their annotation status and source.

Table 1
Genomes in ToxoDB

Organism	Annotation available?	Total number of genes	Genome size Mbps	Total number of contigs	Organellar genome	Data source
Toxoplasma gondii ME49	Yes	8920	65.67	2265	Apicoplast	[8]
Toxoplasma gondii VEG	Yes	8563	64.52	1323	Apicoplast	[8]
Toxoplasma gondii GT1	Yes	8637	63.95	2063	Apicoplast	[8]
Toxoplasma gondii GAB2-2007-GAL-DOM2	Yes	9296	63.55	2511	Apicoplast	[8]
Toxoplasma gondii TgCatPRC2	Yes	10,300	64.19	3064	Apicoplast	[8]
Toxoplasma gondii ARI	Yes	10,148	64.69	2745	Apicoplast	[8]
Toxoplasma gondii FOU	Yes	10,297	64.53	2871	Apicoplast	[8]
Toxoplasma gondii VAND	Yes	9426	64.27	2141	Apicoplast	[8]
Toxoplasma gondii RUB	Yes	10,213	64.96	2431	Apicoplast	[8]
Toxoplasma gondii MAS	Yes	10,176	63.32	2183	Apicoplast	[8]
Toxoplasma gondii p89	Yes	9874	64.16	2153	Apicoplast	[8]
Toxoplasma gondii RH	Partial	63	4.03	3	Apicoplast	[8]
Toxoplasma gondii TgCATBr9	No	0	61.82	6287	Apicoplast	[8]
Toxoplasma gondii TgCATBr5	No	0	61.64	6995		[8]
Toxoplasma gondii CAST	No	0	63.05	5717		[8]
Toxoplasma gondii COUG	No	0	63.70	8562		[8]

(continued)

Table 1
(continued)

Organism	Annotation available?	Total number of genes	Genome size Mbps	Total number of contigs	Organellar genome	Data source
Toxoplasma gondii CtCo5	No	0	62.62	6177		[8]
Toxoplasma gondii TgCkUg2	No	0	41.93	36,913		[9]
Neospora caninum Liverpool	Yes	7276	59.10	66		[10]
Hammondia hammondi H. H.34	Yes	8178	67.70	14,861	Apicoplast	[8]
Cyclospora cayetanensis CHN_HEN01	Yes	7901	44.03	2297		[11]
Cystoisospora suis Wien I	Yes	11,785	83.64	14,630		{[12]
Sarcocystis neurona SN3	Yes	7089	124.41	873	Apicoplast	[13]
Sarcocystis neurona SO SN1	Yes	7177	130.22	3066		[13]
Eimeria tenella Houghton	Yes	8634	51.86	4664		[14]
Eimeria acervulina Houghton	Yes	7045	45.83	3415		Pain unpublished
Eimeria brunetti Houghton	Yes	8898	66.89	8575		Pain unpublished
Eimeria falciformis Bayer Haberkorn 1970	Yes	6102	43.67	753	Apicoplast	[15]
Eimeria maxima Weybridge	Yes	6258	45.98	3564		Pain unpublished
Eimeria mitis Houghton	Yes	10,265	72.24	15,978		Pain unpublished
Eimeria necatrix Houghton	Yes	8872	55.01	3707		Pain unpublished
Eimeria praecox Houghton	Yes	7906	60.08	21,348		Pain unpublished

1.1.2 Transcriptomics   ToxoDB contains a number of datasets that provide information about the transcriptional status of genes. These data come from a variety of experimental types including expressed sequence tags (ESTs), DNA microarrays, RNA sequence (RNAseq), and chromatin immunoprecipitation microarrays (ChIP-chip).

EST data are retrieved periodically from the GenBank dbEST resource. While this data type is considered antiquated, it still contains valuable information from different developmental life-stages and strains, and offers additional support for gene structure. Release 39 of ToxoDB contains 94 EST libraries from *Toxoplasma*, *Eimeria*, *Neospora*, and *Sarcocystis* species. EST sequences are mapped to the reference genomes and made available for searching. For example, genes may be identified based on their homology to ESTs in chosen libraries or ESTs may be identified based on their extent of gene overlap.

Microarray data is available from ten published or unpublished experiments for *Toxoplasma gondii*. Each experiment can be searched based on fold change differences between samples within an experiment or based on percentile expressions within an experiment. In addition, experiments with sufficient time points can be queries using an expression similarity search. Table 2 includes all available microarray experiments with information about the strains they were conducted on and the developmental stage. All microarray searches can be accessed by following this link: http://toxodb. org/toxo/showQuestion.do?questionFullName=InternalGene DatasetQuestions.GenesByMicroarrayEvidence.

Table 2
List of microarray experiments available in ToxoDB

Experiment	Strains	Stages	Reference
Expression profiling of 3 archetypal lineages	RH, GT1, Pru, ME49, CTG, VEG	Tachyzoite	Roos et al. (unpublished)
Transcriptome during invasion	RH	Tachyzoite	[16]
Cell cycle	RH	Tachyzoite	[17]
GCN5-A mutant	RH	Tachyzoite	[18]
Bradyzoite differentiation	Pru	Tachyzoite, Bradyzoite	Boothroyd et al. (unpublished)
Bradyzoite differentiation	Pru, RH	Tachyzoite, Bradyzoite	Roos et al. (unpublished)
Bradyzoite differentiation	GT1, ME49	Tachyzoite, Bradyzoite	[19]
Bradyzoite differentiation	RH	Tachyzoite, Bradyzoite	[20]
Oocyst, tachyzoite, and bradyzoite developmental expression	M4	Tachyzoite, Bradyzoite, oocyst	[21]
Merozoite	TgNmBr1	Tachyzoite, Merozoite	[22]

RNA sequencing data from 14 experiments (both stranded and unstranded), 11 from *Toxoplasma*, 2 from *Eimeria* and 1 from *Neospora* have been loaded and mapped to the reference genomes (Table 3). RNAseq data can be queried using a number of searches including a fold change search that allows for the identification of genes based on their expression, a percentile search, and profile similarity. In addition to available searches, RNAseq data is used by ToxoDB to provide evidence for gene structure in the form of intron spanning reads (ISRs). ISRs are available individually for each experiment or as cumulative support from all experiments. A track of ISRs is available on gene pages in the gene models section. Mousing over ISRs provides a summary of the supporting RNAseq evidence and the originating experiment(s) (*see* below).

1.1.3 High Throughput Sequencing Data

ToxoDB includes high throughput genome sequencing data from 64 *Toxoplasma* strains and two *Hammondia* strains [8]. ToxoDB integrates sequencing data and enables searches to identify single nucleotide polymorphisms (SNPs) between strains and to determine copy number variation (CNV). SNP searches can be accessed from two places: (1) Under "Search for Genes"—enabling the identification of genes with specific SNP characteristics within a group of isolates. (2) Under "Search for other data types" SNPs may be identified regardless of their presence within gene or not. Genes by copy number searches allow a user to identify genes that are present in regions of the genome that exhibit CNV based on the selected strains or based on copy number comparison with the reference genome assembly.

1.1.4 Proteomics

ToxoDB contains 21 proteomics datasets (Table 4), which depending on the type of experiment, include evidence for peptides, levels of expression or post-translational modifications (PTMs). All data from proteomics experiments are available for searching or viewing on gene pages. Searches enable defining genes based on the number of mapped peptides, fold-change or direct comparison for quantitative data or type and number of PTMs. Results from all proteomics data are displayed graphically and in tables in the proteomics section of gene pages.

1.1.5 Phenotypic Data

ToxoDB includes a whole-genome CRISPR screen providing evidence of possible effect of gene disruption on parasite fitness [48]. The experiments in this study were carried out using the GT1 strain hence the data in ToxoDB was loaded against the *T. gondii* GT1 genome. A graphical representation of this data is available on each gene page in the phenotype section (*see* for example: http://toxodb.org/toxo/app/record/gene/TGGT1_232430#phenomics). In addition, searches can be run against this

Table 3
List of RNA sequencing experiments available in ToxoDB

Experiment	Strains	Stages	Reference
Tachyzoite	ME49	Tachyzoite	[10]
Transcriptome during infection in four mouse cell types**	NTE 3	Tachyzoite	[23]
Tachyzoite time series	ME49, GT1, VEG, RH	Tachyzoite	Roos and Gregory (unpublished)
Transcriptomes of 29 strains during murine macrophage infection**	ARI, B41, B73, BOF, CAST, CASTELLS, CEP delta HXGPRT, COUGAR, DEG, FOU, GPHT, GT1, GUYDOS, GUYKOE, GUYMAT, MAS, ME49, P89, PRU delta HXGPRT, RAY, RH delta HXGPRT, ROD, RUB, TgCATBr44, TgCATBr5, TgCATBr9, VAND, VEG, WTD3	Tachyzoite	[24]
Alternative-splicing factor TgSR3 overexpression	ME49	Tachyzoite	[25]
Ribosome profiling of intracellular and extracellular parasites	RH	Tachyzoite	[26]
Acute or chronic infection in mouse brain	ME49	In vivo tachyzoite & bradyzoite	[27]
In vitro bradyzoite	ME49	Bradyzoite	Sibley et al. (unpublished)
In vivo bradyzoite	M4	Bradyzoite	Boothroyd et al. (unpublished)
Feline stages	CZ	Enterocyte, Tachyzoite, Bradyzoite	Hehl et al. (unpublished)
Oocyst	M4	Oocyst	[21]
Tachyzoite	*N. caninum* Liverpool	Tachyzoite	[10]
Gametocytes vs. asexual stages	*E. tenella* Houghton	Gametocyte, asexual	[28]
Life cycle stages	*E. tenella* Houghton	Oocyst, sporozoite, and second generation merozoite	[14]

**These experiments have also been loaded into HostDB http://hostdb.org where host response data may be searched

Table 4
List of proteomics experiments available in ToxoDB

Experiment	Strains	Stages	Reference
Infection time course [+++]	ME49, GT1, RH, VEG	Tachyzoites	[29]
In vitro proteome	RH	Tachyzoites	[30]
Membrane and cytosolic	RH	Tachyzoites	[31]
Subcellular fractions	RH	Tachyzoites	Moreno et al. (unpublished)
Conoid	RH	Tachyzoites	[32]
Mitochondrial matrix [+++]	RH	Tachyzoites	[33]
Rhoptry	RH	Tachyzoites	[34]
Secretome	RH	Tachyzoites	[35]
Extracellular vesicles	RH	Tachyzoites	[36]
Calcium-dependent phosphoproteome	RH	Tachyzoites	[37]
Phosphoproteome	RH	Tachyzoites	[38]
Monomethylarginine	RH	Tachyzoite	[39]
Lysine-Acetylome	RH	Tachyzoites	[40, 41]
Ubiquitome	RH	Tachyzoites	[42]
N-terminal	RH	Tachyzoite	[43]
TAILS peptides	RH	Tachyzoites	[44]
Partially sporulated oocyst	VEG	Oocyst	[45]
Oocyst	M4	Oocyst	[29]
Fractionated oocyst	M4	Oocyst, Sporozoite	[46]
Infection time course [+++]	N. caninum Liverpool	Tachyzoites	[29]
Rhoptry	E. tenella Wisconsin	Sporozoites	[47]

[+++] These datasets contain quantitative data which can be queried using the specialized quantitative proteomics searches in ToxoDB

data by specifying the desired fitness score: http://toxodb.org/toxo/showQuestion.do?questionFullName=GeneQuestions.GenesByPhenotype_tgonGT1_crisprPhenotype_CrisprScreen_RSRC.

1.1.6   Isolates

Single and multilocus typed isolates from GenBank are integrated into ToxoDB on a periodic basis. Information about the isolates is extracted from structured field sin the GenBank records and made available for searching in ToxoDB. This, for example, allows for the identification of isolates based on geographic location, locus used for typing, and isolation source or host. Currently the integrated isolates belong to the *Eimeriidae*, *Sarcocystidae*, and environmental samples. As a result, ToxoDB includes typed isolates from 417 species covering 7516 isolates.

*1.1.7   Restriction
Fragment Length
Polymorphism (RFLP)*
.

Genotyping data based on RFLP analysis is provided as a reference and is available using a number of searches [49]. This section of ToxoDB includes reference images of RFLP results and searches to identify genotypes based on isolate ID, RFLP genotype, or RFLP genotype number. To access these searches, explore the "Search for Other Data Types" section from the home page and select the "RFLP Genotype Isolates" category.

*1.1.8   Metabolic
Pathways and Compounds*

Metabolic pathways from the Kyoto Encyclopedia of Genes and Genomes (KEGG) [50] and MetaCyc [51] have been integrated into ToxoDB. Pathways are populated and linked to genes based on enzyme commission numbers available both as part of the official annotation and inferred by orthology. In addition, metabolites and small molecules have been obtained from the chemical entities of biological interest (ChEBI) database [52]. Compounds are integrated into pathways and linked to genes through chemical reactions orchestrated by enzymes—that is, Substrates and products. Searches in ToxoDB allow for the identification of pathways or compounds based on a number of searches available under the "Search for Other Data Types" panel on the home page and include finding metabolic pathways based on genes, compounds or pathway name, and finding compounds based on compound ID, metabolic pathway, molecular formula, etc.

All metabolic pathways are available as interactive graphical displays using a cytoscape interface [53]. Figure 1a shows the KEGG pathway for glycolysis, zooming in reveals EC numbers in rectangles and metabolite chemical structures (Fig. 1b). Rectangles colored in orange indicate the presence of the enzyme in at least one of the genomes in ToxoDB. Clicking on the rectangles or compounds reveals a pop-up window with additional information (Fig. 1c, d). Metabolic pathways can also be decorated with additional information based on phylogeny or experiments (Fig. 1e). Painting pathways with experimental data reveals a minigraph in place of the enzymes and clicking on the graph opens a pop-up with a larger image of the experiment results (Fig. 1f). Painting a metabolic pathway by phylogeny replaces each enzyme with a mini–bar graph with each bar representing one of the organisms chosen. Clicking on this graph expands it for a more detailed examination (Fig. 1g).

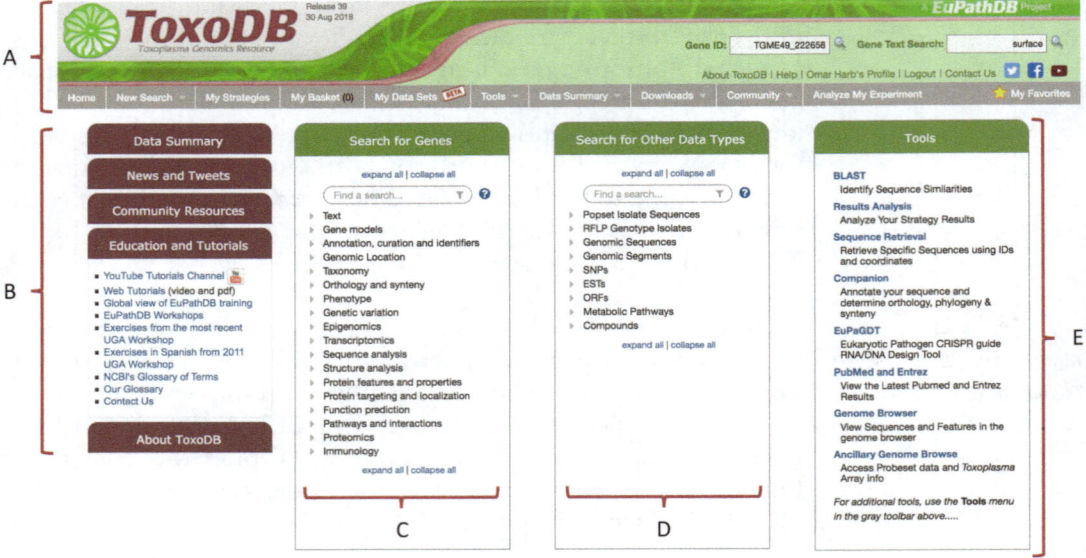

Fig. 1 Metabolic pathways in ToxoDB. (**a**) Screenshot of a KEGG pathways representing glycolysis. Orange boxes represent enzymes that have at least one representative in ToxoDB. (**b**) A zoomed-in section of glycolysis showing how zooming in reveals EC numbers for enzymes in rectangles and chemical structures of metabolites. (**c**) Clicking on chemical structures reveals a pop-up window with additional information including metabolite name, ChEBI ID and link to the compound page. (**d**) Clicking on the EC number reveals a pop-up window with additional information about the enzyme such as the name and a link to the genes in ToxoDB that match the EC number. (**e**) The paint pathway drop-down menu allows for decorating the pathway with phylogenetic or experimental evidence for the represented enzymes. (**f**) Screenshot showing experimental evidence painted on pathways. (**e**) Screenshot showing phylogenetic evidence painted on pathways

1.1.9 Analysis Pipeline Results

All genomes loaded in ToxoDB are analyzed using a number of standard tools which provide additional information about gene function. Results from the analyses are available on gene pages, as columns that can be added to search results and as dedicated searches that allow for the identification of genes based on analysis specific criteria. Table 5 lists some of the key analysis tools and their use.

1.2 Using ToxoDB

1.2.1 The Home Page

The ToxoDB home page is organized to easily provide users with access to all searches, tools, and documentation.

The header section (Fig. 2a) appears on all ToxoDB gene pages and provides quick access to gene ID and text searches, information about the release version and date, access to EuPathDB social media and YouTube tutorials, help documentation, registration, and log-in links and a link to the "contact us" form. In addition, the banner includes a gray menu bar providing drop down menus with access to all searches, tools, and downloads in ToxoDB. The latter feature enables users to access this information from anywhere in ToxoDB without requiring them to return to the home page.

Table 5
Key analysis tools and their use

Analysis	Output	Use	Reference
OrthoMCL	Groups of genes mapped to OrthoMCL groups or unique groups if no mapping to OrthoMCL exists	Orthology group table on gene pages. Searches that allow for the identification of genes based on a desired phyletic pattern. Transform genes from one species to another based on orthology. Identify paralogs	[54]
InterPro Scan	InterPro domains such as PFAM mapped to genes	Graphical display of InterPro domains on gene pages. Search that allows for the identification of genes based on chosen InterPro domains(s)	[55, 56]
InterPro to GO	GO terms associated with genes	GO term searches. GO terms table on gene pages. GO term enrichment	[55]
SignalP	Predicted secretory signal peptides	Graphical display of signal peptides on genes pages. Search that allows for the identification of possible secreted proteins	[57]
THMM	Predicted transmembrane domains	Graphical display of transmembrane domains on genes pages. Search that allows for the identification of genes based on chosen number of transmembrane domains	[58]
BLAST	Top BlastP results against the nonredundant database	Graphical display of Blast results on gene pages	
PDB	Mapping to 3D structures in the protein databank	Table on gene pages with best matches to PDB. Searches that allow for the identification of genes based on their matches to PDB	
IEDB	Mapping to epitopes in the Immune Epitope Data Base	Table on gene pages with best-matched epitopes in IEDB. Searches that allow for the identification of genes with matched epitopes in IEDB	

The side bar (Fig. 2b) contains expandable subsections with access to a summary of all genomes and data in ToxoDB, release news and the live EuPathDB Twitter feed, community resources, education and tutorials, and about section which includes general information about ToxoDB.

Searches and tools (Fig. 2c–e) are located in the central portion of the home page and are categorized into gene searches (Fig. 2c), searches of other data types (Fig. 2d), and Tools (Fig. 2e).

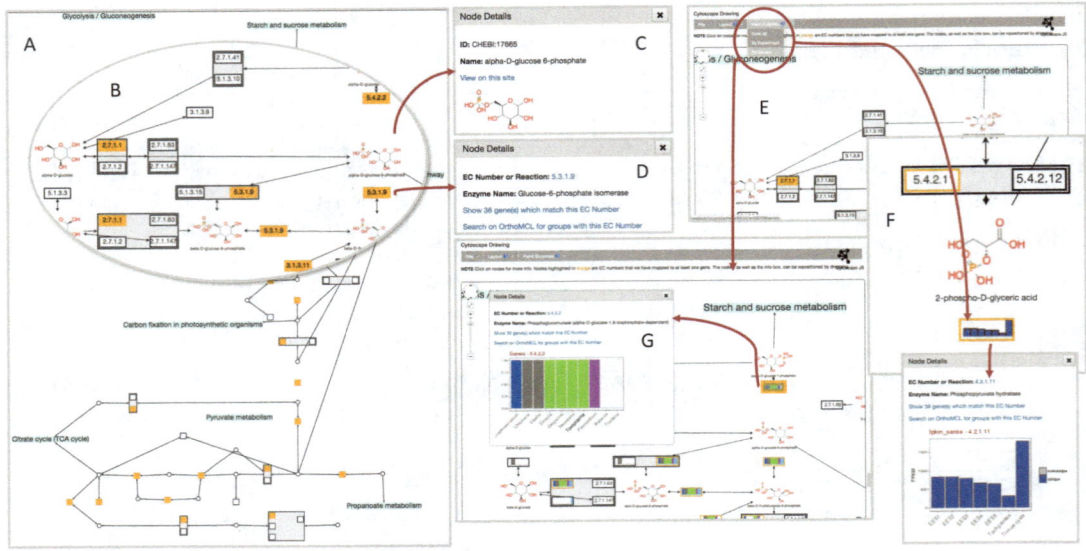

Fig. 2 Screenshot of the ToxoDB home page (http:/ToxoDB.org). (**a**) The banner section which includes text and ID search boxes, registration and login links, contact us link, and the gray menu bar with access to all searches and tools in the database. (**b**) This section includes access to the ToxoDB data summary, news and tweets, community resources, education and tutorials, and the about ToxoDB section. (**c**) This section includes all the searches that return genes. (**d**) This section includes searches that return other data types such as popset isolates, RFLP genotypes isolates, genomic sequence data, SNP data, metabolic pathways, and compounds. (**e**) This section includes links to tools useful to the community

1.2.2 Searches in ToxoDB

A search in ToxoDB starts by selecting one of the over 80 available searches. All searches have been categorized to facilitate finding them. However, to make it even easier to locate a search of interest a "Find a search" search is available right above the list of categories on the home page (Fig. 3a, b). Typing a key word in the "Find a search" box will filter the searches below (Compare Fig. 3a, b). Once a search is located, clicking on the search link offers a user a search page where they can configure various parameters depending on the selected search. In the example in Fig. 3, the search for genes with a predicted secretory signal peptide is selected (Fig. 3c). The search page allows a user to select the organism(s) of interest (Fig. 3c) and in many cases advanced parameters (Fig. 3d). Once the parameters are configured, clicking on the "Get Answer" button (Fig. 3e) will return the results as a step in a search strategy, where the number of returned genes is displayed within the step (Fig. 3f). Right below the search strategy is an organism filter table which allows a user to quickly filter the results based on the organism of interest (Fig. 3g). The results are displayed in tabular format below the organism filter (Fig. 3h). The results table can be configured by adding, removing, or moving columns. In addition,

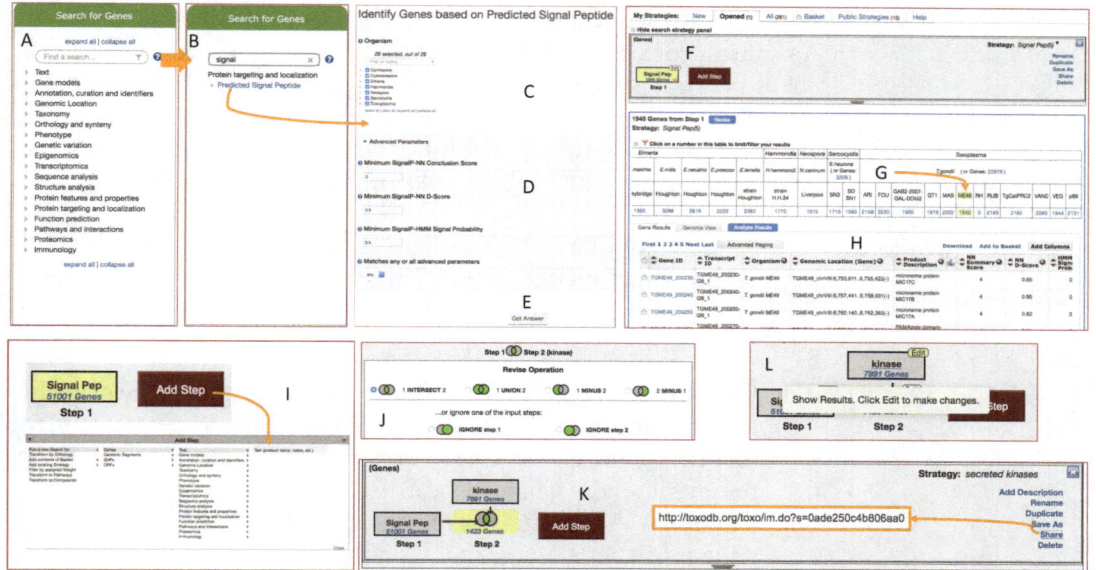

Fig. 3 Running searches in ToxoDB. (**a**) Searches for genes are categorized in expandable menus. (**b**) A search window is available to facilitate finding searches. In the example shown, typing signal reveals the search for genes based on predicted signal peptides. (**c**) Screenshot showing the signal peptide search page with the top portion that includes the organism selection section. (**d**) The search parameter section. (**e**) The search submit button. (**f**) Results of a search appear as a step in a search strategy with the number of results highlighted in a rectangle. (**g**) An organism filter table shows the number of results in each organism present within ToxoDB. Clicking on any of the numbers filters the results to the selected organism. (**h**) The results of a search are displayed in the lower section of the page. (**i**) Searches in ToxoDB can be added to a strategy by clicking on the "Add Step" button. This reveals a pop-up window with all the available searches. (**j**) Once a new search is configured, the operation describing how to combine results is chosen (e.g., intersect, union, or minus operations). (**k**) Combined results are graphically represented as a growing search strategy. Strategies can be saved and shared with others using a unique URL. (**l**) The steps in a strategy may be revised by clicking on the edit link that appears on a step upon mousing over

results of any search may be further analyzed (*see* below). A search strategy may be expanded by clicking on the "Add Step" button then selecting any of the available searches in the pop-up window (Fig. 3i). Once the parameters of the new search are configured, a user has to choose how to combine the two searches using options such as intersect, union, or minus operations (Fig. 3j). The combined results are displayed in an expanding search strategy that can be saved and shared with other users using a private link (Fig. 3k). Any step in a strategy may be revised by clicking on the step edit link then choosing from a list of options (Fig. 3l).

1.2.3 Exercises

Detailed step-by-step instructions on how to use EuPathDB resources including ToxoDB have been published elsewhere [3, 59–61]. In addition, to facilitate understanding how to access and use the available tools and features in ToxoDB, the authors recommend that users explore workshop exercises available through the education and tutorials section of ToxoDB. These exercises from previously held workshops are updated on a regular basis hence it is recommended that a user start with the most recent available workshop exercises. All EuPathDB workshop material can be accessed here: https://workshop.eupathdb.org (select the most recent workshop then follow links to the workshop schedule).

1.2.4 Tools and Features in ToxoDB

Over the years EuPathDB sites have accumulated a number of tools and features that enable users to interrogate data within the databases or to analyze their own primary data. Below is a list of a few of these features:

1. Genome view: this feature allows a user to quickly inspect the genomic location of genes in a result set. This is tool is useful to identify gene clusters or location bias of genes such as at telomeric ends. This tool can be accessed by clicking on the "Genome View" tab (red rectangle in Fig. 4) available with any gene result set (Fig. 4).

2. Gene enrichment tools: this feature allows a user to determine if there is a statistical enrichment of gene ontology (GO), metabolic pathway or product description key words in a result set. These enrichment tools can be accessed by clicking on the

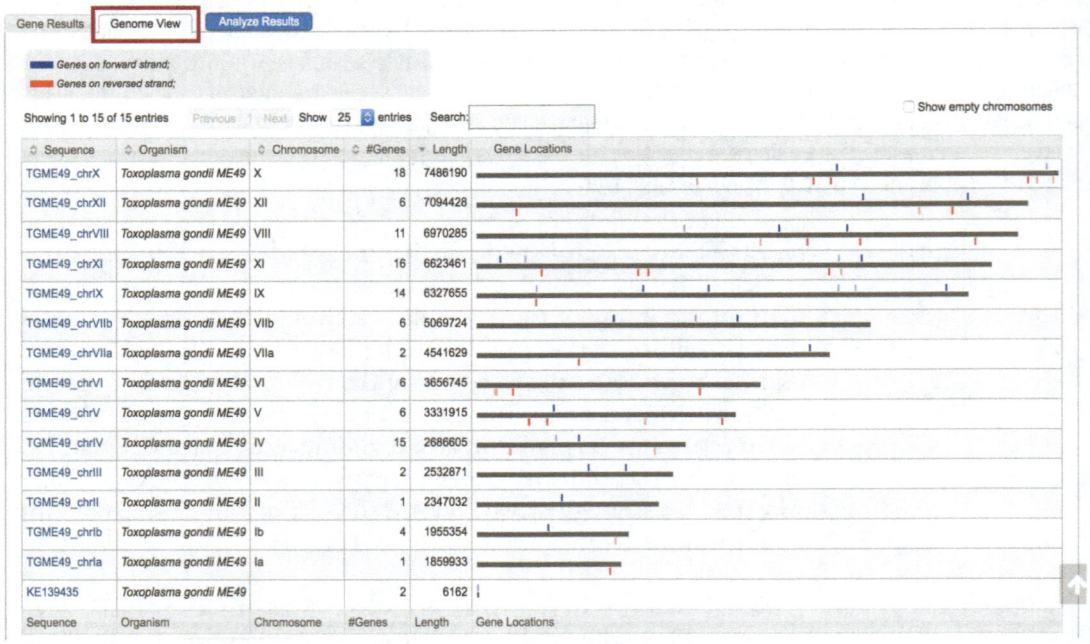

Fig. 4 Screenshot depicting the genome view. Clicking on the genome view tab displays gene results graphically. Blue and red boxes highlight locations of genes from a search and clicking on these boxes reveals a list of the underlying gene(s)

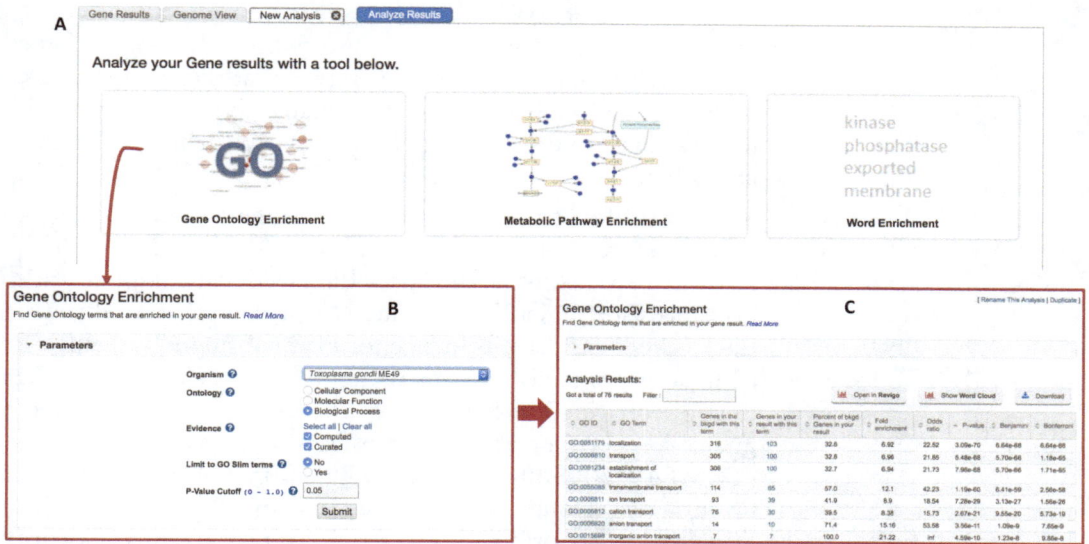

Fig. 5 Screenshot of the analyze results section. (**a**) Clicking on the "Analyze Results" tab reveals the available analysis options which include GO, metabolic pathways, and text enrichment. (**b**) Screenshot showing the GO enrichment configuration panel. Clicking on the GO enrichment box in **a** reveals the configurable parameters. (**c**) Results of a GO enrichment analysis. Columns include GO IDs and terms, number of genes with the GO term in the results, number of genes with the GO term in the background (whole genome), and various columns with the results of statistical enrichment

"Analyze Results" tab available with any gene result set (Fig. 5).

3. Favorites: This tool allows a user to create bookmarks to their favorite genes of interest. To add a gene to the favorites, a user can click on the "Add to Favorites" link at the top of any gene page. The favorites page can be accessed by clicking on the "My Favorites" link at the right of the gray menu bar (Fig. 2a). The "favorites" page allows a user to include notes and organize genes by user defined projects.

4. The basket: This tool allow a user to cherry-pick genes from searches by clicking on the "Add to Basket" icon or link at the top of gene pages or next to IDs in a results page. The basket serves as a temporary holding place for genes. Once a user is ready to work with the genes in a basket they can be easily converted to a step in a search strategy for additional analysis.

5. Analyze my experiment: This feature provides users with access to a EuPathDB Galaxy platform which enables them to upload and analyze their primary data in a private and secure workspace. While Galaxy tools are extensively described elsewhere [62], users can analyze their RNA or genomic sequencing data using predefined workflows. In addition, users have access to

the hundreds of bioinformatics tools to run directly or create their own custom workflows. One major advantage of the EuPathDB Galaxy platform is that all EuPathDB genomes are preloaded and available with the available tools. To access this feature, click on the "Analyze My Experiment" link in the gray menu bar.

6. Splice Junction tracks: In order to facilitate analysis of gene models, all RNA sequence data in ToxoDB is used to identify reads that span introns, thus providing evidence for an intron's existence (*see* Table 3). This data is represented as a GBrowse track called "RNAseq evidence for introns" and is available on all gene pages for organisms with mapped RNAseq data. The example provided in Fig. 5 is for the hypoxanthine-xanthine-guanine phosphoribosyl transferase (HXGPRT) gene (TGME49_200320). The splice junction tracks are divided up into two groups called filtered and inclusive (Fig. 6a, b). Filtering is performed in order to display high-confidence intron spanning evidence. In addition, each track is further subdivided into a "Matches Transcript annotation" track and "Novel" track as indicated by red arrows in Fig. 6a, b. The "Matches Transcript annotation" track shows evidence of intron spans from RNAseq data that matches the official structural annotation. The "Novel" track shows evidence of intron

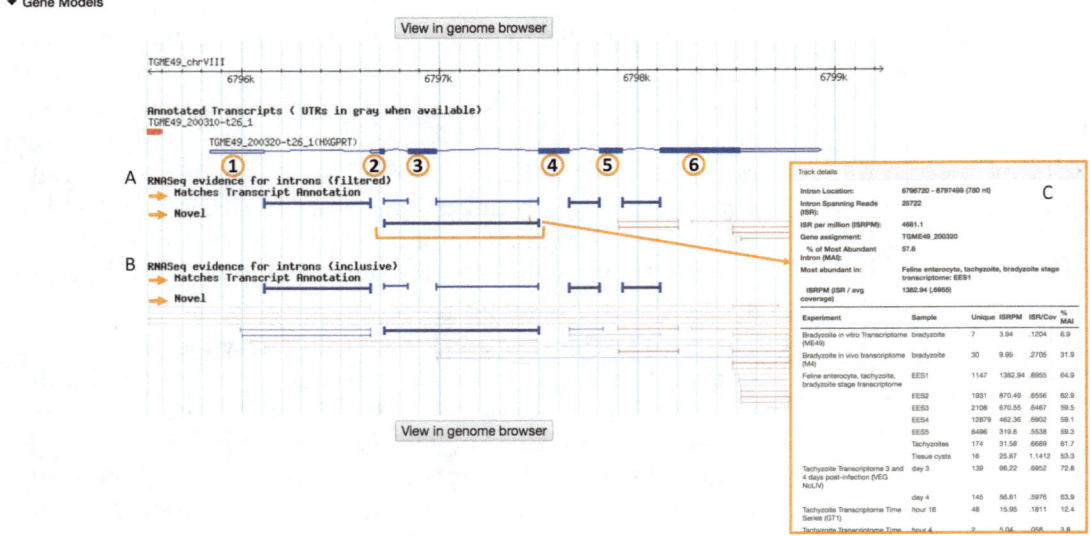

Fig. 6 Screenshot showing the intron evidence tracks available in ToxoDB for the HXGPRT gene. This gene has six annotated exons labeled one through six. (**a**) Filtered splice junctions showing only high-confidence evidence. Orange arrows point to the "matches transcript annotation" and "novel" subtracts. (**b**) Inclusive splice junctions do not include any filtering and thus may include noise. Orange arrows point to the "matches transcript annotation" and "novel" subtracts. (**c**) Mousing over splice junctions reveals the underlying evidence for that junction in a pop-up window

spans from RNAseq data that match the official annotation and those that do not representing possible alternative introns and may provide evidence for alternative gene models or in some cases more accurate gene models than the official annotation. In addition, the stronger the evidence for an intron span, the darker the color of the intron spanning graphics. In the case of HXGPRT, a clear alternative splice variant is formed by skipping exon 3 (exons numbers in circles in Fig. 6) and the evidence is indicated by the dark line that spans intron three highlighted by a red curved line in Fig. 6. Note that hovering over any of the intron spanning graphics provides information about the number of detected reads and the experiment they originated from (Fig. 6c). Note that the experiment providing the most abundant evidence for an intron span is indicated, in this case the feline enterocyte stage experiment (Hehl et al. unpublished).

2 Conclusions and Future Directions

Over the next few years, ToxoDB will continue to expand both in data content and in functionality. The rapid access to whole-genome sequencing platforms and genetic accessibility of the parasites with new mutagenesis techniques such as CRISPR will result in the availability of higher-throughput datasets. Integration of these datasets into ToxoDB will require additional development and tools to enable users to easily and accurately interrogate the underlying data. Expected advances include more effective integration of population biology data with associated searches and visualization tools, functional data summarization tools that allow a user to explore multiple datasets at the same time and better metabolic pathway representations with tools to explore functional data within pathways. In addition, tools that would allow users to integrate their own data into ToxoDB will be developed. An example of this is enabling users to upload their own expression data in their private dataset section and running searches on their data using the standard ToxoDB query interface.

References

1. Wattam AR, Abraham D, Dalay O, Disz TL, Driscoll T, Gabbard JL et al (2014) PATRIC, the bacterial bioinformatics database and analysis resource. Nucleic Acids Res 42: D581–D591. https://doi.org/10.1093/nar/gkt1099

2. Pickett BE, Sadat EL, Zhang Y, Noronha JM, Squires RB, Hunt V et al (2011) ViPR: an open bioinformatics database and analysis resource for virology research. Nucleic Acids Res 40: D593–D598. https://doi.org/10.1093/nar/gkr859

3. Aurrecoechea C, Barreto A, Basenko EY, Brestelli J, Brunk BP, Cade S et al (2017) EuPathDB: the eukaryotic pathogen genomics database resource. Nucleic Acids Res 45: D581–D591. https://doi.org/10.1093/nar/gkw1105

4. Megy K, Emrich SJ, Lawson D, Campbell D, Dialynas E, Hughes DST et al (2011) Vector-Base: improvements to a bioinformatics resource for invertebrate vector genomics. Nucleic Acids Res 40:D729–D734. https://doi.org/10.1093/nar/gkr1089

5. Oliveira FS, Brestelli J, Cade S, Zheng J, Iodice J, Fischer S et al (2018) MicrobiomeDB: a systems biology platform for integrating, mining and analyzing microbiome experiments. Nucleic Acids Res 46:D684–D691. https://doi.org/10.1093/nar/gkx1027

6. Kissinger JC, Gajria B, Li L, Paulsen IT, Roos DS (2003) ToxoDB: accessing the *Toxoplasma gondii* genome. Nucleic Acids Res 31:234–236. https://doi.org/10.1093/nar/gkg072

7. Ajioka JW, Boothroyd JC, Brunk BP, Hehl A, Hillier L, Manger ID et al (1998) Gene discovery by EST sequencing in *Toxoplasma gondii* reveals sequences restricted to the apicomplexa. Genome Res 8:18–28. https://doi.org/10.1101/gr.8.1.18

8. Lorenzi H, Khan A, Behnke MS, Namasivayam S, Swapna LS, Hadjithomas M et al (2016) Local admixture of amplified and diversified secreted pathogenesis determinants shapes mosaic *Toxoplasma gondii* genomes. Nat Commun 7:10147. https://doi.org/10.1038/ncomms10147

9. Bontell IL, Hall N, Ashelford KE, Dubey JP, Boyle JP, Lindh J et al (2009) Whole genome sequencing of a natural recombinant *Toxoplasma gondii* strain reveals chromosome sorting and local allelic variants. Genome Biol 10 (5):R53. https://doi.org/10.1186/gb-2009-10-5-r53

10. Reid AJ, Vermont SJ, Cotton JA, PLoS DH (2012) Comparative genomics of the apicomplexan parasites *Toxoplasma gondii* and Neospora caninum: coccidia differing in host range and transmission strategy. Plos Pathog 83:e1002567. https://doi.org/10.1371/journal.ppat.1002567

11. Liu S, Wang L, Zheng H, Xu Z (2016) Comparative genomics reveals Cyclospora cayetanensis possesses coccidia-like metabolism and invasion components but unique surface antigens. BMC Genomics 17(2016):218. https://doi.org/10.1186/s12864-016-2632-3

12. Palmieri N, Shrestha A, Ruttkowski B, Beck T (2017) The genome of the protozoan parasite Cystoisospora suis and a reverse vaccinology approach to identify vaccine candidates. Int J Parasitol 47:189–202. https://doi.org/10.1016/j.ijpara.2016.11.007

13. Blazejewski T, Nursimulu N, MBio VP (2015) Systems-based analysis of the Sarcocystis neurona genome identifies pathways that contribute to a heteroxenous life cycle. Am Soc Microbiol 6:1. https://doi.org/10.1128/mBio.02445-14

14. Reid AJ, Blake DP, Ansari HR, Billington K, Browne HP, Bryant J et al (2014) Genomic analysis of the causative agents of coccidiosis in domestic chickens. Genome Res 24:1676–1685. https://doi.org/10.1101/gr.168955.113

15. Heitlinger E, Spork S, Lucius R, Dieterich C (2014) The genome of Eimeria falciformis—reduction and specialization in a single host apicomplexan parasite. BMC Genomics 15:696. https://doi.org/10.1186/1471-2164-15-696

16. Gaji RY, Behnke MS, Lehmann MM, White MW, Carruthers VB (2010) Cell cycle-dependent, intercellular transmission of *Toxoplasma gondii* is accompanied by marked changes in parasite gene expression. Mol Microbiol 79:192–204. https://doi.org/10.1111/j.1365-2958.2010.07441.x

17. Behnke MS, Wootton JC, Lehmann MM, Radke JB, Lucas O, Nawas J et al (2010) Coordinated progression through two subtranscriptomes underlies the tachyzoite cycle of *Toxoplasma gondii*. PLoS One 5:e12354. https://doi.org/10.1371/journal.pone.0012354

18. Naguleswaran A, Elias EV, McClintick J, Edenberg HJ, Sullivan WJ (2010) *Toxoplasma gondii* lysine acetyltransferase GCN5-A functions in the cellular response to alkaline stress and expression of cyst genes. PLoS Pathog 6:e1001232. https://doi.org/10.1371/journal.ppat.1001232

19. Behnke MS, Radke JB, Smith AT, Sullivan WJ, White MW (2008) The transcription of bradyzoite genes in *Toxoplasma gondii* is controlled by autonomous promoter elements. Mol Microbiol 68:1502–1518. https://doi.org/10.1111/j.1365-2958.2008.06249.x

20. Lescault PJ, Thompson AB, Patil V, Lirussi D, Burton A, Margarit J et al (2010) Genomic data reveal *Toxoplasma gondii* differentiation mutants are also impaired with respect to switching into a novel extracellular tachyzoite state. PLoS One 5:e14463. https://doi.org/10.1371/journal.pone.0014463

21. Fritz HM, Buchholz KR, Chen X, Durbin-Johnson B, Rocke DM, Conrad PA et al (2012) Transcriptomic analysis of *Toxoplasma* development reveals many novel functions and structures specific to sporozoites and oocysts. PLoS One 7:e29998. https://doi.org/10.1371/journal.pone.0029998

22. Behnke MS, Zhang TP, Dubey JP, Sibley LD (2014) *Toxoplasma gondii* merozoite gene expression analysis with comparison to the life cycle discloses a unique expression state during enteric development. BMC Genomics 15:350. https://doi.org/10.1186/1471-2164-15-350

23. Swierzy IJ, Händel U, Kaever A, Jarek M, Scharfe M, Schlüter D et al (2017) Divergent co-transcriptomes of different host cells infected with *Toxoplasma gondii* reveal cell type-specific host-parasite interactions. Sci Rep 7:7229. https://doi.org/10.1038/s41598-017-07838-w

24. Minot S, Melo MB, Li F, Lu D, Niedelman W, Levine SS et al (2012) Admixture and recombination among *Toxoplasma gondii* lineages explain global genome diversity. Proc Natl Acad Sci U S A 109:13458–13463. https://doi.org/10.1073/pnas.1117047109

25. Yeoh LM, Goodman CD, Hall NE, van Dooren GG, McFadden GI, Ralph SA (2015) A serine-arginine-rich (SR) splicing factor modulates alternative splicing of over a thousand genes in *Toxoplasma gondii*. Nucleic Acids Res 43:4661–4675. https://doi.org/10.1093/nar/gkv311

26. Hassan MA, Vasquez JJ, Guo-Liang C, Meissner M, Nicolai Siegel T (2017) Comparative ribosome profiling uncovers a dominant role for translational control in *Toxoplasma gondii*. BMC Genomics 18:961. https://doi.org/10.1186/s12864-017-4362-6

27. Pittman KJ, Aliota MT, Knoll LJ (2014) Dual transcriptional profiling of mice and *Toxoplasma gondii* during acute and chronic infection. BMC Genomics 15:806. https://doi.org/10.1186/1471-2164-15-806

28. Walker RA, Sharman PA, Miller CM, Lippuner C, Okoniewski M, Eichenberger RM et al (2015) RNA Seq analysis of the Eimeria tenella gametocyte transcriptome reveals clues about the molecular basis for sexual reproduction and oocyst biogenesis. BMC Genomics 16:94. https://doi.org/10.1186/s12864-015-1298-6

29. Krishna R, Xia D, Sanderson S, Shanmugasundram A, Vermont S, Bernal A, Daniel-Naguib G, Ghali F, Brunk BP, Roos DS, Wastling JM, Jones AR (2015) A large-scale proteogenomics study of apicomplexan pathogens-*Toxoplasma gondii* and Neospora caninum. Proteomics 15:2618–2628. doi: https://doi.org/10.1002/pmic.201400553

30. Xia D, Sanderson SJ, Jones AR, Prieto JH, Yates JR, Bromley E, Tomley FM, Lal K, Sinden RE, Brunk BP, Roos D S, Wastling JM (2008) The proteome of *Toxoplasma gondii*: integration with the genome provides novel insights into gene expression and annotation. Genome Biology 2009 10:5 9:R116. doi: https://doi.org/10.1186/gb-2008-9-7-r116

31. Dybas JM, Madrid-Aliste CJ, Che F-Y, Nieves E, Rykunov D, Angeletti RH et al (2008) Computational analysis and experimental validation of gene predictions in *Toxoplasma gondii*. PLoS One 3:e3899. https://doi.org/10.1371/journal.pone.0003899

32. Hu K, Johnson J, Florens L, Fraunholz M, Suravajjala S, DiLullo C et al (2006) Cytoskeletal components of an invasion machine—the apical complex of *Toxoplasma gondii*. PLoS Pathog 2:e13. https://doi.org/10.1371/journal.ppat.0020013

33. Seidi A, Muellner-Wong LS, Rajendran E, Tjhin ET, Dagley LF, Aw VY, Faou P, Webb AI, Tonkin CJ, van Dooren GG (2018) Elucidating the mitochondrial proteome of *Toxoplasma gondii* reveals the presence of a divergent cytochrome c oxidase. eLife 7: D684. doi: https://doi.org/10.7554/eLife.38131

34. Bradley PJ, Ward C, Cheng SJ, Alexander DL, Coller S, Coombs GH et al (2005) Proteomic analysis of rhoptry organelles reveals many novel constituents for host-parasite interactions in *Toxoplasma gondii*. J Biol Chem 280:34245–34258. https://doi.org/10.1074/jbc.M504158200

35. Zhou XW, Kafsack BFC, Cole RN, Beckett P, Shen RF, Carruthers VB (2005) The opportunistic pathogen *Toxoplasma gondii* deploys a diverse legion of invasion and survival proteins. J Biol Chem 280:34233–34244. https://doi.org/10.1074/jbc.M504160200

36. Travier L, Mondragon R, Dubremetz JF, Musset K, Mondragon M, Gonzalez S et al (2008) Functional domains of the *Toxoplasma* GRA2 protein in the formation of the membranous nanotubular network of the parasitophorous vacuole. Int J Parasitol 38:757–773. https://doi.org/10.1016/j.ijpara.2007.10.010

37. Nebl T, Prieto JH, Kapp E, Smith BJ, Williams MJ, Yates JR et al (2011) Quantitative in vivo analyses reveal calcium-dependent phosphorylation sites and identifies a novel component of the *Toxoplasma* invasion motor complex. PLoS Pathog 7:e1002222. https://doi.org/10.1371/journal.ppat.1002222

38. Treeck M, Sanders JL, Elias JE, Boothroyd JC (2011) The phosphoproteomes of Plasmodium falciparum and *Toxoplasma gondii* reveal unusual adaptations within and beyond the parasites' boundaries. Cell Host Microbe 10:410–419. https://doi.org/10.1016/j.chom.2011.09.004

39. Yakubu RR, Silmon de Monerri NC, Nieves E, Kim K, Weiss LM (2017) Comparative mono-methylarginine proteomics suggests that protein arginine methyltransferase 1 (PRMT1) is a significant contributor to arginine mono-methylation in *Toxoplasma gondii*. Mol Cell Proteomics 16:567–580. https://doi.org/10.1074/mcp.M117.066951

40. Jeffers V, Sullivan WJ (2012) Lysine acetylation is widespread on proteins of diverse function and localization in the protozoan parasite *Toxoplasma gondii*. Eukaryot Cell 11:735–742. https://doi.org/10.1128/EC.00088-12

41. Xue B, Jeffers V, Sullivan WJ, Uversky VN (2013) Protein intrinsic disorder in the acetylome of intracellular and extracellular *Toxoplasma gondii*. Mol BioSyst 9:645–657. https://doi.org/10.1039/c3mb25517d

42. Silmon de Monerri NC, Yakubu RR, Chen AL, Bradley PJ, Nieves E, Weiss LM et al (2015) The ubiquitin proteome of *Toxoplasma gondii* reveals roles for protein ubiquitination in cell-cycle transitions. Cell Host Microbe 18:621–633. https://doi.org/10.1016/j.chom.2015.10.014

43. Dogga SK, Mukherjee B, Jacot D, Kockmann T, Molino L, Hammoudi P-M et al (2017) A druggable secretory protein maturase of *Toxoplasma* essential for invasion and egress. eLife 6:223. https://doi.org/10.7554/elife.27480

44. Coffey MJ, Dagley LF, Seizova S, Kapp EA, Infusini G, Roos DS, Boddey JA, Webb AI, Tonkin CJ (2018) Aspartyl Protease 5 Matures Dense Granule Proteins That Reside at the Host-Parasite Interface in *Toxoplasma gondii*. MBio 9:e01796–18. doi: https://doi.org/10.1128/mBio.01796-18

45. Possenti A, Fratini F, Fantozzi L, Pozio E, Dubey JP, Ponzi M et al (2013) Global proteomic analysis of the oocyst/sporozoite of *Toxoplasma gondii* reveals commitment to a host-independent lifestyle. BMC Genomics 14:183. https://doi.org/10.1186/1471-2164-14-183

46. Fritz HM, Bowyer PW, Bogyo M, Conrad PA, Boothroyd JC (2012) Proteomic analysis of fractionated *Toxoplasma* oocysts reveals clues to their environmental resistance. PLoS One 7:e29955. https://doi.org/10.1371/journal.pone.0029955

47. Oakes RD, Kurian D, Bromley E, Ward C, Lal K, Blake DP et al (2013) The rhoptry proteome of *Eimeria tenella* sporozoites. Int J Parasitol 43:181–188. https://doi.org/10.1016/j.ijpara.2012.10.024

48. Sidik SM, Huet D, Ganesan SM, Huynh M-H, Wang T, Nasamu AS et al (2016) A genome-wide CRISPR screen in *Toxoplasma* identifies essential apicomplexan genes. Cell 166:1423–1435.e12. https://doi.org/10.1016/j.cell.2016.08.019

49. Su C, Zhang X, Dubey JP (2006) Genotyping of *Toxoplasma gondii* by multilocus PCR-RFLP markers: a high resolution and simple method for identification of parasites. Int J Parasitol 36:841–848. https://doi.org/10.1016/j.ijpara.2006.03.003

50. Kanehisa M, Furumichi M, Tanabe M, Sato Y, Morishima K (2017) KEGG: new perspectives on genomes, pathways, diseases and drugs. Nucleic Acids Res 45:D353–D361. https://doi.org/10.1093/nar/gkw1092

51. Caspi R, Billington R, Ferrer L, Foerster H, Fulcher CA, Keseler IM et al (2016) The Meta-Cyc database of metabolic pathways and enzymes and the BioCyc collection of pathway/genome databases. Nucleic Acids Res 44:D471–D480. https://doi.org/10.1093/nar/gkv1164

52. Hastings J, de Matos P, Dekker A, Ennis M, Harsha B, Kale N et al (2013) The ChEBI reference database and ontology for biologically relevant chemistry: enhancements for 2013. Nucleic Acids Res 41:D456–D463. https://doi.org/10.1093/nar/gks1146

53. Lopes CT, Franz M, Kazi F, Donaldson SL, Morris Q, Bader GD (2010) Cytoscape Web: an interactive web-based network browser. Bioinformatics 26:2347–2348. https://doi.org/10.1093/bioinformatics/btq430

54. Chen F (2006) OrthoMCL-DB: querying a comprehensive multi-species collection of ortholog groups. Nucleic Acids Res 34:D363–D368. https://doi.org/10.1093/nar/gkj123

55. Zdobnov EM, Apweiler R (2001) InterProScan—an integration platform for the signature-recognition methods in InterPro. Bioinformatics 17:847–848

56. McDowall J, Hunter S (2010) InterPro protein classification, in: yeast functional genomics. Humana Press, Totowa, NJ, pp 37–47. https://doi.org/10.1007/978-1-60761-977-2_3

57. Emanuelsson O, Brunak S, von Heijne G, Nielsen H (2007) Locating proteins in the cell using TargetP, SignalP and related tools. Nat Protoc 2:953–971. https://doi.org/10.1038/nprot.2007.131

58. Predicting transmembrane protein topology with a hidden markov model: application to complete genomes (2000)

59. Harb OS, Roos DS (2015) The eukaryotic pathogen databases: a functional genomic

resource integrating data from human and veterinary parasites. Methods Mol Biol 1201:1–18. https://doi.org/10.1007/978-1-4939-1438-8_1

60. Warrenfeltz S, Basenko EY, Crouch K, Harb OS, Kissinger JC, Roos DS et al (2018) EuPathDB: the eukaryotic pathogen genomics database resource. In: Eukaryotic genomic databases. Humana Press, New York, NY, pp 69–113. https://doi.org/10.1007/978-1-4939-7737-6_5

61. Basenko EY, Pulman JA, Shanmugasundram A, Harb OS, Crouch K, Starns D et al (2018) FungiDB: an integrated bioinformatic resource for fungi and oomycetes. J Fungi (Basel) 4:39. https://doi.org/10.3390/jof4010039

62. Afgan E, Baker D, Batut B, van den Beek M, Bouvier D, Čech M et al (2018) The Galaxy platform for accessible, reproducible and collaborative biomedical analyses: 2018 update. Nucleic Acids Res 46:W537–W544. https://doi.org/10.1093/nar/gky379

Chapter 3

Isolation and Genotyping of *Toxoplasma gondii* Strains

Chunlei Su and Jitender P. Dubey

Abstract

Toxoplasma gondii is a protozoan parasite that infects mammals and birds. Molecular epidemiology and population genetic studies have revealed widespread and distinct distribution of different *T. gondii* genotypes globally. Animals (domestic and wild) are the reservoirs for transmission of this parasite to humans. Recent development in molecular genotyping methods allowed us to identify parasite strains with high resolution and to dissect transmission patterns among different hosts. However, current data in the literature is still limited and fragmented. Here, we summarize a set of protocols that can be used to identify *T. gondii* infection in clinically normal animals, isolate the parasite by bioassay using animal tissues, extract parasite DNA from tissue samples, and finally identify the parasite by multilocus PCR-RFLP genotyping. We hope these protocols provide essential tools to study genetic diversity, population structure and transmission dynamics of *T. gondii*. Accumulation of the information will allow us to better understand, control, and prevent *T. gondii* infection in the future.

Key words *Toxoplasma*, Modified agglutination test (MAT), PCR, RFLP, Genotype, Genetic diversity

1 Introduction

Toxoplasma gondii is a widespread protozoan parasite that infects mammals and birds [1]. Felids (domestic and wild cats) are the definitive hosts in which the parasite undergoes sexual reproduction and release many environmentally resistant *T. gondii* in the form of oocysts in cat feces. Other animals can be infected by ingesting oocysts from contaminated environment. Most animal species are resistant to *T. gondii*, which leads to chronic infection with the parasites encysting (tissue cysts) in many organs, primarily in muscle and neural tissues. Humans can be infected by ingesting food and water contaminated with oocysts, or under cooked meat that contains *T. gondii* tissue cysts. Approximately one-third of human population is infected with this parasite [1]. Though most infections in humans are asymptomatic, some may progress to severe ocular infection and cause retinochoroiditis, and even total blindness. In immunocompromised patients such as those with AIDS, reactivation of chronic *T. gondii* infection may lead to fatal

Christopher J. Tonkin (ed.), *Toxoplasma gondii: Methods and Protocols*, Methods in Molecular Biology, vol. 2071,
https://doi.org/10.1007/978-1-4939-9857-9_3, © Springer Science+Business Media, LLC, part of Springer Nature 2020

encephalitis. In addition, primary infection in pregnant women may cause severe congenital toxoplasmosis in developing fetus, leading to hydrocephalus, microcephaly, microphthalmia, intracerebral calcification, and blindness [2].

Recent molecular and population genetic studies revealed high diversity of *T. gondii* worldwide. Among hundreds of genotypes identified from thousands of *T. gondii* samples, a strong population structure was revealed [3]. Whereas *T. gondii* populations in north hemisphere are dominated by a few clonal genotypes, it is highly diverse in South America. In addition, the parasite strains from the latter are likely to be more virulent to laboratory mice than the clonal types in north hemisphere. Coincidently, severe disseminated acute toxoplasmosis cases in humans are often associated with unique genotypes in South America [4], suggesting potential link of *T. gondii* genotypes with their virulence.

Given a large number of animal species serve as the hosts for *T. gondii*, as well as the genetic and phenotypic diversity of this parasite, it is important to understand the transmission dynamics of *T. gondii*. To this end, identify infection, isolate the parasites and distinguish different parasite strains are essential. There are a variety of reports that are published in the literature and used for these purposes. Here we provide a collection of protocols that have been tested and adopted in our laboratories. We hope these protocols are useful in providing basic information regarding how to identify *T. gondii* infection in animals, to isolate the parasite by bioassay, to extract DNA, and to genotype the parasites.

2 Materials

There are four major steps for isolation and genotyping *T. gondii* strains, including: (1) identify chronic infection of *T. gondii* in animals; (2) bioassay in mice to isolate *T. gondii*; (3) extract DNA from blood or tissues of infected animals; and (4) genotype *T. gondii* isolates. Materials described here are divided into four sections accordingly. Given *T. gondii* is a zoonotic pathogen, all procedures involved in handling animal tissues potentially containing the parasite must be performed with caution, and using a biosafety hood is highly recommended. In addition, these protocols also apply to the isolation of *T. gondii* from human samples. To this end, proper training of biosafety and handling of human derived materials are necessary.

2.1 Identify Infection of T. gondii in Animals— Serological Diagnosis Using the Modified Agglutination Test (MAT)

1. Alkaline Buffer. Dissolve 7.01 g sodium chloride (NaCl), 3.09 g boric acid (H_3BO_3), and 1 g sodium azide in 900 ml distilled water, add 20 ml 1 N sodium hydroxide (NaOH) and adjust pH to 8.95. Add 4 g bovine albumin, bring volume to 1 l with distilled water. Store at 4 °C.

2. Phosphate Buffered Saline (PBS). Dissolve 7.20 g NaCl, 1.48 g sodium phosphate dibasic (Na_2HPO_4, anhydrous), and 0.43 g potassium phosphate monobasic (KH_2PO_4, anhydrous) in 1 l distilled water (*see* **Note 1**). Autoclave to sterilize, and store at 4 °C.

3. *Toxoplasma gondii* whole-cell antigen containing 2×10^8 tachyzoites/ml, store at 4 °C (*see* **Note 2**). Mix well before use, the resuspension should be cloudy but without clumps.

4. Positive and negative control sera, store at −20 °C (*see* **Note 3**).

5. 2% Evans blue dye. Dissolve 2 g of Evans blue in 100 ml distilled H_2O, store at 4 °C.

6. 2-mercaptoethanol.

7. 96-well U-bottom microtiter plates.

8. 96-well microtiter plate sealing film or duct tape. This is to seal the plate to prevent evaporation during incubation at 37 °C.

9. 37 °C incubator.

10. Serum, plasma or tissue fluid samples to be tested. A minimum of 3 μl of sample is needed for a MAT test for mammals, 12 μl for birds.

11. 0.5-ml microcentrifuge tubes.

2.2 Bioassay to Isolate T. gondii from Infected Animals

1. Blood (coagulant-treated) or tissues (lung, mesenteric lymph node, heart, spleen, etc.) collected from animals with acute toxoplasmosis, or heart or brain tissues collected from animals chronically infected with *T. gondii* (MAT positive).

2. IFN-γ knock-out mice or CD1 (ICR) outbred mice for bioassay.

3. (Optional) 15 μg/ml dexamethasone phosphate. Dissolve 30 mg dexamethasone phosphate in 200 ml distilled H_2O.

4. IKA ULTRA-TURRAX disperser and 15-ml IKA DT tubes (or other suitable tissue homogenizer).

5. Saline (0.85% NaCl). Dissolve 4.25 g NaCl in 500 ml double distilled water. Autoclave to sterilize.

6. Acid pepsin solution (pH ~1.1–1.2). Dissolve 0.85 g NaCl in 100 ml distilled water, add 1.4 ml 12 N hydrochloric acid, mix well, and add 0.52 g pepsin. Note: At low pH, pepsin also digests bacteria. When acid is neutralized, pepsin is inactivated.

7. 1.2% sodium bicarbonate (pH ~8.3). Dissolve 1.2 g sodium bicarbonate ($NaHCO_2$) in 100 ml double distilled water, add

2 mg phenol red as the pH indicator. Filter through 0.22 μm filter to sterilize.

8. Phosphate buffered saline (PBS) *see* Subheading 2.1.

9. PBS containing 10 μg/ml of gentamicin: Add 0.1 ml 10 mg/ml gentamicin to 100 ml PBS.

10. 70% ethanol.

11. Mortars and pestles, autoclaved.

12. Medium A: 50% fetal bovine serum (FBS) in Dulbecco's Modified Eagle Media (DMEM). Mix 15 ml FBS with 15 ml DMEM, filter-sterilize using 0.22 μm filter. This medium can be stored at 4 °C for a few months.

13. Medium B: 20% DMSO in DMEM. Mix 5 ml DMSO with 20 ml DMEM, filter sterilize using 0.22 μm filter. This medium can be stored at 4 °C for a few months.

14. 15-ml and 50-ml centrifuge tubes, sterile.

15. 3-ml, 5-ml, 10-ml syringes, 20 G, 22 G needles.

16. Sterile gauze.

17. 1-ml cryovials for preservation of *T. gondii* strains.

18. Nalgene Cryo 1 °C Freezing Container.

19. −80 °C freezer.

20. −140 °C freezer or liquid N_2 tank for long-term storage of *T. gondii* stocks.

21. 1.5-ml microcentrifuge tubes.

2.3 Extract DNA from Blood and Tissues of Infected Animals

1. Qiagen DNeasy Blood & Tissue Kit: Buffer AL, ATL, AW1, AW2, AE, proteinase K, Mini spin columns, 2-ml collection tubes.

2. Blood or homogenized tissue samples.

3. Ethanol (96%–100%).

4. Microcentrifuge.

5. 1.5-ml microcentrifuge tubes.

2.4 Genotype T. gondii Isolates

1. FastStart DNA polymerase kit (Roche Applied Science) or similar reagents.

2. dNTPs mix, 2.5 mM each.

3. External primers each at 500 μM (Table 1).

4. Internal (nested) primers each at 50 μM (Table 1).

5. Thermocycler.

6. 0.2-ml PCR tubes.

7. 0.5-ml microcentrifuge tubes.

8. Gel electrophoresis apparatus.

Table 1
Summary of primers for multilocus PCR-RFLP markers (Su et al. [5])

Markers	External primers (multiplex PCR)	Internal primers (nested PCR)	Nested PCR (bp)	Restriction enzymes, NEB buffers, incubation temperature and time
SAG1	SAG1-Fext: GTTCTAACCACGCACCCTGAG SAG1-Rext2: AAGAGTGGGAGGCTCTGTGA	SAG1-S2: CAATGTGCACCTGTAGGAAGC SAG1-Rext: GTGGTTCTCCGTCGGTGTGAG	390	Sau96I + HaeII (double digest) NEB4, BSA, 37 °C 1 h. 2.5% gel
5'-SAG2	Not needed	5-SAG2F: GAAATGTTTCAGGTTGCTGC 5-SAG2R: GCAAGAGCGAACTTGAACAC	242	MboI, NEB4, BSA, 37 °C 1 h. 2.5% gel
3'-SAG2	3'-SAG2-Fext: TCTGTTCTCCGAAGTGACTCC 3'-SAG2-Rext: TCAAAGCGTGCATTATCGC	3-SAG2F: ATTCTCATGCCTCCGCTTC 3-SAG2R: AACG TTTCACGAAGGCACAC	222	HhaI, NEB4, BSA, 37 °C 1 h. 2.5% gel
SAG3	SAG3-Fext: CAACTCTCACCATTCCACCC SAG3-Rext: GCGCGTTGTTAGACAAGACA	P43S2: TCTTGTCGGGTGTTCACTCA P43AS2: CACAAGGAGACCGAGAAGGA	225	NciI, NEB4, BSA, 37 °C 1 h. 2.5% gel
BTUB	BTUB-Fext: TCCAAAATGAGAGAAATCGT BTUB-Rext: AAATTGAAATGACGGAAGAA	Btub-F: GAGGTCATCTCGGACGAACA BtubR: TTGTAGGAACACCCGGACGC	411	BsiEI + TaqI (double digest), NEB4, BSA, 60 °C 1 h. 2.5% gel
GRA6	GRA6-Fext: ATTTGTGTTTCCGAGCAGGT GRA6-Rext: GCACCTTCGCTTGTGGTT	GRA6-F1: TTTCCGAGCAGGTGACCT GRA6-R1x: TCGCCGAAGAG TTGACATAG	344	MseI, NEB2, BSA, 37 °C 1 h. 2.5% gel Note: use 0.2 μl/rxn of MseI
c22-8	c22-8-Fext: TGATGCATCCATGCGTTTAT c22-8-Rext: CCTCCACTTCTTCGGTCTCA	C22-8F: TCTCTCTACGTGGACGCC C22-8R: AGGTGCTTGGATATTCGC	521	BsmAI (or BCoDI) + MboII (double digest), NEB2, BSA, 37 °C 30 min, 55 °C 30 min. 2.5% gel

(continued)

Table 1
(continued)

Markers	External primers (multiplex PCR)	Internal primers (nested PCR)	Nested PCR (bp)	Restriction enzymes, NEB buffers, incubation temperature and time
c29-2	c29-2-Fext: ACCCACTGAGCGAAAAGAAA c29-2-Rext: AGGGTCTCTTGCGCATACAT	C29-2F: AGTTCTGCAGAGTGTCGC C29-2R: TGTCTAGGAAAGAGGGCGC	446	HpyCH4IV + RsaI (double digest), NEB1, BSA, 37 °C 1 h. 2.5% gel. Note: may use 0.2 μl/rxn of both enzymes
L358	L358-Fext: TCTCTCGACTTCGCCTCTTC L358-Rext: GCAATTTCCTCGAAGACAGG	L358-F2: AGGAGGCGTAGCGCAAGT L358-R2: CCCTCTGGCTGCAGTGCT	418	HaeIII + NlaIII (double digest), NEB4, BSA, 37 °C 1 h. 2.5% gel. Note: use 0.2 μl/rxn of NlaIII
PK1	PK1-Fext: GAAAGCTGTCCACCCTGAAA PK1-Rext: AGAAAGCTCCGTGCAGTGAT	PK1-F: CGCAAAGGGGAGACAATCAGT PK1-R: TCATCGCTGAATCTCATTGC	903	AvaI + RsaI (double digest), NEB4, BSA, 37 °C 1 h. 2.5% gel
Alt. SAG2	Alt. SAG2-Fext: GGAACGGCGAACAATGAGTTT Alt. SAG2-Rext: GCACTGTTGTCCAGGGTTTT	SAG2-Fa: ACCCATCTGCGAAGAAAACG SAG2-Ra: ATTTCGACCAGCGGGGAGCAC	546	HinfI + TaqI, NEB3, BSA, 37 °C 30 min, 65 °C 30 min. 2.5% gel
Apico	Apico-Fext: TGGTTTTAACCCTAGATTGTGG Apico-Rext: AAACGGAATTAATGAGATTTGAA	Apico-F: TGCAAATTCTTGAATTC TCAGTT Apico-R: GGGATTCGAACCCTTGATA	640	AflII + DdeI (double digest), NEB2, BSA, 37 °C 1 h. 3% gel. Note: may use 0.2 μl/rxn of both enzymes

9. Restriction enzymes, buffers, bovine serum albumin (BSA) (Table 1).

10. Agarose.

11. RedSafe nucleic acid staining dye, 20,000×.

12. SB electrophoresis buffer (Dissolve 2.25 g boric acid (H_3BO_3), 0.4 g sodium hydroxide (NaOH) in 1 l double distilled H_2O).

13. DNA loading dye, 6×.

14. DNA size marker.

15. UV box and image system to take and record results from gel electrophoresis.

3   Methods

3.1   Identify Infection of T. gondii in Animals by MAT Test

The MAT test is the most widely used method for the diagnosis of *T. gondii* infection in animals. It can be used for mammals and birds. The advantage of this method is its high sensitivity and specificity, as well as its ease of performance, and there is no need for specific equipment [6, 7].

1. For mammals, make 1:25 dilution of serum, plasma, or tissue fluid samples and the controls in PBS in 0.5-ml microcentrifuge tubes as below:

PBS	72.0 µl
Sample or control	3.0 µl
Total volume	75.0 µl
Mix well	

For birds, make 1:5 dilution of serum, plasma or tissue fluid samples in PBS in 0.5-ml microcentrifuge tubes as below. For the positive and negative controls, start with 1:25 dilution as above.

PBS	48.0 µl
Sample	12.0 µl
Total volume	60.0 µl
Mix well	

2. To a 96-well U-bottom microtiter plate, transfer 50 µl of diluted samples to the first row from column 1 to column 10 of the plate. Transfer 50 µl of diluted negative and positive controls to the first wells of columns 11 and 12, respectively (10 samples, one negative and one positive control) *see* Fig. 1 for sample layout.

	Sample 1	Sample 2	Sample 3	Sample 4	Sample 5	Sample 6	Sample 7	Sample 8	Sample 9	Sample 10	Negative control	Positive control	
1:25	50 µl	50 µl	50 µl	50 µl	50 µl	50 µl	50 µl	50 µl	50 µl	50 µl	50 µl	50 µl	25 µl
1:50	25 µl PBS	25 µl PBS	25 µl PBS	25 µl PBS	25 µl PBS	25 µl PBS	25 µl PBS	25 µl PBS	25 µl PBS	25 µl PBS	25 µl PBS	25 µl PBS	25 µl
1:100	25 µl PBS	25 µl PBS	25 µl PBS	25 µl PBS	25 µl PBS	25 µl PBS	25 µl PBS	25 µl PBS	25 µl PBS	25 µl PBS	25 µl PBS	25 µl PBS	25 µl
1:200	25 µl PBS	25 µl PBS	25 µl PBS	25 µl PBS	25 µl PBS	25 µl PBS	25 µl PBS	25 µl PBS	25 µl PBS	25 µl PBS	25 µl PBS	25 µl PBS	25 µl
1:400	25 µl PBS	25 µl PBS	25 µl PBS	25 µl PBS	25 µl PBS	25 µl PBS	25 µl PBS	25 µl PBS	25 µl PBS	25 µl PBS	25 µl PBS	25 µl PBS	25 µl
1:800	25 µl PBS	25 µl PBS	25 µl PBS	25 µl PBS	25 µl PBS	25 µl PBS	25 µl PBS	25 µl PBS	25 µl PBS	25 µl PBS	25 µl PBS	25 µl PBS	25 µl
1:1,600	25 µl PBS	25 µl PBS	25 µl PBS	25 µl PBS	25 µl PBS	25 µl PBS	25 µl PBS	25 µl PBS	25 µl PBS	25 µl PBS	25 µl PBS	25 µl PBS	25 µl
1:3,200	25 µl PBS	25 µl PBS	25 µl PBS	25 µl PBS	25 µl PBS	25 µl PBS	25 µl PBS	25 µl PBS	25 µl PBS	25 µl PBS	25 µl PBS	25 µl PBS	

Discard 25 µl

Fig. 1 MAT test to identify *T. gondii* positive samples. Serum, plasma, or tissue fluid samples and the controls are diluted from 1:25 to 1:3200 in columns

3. Add 25 µl of PBS to the rest of the wells.

4. Using a multichannel pipette, take 25 µl of diluted samples and the controls from row 1, make serial 1:2 dilution, remove 25 µl from the last dilution (1:3200) and discard.

5. Prepare antigen mixture (each 96-well plate):

Alkaline buffer	2.5 ml
2-mercaptoethanol	35 µl
Evans blue dye (2 mg/ml in H_2O)	50 µl
TgMAT antigen	150 µl
Total	2.735 ml

6. Mix antigen well by pipetting, immediately transfer 25 µl antigen mixture to each well using multichannel pipette. To prevent carryover of samples, the pipette tips should not touch the bottom of wells. Tap the plate lightly to bring the liquid to the bottom of the wells. Note: Each well has 3×10^5 tachyzoites.

7. Cover the plate with sealing film or duct tape and incubate at 37 °C for 16–24 h. A clear pellet at the bottom of the well means negative. The wells without pellets (form diffused mats) are positive. An example of a MAT test is presented in Fig. 2.

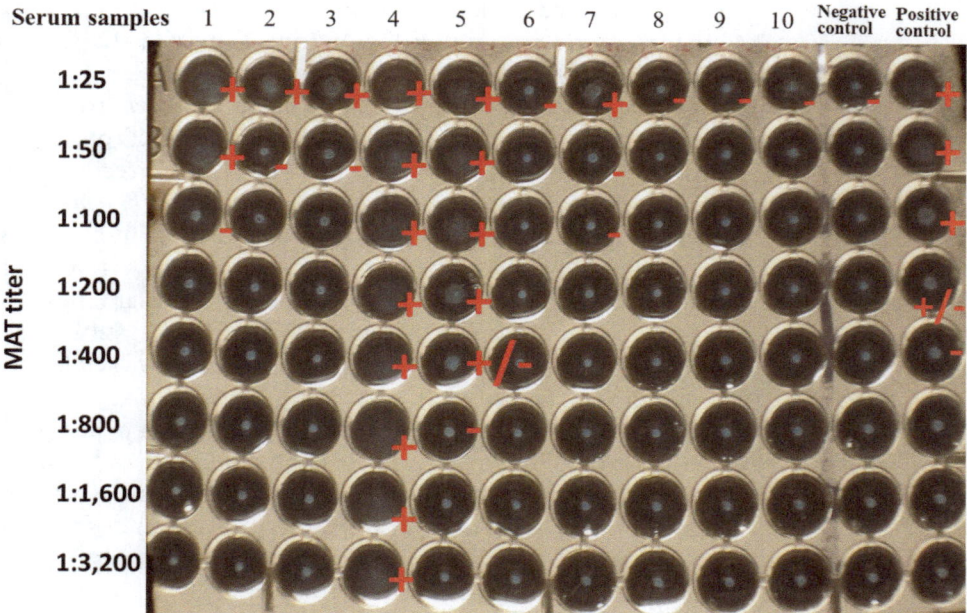

Fig. 2 Example of MAT test results. Wells that have a layer of mat (no distinct pellet) are considered positive. Wells with clear pellets are negative

8. For mammals, serum samples with MAT titer ≥1:25 are considered positive. For birds, MAT titer ≥1:5 are considered positive.

9. For positive mammal samples with titers ≥1:3200, further test is needed to determine titers. Start with making 1:100 dilution of the original samples in 0.5-ml microcentrifuge tubes (1 µl sample in 99 µl PBS), then make three serial 1:2 dilutions (25 µl of the diluted + 25 µl PBS) to 1:800. Take the 1:800 dilutions, proceed as in **step 2** above using a 96-well U-bottom microtiter plate, the final dilution is 1:102,400. For negative and positive controls, start with 1:25 dilution as in **step 2** above, the final dilution is 1:3200.

For positive bird samples with titers ≥1:640, further test is performed to determine titers. Start with making 1:80 dilution of the original samples in 0.5-ml microcentrifuge tubes (mix 1 µl sample with 79 µl PBS), then proceed as in **step 2** above using a 96-well U-bottom microtiter plate, the final dilution is 1:10,240. For negative and positive controls, start with 1:25 dilution as in **step 2** above, and the final dilution is 1:3200.

3.2 Bioassay to Isolate T. gondii from Infected Animals

Samples used to isolate *T. gondii* by bioassay can be divided into two groups. Group I samples include blood (anticoagulant-treated) and tissues (lung, mesenteric lymph node, heart, spleen, etc.) from animals that died from acute toxoplasmosis (*see* **Note 4**). DNA directly extracted from blood or tissues from this group often contains a good amount of DNA from *T. gondii*; therefore, it is worth the effort to extract DNA for genotyping.

Group II samples include heart or brain tissues from animals that are chronically infected with *T. gondii* (MAT positive) but there are no clinical symptoms of infection. DNA directly extracted from tissues of this group contains little or none *T. gondii* DNA, therefore, isolating the parasites by bioassay is absolutely necessary.

For bioassay, the collected animal blood or tissue samples should be stored at 4 °C but not to be frozen at any time, since freezing can kill *T. gondii* in tissue cysts [1]. If possible, enclose tissue samples in vacuum bags and remove the air by vacuum pump, which seems to be beneficial in keeping *T. gondii* viable for several weeks [8]. The success rates of isolating *T. gondii* in mice vary from 0% to approx. 90%. Many factors influence the outcome. The amount of tissues used, the period of time that tissues were refrigerated, and the MAT titer. In general, larger amount of tissues and short storage time are better. Higher MAT titer is positively associated with higher rate in isolating the parasite by bioassay [9]. Different laboratory mouse strains have been used for bioassay of *T. gondii*. IFN-γ knock-out mice are excellent for bioassay as they are completely susceptible to *T. gondii*, and infection of the parasite will lead to acute toxoplasmosis and death of mice within 2–3 weeks, regardless the genotypes of the parasites. This makes it easier to isolate *T. gondii* and collect large amount of parasites for genotyping. However, due to the high cost of IFN-γ knock-out mice, many laboratories are using outbred CD1 (ICR) mice as the alternative. The CD1 mice are relatively resistant to *T. gondii*. Whereas infection with highly virulent *T. gondii* strains will lead to acute toxoplasmosis and death of mice, the less virulent strains will establish chronic infection which may not present obvious clinical symptoms. For the latter, the parasites form tissue cysts in mouse brain or muscle. DNA may be extracted from these tissues but parasite yield may not be high enough to give adequate amount of *T. gondii* DNA for genotyping.

1. For each sample, two IFN-γ knock-out mice or three outbred mice may be used. If outbred mice are used, it is optional to treat mice with 15 μg/ml dexamethasone phosphate in drinking water to make them more susceptible to *T. gondii* infection. The treatment can be administered for up to 10 days, starting the day of inoculation of tissues or 2 days prior. Longer treatment is not recommended, as it may cause complications.

2. Group I samples (acute toxoplasmosis). For anticoagulant-treated blood, transfer 100 μl to each of two 1.5-ml microcentrifuge tubes, proceed to Subheading 3.3 to extract DNA for genotyping. Transfer up to 5 ml blood to a 15-ml centrifuge tube, spin down at 800 × *g* for 10 min, remove and keep

serum, resuspend cells in up to 5 ml PBS containing 10 μg/ml of gentamicin, proceed to **step 10** to inoculate mice to isolate the parasite. For tissues, take 1 to 2 g of samples, cut into small pieces, place into a 15-ml IKA DT tube, and add 10 ml PBS. Homogenize by IKA ULTRA-TURRAX disperser (30 s at 6× speed, 3 times, or until tissue is homogenized). Transfer 50 μl tissue homogenate to each of two 1.5-ml microcentrifuge tubes, proceed to Subheading 3.3 to extract DNA for genotyping. Filter the homogenate through two layers of sterile gauze into a 50-ml centrifuge tube. Spin at 800 × *g* for 10 min. Discard the supernatants. Resuspend pellet in 5 ml PBS containing 10 μg/ml of gentamicin. Proceed to **step 10** to inoculate mice with up to 0.5 ml processed samples to isolate the parasite.

3. Group II samples. Weigh 3–5 g of the heart or brain sample, cut into small pieces. Place into a 15-ml IKA DT tube, add 10 ml saline. Homogenize by IKA ULTRA-TURRAX disperser (30 s at 6× speed, three times, or until tissue is homogenized).

4. Transfer into 50-ml centrifugation tube. Rinse the DT tube with 5 ml saline and add to the homogenate.

5. Add 15 ml of freshly prepared, prewarmed (37 °C) acid pepsin solution and incubate at 37 °C for 30–40 min with shaking.

6. After incubation, filter the homogenate through two layers of sterile gauze into a 50-ml centrifuge tube. Spin at 800 × *g* for 10 min. Discard the supernatants.

7. Resuspend the pellet in 10 ml PBS, if see fat adhere to the tubes, transfer the homogenate to a new 50-ml centrifugation tube, add 8 ml of freshly prepared 1.2% sodium bicarbonate with phenol red as a pH indicator. If the color changes to orange, add more 1.2% sodium bicarbonate until the color becomes red.

8. After mixing, centrifuge at 800 × *g* for 10 min. Discard the supernatant.

9. Add 3 ml of PBS containing 10 μg/ml gentamicin. Mix well (*see* **Note 5**).

10. Use a 3-ml syringe with 22 G needle, inoculate 0.5–1.0 ml of samples to each of two IFN-γ knockout mice or three outbred mice by intraperitoneal injection.

11. Observe mice daily. If mice show clinical signs of acute toxoplasmosis, such as rough fur or lethargic between day 6 and day 12 postinfection, euthanize the animals. Lay down the mouse on a flat surface, abdomen facing up, spray 70% ethanol to sterilize fur and skin. Cut open skin and tear open to expose the abdomen. Use a 5-ml syringe to inject up to 5 ml PBS

containing 10 μg/ml gentamicin into mouse peritoneal cavity, tap the abdomen to mix, collect peritoneal lavage into 15-ml centrifuge tube. Usually 3–5 ml of peritoneal lavage can be collected. In addition (optional), take 1/4 of the lung tissue, grind into small pieces using a sterile mortar and pestle.

12. Centrifuge peritoneal lavage at $800 \times g$ for 10 min. Discard the supernatant. Resuspend cells (mixture of mouse inflammatory cells and *T. gondii*) in 3 ml Medium A. For ground lung tissue, resuspend in 3 ml Medium A as well.

13. Cryopreserve *T. gondii*. Take 1 ml cell mixture (peritoneal lavage or ground lung), mix with 1 ml Medium B. Transfer 1 ml of mixture to two 1-ml cryovials. Put all vials into Nalgene Cryo 1 °C Freezing Container and place in −80 °C freezer overnight. Transfer cryovials to −140 °C freezer (or liquid N_2) for long-term storage.

14. Extract DNA: Transfer 0.5 ml of cell mixture to each of two 1.5-ml microcentrifuge tubes, centrifuge at $10,000 \times g$ for 2 min, discard supernatant, wash with 0.5 ml PBS, spin down cells, discard supernatant. Resuspend in 50 μl PBS, proceed to Subheading 3.3 to extract DNA for genotyping.

15. If outbred mice show no symptom of *T. gondii* infection after 12 days postinoculation, keep observing up to 4 weeks. Collect mouse blood samples, and determine if they are MAT positive (usually ≥1:200). MAT positive mice are chronically infected with *T. gondii*. IFN-γ knockout mice that did not show any symptoms by 4 weeks postinoculation are not expected to be infected and can be terminated.

16. Euthanize mice chronically infected with *T. gondii*, collect brain tissues in 50-ml centrifuge tubes, and add 5 ml PBS. Using a 10-ml syringe with 20 G needle to repeatedly pass brain tissue through the needle until it is homogenized. Transfer 10 μl of the homogenate to a glass slide, put on a cover slip and observe under a microscope. *T. gondii* tissue cysts may be observed (Fig. 3). Note: for some mice with low number of brain tissue cysts, the cysts may be difficult to find.

17. Cryo preserve mouse brain tissue. Transfer 2 ml brain homogenate into a 15-ml centrifuge tube, spin at $800 \times g$ for 10 min. Discard the supernatant. Add 1 ml Medium A and 1 ml Medium B, mix well. Transfer 1 ml mixture to two 1-ml cryovials. Cryopreserve as in **step 13** above.

18. Extract DNA. Take 0.5 ml brain homogenate from **step 16**, add to each of two 1.5-ml microcentrifuge tubes, spin at $10,000 \times g$ for 2 min, discard supernatant, wash with 0.5 ml PBS, spin down cells again, discard supernatant. Resuspend in 50 μl PBS, proceed to Subheading 3.3 to extract DNA for genotyping.

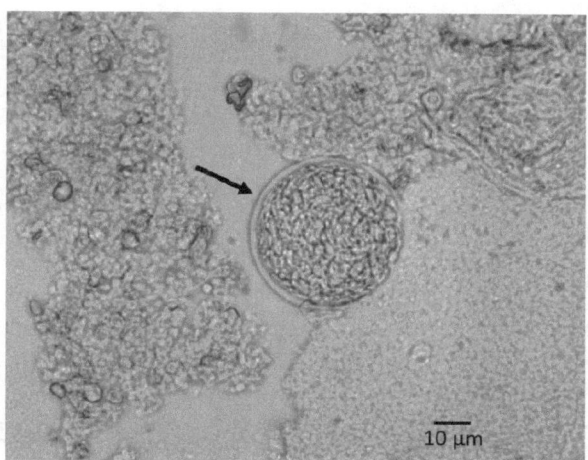

Fig. 3 *Toxoplasma gondii* tissue cyst from mouse brain. The image shows a tissue cyst with *T. gondii* bradyzoite enclosed (indicated by the arrow). The mouse was experimentally infected with a *T. gondii* strain, tissue cysts observed 6 weeks postinfection

19. (Optional) Given that parasite load in brain tissues of chronically infected mice is often low, *T. gondii* DNA concentration may be too low for genotyping. To overcome this limitation, it is highly recommended to isolate the parasites from a second round of bioassay, and then collect peritoneal lavage and the lung tissue during acute phase of toxoplasmosis. To accomplish this, inoculate 1 ml brain homogenate from **step 16** to each of two INF-γ knockout mice, and collect samples when symptoms of toxoplasmosis is obvious. Alternatively, treat three outbred mice with 15 μg/ml dexamethasone phosphate in drinking water 3 days before inoculating mouse brain homogenate (and continue to treat for additional 7 days). This treatment will make mice more susceptible to *T. gondii* and likely to develop acute toxoplasmosis when infected. Inoculate 1 ml brain homogenate to each of the three dexamethasone-treated outbred mice, obverse daily and collect samples when symptoms of toxoplasmosis is obvious between day 6 to day 12 post-inoculation. Following the **steps 11–14** above.

3.3 Extract DNA from Tissues of Infected Mice

Samples prepared from Subheading 3.2 are used to extract DNA. This protocol is adopted based on the manufacturer's instructions (Qiagen).

1. To the 1.5-ml microcentrifuge tubes containing 100 μl blood samples (from Subheading 3.2, **step 2**), add 20 μl proteinase K, 100 μl PBS, and 200 μl Buffer AL, mix well, incubate at 56 °C for 10 min, proceed to **step 2** below. To the 1.5-ml tubes

containing 50 μl tissue homogenates (from Subheading 3.2, steps **2**, **14**, **18**, and **19**), add 20 μl proteinase K and 180 μl Buffer ATL, mix by vortexing, and incubate at 56 °C until completely lysed. Vortex occasionally during incubation. Add 200 μl Buffer AL and mix by vortexing.

2. Add 200 μl ethanol (96%–100%). Mix thoroughly by vortexing.

3. Pipet the mixture into a DNeasy Mini spin column placed in a 2-ml collection tube. Centrifuge at ≥6000 × g for 1 min. Discard the flow-through and collection tube.

4. Place the spin column in a new 2-ml collection tube. Add 500 μl Buffer AW1. Centrifuge for 1 min at ≥6000 × g. Discard the flow-through and collection tube.

5. Place the spin column in a new 2-ml collection tube and add 500 μl Buffer AW2. Centrifuge for 3 min at 20,000 × g. Discard the flow-through and collection tube.

6. Transfer the spin column to a new 1.5-ml or 2-ml microcentrifuge tube.

7. Elute the DNA by adding 50 μl Buffer AE to the center of the spin column membrane. Incubate for 1 min at room temperature. Centrifuge for 1 min at ≥6000 × g.

8. To increase DNA yield, transfer the flow through back to the spin column membrane, centrifuge for 1 min at ≥6000 × g, and store DNA at −20 °C before use.

3.4 Genotype T. gondii Isolates by Multilocus PCR-RFLP

Multilocus restriction fragment length polymorphism (RFLP) and microsatellite markers are often used to reveal genetic diversity in *T. gondii* [5, 10]. Here we focus on the RFLP typing method. Ten PCR-RFLP markers, namely, SAG1, SAG2, SAG3, BTUB, GRA6, c22-8, c29-2, L358, PK1, and Apico, have been widely used to identify *T. gondii* isolates from a variety of hosts in different geographical regions, and revealed different population structure [3, 5, 11]. Applying this method for future molecular epidemiology and population studies will help us build up a larger database for better understanding transmission dynamics for this important parasite.

3.4.1 Multiplex PCR

1. Mix 10 μl of 500 μM external forward primers (SAG1, 3′-SAG2, alt.SAG2, SAG3, BTUB, GRA6, c22-8, c29-2, L358, PK1, and Apico), bring final volume to 200 μl by H₂O. The final concentration for each external forward primer is 25 μM. Prepare external reverse primers the same way. Note: 5′-SAG2 external primers are not needed because 5′-SAG2 sequence is covered by the alt. SAG2 external primers.

2. Assemble multiplex PCR mix (number of reactions + 1):

H$_2$O	16.5 µl
10× PCR buffer (Mg−)	2.5 µl
dNTPs (2.5 mM each)	2.0 µl
25 mM MgCl$_2$	2.0 µl
Mixed external forward primer (25 µM each)	0.15 µl
Mixed external reverse primer (25 µM each)	0.15 µl
FastStart Taq (5 U/µl)	0.20 µl
Total	23.5 µl

Note: For better results from Multiplex PCR, using FastStart Taq polymerase. It is a hot-start enzyme which eliminates nonspecific amplification of DNA in PCR reaction. If FastStart polymerase is not available, then other hot-start DNA polymerases will work.

3. Aliquot 23.5 µl of PCR mix to 0.2-ml PCR tubes. Add 1.5 µl of extracted DNA sample. Negative and positive controls should be included for each batch of PCR. Spin briefly if necessary.

4. In a thermocycler, heat samples at 95 °C for 4 min, then PCR 30 cycles of 94 °C for 30 s, 55 °C for 1 min, 72 °C for 2 min. Soak at 15 °C.

5. Add 25 µl of H$_2$O to dilute amplified PCR products.

3.4.2 Nested PCR

1. Prepare nested PCR mix for each individual marker (rxns + 1):

H$_2$O	16.5 µl
10× PCR buffer (Mg−)	2.5 µl
dNTPs (2.5 mM each)	2.0 µl
25 mM MgCl$_2$	2.0 µl
Nested forward primer (50 µM)	0.15 µl
Nested reverse primer (50 µM)	0.15 µl
FastStart Taq (5 U/µl)	0.20 µl
Total	23.5 µl

2. Aliquot 23.5 µl of PCR mix to 0.2-ml PCR tubes. Add 1.5 µl of multiplex PCR products. Spin briefly if necessary.

3. Heat samples at 95 °C for 4 min, then PCR 35 cycles of 94 °C for 30 s, 60 °C for 1 min, 72 °C for 1.5 min. Soak at 15 °C.

Note: For marker Apico, PCR 35 cycles of 94 °C for 30 s, 55 °C for 1 min, 72 °C for 2 min. Soak at 15 °C.

4. Prepare 1.5% agarose gel. Add appropriate amount of agarose to the volume of 1× SB buffer needed, microwave to dissolve agarose completely. Cool down to about 50 °C, add 10 µl of RedSafe nucleic acid staining dye to every 100 ml of 1× SB buffer, swirling to mix well. Pour gel to the tray and let cool down and solidify. Take 5 µl of PCR products, mix with 1 µl of 6× loading buffer, also prepare the DNA size marker, and run gel electrophoresis at 80–120 V for ~1.5 h. Exam gel under UV box. Take gel picture to record the results. If PCR successfully amplified the target sequences, then proceed to digest PCR products by restriction enzymes.

5. Prepare Digestion Mix (number of reactions + 1):

H₂O	14.6 µl
10× NEB buffer	2.0 µl
100× BSA	0.2 µl
Rest. Enzyme 1	0.1 µl
Rest. Enzyme 2 (if apply)	0.1 µl
Total	17.0 µl

6. Aliquot 17 µl Digestion Mix to 0.5 ml microcentrifuge tubes, add 3 µl PCR products, incubate for 1 h at the corresponding temperature (Table 1).

7. Prepare 2.5% agarose gel as in **step 4** above.

8. Add 4 µl of 6× loading dye to the digestion mix, run 2.5% agarose gel (containing RedSafe nucleic acid staining dye) in 1× SB buffer at 80–120 V for ~1.5 h. Note: marker Apico needs 3% gel. Take gel pictures and record results. An example of genotyping results for marker c22-8 is presented in Fig. 4.

9. Determine genotype results by comparing samples with the positive controls (*see* Table 2, **Note 6**). Examples of RFLP

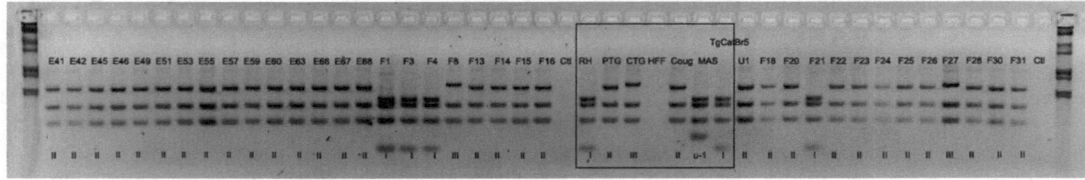

Fig. 4 An example of genotyping results for PCR-RFLP marker c22-8. Samples outlined in the square are positive controls (RH, PTG, CTG, Coug, MAS, and TgCaBr5). HFF is human DNA, Ctl is negative control without DNA added. Allele types (I, II, III, and u–1) for all samples are listed at the bottom. It is highly recommended to include positive and negative controls in each row of samples on the gel. This is because each enzyme digestion or agarose gel maybe slightly different from the others. Sometimes, incomplete digestion also occurs. Also, some DNA fragment patterns are very similar, it will be difficult to call alleles without positive controls in the same row on the same gel

Table 2
Summary of multilocus PCR-RFLP genotyping for *T. gondii* positive controls (Su et al. [5])

	Genetic markers											ToxoDB PCR-RFLP genotype
	SAG1	(5′ + 3′) SAG2	alt. SAG2	SAG3	B TUB	GRA6	C22-8	C29-2	L358	PK1	Apico	
GT1, RH (type I)	I	I	I	I	I	I	I	I	I	I	I	#10
PTG (type II)	II or III	II	II	II	II	II	II	II	II	II	II	#1
CTG (type III)	II or III	III	III	III	III	III	III	III	III	III	III	#2
TgCgCa1 (Coug)	I	II	II	III	II	II	II	u–1	I	u–2	I	#66
MAS	u–1	I	II	III	III	III	u–1	I	I	III	I	#17
TgCatBr5	I	III	III	III	III	III	I	I	I	u–1	I	#19
TgCatBr64	I	I	u-1	III	III	III	u–1	I	III	III	I	#111
TgRsCr1	u–1	I	II	III	I	III	u–2	I	I	III	I	#52

patterns for *T. gondii* reference strains can be found in previous published report [5].

10. Compare with existing ToxoDB PCR-RFLP genotypes to determine if there are matches (Table 3).

4 Notes

1. PBS from commercial vendors works well.

2. The whole-cell antigen can be prepared in-house in cell culture or purchased from other source (e.g., https://utrf.tennessee.edu/product-category/tgmat/). Freezing whole-cell antigen will destroy the tachyzoites, which makes the antigen unsuitable for MAT test.

3. The positive control can be serum from animals experimentally infected with *T. gondii* or animals known to be positive with *T. gondii* infection. The negative control serum can be fetal bovine serum or serum from animals known to be negative with *T. gondii* infection. Dilute positive serum to a titer of 1:200 in fetal bovine serum. Aliquot positive control serum in small volume (e.g., 50 ul) and store at −20 °C.

4. If tissue samples (lung, liver, muscle, etc.) collected from animals were frozen during storage, then they are not suitable to

Table 3
Identified PCR-RFLP genotypes

ToxoDB Genotypes	PCR-RFLP markers										
	SAG1	3′, 5′-SAG2	alt. SAG2	SAG3	BTUB	GRA6	C22-8	C29-2	L358	PK1	Apico
#1	II or III	II	II	II	II	II	II	II	II	II	II
#2	II or III	III	III	III	III	III	III	III	III	III	III
#3	II or III	II	II	II	II	II	II	II	II	II	I
#4	II or III	II	II	II	II	II	II	II	I	II	I
#5	u-1	II	II	II	II	II	I	II	II	II	I
#6	I	I	I	I	I	I	u-1	I	I	I	I
#7	I	III	III	III	III	III	III	III	III	III	III
#8	I	III	III	III	III	II	II	III	III	II	I
#9	u-1	II	I	I	I	I	I	I	I	I	I
#10	I	III	III	III	III	III	III	III	III	II	III
#11	I	I	I	I	I	I	I	I	I	I	I
#12	I	III	III	III	III	III	III	III	III	III	III
#13	I	I	I	I	I	I	I	III	III	I	III
#14	I	III	III	III	III	III	III	III	III	III	III
#15	u-1	I	II	III	III	I	III	I	I	I	I
#16	I	I	III	III	III	III	III	III	III	I	I
#17	u-1	I	II	III	I	I	u-1	III	I	III	I
#18	I	I	I	III	II	III	II	I	III	III	I
#19	I	III	III	III	II	I	I	I	I	u-1	I

Sample											
#20	II	u-1	II	II	III	III	II	III	II	u-2	I
#21	III	I	III	III	III	III	III	III	I	III	III
#22	I	u-1	I	II	III	II	III	III	u-1	III	III
#23	I	I	I	I	I	III	III	III	III	u-1	III
#24	I	I	I	I	I	I	I	I	I	I	I
#25	III	I	III	III	III	I	III	III	III	I	III
#26	III	II or III	III	III	III	III	III	III	III	III	III
#27	III	I	I	I	I	I	I	I	I	I	III
#28	I	I	II	I	III	III	III	III	I	III	III
#29	II	I	III	I	I	III	III	I	II	I	I
#30	III	I	III	I	III	III	III	III	III	I	III
#31	III	III	III	III	III	III	III	III	III	I	III
#32	III	III	I	I	I	I	I	I	I	I	I
#33	III	u-1	I	III	III	III	III	I	u-1	I	I
#34	I	u-1	I	III	I	III	III	III	I	u-1	I
#35	II	I	II	I	I	I	I	I	I	I	III
#36	III	I	III	III	III	III	III	III	I	III	III
#37	III	I	III	III	I	III	III	III	u-1	I	I
#38	I	I	I	I	III	III	III	III	I	III	III
#39	II	II or III	II	II	III	II	III	I	II	III	II
#40	II	u-1	I	III	III	III	III	III	I	III	I
#41	I	I	I	I	III	I	I	I	I	I	I
#42	I	I	III	I	III	III	III	I	I	u-1	I

(continued)

Table 3
(continued)

ToxoDB Genotypes	PCR-RFLP markers										
	SAG1	3′, 5′-SAG2	alt. SAG2	SAG3	BTUB	GRA6	C22-8	C29-2	L358	PK1	Apico
#43	I	I	II	I	II	I	I	I	I	u-1	I
#44	I	I	II	III	I	III	II	I	I	u-3	I
#45	I	III	III	III	I	II	II	III	I	I	III
#46	I	III	III	III	I	III	II	I	III	III	I
#47	I	III	III	III	III	III	u-1	I	I	II	I
#48	I	III	III	III	III	III	III	III	III	III	III
#49	II or III	II	II	I	II	I	II	II	III	II	nd
#50	II or III	III	III	III	III	III	III	III	III	III	III
#51	u-1	I	II	III	I	III	II	I	I	I	I
#52	u-1	I	II	II	I	III	u-2	I	I	III	I
#53	u-1	I	II	III	III	III	III	III	III	III	I
#54	II or III	II	II	III	III	III	III	III	III	III	II
#55	I	I	I	I	II	II	u-1	I	I	I	I
#56	I	I	I	III	III	II	u-1	I	I	I	I
#57	I	I	I	III	I	II	u-1	I	III	III	III
#58	I	I	I	III	I	III	u-1	II	III	III	I
#59	I	I	I	III	III	III	u-1	I	I	I	I
#60	I	I	II	I	I	III	III	I	I	III	I
#61	I	I	II	III	I	III	II	III	I	u-2	I

#62	I	I	II	III	I	III	II	III	III	III	I
#63	I	I	II	III	III	III	I	III	I	III	I
#64	I	I	II	III	III	III	u-1	I	I	u-2	I
#65	I	I	III	III	III	III	u-1	I	I	III	I
#66	II	II	II	I	I	III	I	u-1	I	u-2	I
#67	I	III	III	I	I	III	I	III	III	u-1	III
#68	I	III	III	I	I	III	I	III	III	III	III
#69	I	III	III	III	III	III	I	III	I	III	I
#70	I	III	III	II	III	II	III	I	I	I	III
#71	I	III	III	I	III	III	I	III	III	III	I
#72	u-2	III	III	I	I	I	u-1	I	III	u-2	III
#73	II or III	III	III	III	I	III	III	III	III	I	I
#74	II or III	III	III	III	III	III	III	III	I	III	I
#75	u-1	I	II	I	III	III	II	I	I	III	III
#76	u-1	III	III	I	I	III	II	I	I	III	I
#77	I	I	I	III	I	I	u-1	III	III	I	III
#78	I	I	I	III	III	III	u-1	III	I	I	III
#79	I	I	I	I	I	III	II	III	I	I	III
#80	I	I	III	III	I	I	I	I	I	u-1	I
#81	I	I	I	III	I	III	u-1	I	I	III	III
#82	I	I	I	III	I	III	II	III	I	I	III
#83	I	I	I	III	I	III	II	I	III	I	III
#84	I	I	I	III	I	III	u-1	I	I	III	I

(continued)

Table 3
(continued)

ToxoDB Genotypes	PCR-RFLP markers										
	SAG1	3′, 5′-SAG2	alt. SAG2	SAG3	BTUB	GRA6	C22-8	C29-2	L358	PK1	Apico
#85	I	I	I	III	III	II	u–1	I	I	II	I
#86	I	I	I	III	III	II	u–1	I	I	III	I
#87	I	I	I	III	III	III	I	I	III	I	III
#88	I	I	I	III	III	III	II	I	III	I	III
#89	I	I	I	III	III	II	II	III	III	III	III
#90	I	I	I	III	III	II	III	III	III	I	III
#91	I	I	II	I	I	I	II	I	I	I	I
#92	I	I	II	I	III	II	II	I	I	II	I
#93	I	I	II	I	III	III	u–1	I	I	III	I
#94	I	I	II	I	III	III	I	I	I	II	I
#95	I	I	II	I	III	III	II	I	I	III	I
#96	I	I	II	I	III	III	II	III	I	III	III
#97	I	I	II	I	III	III	II	III	I	III	I
#98	I	I	II	I	III	III	III	III	I	III	III
#99	I	I	II	I	III	III	u–1	I	I	III	I
#100	I	I	II	III	I	III	u–1	I	III	III	I
#101	I	I	II	III	I	III	II	I	I	u–2	I
#102	I	I	II	III	I	III	II	I	III	u–1	III
#104	I	I	II	III	I	III	u–1	I	I	III	I

Sample											
#105	I	III	III	III	u-1	II	III	III	II	III	I
#106	I	II	I	I	u-1	II	III	III	II	III	I
#107	I	III	I	I	u-1	II	III	III	II	I	I
#108	I	III	I	I	III	III	III	III	II	I	I
#109	III	III	III	I	III	III	III	III	II	III	I
#110	I	III	I	III	u-1	III	III	III	II	I	I
#111	I	I	III	I	u-1	I	I	III	u-1	II	I
#112	nd	I	III	II	III	II	I	I	II	I	I
#113	nd	II	II	nd	III	II	II	I	II	II	nd
#114	I	I	III	I	III	III	III	III	III	III	I
#115	I	III	III	III	III	III	III	III	III	III	I
#116	III	III	III	III	III	I	I	I	III	I	III
#117	III	u-1	I	I	u-1	II	I	I	III	I	III
#118	nd	I	III	III	III	III	III	III	II	III	I
#119	I	u-1	I	I	u-1	I	I	I	III	I	III
#120	III	III	III	I	I	III	III	III	III	III	III
#121	III	III	I	III	I	III	III	III	III	III	III
#122	III	I	III	III	I	III	III	III	III	III	III
#123	III	III	I	III	I	III	III	III	III	III	III
#124	I	u-1	I	III	I	III	III	III	III	III	III
#125	III	u-2	III	III	I	III	III	III	III	III	III
#126	I	u-1	I	I	u-1	II	III	III	I	I	I
#127	III	III	III	II	II	II	II	II	II	II	II or III

(continued)

Table 3
(continued)

ToxoDB Genotypes	PCR-RFLP markers										
	SAG1	3′, 5′-SAG2	alt. SAG2	SAG3	BTUB	GRA6	C22-8	C29-2	L358	PK1	Apico
#128	II or III	II	II	II	II	II	II	III	II	II	I
#129	II or III	II	II	II	III	II	II	II	II	II	II
#130	II or III	III	III	I	III	III	II	I	III	III	III
#131	II or III	III	III	II	II	I	III	III	II	II	I
#132	II or III	III	III	III	III	III	II	II	III	II	III
#133	II or III	III	III	III	III	II	III	III	III	I	III
#134	u–1	I	II	III	I	III	II	III	III	I	III
#135	u–1	I	I	III	III	III	II	II	II	III	I
#136	u–1	I	u–1	III	III	III	II	I	II	III	I
#137	u–1	II	II	III	II	III	III	II	III	III	I
#138	u–1	III	III	III	III	II	II	I	III	III	III
#139	II or III	II	II	III	III	III	III	II	III	III	I
#140	II or III	III	III	III	III	II	III	I	III	I	III
#141	II or III	III	III	III	III	II	II	III	III	III	III
#142	I	I	I	I	I	II	II	III	II	III	I
#143	I	I	III	III	I	III	II	I	I	III	III
#144	I	I	I	III	I	III	u–1	III	I	I	I
#145	I	I	I	II	I	II	I	I	I	I	III
#146	I	I	I	III	II	II	I	III	III	II	III

Sample										
#147	I	III	I	I	I	III	III	I	II	I
#148	I	III	I	I	II	III	I	III	III	I
#149	I	I	I	I	II	III	III	III	II	I
#150	I	I	I	III	II	III	II	III	II	I
#152	I	III	I	I	I	III	I	III	I-u	I
#153	III	III	III	III	III	III	I	III	II	II
#154	I	II	III	I-u	III	I	III	III	III	III
#155	nd	I	III	III	I	III	I	I	III	I
#156	III	I	III	III	III	I	I	III	III	I
#157	III	III	III	III	III	III	I	III	III	III
#158	I	III	I	III	I-u	III	I	III	III	I
#159	III	III	III	III	I	I	III	III	III	III
#160	III	I-u	III	I	I	III	III	III	III	I
#161	I	III	I	III	I	III	III	III	III	I
#162	I	III	III	I	II	III	III	III	III	I
#163	III	III	I	III	II	III	III	III	III	I
#164	I	III	III	I	III	III	III	III	III	I
#165	III	III	I	III	I-u	III	I	I	I	III
#166	III	III	III	I	I-u	I	III	III	II	I
#167	III	III	III	III	I	III	III	III	II	II or III
#168	I	I	III	III	II	III	III	III	II	II or III
#169	III	II	II	III	III	III	III	III	III	II or III
#170	III	III	III	III	III	III	I	III	III	II or III

(continued)

Table 3
(continued)

ToxoDB Genotypes	PCR-RFLP markers										
	SAG1	3′, 5′-SAG2	alt. SAG2	SAG3	BTUB	GRA6	C22-8	C29-2	L358	PK1	Apico
#171	u–1	I	I	III	III	I	u–1	III	III	I	III
#172	u–1	I	II	I	III	I	u–1	III	III	III	III
#173	u–1	I	II	III	II	II	u–1	I	I	II	I
#174	u–1	I	II	III	III	III	u–1	III	I	III	I
#175	u–1	I	II	III	III	III	III	I	I	u–1	I
#176	u–1	II	II	II	III	III	II	III	II	III	I
#177	I	I	I	I	I	II	I	III	I	I	III
#178	I	I	III	III	I	II	II	I	I	I	III
#179	I	I	III	III	I	III	II	III	III	III	III
#180	I	III	III	I	I	II	II	III	I	I	I
#181	I	III	III	III	I	II	u–1	I	I	u–1	I
#182	I	III	III	III	III	III	III	III	III	III	III
#183	I	III	III	III	III	III	III	I	I	I	III
#184	I	III	III	III	III	III	u–1	I	III	III	I
#185	II or III	II	II	III	III	I	III	III	III	u–2	III
#186	II or III	III	III	III	III	III	I	I	III	III	III
#187	II or III	III	III	III	III	III	III	III	III	III	III
#188	II or III	III	III	III	III	III	III	III	I	I	III
#189	u–n	I	II	I	I	III	III	I	I	III	I

#190	I	III	III	III	I	I	II	III	III	I	I	III
#191	I	I	I	I	I	I	II	III	III	I	I	III
#192	I	I	I	III	III	III	II	III	III	I	I	I
#193	I	I	II	I	III	III	II	III	I	III	III	III
#194	I	I	II	I	III	III	II	I	II	III	III	III
#195	I	I	II	I	III	III	II	I	II	III	III	III
#196	I	I	II	I	III	III	II	III	III	u–2	u–2	I
#197	I	II	II	I	I	I	II	II	I	I	I	I
#198	I	II	II	III	III	III	II	II	II	III	III	II
#199	II or III	II	II	III	II	II	II	III	II	II	II	I
#200	II or III	II	II	III	III	II	II	II	II	III	III	III
#201	II or III	III	III	III	I	II	III	III	I	I	I	III
#202	u–1	I	II	I	III	II	u–1	I	II	III	III	I
#203	I	I	I	I	I	II	III	III	III	II	I	III
#204	u–2	II	II	II	II	II	II	II	II	II	II	II
#205	II or III	II	II	I	I	II	II	I	I	II	I	II
#206	u–1	u–1	II	III	I	II	II	III	I	III	III	I
#207	I	I	u–1	III	I	II	III	II	I	III	I	I
#208	I	I	II	I	III	II	II	I	I	III	I	I
#209	u–1	u–1	II	II	III	II	II	III	I	I	III	III
#210	u–1	u–1	II	III	I	II	II	III	I	III	I	III
#211	I	I	I	III	III	I	I	III	III	I	I	III
#212	I	I	I	III	III	I	I	III	I	II	II	III

(continued)

Table 3
(continued)

ToxoDB Genotypes	PCR-RFLP markers										
	SAG1	3′, 5′-SAG2	alt. SAG2	SAG3	BTUB	GRA6	C22-8	C29-2	L358	PK1	Apico
#213	I	I	II	III	III	III	u-1	III	I	III	III
#214	u-1	I	I	III	I	II	II	I	I	I	I
#215	u-1	I	II	u-1	III	III	II	II	I	III	I
#216	I	I	I	III	III	I	II	III	III	I	III
#217	I	III	III	III	I	III	II	II	III	III	I
#218	I	III	III	III	III	III	II	II	III	II	III
#219	II or III	III	III	III	III	III	II	I	I	III	I
#220	II or III	II	II	II	II	II	III	III	III	III	I
#221	u-1	II	II	II	II	II	II	II	I	II	II
#222	I	II	II	III	I	III	II	u-1	II	III	I
#223	I	III	III	III	I	III	II	III	III	III	II
#224	II or III	III	III	III	III	III	II	I	III	I	III
#225	I	I	I	III	I	III	I	I	I	I	I
#226	I	I	u-1	III	III	III	II	III	II	III	I
#227	I	I	II	III	III	II	u-1	I	III	III	II
#228	I	III	III	III	III	III	u-1	I	III	III	I
#229	I	I	III	III	II	II	I	I	I	III	I
#230	I	II	II	III	III	III	III	III	III	III	III
#231	I	I	II	I	III	II	II	III	I	III	I

Sample	1	2	3	4	5	6	7	8	9	10
#232	I	I	II	I	III	III	II	III	u-1	III
#233	I	I	III	I	III	III	III	I	III	III
#234	I	I	III	III	III	I	III	III	III	I
#235	I	III	II	I	I	III	I	III	I	III
#236	u-1	I	III	III	III	III	III	I	III	III
#237	I	III	II	III	III	III	I	III	u-1	III
#238	I	I	II	I	III	III	III	III	III	I
#239	I	I	I	III	III	III	I	I	III	III
#240	I	I	II	I	III	III	I	I	u-2	III
#241	I	I	II	III	III	III	I	I	III	III
#242	II or III	I	u-1	III	III	III	III	III	u-1	III
#243	III	III	II	III	III	III	III	III	u-1	III
#244	I	I	III	III	III	III	I	I	u-1	I
#245	I	I	II	I	III	III	I	I	III	III
#246	u-1	I	III	III	III	III	I	II	III	I
#247	u-1	I	II	III	III	III	I	III	III	III
#248	I	III	I	III	III	III	I	III	u-2	III
#249	I	III	III	III	III	III	III	III	III	III
#250	II or III	III	III	I	III	III	III	III	I	III
#251	I	I	u-1	I	I	I	III	II	I	I
#252	I	I	I	III	III	III	III	I	I	III
#253	I	I	u-1	III	III	III	u-1	III	III	III
#254	II or III	III	III	II	II	II	III	II	III	I

(continued)

Table 3
(continued)

ToxoDB Genotypes	PCR-RFLP markers										
	SAG1	3′, 5′-SAG2	alt. SAG2	SAG3	BTUB	GRA6	C22-8	C29-2	L358	PK1	Apico
#255	u-1	I	II	III	III	II	II	I	I	I	I
#256	u-1	I	II	III	II	III	u-1	I	I	III	I
#257	I	I	I	I	III	II	I	III	III	u-1	I
#258	I	I	II	I	I	III	II	III	I	III	I
#259	II or III	III	III	III	I	III	II	III	III	III	III
#260	I	I	I	I	III	III	II	III	III	I	nd
#261	I	I	I	III	III	I	II	III	III	I	nd
#262	I	III	III	III	I	III	II	III	III	u-2	nd
#263	I	I	II	III	III	II	II	III	III	I	III
#264	II or III	II	II	II	III	II	II	III	II	II	I
#265	II or III	II	II	III	III	II	II	III	II	II	III
#266	II or III	III	III	III	III	III	II	III	I	III	III
#267	I	I	I	I	I	III	II	I	III	III	III
#269	I	III	III	III	I	II	II	III	I	III	III
#270	u-1	I	u-1	III	III	I	u-1	I	I	u-2	I
#271	I	I	I	III	I	II	II	III	III	I	III
#272	I	I	I	III	III	III	II	III	III	III	III
#273	I	I	I	III	I	II	u-1	III	III	I	III
#274	I	III	III	III	I	II	II	I	III	III	III

#275	I	III	III	III	I	III	III	I	III	I	III
#276	I	III	III	III	III	I	I–s	I	III	III	I
#277	I	III	III	I	III	III	II	I	III	I	III
#278	I	I	I	III	III	III	III	III	I	I	I
#279	I	III	III	I	III	III	I	III	I	I	III
#280	I	I	I	III	I	III	II	III	III	I	III
#281	I	I	I	III	I	II	III	I	II	I	III
#282	I	I	I	III	III	III	II	III	III	I	III

nd no data

There are no genotypes #103, #151, and #268

isolate the parasites by bioassay, as freezing will kill *T. gondii* in tissue cysts. However, these frozen tissues can be used to extract DNA for genotyping (*see* Subheading 3.2, **step 2**). To isolate *T. gondii* by bioassay, blood samples should be collected before animals die and fresh tissues should be collected immediately after animals died of acute toxoplasmosis. Diagnosis of acute toxoplasmosis may be confirmed by tissue smear revealing crescent shaped protozoan parasite under microscope. All samples should be stored at 4 °C. Bioassay should be performed as soon as possible, preferably within a week.

5. Acid pepsin treated tissue samples have very few *T. gondii* parasite, DNA extracted from these samples are not suitable for genotyping.

6. To monitor contamination of PCR amplification, negative controls without DNA template should be included in each batch of experiment. In addition, a set of positive controls are also included to monitor efficiency of PCR amplification and genotyping. The suggested positive controls include GT1 (or RH88), PTG, CTG, TgCgCa1, MAS, TgCatBr5, TgCatBr64, and TgRsCr1. The genotyping data for these controls is summarized in Table 2. Currently identified PCR-RFLP genotypes are summarized in Table 3.

References

1. Dubey JP (2010) Toxoplasmosis of animals and humans, 2nd edn. CRC Press, Boca Raton, FL, p 313

2. Montoya JG, Liesenfeld O (2004) Toxoplasmosis. Lancet 363:1965–1976

3. Shwab EK, Zhu X-Q, Majumdar D, Pena HFJ, Gennari SM, Dubey JP, Su C (2014) Geographical patterns of *Toxoplasma gondii* genetic diversity revealed by multilocus PCR-RFLP genotyping. Parasitology 141:453–461

4. Behnke MS, Dubey JP, Sibley LD (2016) Genetic mapping of pathogenesis determinants in *Toxoplasma gondii*. Annl Rev Microbiol 70:63–81

5. Su C, Shwab EK, Zhou P, Zhu XQ, Dubey JP (2010) Moving towards an integrated approach to molecular detection and identification of *Toxoplasma gondii*. Parasitology 137:1–11

6. Desmonts G, Remington JS (1980) Direct agglutination test for diagnosis of *Toxoplasma* infection: method for increasing sensitivity and specificity. J Clin Microbiol 11:562–568

7. Dubey JP, Desmonts G (1987) Serological responses of equids fed *Toxoplasma gondii* oocysts. Equine Vet J 19:337–339

8. Neumayerová H, Juránková J, Saláková A, Gallas L, Kovařčík K, Koudela B (2014) Survival of experimentally induced *Toxoplasma gondii* tissue cysts in vacuum packed goat meat and dry fermented goat meat sausages. Food Microbiol 39:47–52

9. Gerhold RW, Saraf P, Chapman A, Zou X, Hickling G, Stiver WH, Houston A, Souza M, Su C (2017) *Toxoplasma gondii* seroprevalence and genotype diversity in select wildlife species from the southeastern United States. Parasit Vectors 10:508

10. Ajzenberg D, Collinet F, Mercier A, Vignoles P, Dardé M-L (2010) Genotyping of *Toxoplasma gondii* isolates with 15 microsatellite markers in a single multiplex PCR assay. J Clin Microbiol 48:4641–4645

11. Pena HFJ, Gennari SM, Dubey JP, Su C (2008) Population structure and mouse-virulence of *Toxoplasma gondii* in Brazil. Int J Parasitol 38:561–569

Chapter 4

Generation of *Toxoplasma gondii* and *Hammondia hammondi* Oocysts and Purification of Their Sporozoites for Downstream Manipulation

Sarah L. Sokol, Zhee Sheen Wong, Jon P. Boyle, and Jitender P. Dubey

Abstract

Toxoplasma gondii tachyzoites and bradyzoites are studied extensively in the laboratory due to the ease with which they can be cultured. In contrast, oocysts and the sporozoites within them are more difficult to work with, in that cat infections are required for their generation and isolating sporozoites requires a laborious excystation procedure. More over some parasite species such as *Hammondia hammondi* are obligately heteroxenous and require passage through a cat for completion of the life cycle. There is no debate that there is great value in studying this important life cycle stage, and we present here a detailed description of the current protocols used in our laboratories to generate and isolate *T. gondii* and *H. hammondi* oocysts, and to excyst and purify the sporozoites within them for use in downstream experimental applications.

Key words Oocyst, Sporozoite, Forward genetics, *Toxoplasma gondii*, *Hammondia hammondi*

1 Introduction

Toxoplasma gondii is an exceptional model of intracellular parasitism, and a large body of research has been generated using in vitro cultivated parasites, including both tachyzoites and bradyzoites [1]. In contrast, the sporozoite stage is less studied, most certainly due at least in part to the logistical difficulties, costs, and hazards associated with producing and working with oocysts. To date there are no means of producing oocysts in tissue or cell culture, and therefore production of these life stages requires cat infections. Work with cat life cycle stages have had an enormous impact on the field.

Most notably, sexual crosses can only be carried out in cats, and coinfections with phenotypically distinct strains has resulted in the generation of recombinant progeny that have been crucial for the

Sarah L. Sokol and Zhee Sheen Wong contributed equally to this work.

Christopher J. Tonkin (ed.), *Toxoplasma gondii: Methods and Protocols*, Methods in Molecular Biology, vol. 2071, https://doi.org/10.1007/978-1-4939-9857-9_4, © Springer Science+Business Media, LLC, part of Springer Nature 2020

identification of key virulence determinants (e.g., [2–11]). Moreover, for parasites such as *Hammondia hammondi* for which no methods of long-term in vitro cultivation exist, cat infections are essential for its propagation [12–14] and are key to work aimed at understanding the dramatic developmental and virulence differences between *T. gondii* and *H. hammondi* [15–17]. Moreover, oocyst shedding provides a remarkably sensitive bioassay for determining the presence of viable tissue cysts in meat, lending great importance to such methods in establishing that curing, freezing, cooking and irradiation are important measures to safeguard food safety and public health [18–21]. By identifying antigens exclusively expressed by the sporozoites encased by oocysts, it has been further established that oocysts represent the principal route by which people become exposed to *T. gondii* [22] which ranks among the most costly foodborne infections [23].

Before describing the means to purify oocysts of *Toxoplasma gondii* from cat feces, we hasten to underscore the significant health risks inherent in this activity. Conducting this important work requires the highest level of personal and institutional commitment to biosafety and occupational health, and must only be conducted under rigorous regimes of testing, training, oversight, and documentation regarding occupational health, environmental safety, and animal welfare.

A brief review of clinical toxoplasmosis is therefore warranted. Infections are widely prevalent in humans and animals. All three stages of *Toxoplasma* (oocysts/sporozoites, tachyzoites, and bradyzoites) are infective to humans. In human hosts with a competent immune system, *T. gondii* infection generally develops into an asymptomatic chronic infection, with the organism sequestered in dormant tissue cysts, often for the lifetime of the host. However, in immunocompromised hosts, such as AIDS patients, cancer patients receiving chemotherapy, or organ transplant recipients receiving immunosuppressive therapy, infection can lead to toxoplasmosis, with serious consequences including potential damage to the central nervous system. This can result from a new infection or more commonly from reactivation of a latent infection. In pregnant women who first become infected during pregnancy, the newborn may develop congenital toxoplasmosis, which can result in blindness or mental retardation. In addition, *T. gondii* is now recognized as a cause of ocular disease in both immunocompetent and immunosuppressed persons. Unlike tachyzoites and bradyzoites, oocysts are environmentally resistant and highly infectious for humans [24]. Therefore, extra precautions are needed while working with oocysts. It is highly recommended that immunocompromised individuals or pregnant women do not work directly with sporulated oocysts. However, in our experience this does not require that these individuals stop working on the project in question as long as nonpregnant or nonimmunocompromised lab members can manipulate the infectious stages and then pass them off once they are no longer in their most infectious form.

Our experience with generating and excysting oocysts of both *T. gondii* and *H. hammondi* has led to some recent improvements in sporozoite isolation and purification, including a new method to directly generate transgenic *H. hammondi* using sporozoites as input [17]. The mouse infection and oocyst infection protocols described have been used for decades in the Dubey Lab, while the sporozoite purification protocols are in use in the Boyle Lab and are based on methods that were originally developed by others, most notably those in the laboratory of Michael White (now at the University of South Florida; e.g., [25–27]). For completeness we have included the entire process, starting with mouse infections, cat infections and feces collection, and oocyst purification, sporulation and excystation. We also include general comments on the biosafety precautions that we practice when working with oocysts.

2   Materials

2.1   General Lab Equipment and Personal Protective Equipment

1. Centrifuge with biocertified, transparent lids.
2. Shaker.
3. Vortexer.
4. Biosafety Level 2 cabinet.
5. N95 facemask.
6. Foot covers.
7. General use needles and syringes for mouse infections.

2.2   Cat Infections and Oocyst Isolation

1. Tongue depressors.
2. Disposable cups with lids (Specimen cups such as McKesson-569).
3. Laxatone (optional).
4. Sucrose solution in water (1.1 M).
5. Plastic Pasteur pipettes.

2.3   Sporozoite Excystation

1. Hank's balanced salt solution (Corning; 21-021-CV).
2. Phosphate buffered saline (Lonza; 17-516).
3. Clorox® Regular-Bleach.
4. 50 mL Corning™ polyethylene terephthalate (PET) centrifuge tubes.
5. 15 mL polystyrene centrifuge tubes.
6. 15 mL polypropylene centrifuge tubes.
7. 1 M sodium hydroxide solution (NaOH).

8. Disposable hemocytometers (Incyto; DHC-N01-5).

9. Nail polish.

10. Sterile disposable serological pipettes (5, 10, and 25 mL).

11. Glass beads, acid-washed: 710-1,180 μm (Sigma; G1152).

12. Parafilm.

13. Dulbecco's Modified Eagle Medium with 100 U/mL penicillin, 100 μg/mL streptomycin, 2 mM L-glutamine, 10% FBS, 3.7 g NaH_2CO_3/L, pH 7.2 (cDMEM).

14. 3 mL syringe.

15. 25 5/8 gauge needles.

16. Trypsin from porcine pancreas (Sigma; T4799).

17. Taurocholic acid sodium salt hydrate (Sigma; T4009).

18. 0.22 μm 50 mL Steriflip® filter (Millipore; SCGP00525).

2.4 Sporozoite Purification

1. Autoclavable (or disposable) cell scrapers.

2. Sealable autoclave bags.

3. Disposable transfer pipettes.

4. 5 μm filters (Millex®; SLSV025LS).

5. 10 mL syringes.

6. PD-10 desalting column with Sephadex G-25 resin (GE Healthcare; 17085101).

3 Methods

3.1 Safety Precautions When Working with Oocysts

3.1.1 During Cat Infections

During the period of oocyst shedding by cats, *T. gondii*- and *H. hammondi*-infected cats are housed individually in stainless steel cages in a room with limited access. In our facility, each cage has a 2-kg stainless steel litter pan with a heavy bottom so that cats cannot tip it and a bottom tray to catch the spilled material. Feces are collected daily from each litter pan using disposable gloves and disposable fecal scoop. The litter pan is filled to about ½ the depth (~1 in.) with crushed corn cobs as bedding. During the period of oocyst shedding, the floor under, and in front of, the cages is covered with plastic sheets to catch any material that may be shed by cats; the plastic sheets are replaced daily and used sheets are incinerated. Care should be exercised to avoid aerosolization. Masks (N95) are to be worn at all times during work with infected materials. During the period of oocyst shedding, the litter pans and bottom trays are not washed to avoid the spread of oocysts. When cats have stopped shedding oocysts, they are euthanized or transferred to clean cages.

There is a public debate concerning whether cats that have been experimentally infected, and which have resolved their initial episode of oocyst shedding, should be euthanized or could instead be candidates for adoption. The historical case for euthanasia derives from the fact that asymptomatic cats may resume oocyst shedding. Persistent antibody titers attest to lifelong latent infections in cats. Such asymptomatic cats have been shown prone to resheddinng millions of oocysts once exposed to another common coccidian infection of cats, *Cystoisospora* (*Isospora*) *felis* [28]. It is not known whether natural immunosuppressive conditions (i.e., those mediated by nutritional status, viral infection, or chemotherapy) might similarly provoke renewed oocyst shedding, although in one study experimental immunosuppression of cats that had stopped shedding oocysts *did* result in the resumption of oocyst shedding [29]. Immunity to secondary challenge with *T. gondii*, especially to heterologous strains, does wane over time [30, 31] and it remains to be determined whether such waning immunity predisposes a cat to undergo subsequent rounds of oocyst shedding in the absence of secondary exposure. At the very least, newfound susceptibility to new infections creates liability for a donor of such cats, because it may be difficult or impossible to establish whether infections derived from an older cat derived from new or prior (experimental) exposure. Any prospective adoptive home must be made aware of risks that doing so may result in serious harms to health.

The contaminated cages, including bottom trays, food and water dishes, and litter pans, are first run through a steam cage washer (internal temperature of >70 °C) to kill oocysts before cages are scrubbed. The cage washer must have a final rinse temperature of at least 82 °C. All bedding and waste from the room housing infected cats are incinerated. Feces are stored in a refrigerator (4 °C) to prevent sporulation prior to being processed in a separate building.

3.1.2 During Fecal Flotation

Special precautions are taken to properly dispose of liquid feces or fecal wash. All liquids are poured in plastic containers, tightly capped, and sealed in 12 × 9.5 in., heat sealable special pouches (Kapak/Scotchpak) designed for the electric sealer. The sealed pouches are enclosed in a biohazard bag, and resealed in another biohazard bag for extra security. The biohazard bag is enclosed in a plastic bucket with absorbent material, and labeled.

All contaminated materials from the fecal room are incinerated or boiled. Large bottles, and metal cups used in the centrifuge are boiled in water to kill any oocysts present. Boiling water is poured on the sink surface to kill any infectious *Toxoplasma* oocysts—precautions should be taken while handling boiled water to prevent burns. All protective coverings/PPE and plastic sheets used to cover the sink are sealed in a red-biohazard bag, enclosed in a cardboard box with a biohazard sign, and properly labeled. All waste is disposed in accordance with the SOP requirements for Special (Regulated) Medical waste disposal. These boxes are transported to the incinerator. Glass slides, coverslips, and pipettes used for fecal examination are placed in an OSHA-approved sharps container, enclosed in red bag, and finally enclosed in a box, labeled biohazard, and incinerated.

3.1.3   During Excystation and Sporozoite Isolation

Sporulated oocysts are highly infectious and environmentally stable, even when treated with common laboratory disinfectants. Therefore, anyone working with oocysts should be properly trained and should exhibit extreme caution to prevent accidental exposure. To minimize the exposure risk, all individuals working with oocysts should wear proper personal protection equipment, including a lab coat and disposable gloves. Gloves should be changed often and immediately if contamination occurs. To minimize contamination of laboratory equipment, all oocyst work should be conducted in a biological safety cabinet that contains its own biohazard waste disposable bag and liquid oocyst waste container (Fig. 1a). Any time a vessel containing oocysts is manipulated outside the hood, the lid should be sealed with Parafilm and the vessel should be transported in a secondary container. When centrifuging vessels containing oocysts, transparent biocertified covers should be used to prevent contamination in case vessel rupture occurs. When vessels containing oocyst material are opened, their caps should be visually inspected for any liquid contamination. If contamination occurs, the cap should be immediately discarded in the biohazard waste bag within the biosafety cabinet. Anything that comes into contact with oocyst material should be discarded in this way after use (serological pipette tips, transfer pipettes, etc.). After oocyst manipulation has been completed, the biosafety cabinet should be first cleaned liberally with a 10% bleach solution (no more than 1 month in age). Allow bleach to sit for 10–30 min before wiping away. After cleaning with bleach, the biosafety cabinet should be cleaned with a hospital grade disinfectant, such as CaviCide, followed by 70% ethanol. The UV light source of the biosafety cabinet should be turned on for at least 1 h prior to additional work. Gloves should be changed frequently during this cleaning process. All liquid waste and any reusable supplies, such as autoclavable cell scrapers, must be autoclaved prior to being discard or reused. If a spill occurs, first alert all personal of the spill and clean the area liberally with a freshly prepared 10% bleach solution, being sure to allow the bleach to sit for 30 min. The spill area should then be liberally cleaned with CaviCide followed by 70% ethanol. All waste products (paper towel, Kimwipes, etc.) used in the cleaning process should be discarded in the biohazard waste bag inside the biosafety cabinet since none of these treatments will completely inactivate the oocysts.

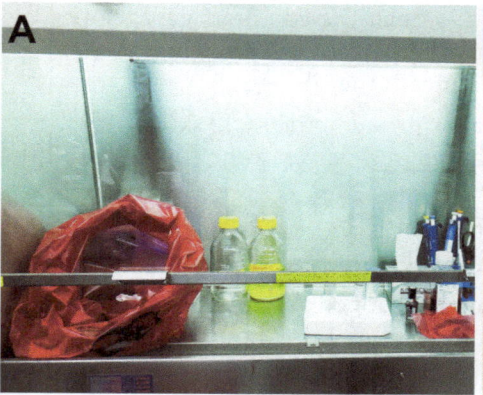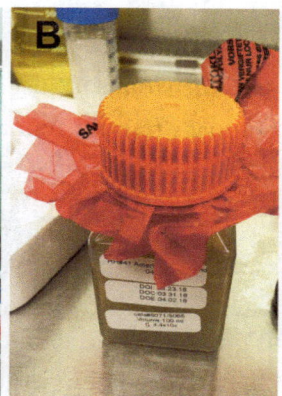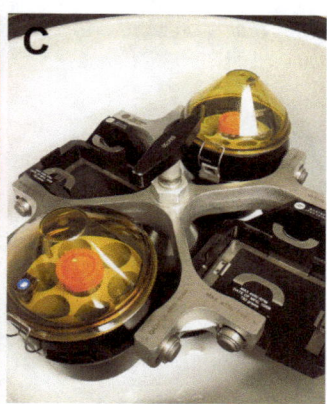

Fig. 1 Safety precautions to utilize when working with oocysts. (**a**) Biosafety cabinet set up with biohazard waste bag and oocyst waste containers. (**b**) A piece of plastic is placed between oocyst stock container and cap to shield cap from oocyst exposure and to prevent leaks. (**c**) Transparent biocertified covers for centrifuge buckets are used to contain spills that may occur as a result of container damage. This can also be accomplished by vacuum sealing tubes in plastic bags prior to centrifugation

3.2 Infection of Mice for Use in Oocyst Production

General notes: In our own work we have found that *T. gondii* strains grown extensively in vitro as tachyzoites lose their ability to produce oocysts in cats despite being very competent at forming bradyzoite cysts in vitro and in mice (Boyle, Boothroyd and White, Unpublished observations). While the reasons for this are unclear, given the costs of cat infections it is important that "cat competent" strains are used to produce oocysts. We recommend "resetting" any strains of interest by infecting mice with low passage samples and feeding those mice to cats. Oocysts collected from these cats can be used as a seed strains to perform further experiments. Mice can be infected parenterally with tachyzoites or tissues cysts or using oocysts (oral or subcutaneous). If oocysts are the starting material, we prefer the subcutaneous route for inoculating mice with *T. gondii* and *H. hammondi* if the main goal is the production of oocysts for use in downstream experiments.

3.2.1 Subcutaneous Infection of Mice with Oocysts

1. Using oocysts isolated as described below, quantify and take an appropriate volume and neutralize the 2% H_2SO_4 using 3.3% NaOH (add drops until neutral red is the appropriate hue).

2. Place the animal on top of a screen or wire-top cage lid and manually restrain it by grasping the base of the tail and slightly lifting the hind limbs off the surface.

3. As the animal pulls forward with the front feet, insert a 0.5 mL syringe with a 1-in., 21-gauge needle into the loose skin located over the back of the neck at a 15° to 30° angle on either side of the spine.

4. Inject up to 0.5 mL and return the animal to the cage.

3.2.2 Oral Inoculation
with Oocysts

1. Premeasure and mark a ball-tipped oral gavage needle (8–10 mm) to indicate where shaft will be when the ball is near the stomach (just beneath the ribcage).

2. Manually restrain animal by grasping the loose skin on the back of the neck with the tail secured between the fourth and fifth fingers of the same hand.

3. Hold the mouse in an upright position with the head tilted slightly back to straighten the esophagus as much as possible.

4. Introduce an 8 to 10-mm ball-tipped gavage needle attached to a 1 to 3-mL syringe into the side of the mouse's mouth.

5. Pass the needle over the tongue and into the esophagus to the mark on the shaft.

   Slowly expel the contents (0.5 mL to 1 mL buffered oocyst prep) into the mouse using the syringe plunger. Carefully withdraw the gavage needle.

6. Return the animal to the home cage and observe frequently for at least 5 min for signs of complications.

   Note: When mice are orally inoculated with T. gondii or H. hammondi oocysts special instructions are posted on each cage because some of the oocysts may pass "undigested" in feces for the first 2 to 3 days. In addition, bedding and feces are incinerated and the caretakers are instructed to use gloves and facemasks while changing or cleaning these cages for the first 7 days after oral oocyst challenge.

   Note: It is sometimes necessary to treat these mice with anti-Toxoplasma therapy following challenge (1–4 mg/mL sulfadiazine per mL of drinking water) until they have recovered from the initial stages of infection.

3.2.3 Collection of
Tissues for Infection of Cats

T. gondii and *H. hammondi* begin to encyst in mouse tissues within a week of inoculation irrespective of the stage inoculated or the route. *T. gondii* cysts are formed in many tissues but are concentrated in the brain after 4 weeks post infection. In contrast *H. hammondi* cysts are not found in significant numbers in the brain. For infection of cats with *T. gondii*, mice are euthanized and brain is collected. The brain can be fed to cats by placing the brain tissue on the back of the tongue with mouth open by firmly holding the cat. If necessary, the entire carcass can be fed to the cat afterward. For this the mouse is skinned, the feet and intestines are removed, and the rest of the mouse is chopped up with scissors. The chopped mouse tissues can be mixed with canned cat food and offered to the cats. Adding fish or watermelon flavors increases palatability. For *H. hammondi* infections, the entire carcass is fed to the cat in this manner.

**3.3   Cat Infections
and Feces Collection**

1. Acquire specific pathogen-free (SPF) cats, raised in biosecurity facilities with no exposure to raw meat. These cats should have available data with respect to date born, sex and their parents (queen, tom). Each cat should have a unique identification (ID), preferably, microchipped. The cats should be *Toxoplasma*-free, based on antibody titers determined by modified agglutination test (MAT) in 1:25 dilution of serum.

2. Infect *Toxoplasma*-free weaned cats; optimal oocyst excretion occurs in 10–20 week old cats. Allow cats to consume infected animal tissues (up to 500 g) ad libitum over a period of 2–4 days.

3. All personnel should wear protective gear including hood covers, a coverall and a ventilation mask (N95). When collecting feces, change gloves between each cage to prevent cross-contamination.

4. Collect all feces in plastic cups from the litter box daily on day 3–14 post-feeding and refrigerate them immediately to prevent the sporulation of oocysts.

5. Label each cup with the cat identification number and the date.

6. Use a double gloved hand (or disposable fecal scoop) to collect ALL the fecal material from the litter box.

7. Add 50 mL of DI water to each fecal cup before closing.

8. Cups are to be placed in the designated refrigerator after collection.

9. If a cat does not defecate, do the following:
   (a) Administer LAXATONE (a petroleum based lubricant) by smearing a 1 in. long streak on either their face or front paws—do not put it in the food dish because they will not eat it.

   (b) Record the date, number and problem in the animal health log book.
      Note: It is important that once the collection period has begun, DO NOT empty the bottom cage pans until the cat is euthanized to minimize spread of oocysts in the feces that might have fallen in the bottom tray.

10. Empty all bedding into biohazard boxes.

11. Determine infection by the identification of oocysts in the feces (*see* "Fecal Examination" below). During the period of oocyst shedding (between 3 and 14 days after feeding test tissue), take special care in handling cages and cats to avoid inadvertent exposure of personnel.

12. Euthanize cats at the end of oocyst shedding period (usually 2 weeks after infection) using the following AVMA approved methods of euthanasia. Administer Ketamine at 10 mg/kg body

weight in combination with Dexdomitor (dexmedetomidine hydrochloride, 0.5 mg/1 mL) intramuscularly or subcutaneously to anesthetize cats before intracardiac administration of Beuthanasia (Schering, Plough Animal Health) at 1 mg/10 lb. body weight.

13. Incinerate all cat remains to prevent the spread of *Toxoplasma gondii* or *Hammondia hammondi*.

3.4 Fecal Examination for Oocysts

1. Wear protective disposable coveralls (covering the whole body), a face mask, face shield, boot covers, N95 mask and gloves.

2. Put fecal cups (securely lidded) with enough water to just cover the feces on the shaker to soften feces and partly emulsify them.

3. For initial examination (screening), mix approximately 10 g (10 mL) of feces from each cat with 5 volumes of sucrose solution (specific gravity 1.15 or higher).

4. Filter by pouring the liquid through two layers of gauze in a cup (layers can be made by folding large pieces of gauze).

5. Squeeze the feces retained on the gauze to extract as many oocysts and then dispose of the gauze/fecal material in a biohazard bag (to be incinerated).

6. Pour the filtered liquid/feces mixture into a 50-mL conical tube, close cap, and centrifuge at $1180 \times g$ for 10 min.
   Note: Enclose tubes in a sealable bag or use approved centrifuge bucket covers to avoid contamination of the centrifuge in the rare event of tube breakage or cap leakage.

7. Using a disposable Pasteur pipette (we prefer plastic since they are sealed and easier to dispose of than glass), take a drop of the fecal float from the top of the tube and examine microscopically for *T. gondii* oocysts. If no oocysts are found, incinerate the remaining cat feces from that cat and that day of collection and discard by incineration. For this, enclose feces in a plastic container, seal in a biohazard bag, and enclose in a plastic disposable hard plastic bucket for incineration.

8. For positive samples, mix the remainder of each feces/water mixture with a few drops of detergent (household soap) and place on rotary shaker until feces are completely broken.

9. Filter the mixture through gauze as above and centrifuge in 250-mL bottles at low speed ($300 \times g$, 15 min). Discard the supernatant.

10. Mix the sediment with water (up to 150 mL) and centrifuge 2–3 times, decanting the supernatant each time and replacing with clean water. Remove the water from the final wash.

Note: it is important to collect all waste from these procedures into autoclavable glass or plastic containers rather than pouring down the drain. Autoclave all liquid waste.

11. Mix the sediment with 5 volumes of sucrose solution of 1.15 specific gravity (530 g/L) and centrifuge for 10 min at $1180 \times g$ in 50-mL tubes with a conical bottom. Most oocysts float to the top of the tube and can be aspirated using a Pasteur pipette.

12. Pellet these oocysts by spinning for 10 min at $1180 \times g$, and resuspend in 2% H_2SO_4 precautions should be taken while handling sulfuric acid—never add water to acid while making dilution.

13. Since not all oocysts rise to the top, take the entire supernatant (40–45 mL) and centrifuge it at $1180 \times g$ for 15 min. Wash the sediment containing the oocysts one more time with water and then resuspend it in 2% H_2SO_4.

14. Pour the isolated oocysts from **steps 12** and **13** above into a 500 mL flat bottom bottle with a sturdy cap (e.g., a HyClone RPMI-1640 Medium bottle). Aerate them on a shaker (Labnet shaker, 150 RPM) for 7 days at room temperature (20–22 °C) to induce sporulation.

15. Sporulation efficiency can be assessed using a hemacytometer.

3.5 Sporozoite Excystation

1. Fill appropriately sized beaker with DI water and place beaker in 37 °C incubator to serve as a water bath at least 4 h prior to excystation incubation.

2. Set up by placing a biohazard bag and liquid oocyst waste bottle in biosafety cabinet (Fig. 1a).

3. Calculate volume of oocysts needed based on the number of sporozoites desired. Assume about a 5% yield unless additional data for a given preparation is available. Calculate volume of HBSS needed for first wash and the volume of 1 M NaOH needed for neutralization (Total volume can range between 25 and 45 mL. Neutralization step is optional.)

4. Cut approximately a 5×5 cm^2 out of a biohazard bag (prepare one for each stock of oocysts used).

5. Remove the cap from the oocyst/cat feces storage container and immediately discard plastic between cap and container (Fig. 1b).

6. Pipette to mix oocyst/cat feces prep to obtain a homogenous mixture. Transfer the calculated volume of the oocyst stock into a 50 mL PET tube.

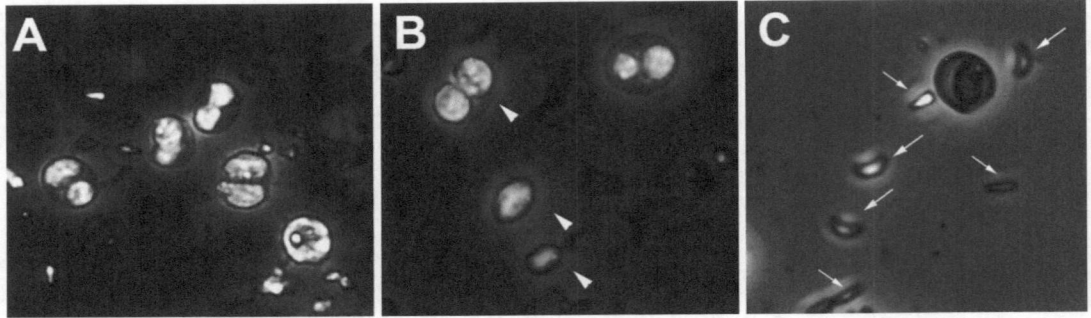

Fig. 2 Progression of excystation process. (**a**) Image of oocyst sucrose float containing both sporulated and unsporulated oocysts. (**b**) Image of sporocysts (arrowheads) released from oocysts after vortexing with glass beads. (**c**) Image of sporozoites (arrows) following 45 min incubation in excystation media and needle passage

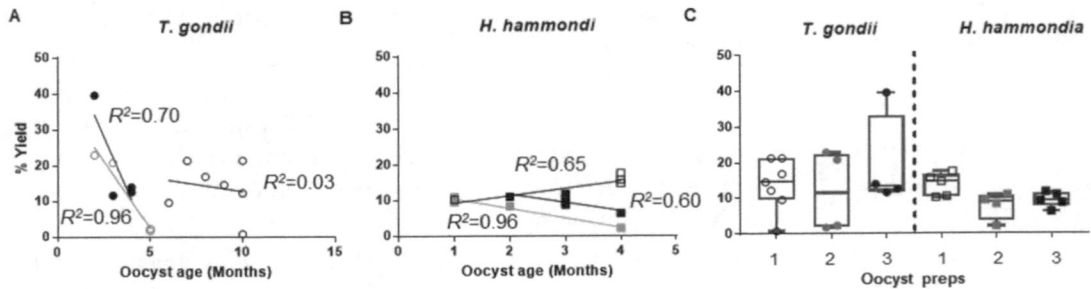

Fig. 3 Excystation rates (% yield) of *T. gondii* and *Hammondia hammondi* oocysts according to age and oocyst batches. (**a, b**) Scatter plots of sporozoite yields (in percentage) of *T. gondii* (**a**) and *H. hammondi* (**b**) from oocysts of different ages (in months). Each shade/shape represents a different oocyst preparation and each data point represents an independent excystation experiment. R^2 values for each oocyst batch were calculated separately. (**c**) Box and whisker plots show min to max of sporozoite yields from three different batches of *T. gondii* and *H. hammondi* oocysts. Each point represents the percent yield of sporozoites from one excystation experiment. Sporozoite yields were not significantly different between *T. gondii* and *H. hammondi* (One-way ANOVA, Tukey's multiple comparison posttest, $P > 0.05$)

7. Place the square of biohazard bag prepared in **step 4** on the opening of the oocyst storage container before replacing the original cap (Fig. 1b).

8. Add 10 μL of each oocyst sample to a disposable hemocytometer. Seal the opening with nail polish. Allow the nail polish to drip off of the applicator (e.g., do not touch the applicator to the opening).

    Note: Allow the hemocytometer to settle for 3 to 5 min before observation.

9. Add appropriate volume of HBSS to the PET tube, pipette up and down to mix. The solution should be yellow in color.

10. If neutralization is desired, add appropriate volume of 1 M NaOH (3/5 volume of oocyst sample) to neutralize the

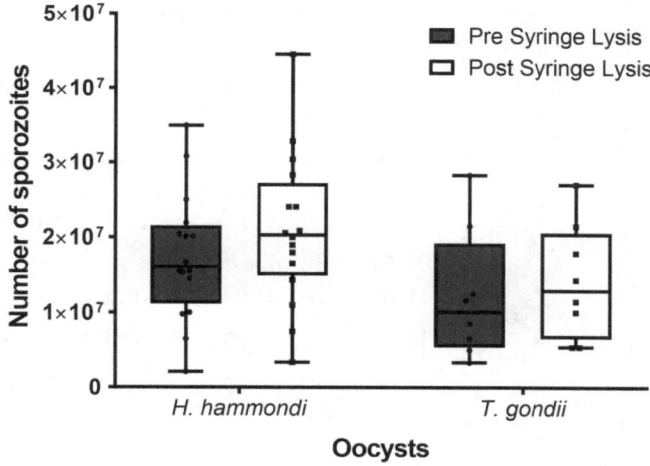

Fig. 4 Syringe lysis in excystation media may slightly improve sporozoite yield. The box and whisker plots show the min to max number of sporozoites excysted prior to and after syringe lysis in excystation media for *H. hammondi* and *T. gondii*. Each point represents the number of sporozoites excysted for a given experiment. This data shows a general, but not significant, increase in the number of sporozoites excysted after syringe lysis. (Two-way ANOVA, Sidak's multiple comparison test, *H. hammondi* $P = 0.47$, *T. gondii* $P = 0.88$)

solution. Pipette up and down to mix. The solution should be red/pink color.

Note: The 3/5 volume is an approximation. The exact amount needed for neutralization will vary.

11. Pellet oocysts by centrifuging at $1000 \times$ g for 8 min at room temperature. Be sure to use transparent biocertified lids when spinning oocyst material (Fig. 1c).

12. Count the number of sporulated and nonsporulated oocysts. Record results and verify that you have added enough of the stock oocyst preparation in order to achieve the desired sporozoite yield (Fig. 2a).

13. Remove supernatant with disposable 25 mL pipette. Dispose of supernatant is appropriately labeled oocyst waste container (1000 mL glass bottle works well).

14. Resuspend pelleted material in 25 mL of HBSS.

15. Pellet oocysts by centrifuging at $1000 \times g$ for 8 min at room temperature.

16. If the supernatant remains a neutral red/pink color, discard supernatant as directed in **step 13**. If the supernatant remains an acidic yellow color, repeat **steps 14–17** until a neutral red/pink color is obtained.

17. Prepare a 10% bleach solution in PBS.

Note: Prepare 10 mL of 10% bleach solution for each 50 mL PET tube used.

18. Resuspend oocyst solution in 10mL of 10% bleach in PBS solution.

19. Secure cap on the 50 mL conical tube by wrapping in Parafilm. Transfer tube into a secondary container and place on shaker for 30 min at room temperature with gentle shaking.

20. After 30 min, remove the tubes from the shaker and verify that the tubes are not leaking.

21. Remove the Parafilm from the caps of the tubes.

22. Pellet the oocyst by centrifuging at $1000 \times g$ for 8 min.
    Note: Use caution when manipulating the tubes after the bleach step because the pellet is fragile.

23. Prepare excystation media by adding 0.1 g Trypsin (Sigma; T4799) and 2 g Taurocholic acid (Sigma; T4009) to 40 mL of PBS. Adjust the pH to 7.5 with 1 M NaOH. Sterilize using a 0.22 μm 50 mL Steriflip® filter. Aliquot ~6 mL of sterile excystation media into 15 mL polypropylene centrifuge tubes. Place in the 37 °C water bath in the incubator to prewarm.

24. After centrifugation, remove the supernatant and discard it in the liquid oocyst waste container.

25. Resuspend the pellet in 25 mL of HBSS. The solution will turn purple.

26. Pellet the oocyst by centrifuging at $1000 \times g$ for 8 min.

27. Repeat **steps 24–26** until solution turns to a neutral red/pink color.

28. Add 4 g of sterile glass beads (prealiquoted into glass tubes and autoclaved) to a 15 mL polystyrene centrifuge tube.

29. Resuspend the final pellet in 3 mL of HBSS and transfer into the 15 mL polystyrene centrifuge tube containing the glass beads.
    Note: When working with large numbers of oocysts (~ten million or more) it is best to divide oocyst mixture into multiple tubes. (e.g., For 60 million oocysts, resuspend in 9 mL of HBSS and transfer 3 mL each to three polystyrene tubes containing 4 g of sterile glass beads.)

30. Cap the tube and seal it by wrapping Parafilm around the tube and cap.

31. Vortex the tube on high for 15 s on and 15 s off for a total vortex time of 1 min.

32. Transfer the supernatant into a new 15 mL conical polystyrene tube.

33. Add 10 µL of the supernatant to a disposable hemocytometer and seal with nail polish as done in **step 8** (Fig. 2b).

34. Wash remaining beads with 3mL of HBSS and transfer into the new conical tube. Conduct a total of 2 washes for a total volume of 9 mL.

35. Pellet the oocysts by centrifuging at $800 \times g$ for 10 min at room temperature.

36. Replace cap on tube containing glass beads and discard in biohazard waste.

37. Count number of freed sporocysts using the hemocytometer prepared in **step 34**.

38. Remove supernatant and discard in oocyst waste container.

39. Resuspend pellet in 5 mL of prewarmed excystation media prepared in **step 24**.

40. Place tubes in water bath in 37 °C incubator. Untwist the cap to allow airflow and incubate for 45 min.
    Note: Be sure that tubes will not be disturbed or tipped during incubation.

41. *Optional: To verify that sporozoites are emerging from sporocysts, after 30 min, remove tubes from incubator, tighten caps, invert once to mix. Remove and discard cap in biohazard waste. Place 10 µL on a hemocytometer and seal it with nail polish. Add a new cap and return tubes to the water bath in incubator. Untwist caps slightly to allow for airflow. Incubate for the remaining 45 min.*

42. After a 45 min incubation, transfer the parasite preparation to an empty T25 flask, syringe lyse the parasite preparation 5 times with 25 5/8 gauge needle and 3 mL syringe, and place 10 µL on hemocytometer, seal with nail polish, and count (Fig. 2c).
    Note: Change gloves after each round of syringe lysis. Be extremely cautious with needles, especially when discarding in biohazard sharps container.

43. Add 7 mL of cDMEM to the tube and gently pipette to mix and quench the reaction.

44. Pellet sporozoites by centrifuging at $800 \times g$ for 10 min at room temperature.

45. Remove supernatant and resuspend pellet in 5 mL of cDMEM to wash the sporozoites.

46. Pellet sporozoites by centrifuging at $800 \times g$ for 10 min at room temperature.

47. Resuspend sporozoites in an appropriate amount of cDMEM. Quantify using a hemacytometer (Fig. 2c). Expected yields from this protocol are shown below in Figs. 3 and 4.

3.6 Optional Overnight Infection

1. Infect a confluent monolayer of HFF's grown in a T-25 with sporozoites.

    Note: It is best to allocate the sporozoites between multiple flasks. We find splitting dirtier preps into 3 or more T-25's improves our parasite yield following filtering.

2. Incubate overnight at 37 °C, 5% CO_2.

3. After overnight incubation, set up biosafety cabinet with biohazard bag and oocyst waste bottle (Fig. 1a).

4. Dislodge cells from the T-25 using a cell scraper.

    Note: for reusable cell scrapers, place used scrapers that have come in contact with oocysts in a sealable autoclave bag. Seal and autoclave prior to reuse.

5. Syringe lyse the media in the T-25 (5 mL) 5 times with 25 gauge needle and 3 mL syringe and place 10 μL on hemocytometer, seal with nail polish, and count

    Note: Change gloves after each round of syringe lysis. Be extremely cautious with needles, especially when discarding in biohazard sharps container.

6. Remove oocyst debris using 5 μm syringe-driven filter or PD-10 desalting column (*see* below).

3.7 Parasite Purification with 5 μm Syringe-Driven Filter

1. Pre-equilibrate a 5 μM filter with 2 mL of cDMEM.

2. To prepare parasites for purification, rinse monolayer with PBS. Syringe lyse HFF monolayer by five passages through a 25-gauge needle.

3. Centrifuge at $100 \times g$ for 5 min to remove large debris.

4. Transfer supernatant to a new Eppendorf tube and centrifuge at $800 \times g$ for 10 min at RT.

5. Resuspend the pellet (contains parasites) with 5 mL of cDMEM and load onto the pre-equilibrated 5 μM syringe-driven filter (10 mL syringe) and filter.

6. Replace the syringe with a new syringe (5 mL syringe), add 5 mL of cDMEM and re-elute through the same filter to collect any trapped parasites.

3.8 Parasite Purification with PD-10 Desalting Column

1. Pre-equilibrate PD-10 column with chilled cDMEM. The PD10-column hold ~5 mL of media, equilibrate column with a total of 30 mL chilled cDMEM. Discard the flow-through

    Note: It typically takes ~20 min for the equilibration step. Keep column at 4 °C if not used immediately

2. While column is equilibrating, prepare parasites for purification. Rinse monolayer with PBS, scrape, and then syringe lyse the HFF monolayer by five passages through a 25-gauge needle.

3. Centrifuge at $100 \times g$ for 5 min at 10 °C to remove large debris.

4. Transfer supernatant to a new eppendorf tube and centrifuge at $800 \times g$ for 10 min at RT. Discard supernatant.

5. Resuspend the pellet (which contains parasites) with 2.5 mL cDMEM and load onto a pre-equilibrated PD-10 column.

6. Add an additional 3.5 mL of cDMEM to the column. Collect the eluate (~6 mL).

Note: If the initial suspension was particularly dark in color, it may be necessary to add another 3 mL of cDMEM and collect a second eluate. Combine with first eluate.

References

1. Weiss LM, Kim K (eds.) (2014) *Toxoplasma gondii*: the model apicomplexan - perspectives and methods, 2nd edn. Elsevier/AP, Amsterdam

2. Behnke MS, Khan A, Sibley LD (2015) Genetic mapping reveals that sinefungin resistance in *Toxoplasma gondii* is controlled by a putative amino acid transporter locus that can be used as a negative selectable marker. Eukaryot Cell 14(2):140–148. https://doi.org/10.1128/EC.00229-14

3. Behnke MS, Khan A, Wootton JC, Dubey JP, Tang K, Sibley LD (2011) Virulence differences in *Toxoplasma* mediated by amplification of a family of polymorphic pseudokinases. Proc Natl Acad Sci U S A 108(23):9631–9636. https://doi.org/10.1073/pnas.1015338108

4. Taylor S, Barragan A, Su C, Fux B, Fentress SJ, Tang K, Beatty WL, Hajj HE, Jerome M, Behnke MS, White M, Wootton JC, Sibley LD (2006) A secreted serine-threonine kinase determines virulence in the eukaryotic pathogen *Toxoplasma gondii*. Science 314 (5806):1776–1780

5. Pernas L, Adomako-Ankomah Y, Shastri AJ, Ewald SE, Treeck M, Boyle JP, Boothroyd JC (2014) *Toxoplasma* effector MAF1 mediates recruitment of host mitochondria and impacts the host response. PLoS Biol 12(4):e1001845. https://doi.org/10.1371/journal.pbio.1001845

6. Reese ML, Zeiner GM, Saeij JP, Boothroyd JC, Boyle JP (2011) Polymorphic family of injected pseudokinases is paramount in *Toxoplasma* virulence. Proc Natl Acad Sci U S A 108 (23):9625–9630. https://doi.org/10.1073/pnas.1015980108

7. Bontell IL, Hall N, Ashelford KE, Dubey JP, Boyle JP, Lindh J, Smith JE (2009) Whole genome sequencing of a natural recombinant *Toxoplasma gondii* strain reveals chromosome sorting and local allelic variants. Genome Biol 10(5):R53

8. Boyle JP, Saeij JP, Harada SY, Ajioka JW, Boothroyd JC (2008) Expression quantitative trait locus mapping of *Toxoplasma* genes reveals multiple mechanisms for strain-specific differences in gene expression. Eukaryot Cell 7 (8):1403–1414. https://doi.org/10.1128/EC.00073-08

9. Saeij JP, Coller S, Boyle JP, Jerome ME, White MW, Boothroyd JC (2007) *Toxoplasma* co-opts host gene expression by injection of a polymorphic kinase homologue. Nature 445 (7125):324–327. https://doi.org/10.1038/nature05395

10. Saeij JP, Boyle JP, Coller S, Taylor S, Sibley LD, Brooke-Powell ET, Ajioka JW, Boothroyd JC (2006) Polymorphic secreted kinases are key virulence factors in toxoplasmosis. Science 314(5806):1780–1783. https://doi.org/10.1126/science.1133690

11. Rosowski EE, Lu D, Julien L, Rodda L, Gaiser RA, Jensen KD, Saeij JP (2011) Strain-specific activation of the NF-kappaB pathway by GRA15, a novel *Toxoplasma gondii* dense granule protein. J Exp Med 208(1):195–212. https://doi.org/10.1084/jem.20100717

12. Riahi H, Darde ML, Bouteille B, Leboutet MJ, Pestre-Alexandre M (1995) Hammondia hammondi cysts in cell cultures. J Parasitol 81 (5):821–824

13. Dubey JP, Sreekumar C (2003) Redescription of Hammondia hammondi and its differentiation from *Toxoplasma gondii*. Int J Parasitol 33 (13):1437–1453

14. Heydorn AO, Mehlhorn H (2001) Further remarks on Hammondia hammondi and the taxonomic importance of obligate heteroxeny. Parasitol Res 87(7):573–577

15. Walzer KA, Wier GM, Dam RA, Srinivasan AR, Borges AL, English ED, Herrmann DC, Schares G, Dubey JP, Boyle JP (2014) Hammondia hammondi harbors functional orthologs of the host-modulating effectors GRA15 and ROP16 but is distinguished from *Toxoplasma gondii* by a unique transcriptional profile. Eukaryot Cell 13(12):1507–1518. https://doi.org/10.1128/EC.00215-14

16. Walzer KA, Adomako-Ankomah Y, Dam RA, Herrmann DC, Schares G, Dubey JP, Boyle JP (2013) Hammondia hammondi, an avirulent relative of *Toxoplasma gondii*, has functional orthologs of known *T. gondii* virulence genes. Proc Natl Acad Sci U S A 110(18):7446–7451. https://doi.org/10.1073/pnas.1304322110

17. Sokol SL, Primack AS, Nair SC, Wong ZS, Tembo M, Verma SK, Cerqueira-Cezar CK, Dubey JP, Boyle JP (2018) Dissection of the in vitro developmental program of Hammondia hammondi reveals a link between stress sensitivity and life cycle flexibility in *Toxoplasma gondii*. eLife 7. https://doi.org/10.7554/eLife.36491

18. Dubey JP, Brake RJ, Murrell KD, Fayer R (1986) Effect of irradiation on the viability of *Toxoplasma gondii* cysts in tissues of mice and pigs. Am J Vet Res 47(3):518–522

19. Dubey JP, Kotula AW, Sharar A, Andrews CD, Lindsay DS (1990) Effect of high temperature on infectivity of *Toxoplasma gondii* tissue cysts in pork. J Parasitol 76(2):201–204

20. Kotula AW, Dubey JP, Sharar AK, Andrews CD, Shen SK, Lindsay DS (1991) Effect of freezing on infectivity of *Toxoplasma gondii* tissue cysts in pork. J Food Protection 54:687–690

21. Hill DE, Benedetto SM, Coss C, McCrary JL, Fournet VM, Dubey JP (2006) Effects of time and temperature on the viability of *Toxoplasma gondii* tissue cysts in enhanced pork loin. J Food Prot 69(8):1961–1965

22. Boyer K, Hill D, Mui E, Wroblewski K, Karrison T, Dubey JP, Sautter M, Noble AG, Withers S, Swisher C, Heydemann P, Hosten T, Babiarz J, Lee D, Meier P, McLeod R (2011) Unrecognized ingestion of *Toxoplasma gondii* oocysts leads to congenital toxoplasmosis and causes epidemics in North America. Clin Infect Dis 53(11):1081–1089. https://doi.org/10.1093/cid/cir667

23. Hoffmann S, Batz MB, Morris JG Jr (2012) Annual cost of illness and quality-adjusted life year losses in the United States due to 14 foodborne pathogens. J Food Prot 75(7):1292–1302. https://doi.org/10.4315/0362-028X.JFP-11-417

24. Dubey JP (2010) Toxoplasmosis of animals and humans, 2nd edn. CRC Press, Boca Raton

25. Radke JR, Gubbels MJ, Jerome ME, Radke JB, Striepen B, White MW (2004) Identification of a sporozoite-specific member of the *Toxoplasma* SAG superfamily via genetic complementation. Mol Microbiol 52(1):93–105

26. Jerome ME, Radke JR, Bohne W, Roos DS, White MW, Veterinary Molecular Biology MSUBMUSA (1998) *Toxoplasma gondii* bradyzoites form spontaneously during sporozoite-initiated development. Infect Immun 66(10):4838–4844

27. Tilley M, Fichera ME, Jerome ME, Roos DS, White MW (1997) *Toxoplasma gondii* sporozoites form a transient parasitophorous vacuole that is impermeable and contains only a subset of dense-granule proteins. Infect Immun 65(11):4598–4605

28. Dubey JP (1976) Reshedding of *Toxoplasma* oocysts by chronically infected cats. Nature 262(5565):213–214

29. Malmasi A, Mosallanejad B, Mohebali M, Sharifian Fard M, Taheri M (2009) Prevention of shedding and re-shedding of *Toxoplasma gondii* oocysts in experimentally infected cats treated with oral clindamycin: a preliminary study. Zoonoses Public Health 56(2):102–104. https://doi.org/10.1111/j.1863-2378.2008.01174.x

30. Dubey JP (1995) Duration of immunity to shedding of *Toxoplasma gondii* oocysts by cats. J Parasitol 81(3):410–415

31. Zulpo DL, Sammi AS, Dos Santos JR, Sasse JP, Martins TA, Minutti AF, Cardim ST, de Barros LD, Navarro IT, Garcia JL (2018) *Toxoplasma gondii*: a study of oocyst re-shedding in domestic cats. Vet Parasitol 249:17–20. https://doi.org/10.1016/j.vetpar.2017.10.021

Chapter 5

Assays for Monitoring *Toxoplasma gondii* Infectivity in the Laboratory Mouse

Qiuling Wang and L. David Sibley

Abstract

Toxoplasma is a widespread parasite of animals including many rodents that are a natural part of the transmission cycle between cats, which serve as the definitive host. Although wild rodents, including house mice, are relatively resistant, laboratory mice are highly susceptible to infection. As such, laboratory mice have been used to compare pathogenesis of natural variants and to evaluate the contributions of both host and parasite genes to infection. Protocols are provided here for evaluating acute and chronic infection with different parasite strains in laboratory mice. These protocols should provide uniform standards for evaluating natural variants and attenuated mutants and for comparing outcomes across different studies and between different laboratories.

Key words Virulence, Bioluminescence, Dissemination, Central nervous system, Pathogenesis

1 Introduction

Toxoplasma gondii is an extremely widespread parasite of animals that also causes zoonotic infections in humans [1]. Strains of *T. gondii* have been grouped into three major clonal lineages that predominate in North America and Europe [2–4]. These lineages differ in their acute virulence in laboratory mice due to the presence of polymorphic secretory effectors, many of which are derived from rhoptry secretion [5] or released from dense granules [6]. Representatives of all three genotypes have been reported as part of a comparative genomes project for *T. gondii*, which provides a framework for comparing strain types within and between major lineages [7]. Strains of *T. gondii* from South America, which differ genetically, also show high levels of virulence in laboratory mice, in part due to similar virulence factors that mediate differences among the clonal lineages [8]. Here we present protocols for monitoring infectivity and pathogenesis of the three major clonal lineages in laboratory mice, although similar methods could be adapted to study other more diverse strains.

Christopher J. Tonkin (ed.), *Toxoplasma gondii: Methods and Protocols*, Methods in Molecular Biology, vol. 2071, https://doi.org/10.1007/978-1-4939-9857-9_5, © Springer Science+Business Media, LLC, part of Springer Nature 2020

Transmission of *T. gondii* normally occurs between cats, which serve as the definitive host, and rodents and many other animals that serve as intermediate hosts [1]. Mice are a natural host for *T. gondii* and as such the laboratory mouse provides an excellent model to study innate and adaptive immunity [9, 10]. Type I strains are acutely virulent and a single viable organism is uniformly lethal in all strains of laboratory mice [11, 12]. Type I strains do not readily differentiate to bradyzoites in mice and their high level of virulence makes it difficult to obtain tissue cysts in chronically infected animals. As a consequence, infections with Type I strains are typically administered by intraperitoneal (IP) injection of tachyzoites. Acute infections progress rapidly by expansion of parasite numbers and dissemination to all organs of the body, leading to death within the first 10–12 days [13]. Parasite expansion and dissemination are prominent features of acute infection, leading to cytokine shock [13, 14], which is likely a contributing cause of death. Genetic crosses have been used to map genes that contribute to acute virulence of Type I strains in laboratory mice [15] and the roles of specific genes in pathogenesis have been confirmed using a variety of techniques to disrupt or modify genes [16].

By contrast, Type II strains display intermediate virulence in laboratory mice where high doses lead to lethal outcome, while lower doses resolve and result in chronic infection, allowing LD_{50} values to be established [13]. Because of their ability to cause nonlethal, chronic infection, Type II strains are often used to explore a range of immunological functions that control infection [9, 10]. Infection protocols vary with some investigators using IP injection of tachyzoites grown in vitro, while others isolate tissue cysts from chronically infected mice and administer them by IP injection or by oral gavage. Oral ingestions of tissue cysts follow the natural route of infection as *T. gondii* is able to transmit between different intermediate hosts by omnivorous or carnivorous feeding [17]. High challenge doses delivered by the oral route result in acute gastroenteritis that can lead to death, and the immunological basis of this form of pathogenesis has been explored through numerous studies [18].

Type III strains are relatively common in animals in North America and yet they are rarely encountered in human cases of toxoplasmosis [4, 19, 20]. Type III strains are highly avirulent in laboratory mice, with high challenge doses leading to low levels of lethal infection [21]. The Type III strain CTG (aka CEP) has been used to study sexual phase transmission in the cat and to develop genetic mapping strategies for *T. gondii* [22, 23]. The basis for the lack of acute virulence in CTG was shown to be due to underexpression of ROP18, a polymorphic virulence determinant of Type I strains [24]. Infection studies with another commonly used Type III strain called VEG revealed that the stage used for infection (i.e., bradyzoite vs. oocyst challenge) greatly influences pathogenesis [25].

Laboratory mice are derived from a few founder lines that represent mixtures of the *Mus musculus musculus*, *M. m. domesticus*, and *M. m. castaneus* lineages, with the majority of loci coming from *M. m. domesticus* [26]. These founders were used to establish outbred Swiss Webster and CD-1 lines, which have been kept in closed colonies and bred to maximize genetic heterozygosity [27]. Inbreeding of founder lineages to minimize heterozygosity gave rise to C57Bl/6 mice and other inbred lines that differ by a small number of polymorphic loci, notably the major histocompatibility complex (MHC). Such inbred lines have been extremely useful for studying the association of genotype with phenotype. However, the total variation within all inbred laboratory mouse lines is far less than that seen in wild caught or wild-derived isolates of *M. musculis* [28]. Although both outbred and inbred strains of laboratory mice are relatively susceptible to *T. gondii* infection, wild strains derived from *M. musculis* are much more resistant [29]. Given their susceptibility to infection, laboratory mice have been extremely useful to highlight pathogenesis differences among parasite strains and to study immune mechanisms involved in control of infection.

2 Materials

2.1 Propagation of Tachyzoite Cultures In Vitro

1. Commonly used strains for mouse challenge studies are shown in Table 1. For type I strains we recommend the lab-adapted RH strain, or GT-1 which undergoes the complete life cycle. Commonly used type II strains include ME49 and Prugniaud

Table 1
Representative strains of *T. gondii* useful for mouse infection

Types	Strains	LD50 values			ATCC #	References
		CD-1[a]	C57BL/6[a]	BALB/c[a]		
I	RHΔhxgΔku80	1	1	1	PRA-319	[40, 41]
	GT-1	1	1	1	50853[b]	[42]
II	ME49Δhxg::FLUC	10^3	100–200	200–500	50611[b]	[33]
	Pru ΔhxgΔku80	10^5	500–1000	500–1000	NA	[44]
III	CTG (CEP)	$>10^6$	$>10^4$	$>10^4$	50842[b]	[22]
	VEG	$>10^6$	$>10^4$	$>10^4$	50861	[45]

[a]These values will vary with local mouse colony and need to be tested
[b]Reference lines are wild type, although FLUC derivatives can be obtained on request

(aka Pru). Type III strains include CTG and VEG. Estimates of the pathogenicity in different mouse strains are also provided, although these can vary with colony and source and so need to be determined locally.

2. Tissue culture incubator for culture at 37 °C, 5% CO_2, and BSL-2 biosafety cabinet.

3. Tissue-culture flasks (25 cm^2), 96-well plates, and cell scrapers.

4. Human foreskin fibroblasts (HFF) cells (ATCC, cat. # SCRC-1041).

5. D10 medium: For 1 L, combine 1 package Dulbecco's Modified Eagle's Medium (DMEM) powder (Thermo Fisher, Gibco cat. # 12100046), 3.7 g $NaHCO_3$, 100 ml fetal bovine serum (FBS), 10 ml of 200 mM L-glutamine, 1 ml of 10 mg/ml gentamycin, and dH_2O to 1 L. Sterilize by 0.45 μm filtration.

6. HHE: 1× Hank's Balanced Salt Solution, 10 mM HEPES, 1 mM EGTA, sterilized by 0.45 μm filtration.

7. Blunt-end needles (20, 23, and 25 gauge), bulb transfer pipettes, 5 and 10 ml pipettes, 5 and 10 ml syringes.

8. Hemocytometer (Thermo Fisher Scientific, cat. # 0267151B) or other cell counting instrument.

9. Inverted tissue culture microscope equipped with 10×, 20× objectives.

10. Swin-Lok filter holder (Whatman, cat. # 420200) and polycarbonate filter membranes (3 μm pore) (Whatman, cat. # 110612). Although larger pore sizes can be used, there is more risk of contaminating host nuclei or debris.

11. Centrifuge capable of holding 15 conical tubes and spinning at 400 × *g*.

2.2 Challenge Studies

1. In vitro tachyzoite cultures of the *T. gondii* strains of interest.

2. Outbred CD-1 and various inbred lines of mice.

3. HHE: 1× Hank's Balanced Salt Solution, 10 mM HEPES, 1 mM EGTA, sterilized by 0.45 μm filtration.

4. Tuberculin syringes for IP injection.

5. Oral gavage needles 22 g × 1½ in., 2.4 mm tip (Patterson Veterinary, cat. # 07-809-7615).

6. Sterile PBS.

7. Sterile plastic 10 ml syringes equipped with 16, 18, 20 g needles.

8. Sulfadiazine (Thermo Fisher Scientific, cat. # S-6387) solution (0.1–0.2 g/l).

2.3 Plaquing Assay

1. Tissue culture incubator for maintaining cell cultures at 37 °C, 5% CO_2 and BSL-2 biosafety cabinet.

2. Human foreskin fibroblasts (HFF) cells (ATCC, cat. # SCRC-1041).

3. D10 medium: For 1 L, combine 1 package Dulbecco's Modified Eagle's Medium (DMEM) powder (Gibco, cat. # 12100046), 3.7 g $NaHCO_3$, 100 ml FBS, 10 ml of 200 mM L-glutamine, 1 ml of 10 mg/ml gentamycin, and dH_2O to 1 L. Sterilize by 0.45 μm filtration.

4. Tissue culture plates (6 well) containing confluent monolayers of HFF cells.

5. Solution of 1% Crystal violet solution water.

6. Inverted tissue culture microscope, equipped with 4×, 10×, 20× objectives.

2.4 ELISA for Monitoring Infection Status

1. High binding ELISA plates (Disposable Sterile ELISA Plates, cat. # 25801).

2. Model 500 Sonic Dismembrator with microprobe (Thermo Fisher Scientific).

3. Tachyzoite culture of *T. gondii*. Most antigens cross-react so RH (Type I) or ME49 (Type II) strains can be used interchangeably for detecting infection with multiple different strain types.

4. Control mouse serum (previously infected positive and noninfected negative animals for reference). Store in aliquots at −80 °C until use.

5. Serum samples from infected mice. BD Microtainer tube with serum separator gel (Thermo Fisher Scientific, cat. # 02-675-185). Typically small volumes (10–100 μl) can be collected from saphenous vein or cheek vein puncture. Store in aliquots at −80 °C until use.

6. Horseradish peroxidase (HRP)-conjugated secondary antibody (HRP goat anti-mouse IgG) (Thermo Fisher Scientific, cat. # 62-6520).

7. Phosphate buffered saline (PBS).

8. Wash solution: PBS/0.05% Tween 20. Plastic squirt bottle for dispensing wash solution.

9. BSA blocking solution: PBS/0.05% Tween 20, 1.0% bovine serum albumin (BSA).

10. BSA incubation solution: PBS/0.05% Tween 20, 0.1% BSA.

11. Substrate: BD OptEIA Substrate Reagent A, Substrate Reagent B (BD Biosciences, cat. # 51-2606KC).

12. Plate reader for absorbance reading at 450 nm.

2.5 Tracking Infection by Bioluminescence

1. D-luciferin, potassium salt (Gold Biotechnology, cat # Luck-1G).

2. Isoflurane (Henry Schein Animal Health, cat. # SKU 029405).

3. IVIS Spectrum BL imager (PerkinElmer) or equivalent instrument capable of detecting bioluminescence.

4. Tuberculin syringes for injection.

2.6 Cyst Harvesting and Staining

1. *Dolichos biflorus* lectin conjugated with FITC (Vector Labs, cat. # FL-1031).

2. Fixating and Permeabilizing Solution: 2× stock consisting of 6% formaldehyde, 0.2% Triton-X-100 in PBS.

3. Blocking solution: 10% normal goat serum in PBS.

4. Glass slides and coverslips.

5. Epifluorescence microscope equipped with phase contrast (10×, 40×) and filter set for detecting FITC.

6. Sterile PBS.

7. Sterile plastic 5, 10 ml syringes equipped with 16, 18, 20 g needles.

8. Polystyrene 15 ml tubes and centrifuge capable of spinning at 400 × *g*.

3 Protocols

3.1 In Vitro Propagation of Tachyzoites

T. gondii are most easily propagated in human foreskin fibroblasts (HFFs) because the host cells reach confluency and stop dividing. These features facilitate passage at high MOI that leads to natural egress at 2–3 day intervals, and also allow for plaque formation on preformed monolayers. Procedures for propagation of HFF monolayers, serial passage of *T. gondii* lines, and harvest of viable tachyzoites have been defined previously [30] and are only briefly summarized here.

1. Passage *T. gondii* tachyzoites by serial passage on HFF monolayers. Typically, strains are inoculated serially using parasites from a freshly egressed culture to inoculate a new monolayer of HFF cells. The flask is inoculated at a high MOI (1:1 or 2:1) to assure uniform infection and host cell lysis in a single round. For Type I stains, natural egress occurs ~2 days after the initial inoculation (or slightly less), while for Type II and III strains it is often 3 days postinoculation.

2. To passage strains, disperse the contents of a recently egressed culture using a 5 ml pipette to resuspend the culture material and remove cells from the surface (it is also possible to mechanically release as described below).

3. Gently pipet the material using 5 ml pipette to draw the liquid in and out several times to disperse and break up clumps. Dispense parasites using five to ten drops from a bulb transfer pipette (1 drop ~ 50 μl) to inoculate a new confluent monolayer of HFF cells grown in a T25^2 flask. For Type I strains, this method results in a 1:10 to 1:20 split by volume (based on a starting volume of 5 ml for culture in a T25^2 flask) every 2 days. Type II and III strains may require a higher inoculum from 10 to 20 drops, equating to a 1:10 to 1:5 split by volume. Return the flask to the incubator, 37 °C, 5%CO_2, for 2–3 days.

4. Prior to inoculating mice, it is important to establish the parasites on a consistent passage cycle every 2–3 days, otherwise viability will be compromised.

5. To prepare parasites for inoculation into animals, harvest tachyzoites at the peak of their natural intracellular replication cycle, either at the point of natural egress or shortly before. Any cells remaining on the monolayer at this time point should be heavily infected and will be easily disrupted by gentle pipetting. If necessary, scrape the monolayer to remove cells

6. Resuspend the contents of the flask and passage sequentially through 20, 23, and 25 g blunt needles attached to a 10 ml syringe. When expelling the material from the needle, keep it submerged below the surface to avoid aerating the sample.

7. Filter to separate host cell debris from tachyzoites using 3 μm polycarbonate filter unit. Flush the filter with 10 ml of HHE collecting the flow-through in a 15 ml conical tube.

8. Centrifuge the filtered culture at $400 \times g$ for 10 min at 18 °C, resuspend the pellet in 10 ml HHE.

9. Count the parasites using a hemocytometer.

10. Dilute the parasites to an appropriate concentration so that injection volumes (typically 0.1–0.2 ml) will contain the desired number of parasites.

11. Maintain the parasite at room temperature throughout, chilling them does not result in better viability. Rather it is important to perform these procedures quickly and immediately before you go the facility to inject animals. Different strains of *T. gondii* also vary on how well tachyzoites survive outside of culture, with type I being the most robust. Type II and III strains loose viability much faster and should be used immediately after harvest. We also find the use of Hank's Balanced Salt Solution based medium is better for resuspending the parasites in compared to PBS, as the former is better for maintaining parasite viability.

3.2 Estimating Viability by Plaquing

1. After returning from the animal facility, use a portion of the unused parasite suspension to perform a plaquing assay and establish the viability of the inoculum.

2. Inoculate 200–500 parasites per well of a 6 well plate containing HFF cells growing in DMEM-10% FBS. For a uniform suspension, it is best to place the parasites in 2 ml of D10 medium and then use this to replace the medium that is in each well. Allow parasites to settle by gravity being careful not to swirl the plate (this action creates a vortex that brings the parasites to the center and skews the count). Use triplicate wells per strain.

3. Incubate at 37 °C, 5% CO_2 for 7–9 days, depending on the strain. Do not move the plate during this time period.

4. Remove the plate from the incubator, rinse in PBS, and stain with 1% Crystal violet (made in dH_2O) followed by rinsing in H_2O.

5. Plaques will appear as clear zone on the stained background. Count by eye or under low power (2–5×). In the event that plaques have not fully lysed, they can be difficult to visualize. In this case, score foci of infection by examining the stained monolayer under low power using an inverted microscope (5–20× depending).

6. Expect maximum viability of 50%, however it can also be as low as 5%, especially if tested more than 1–2 h after initial harvest of the parasites.

3.3 Acute Virulence Model

The following protocol is used to establish "acute virulence" based on serial dilution of parasites and challenge into outbred CD-1 mice. Cumulative survival (or inversely % mortality) is used to evaluate the degree of pathogenicity. This definition of acute virulence has been used to establish the difference between clonal types [11], and map virulence differences between them [12, 24, 31]. Additional readouts that are useful to obtain include weight loss, time to death, and tissue burden by bioluminescence (Fig. 1).

1. Harvest tachyzoites from freshly egressed cultures, count, and dilute in HEE as described above.

2. Infect separate groups of 5 CD-1 mice by IP inoculation with serial dilutions of tachyzoite (i.e., 10, 100, or 1000 tachyzoites/mouse using Type I parasites). Experiments should be repeated two to three times on different days to account for possible variation in the viability of the inoculum.

3. Monitor the animals for weight loss and signs of illness. Use an appropriate end point prior to death, depending on institutional approved protocol.

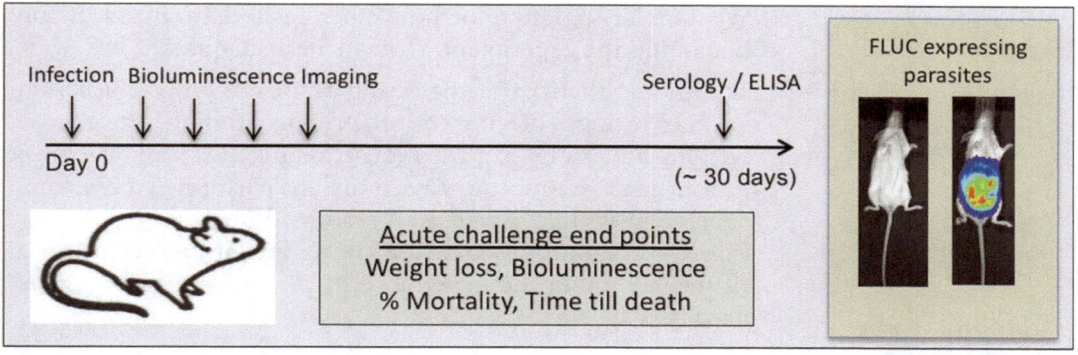

Fig. 1 Acute virulence model in outbred CD-1 mice. Following IP challenge with different doses of tachyzoites, mice are followed for 30 days postinfection. Useful end points include weight loss, bioluminescence imaging for luciferase expressing parasites, percent mortality, and time to death. Example shows control and infected mouse imaged for firefly luciferase (FLUC) expression

4. Animals can be monitored for expansion of parasites using luciferase tagged strains and bioluminescence (*see* Subheading 3.4 protocol).

5. At 30 days postinfection, determine the number of surviving animals. The time point of 30 days is somewhat arbitrary as acutely virulent lineages will generally lead to death prior to day 20.

6. Bleed animals form the saphenous or cheek vein, collecting a small volume (100–200 μl) in a microtainer with serum separator gel. Spin the separator to extract the serum (top) layer from the red cells. Store serum at −20 °C before use.

7. Perform ELISA (*see* Subheading 3.5 protocol below) to determine the titer in comparison to controls. Seropositivity is an outcome of successful infection. At low inoculum, or low viability of the inoculum, some animals may not become infected and they remain serologically negative. Such noninfected animals are removed from the calculation of % survival.

8. Survival % is calculated as: # infected animals that survive/the number of infected animals (dead animals plus seropositive survivors) × 100. Lower survival equates with higher virulence.

3.4 Imaging Infection by Bioluminescence

Bioluminescence provides a powerful way to track infection in vivo with the advantage that the same animals can be imaged over time [32]. Strains of *T. gondii* have been transfected with various luciferase proteins including firefly [33] and click beetle luciferase [34]. These reporters can be imaged by injecting the substrate luciferin in vivo just prior to imaging with very sensitive bioluminescence imagers.

1. Resuspend 1 g of luciferin into 66.7 ml of PBS, filter, dispense in 1.5 ml aliquots, and store in −80 °C. One tube should be sufficient for ~5 mice.

2. Weigh mice to determine how much luciferin to inject. Before beginning the experiment, thaw luciferin aliquots.

3. Lightly anesthetize the mice using isoflurane. Inject mice using 10 μl of luciferin (15 mg/ml stock concentration) per gram of weight. For example, if the mouse weighs 25 g, you will inject 250 μl into the mouse. Injections are performed IP using a tuberculin syringe. Luciferin is readily soluble and rapidly partitions throughout the body, allowing imaging of essentially al tissues, although the penetrance of the signal varies by tissue density.

4. Place the animals in the IVIS chamber using the isoflurane manifold to keep them under light anesthesia to prevent movement during imaging. Image the mice within 20 min of injection for best results.

5. Image the bioluminescence signal following the manufacturer's instructions for operation of the IVIS unit.

6. Analyze your data using Living Image® (PerkinElmer) and graph results using Prism (GraphPad) or Excel. Appropriate statistical analyses typically involve nonparametric tests using adjustments for multiple comparisons.

3.5 ELISA for Monitoring Infection

Antigen preparation:

1. Harvest parasites from a freshly egressed culture grown in HFF cells into a 50 ml polystyrene tube. Centrifuge at $400 \times g$ for 10 min, room temperature. Resuspend the pellet in 10 ml HHE.

2. Count the parasites and resuspend in PBS at a final concentration of 10^8 cells/ml. Sonicate using 15 s on/45 s off cycle for 2 min, power 2.8 unit (Fisher Model 500 Sonic Dismembrator with microprobe).

3. Add glycerol to a final concentration of 10%, aliquot, and store aliquots in $-80\ °C$.

Perform the ELISA:

1. Take an aliquot of parasite lysate from the freezer and dilute in PBS (1×10^6 /ml parasites). Add 100 μl of antigen per well and incubate the plate for 1 h at 37 °C or at 4 °C overnight. Cover the plates with lid or Parafilm.

2. After incubation, rinse wells three times with PBS/0.05% Tween 20, using a squirt bottle.

3. Add 250 μl of 1% BSA blocking solution in each well and incubate for 1 h at room temperature. After incubation, rinse all the wells with PBS/0.05% Tween 20 three times.

4. Dilute primary antibody (unknown mouse sera, positive, or negative controls) to appropriate concentration in BSA

incubation solution (1:500–1:5000). Add 100 μl of primary antibody to each well and incubate for 1 h at room temperature. Test each sample and positive and negative controls in duplicate wells. Rinse three times with PBS/0.05% Tween 20.

5. Dilute HRP-conjugated secondary antibody to 1:2500–1:10,000 in PBS/0.05% Tween 20, 0.1%BSA. Add 150 μl of secondary antibody per well for 1 h at RT°C. Rinse four to five times with PBS/0.05% Tween 20. It is important to wash very carefully with PBS after this incubation to avoid unspecific staining because of free peroxidase-conjugated antibodies.

6. Mix equal volume of substrate-A and substrate-B and immediately add 100 μl of this mixture to each well and incubate for 20–30 min at dark. Stop the reaction with 50 μl of 2M H_2SO_4 added to each well.

7. Measure the Absorbance at 450 nm with a plate reader.

8. The results of ELISA assays from sample of infected mice are compared to known positive and negative controls. Comparisons can be made by ANOVA to compare the average values of positive and negative controls to individual samples. Alternatively, cutoffs for positive values can be determined as described previously [35].

3.6 Chronic Tissue Cyst Bank

Outbred mice are useful to maintain chronic infections that are characterized by low cyst burdens (i.e., 50–200/animal). Cyst numbers can be amplified in strains of inbred mice that develop higher cysts counts (i.e., 500–3000/animal). It is advisable to "bank" strains in CD-1 outbred mice and pass them by subinoculating every ~6 mos. Cysts are then amplified in susceptible inbred strains (e.g., BALB/c, CBA/J) followed by harvest of tissue cysts over a 1–3 mos period for use in experiments. Although this protocol takes longer to establish, it avoids increases in virulence that can occur with frequent passage and also allows for production of high number of cysts for challenge experiments.

1. Inject mice IP with 100–1000 tachyzoites that have been grown in tissue culture, harvested, purified by filtration, and resuspended in HHE. Viability can be a major issue since it will take you some time to prepare the inoculum and walk to the animal house. Use only freshly egressed parasites that have been grown under optimum conditions (i.e., 2–3 day synchronous cultures).

2. Intermediately virulent strains (i.e., ME49) have LD_{50}s around 10^3–10^5 in outbred mice. Therefore it is usually not necessary to treat the mice to prevent death. You want the mice to be heavily infected without dying. Use animals that survive the highest dose possible to obtain higher cyst counts.

3. Virulent Type I strains like GT-1 are more problematic as they will invariably cause death even at low doses. Use an inoculum of 50–100 tachyzoites IP (at lower doses some mice will not become infected).

4. To prevent accidental death with high virulence strains, it is necessary to treat the mice with sulfadiazine (dissolved in the drinking water). Begin treatment with a dose of 0.4–0.5 g/l on day 3 or 4 and treat for 6–10 days or until they recover. Even for less virulent strains (i.e., ME49) it is sometimes necessary to treat with sulfadiazine at lower doses (0.1 or 0.2 g/l as above).

5. Harvest the brain of chronically infected mice at 1–3 months postinfection and determine the cyst burden by homogenizing and counting a fraction of the homogenate (*see* Subheading 3.7 protocol below). It is possible to obtain a sufficient number of cysts from a single animal to use in subsequent challenge studies, depending in the number of animals and desired inoculum.

6. To maintain chronic cysts, establish a bank of CD-1 mice and passage them at 6 mos intervals. Infected animals should be humanely sacrificed, brains removed and homogenized. After staining and counting a proportion of the brain (*see* Subheading 3.7 protocol below) serial passages are done by oral gavage of 5–10 cysts per animal into naïve mice.

7. To expand cyst numbers, inoculate 5–10 cysts IP or PO into inbred CBA/J or BALB/c mice, which are more susceptible and will lead to higher cysts counts. Infections can be passed sequentially for two to three times in inbred mice, but do not use this for long-term passage as the strain will increase in virulence.

3.7 Cyst Harvesting and Staining

This protocol is designed to help visualize tissue cysts that form in the brain of chronically infected animals. Tissue cysts can be recognized by their appearance in phase contrast microscopy (refractive, slightly amber cyst wall with internal granular material). However, it is much easier to identify them based on positive staining with FITC-conjugated *Dolichos biflorus* lectin (DBL) [36].

1. Sacrifice chronically infected animals using an approved method.

2. Remove the brain and place in a sterile conical 15 ml tube containing ~2 ml PBS. Gently mince the brain using a 16 g needle. Draw the tissue into a 5 ml syringe and gently expel. Repeat three times using 16 and 18 g needles to homogenize the tissue.

3. Add an aliquot of brain lysate (typically ¼ of the total or 0.5 ml) to an equal volume of Fixing and Permeabilizing Solution in a 15 ml polystyrene centrifuge tube. Incubate for 20 min at 4 °C.

4. Spin at 400 × *g*, 4 °C, 5 min. Resuspend in 4 ml PBS/10% goat serum. Spin down pellet at 400 × *g* for 5 min and remove supernatant.

5. Retain the pellet and add 1 ml of 10% goat serum in PBS, containing 2~4 μl of FITC-conjugated-lectin stock solution. Incubate at room temperature for 45–60 min.

6. Wash twice by centrifugation at 400 × *g*, 15 °C for 5 min. Resuspend the pellet each time in 4 ml PBS + 10% goat serum.

7. After the final wash, resuspend cysts in PBS at the original volume of tissue homogenate used.

8. Add 12.5 μl of sample to a microscope slide, cover the sample with coverslip, and screen under fluorescence microscope using a 10× objective. Scan the slide at 10× and when you see a possible cyst, confirm by examining at 40×. Measure the diameter of the cysts using a calibrated ocular micrometer. Scan the entire slide and determine the cyst number per 12.5 μl. For each sample, count 4 aliquots and determine the total number of cysts. Calculate the number of cysts per brain (total number of cysts in 4 aliquots (50 μl) × 40 = total number per brain).

3.8   Chronic Infection Model

There are many advantages to working with less virulent strains that readily produce chronic infections in mice as both the acute and chronic phases can be studied (Fig. 2). Type II strains, such as ME49 (popular clones include the B7 clone, and PTG) and Pru, provide convenient lab-adapted strains for this purpose. Susceptibility of different mouse strains to infection with Type II strain parasites varies in large part due to differences in MHC with BALB/c (H-2d) and C3H/HeN (H-2k) mice being more resistant

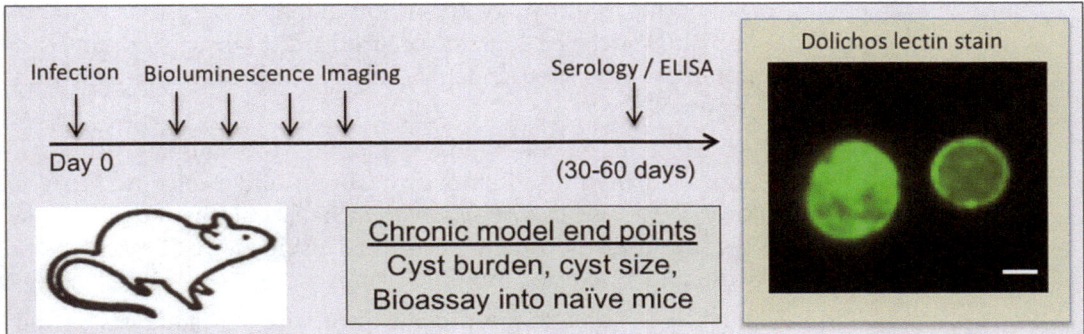

Fig. 2 Chronic infection model in inbred mice. Infections can be administered either by IP injection of tachyzoites or by oral feeding of tissue cysts derived from chronically infected animals. Useful end points include dose-dependent mortality, cyst burden, and cyst size. It is also possible to use bioluminescence imaging to evaluate differences in parasite numbers during the acute phase. The infectivity of tissue cysts can also be tested by subinoculation into naive animals. Example shows tissue cyst stained with *Dolichos biflorus* lectin. Scale bar = 10 μm

than C57Bl/6 (H-2b) [37]. Hence, the combination of Type II strains with different mouse backgrounds can be used to study acute virulence, chronicity and reactivation. Genetic mutants in the Type II strain are particularly useful for studying attenuation as they are more likely to reveal partial phenotypes that may be masked by the extremely high virulence of Type I strains.

1. Inject mice IP with tachyzoites that have been grown in tissue culture, harvested, and resuspended in HHE. Refer to Table 1 for approximate doses depending on the mouse strain being used. Viability can be a major issue since it will take you some time to prepare the inoculum and walk to the animal house. Use only freshly egressed parasites that have been grown under optimum conditions (i.e., 2–3 day synchronous cultures).

2. When testing genetic mutants vs. wild type, it is useful to bracket the inoculum starting at the LD_{50} and increased by half log or log intervals. Typically 5 mice are used per group. It is generally necessary to repeat the experiment at least once since the outcome is influenced by differences in viability. Statistical analysis of Kaplan Meier survival curves is readily performed in Prism (GraphPad).

3. Plaque an aliquot of the parasite suspension after injecting them to assure that the different parasite isolates had approximately equal viability.

4. During the acute phase (day 4–20) monitor expansion of the parasites using the *Imaging infection by bioluminescence* protocol. It is also useful to monitor weight loss and regain as the mice recover following acute infection.

5. Animals are generally followed for 30–60 days, and percent survival is calculated as above. In most cases lethal outcomes will be apparent by day 20, although in rare occasions mutants will show delayed kinetics of death. Use an appropriate end point prior to death, depending on institutionally approved protocol.

6. At the end of 30–60 days, sacrifice the animals using an approved method. Remove the brain and perform the *Cyst harvesting and staining protocol*. Statistical analyses of tissue cyst numbers is usually performed using nonparametric tests with adjustment for multiple comparisons.

7. It is also possible to test the oral infectivity of tissue cysts by oral gavage (or IP injection) into naive animals. Administer tissue cysts in 100–200 μl PBS suspension, inoculating a dose of 5–10 cysts per animal. Progression of infection can be monitored by seroconversion using the *ELISA* protocol.

4   Notes

Strain origins and derivatives: The type I RH strain was originally isolated from an adolescent who succumbed to fatal encephalitis [38]. This lab-adapted strain has been modified to express various transgene reporters including luciferase for bioluminescence imaging [32]. One isolate commonly used for genetic studies has been modified to delete the hypoxanthine, xanthine, guanosine phosphoribosyl transferase gene (*HXGPRT* also known as *HXG*), allowing for positive and negative selection [39], as well as disruption of the *KU80* gene, which results in increased levels of homologous recombination [40, 41]. The RHΔ*hxg*Δ*ku80* strain maintains the full virulence of the wild type RH strain. Another commonly used Type I strain is GT-1, which was isolated from a goat [42], and which maintains the entire life cycle unlike the commonly used RH strain [12]. Type II strains are also widely used for creating chronic infections and for virulence studies where the LD$_{50}$ can be titrated in inbred mice. The most common of these is the ME49 strain, originally isolated from a sheep in California [43]: it readily generates chronic infection in mice and undergoes the entire life cycle in cats [23]. The ME49 strain is also available as a Δ*hxgprt* knockout for facilitating selection and is tagged with firefly luciferase (FLUC) [33]. Another commonly used Type II strain is Prugniaud (aka Pru), originally isolated from a congenital human infection in France, and including a variant that is lacking both *KU80* and *HXGPRT* (Pru Δ*hxg*Δ*ku80)* [44]. Although less commonly used, Type III strains also generate chronic infections in mice but are rarely used for infection studies due to their relative avirulence [4]. The Type III strain CTG was originally isolated from a cat in New Hampshire [22] and the VEG strain was isolated from an immunocompromised patient [45].

Acute virulence: Infection with Type I strains is always lethal in laboratory mice, and any animals surviving at low inoculum are seronegative (i.e., never infected). We favor the use of outbred mice, which are more resistant, as they clearly discriminate from the high virulence of Type I strains in comparison to strains that have intermediate virulence that depends on the mouse strain. This definition of acute virulence has been used to establish the difference between clonal types [11], and map virulence differences between them [12, 24, 31]. With Type II strains, the LD$_{50}$ in outbred and inbred mice differs substantially (Table 1) and aspects of pathogenesis during chronic infection can be evaluated in surviving mice. The LD$_{50}$ of Type II strains is also somewhat dependent on the local mouse colony, so it needs to be titrated in each instance.

Bioluminescence: The sensitivity of bioluminescence detection in vivo is not easy to relate directly to parasite number and it is likely that high tissue burdens (i.e., $>10^5$ parasites/gram) are needed to detect infection. Additionally, it can be more challenging to detect infection in deep tissues in particular in the CNS due to the fact that the cranium partially blocks the signal. Nonetheless, this method has proven highly useful for tracking acute infection and dissemination [8, 31, 46], as well as reactivation of infection in immunocompromised mice [47].

Alternatives for monitoring tissue burdens: Other approaches for monitoring the number of parasites in tissue following acute or chronic infection have been developed based on PCR [48] or plaquing [13]. These methods have the advantage of being quantitative in terms of relating to genome equivalents or infectious units. However, PCR can overestimate the number of parasites due to remnant DNA that is not derived from viable organisms [48]. Using an RNA target and performing qRT-PCR can partially compensate for this possibility [49], although neither method measures viable parasites. The main limitations of these methods are that they are time-consuming and that they do not allow the possibility of sampling the same mouse repeatedly.

Acknowledgments

We thank many former members of the laboratory for developing and refining these protocols over the years, including Mike Behnke, Kevin Brown, Ildiko Dunay, Blima Fux, Dan Howe, Asis Khan, Dana Mordue, and Chunlei Su. We are also grateful to Christopher Hunter and Yasu Suzuki for helpful advice on animal infection models, and to David Bzik, Vern Carruthers, J.P. Dubey, and Laura Knoll for generously providing strains. Supported in part by NIH grants AI118426 and AI034036 to L.D.S.

References

1. Dubey JP (2010) Toxoplasmosis of animals and humans. CRC Press, Boca Raton

2. Ajzenberg D, Cogné N, Paris L, Bessieres MH, Thulliez P, Fillisetti D, Pelloux H, Marty P, Dardé ML (2002) Genotype of 86 *Toxoplasma gondii* isolates associated with human congenital toxoplasmosis and correlation with clinical findings. J Infect Dis 186:684–689

3. Ajzenberg D, Yera H, Marty P, Paris L, Dalle F, Menotti J, Aubert D, Franck J, Bessieres MH, Quinio D, Pelloux H, Delhaes L, Desbois N, Thulliez P, Robert-Gangneux F, Kauffmann-Lacroix C, Pujol S, Rabodonirina M, Bougnoux ME, Cuisenier B, Duhamel C, Duong TH, Filisetti D, Flori P, Gay-Andrieu F, Pratlong F, Nevez G, Totet A, Carme B, Bonnabau H, Darde ML, Villena I (2009) Genotype of 88 *Toxoplasma gondii* isolates associated with toxoplasmosis in immunocompromised patients and correlation with clinical findings. J Infect Dis 199:1155–1167

4. Howe DK, Sibley LD (1995) *Toxoplasma gondii* comprises three clonal lineages: correlation of parasite genotype with human disease. J Infect Dis 172:1561–1566

5. Hunter CA, Sibley LD (2012) Modulation of innate immunity by *Toxoplasma gondii* virulence effectors. Nat Rev Microbiol 10:766–778

6. Hakimi MA, Olias P, Sibley LD (2017) *Toxoplasma* effectors targeting host signaling and transcription. Clin Microbiol Rev 30:615–645

7. Lorenzi H, Khan A, Behnke MS, Namasivayam S, Swapna LS, Hadjithomas M, Karamycheva S, Pinney D, Brunk BP, Ajioka JW, Ajzenberg D, Boothroyd JC, Boyle JP, Darde ML, Diaz-Miranda MA, Dubey JP, Fritz HM, Gennari SM, Gregory BD, Kim K, Saeij JP, Su C, White MW, Zhu XQ, Howe DK, Rosenthal BM, Grigg ME, Parkinson J, Liu L, Kissinger JC, Roos DS, Sibley LD (2016) Local admixture of amplified and diversified secreted pathogenesis determinants shapes mosaic *Toxoplasma gondii* genomes. Nat Commun 7:10147

8. Behnke MS, Khan A, Lauron EJ, Jimah JR, Wang Q, Tolia NH, Sibley LD (2015) Rhoptry proteins ROP5 and ROP18 are major murine virulence factors in genetically divergent south american strains of *Toxoplasma gondii*. PLoS Genet 11:e1005434

9. Dupont CD, Christian DA, Hunter CA (2012) Immune response and immunopathology during toxoplasmosis. Semin Immunopathol 34:793–813

10. Yarovinsky F (2014) Innate immunity to *Toxoplasma gondii* infection. Nat Rev Immunol 14:109–121

11. Sibley LD, Boothroyd JC (1992) Virulent strains of *Toxoplasma gondii* comprise a single clonal lineage. Nature (Lond) 359:82–85

12. Su C, Howe DK, Dubey JP, Ajioka JW, Sibley LD (2002) Identification of quantitative trait loci controlling acute virulence in *Toxoplasma gondii*. Proc Natl Acad Sci U S A 99:10753–10758

13. Mordue DG, Monroy F, La Regina M, Dinarello CA, Sibley LD (2001) Acute toxoplasmosis leads to lethal overproduction of Th1 cytokines. J Immunol 167:4574–4584

14. Gavrilescu LC, Denkers EY (2001) IFN-g overproduction and high level apoptosis are associated with high but not low virulence *Toxoplasma gondii* infection. J Immunol 167:902–909

15. Behnke MS, Dubey JP, Sibley LD (2016) Genetic mapping of pathogenesis determinants in *Toxoplasma gondii*. Annu Rev Microbiol 70:63–81

16. Jacot D, Meissner M, Sheiner L, Soldati-Favre D, Striepen B (2014) Genetic manipulation of *Toxoplasma gondii*. In: Weiss LM, Kim K (eds) *Toxoplasma gondii* the model apicomplexan: perspectives and methods, 2nd edn. Academic Press, Elsevier, New York, pp 578–611

17. Su C, Evans D, Cole RH, Kissinger JC, Ajioka JW, Sibley LD (2003) Recent expansion of *Toxoplasma* through enhanced oral transmission. Science 299:414–416

18. Liesenfeld O (2002) Oral infection of C57BL/6 mice with *Toxoplasma gondii*: a new model of inflammatory bowel disease? J Infect Dis 185:S96–S101

19. Dubey JP (1996) WAAP and Pfizer award for excellence in veterinary parasitology research pursuing life cycles and transmission of cyst-forming coccidia of animals and humans. Vet Parasitol 64:13–20

20. Su CL, Khan A, Zhou P, Majumdar D, Ajzenberg D, Dardé ML, Zhu XQ, Ajioka JW, Rosenthal B, Dubey JP, Sibley LD (2012) Globally diverse *Toxoplasma gondii* isolates comprise six major clades originating from a small number of distinct ancestral lineages. Proc Natl Acad Sci U S A 109:5844–5849

21. Howe DK, Summers BC, Sibley LD (1996) Acute virulence in mice is associated with markers on chromosome VIII in *Toxoplasma gondii*. Infect Immun 64:5193–5198

22. Pfefferkorn ER, Pfefferkorn LC, Colby ED (1977) Development of gametes and oocysts in cats fed cysts derived from cloned trophozoites of *Toxoplasma gondii*. J Parasitol 63:158–159

23. Sibley LD, LeBlanc AJ, Pfefferkorn ER, Boothroyd JC (1992) Generation of a restriction fragment length polymorphism linkage map for *Toxoplasma gondii*. Genetics 132:1003–1015

24. Taylor S, Barragan A, Su C, Fux B, Fentress SJ, Tang K, Beatty WL, Haijj EL, Jerome M, Behnke MS, White M, Wootton JC, Sibley LD (2006) A secreted serine-threonine kinase determines virulence in the eukaryotic pathogen *Toxoplasma gondii*. Science 314:1776–1780

25. Dubey JP (2001) Oocyst shedding by cats fed isolated bradyzoites and comparison of infectivity of bradyzoites of the VEG strain *Toxoplasma gondii* to cats and mice. J Parasitol 87:215–219

26. Frazer KA, Eskin E, Kang HM, Bogue MA, Hinds DA, Beilharz EJ, Gupta RV, Montgomery J, Morenzoni MM, Nilsen GB, Pethiyagoda CL, Stuve LL, Johnson FM, Daly MJ, Wade CM, Cox DR (2007) A sequence-based variation map of 8.27 million SNPs in inbred mouse strains. Nature 448:1050–1053

27. Chia R, Achilli F, Festing MF, Fisher EM (2005) The origins and uses of mouse outbred stocks. Nat Genet 37:1181–1186

28. Yang H, Wang JR, Didion JP, Buus RJ, Bell TA, Welsh CE, Bonhomme F, Yu AH, Nachman MW, Pialek J, Tucker P, Boursot P, McMillan L, Churchill GA, de Villena FP (2011) Subspecific origin and haplotype diversity in the laboratory mouse. Nat Genet 43:648–655

29. Lilue J, Muller UB, Steinfeldt T, Howard JC (2013) Reciprocal virulence and resistance polymorphism in the relationship between *Toxoplasma gondii* and the house mouse. Elife 2:e01298

30. Roos DS, Donald RGK, Morrissette NS, Moulton AL (1994) Molecular tools for genetic dissection of the protozoan parasite *Toxoplasma gondii*. Methods Cell Biol 45:28–61

31. Behnke MS, Khan A, Wootton JC, Dubey JP, Tang K, Sibley LD (2011) Virulence differences in *Toxoplasma* mediated by amplification of a family of polymorphic pseudokinases. Proc Natl Acad Sci U S A 108:9631–9636

32. Saeij JP, Boyle JP, Grigg ME, Arrizabalaga G, Boothroyd JC (2005) Bioluminescence imaging of *Toxoplasma gondii* infection in living mice reveals dramatic differences between strains. Infect Immun 73:695–702

33. Tobin CM, Knoll LJ (2012) A patatin-like protein protects *Toxoplasma gondii* from degradation in a nitric oxide-dependent manner. Infect Immun 80:55–61

34. Jensen KD, Camejo A, Melo MB, Cordeiro C, Julien L, Grotenbreg GM, Frickel EM, Ploegh HL, Young L, Saeij JP (2015) *Toxoplasma gondii* superinfection and virulence during secondary infection correlate with the exact ROP5/ROP18 allelic combination. MBio 6:e02280

35. Khan A, Ajzenberg D, Mercier A, Demar M, Simon S, Darde ML, Wang Q, Verma SK, Rosenthal BM, Dubey JP, Sibley LD (2014) Geographic separation of domestic and wild strains of *Toxoplasma gondii* in French Guiana correlates with a monomorphic version of chromosome1a. PLoS Negl Trop Dis 8:e3182

36. Knoll LJ, Boothroyd JC (1998) Isolation of developmentally regulated genes from *Toxoplasma gondii* by a gene trap with the positive and negative selectable marker hypoxanthine-xanthine-guanine phosphoribosyltransferase. Mol Cell Biol 18:1–8

37. Suzuki Y, Yang Q, Remington JS (1995) Genetic resistance against acute toxoplasmosis depends on the strain of *Toxoplasma gondii*. J Parasitol 81:1032–1034

38. Sabin AB (1941) Toxoplasmic encephalitis in children. J Am Med Assoc 116:801–807

39. Donald RGK, Carter D, Ullman B, Roos DS (1996) Insertional tagging, cloning, and expression of the *Toxoplasma gondii* hypoxanthine-xanthine-guanine phosphoribosyltransferase gene. J Biol Chem 271:14010–14019

40. Fox BA, Ristuccia JG, Gigley JP, Bzik DJ (2009) Efficient gene replacements in *Toxoplasma gondii* strains deficient for nonhomologous end joining. Eukaryot Cell 8:520–529

41. Huynh MH, Carruthers VB (2009) Tagging of endogenous genes in a *Toxoplasma gondii* strain lacking Ku80. Eukaryot Cell 8:530–539

42. Dubey J (1980) Mouse pathogenicity of *Toxoplasma gondii* isolated from a goat. Am J Vet Res 41:427–429

43. Lunde MN, Jacobs L (1983) Antigenic differences between endozoites and cystozoites of *Toxoplasma gondii*. J Parasitol 65:806–808

44. Fox BA, Falla A, Rommereim LM, Tomita T, Gigley JP, Mercier C, Cesbron-Delauw MF, Weiss LM, Bzik DJ (2011) Type II *Toxoplasma gondii* KU80 knockout strains enable functional analysis of genes required for cyst development and latent infection. Eukaryot Cell 10:1193–1206

45. Dubey JP (1996) Infectivity and pathogenicity of *Toxoplasma gondii* oocysts for cats. J Parasitol 82:957–961

46. Reese ML, Zeiner GM, Saeij JP, Boothroyd JC, Boyle JP (2011) Polymorphic family of injected pseudokinases is paramount in *Toxoplasma* virulence. Proc Natl Acad Sci U S A 108:9625–9630

47. Rutaganira FU, Barks J, Dhason MS, Wang Q, Lopez MS, Long S, Radke JB, Jones NG, Maddirala AR, Janetka JW, El Bakkouri M, Hui R, Shokat KM, Sibley LD (2017) Inhibition of calcium dependent protein kinase 1 (CDPK1) by pyrazolopyrimidine analogs decreases establishment and reoccurrence of central nervous system disease by *Toxoplasma gondii*. J Med Chem 60:9976–9989. doi:https://doi.org/10.1021/acs.jmedchem.7b01192

48. Hill RD, Gouffon JS, Saxton AM, Su C (2012) Differential gene expression in mice infected with distinct *Toxoplasma* strains. Infect Immun 80:968–974

49. Jauregui LH, Higgins J, Zarlenga D, Dubey JP, Lunney JK (2001) Development of a real-time PCR assay for detection of *Toxoplasma gondii* in pig and mouse tissues. J Clin Microbiol 39:2065–2071

PCR Screening of *Toxoplasma gondii* Single Clones Directly from 96-Well Plates Without DNA Purification

Federica Piro, Vern B. Carruthers, and Manlio Di Cristina

Abstract

Toxoplasma gondii has become a model for studying the phylum Apicomplexa, and more in general parasite-host interactions, thanks to its ease of growth in culture and availability of a broad array of genetics tools. Assigning gene function typically involves genetic techniques such as gene knockout, conditional expression, or protein tagging. These approaches generally require isolation of single clones that have correctly introduced the desired genetic modification into the target genomic locus. The frequency of positive clones carrying these genetic manipulations depends on the particular parasite strain and the impact that these genome modifications have on parasite fitness. An adverse effect on parasite viability or growth would result in a low abundancy of the correct transgenic parasites within the transfected population. This in turn will account for a low rate of positive clones after population cloning, requiring the genetic analysis of a high number of single clones. We have developed a simple and fast method to screen single clones of *T. gondii* directly from the 96-well plates without previous parasite expansion or time-consuming genomic extraction. This approach permits screening at an earlier point than previously possible, thus allowing for faster movement toward assessing gene function.

Key words *Toxoplasma gondii*, Parasite cloning, PCR screening, Phire Hot Start II DNA Polymerase

1 Introduction

Adoption of CRISPR/Cas9 technology in *T. gondii* [1, 2], coupled with the well-established genetic tools [3–6] and advances in the genome database [7], have greatly extended the capability to successfully and rapidly manipulate the *T. gondii* genome. Successful genome targeting of eukaryotic organisms depends on the prevalent DNA repair mechanism operating in that organism. Nonhomologous end joining (NHEJ) repair is the dominant mechanism used by *T. gondii* to obviate naturally or experimentally induced double strand breaks of its genome. Until recently the low efficiency of homologous recombination (HR) DNA repair has limited targeted genome manipulation in *T. gondii*. Inactivation of the NHEJ pathway by knocking out the critical component Ku80

Christopher J. Tonkin (ed.), *Toxoplasma gondii: Methods and Protocols*, Methods in Molecular Biology, vol. 2071,
https://doi.org/10.1007/978-1-4939-9857-9_6, © Springer Science+Business Media, LLC, part of Springer Nature 2020

[8–10] has largely erased this limitation, thus facilitating gene knock-outs, knock-ins and protein tagging in *T. gondii*. Recently, exploiting CRISPR/Cas9 technology, the Lourido lab has developed a marker-free approach to efficiently generate knockouts or introduce point mutations and epitope tags into the *T. gondii* genome [11]. In our hands, this method shows good reproducibility when ku80-deficient *T. gondii* strains are used, resulting in about 10–80% efficiency of edited or tagged parasites, depending on the impact to parasite fitness of the mutation introduced. On the contrary, in our experience, this approach is very inefficient when using NHEJ-competent strains or the editing impairs partially or completely the function of an essential or growth-controlling gene.

Overall, whatever is limiting the number of parasites carrying the correct genomic modification within the transfect population, this results in laborious and time-consuming screening of clones to obtain the strain containing the desired genetic manipulation. After cloning, single clones are usually analyzed by PCR to identify those carrying the correct substitution, deletion or insertion. This procedure requires the expansion of each single clone in at least a 24-well plate to obtain a critical number of parasites to carry out genomic extraction using a commercial kit. These kits are usually quite expensive and require several passages through a spin column before obtaining the purified genomic DNA appropriate for PCR analysis. To overcome these limitations, we have developed a protocol that allows direct PCR analysis of clones without DNA purification as early as 4–7 days post cloning. DNA is obtained from a portion of the extracellular parasites present in small plaques generated by single parasites in the wells of 96-well plates [12]. This protocol is based on the use of the Phire Tissue Direct PCR Kit commercialized by Thermo Scientific. This kit allows PCR amplification of genomic DNA directly from tissue samples, such as mouse ear or tail, with no prior DNA purification. The Phire Tissue Direct PCR Master Mix employs Phire Hot Start II DNA Polymerase, a specially engineered enzyme with enhanced processivity and resistance to PCR inhibitors commonly found in tissues. Although this kit is designed to perform 250 PCR reactions from tissue samples, our adaptation cost-effectively allows the doubling to 500 PCR analyses by halving the suggested reaction volumes. Prior to PCR amplification, parasites are resuspended in a Thermo Scientific proprietary reagent that requires the use of the Phire Hot Start II DNA Polymerase provided in the Thermo Scientific kit.

Although this protocol represents a great advantage for large-scale screenings, because of its convenience compared to current standard PCR genomic analysis of *T. gondii*, we routinely use it to screen clones regardless of whether the edited parasite desired is expected to be highly represented or not within the population. As for its sensitivity, this protocol allows genomic DNA amplification starting from as few as approximately 10 parasites, as shown in

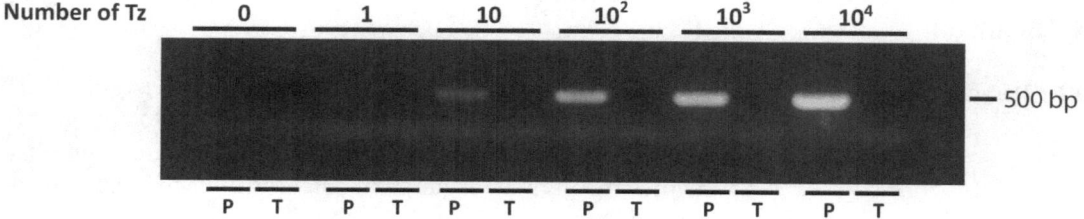

Fig. 1 Direct PCR analysis of a *T. gondii* locus from enumerated parasites. Freshly lysed tachyzoites were counted using a hemocytometer and diluted in growth media to obtain 1, 10, 100, 1000, and 10,000 parasites for PCR analysis using primers designed to amplify a representative 500 bp fragment of the single-copy gene ASP7 (TgME49_261530) from *T. gondii* genome. Parasites were then spun and resuspended in 10.25 μl of Dilution Buffer/DNARelease Additive and 1 μl from each sample was analyzed by PCR using either the Thermo Scientific Phire tissue direct PCR Master kit (P) or a standard Taq polymerase (T) and reagents. Whole PCR reactions were then run on a 1% agarose gel. Standard Taq polymerase does not work when parasites are resuspended in the Thermo Scientific Dilution Buffer/DNARelease Additive. Data are from one representative experiment out of three with similar results. *Tz* Tachyzoites

Fig. 1. Since only one tenth of the sample is used for the PCR reaction, the procedure can amplify from a single parasite genome.

2 Materials

2.1 Cell Culture

1. Human Foreskin Fibroblasts, HFF-1 (ATCC® CRL-1634™) grown in complete media (cDMEM): Dulbecco's Modified Eagle Medium (DMEM) supplemented with 10% fetal bovine serum (FBS), 2 mM L-glutamine, 100 μg/ml penicillin, and 100 U/ml streptomycin.
2. Any *T. gondii* strain.
3. Tissue culture 96-well plates.
4. Tissue culture CO_2 incubators.
5. 5 μm filters and Luer-Lock syringes.
6. Cell scrapers.
7. 26-Gauge needles.
8. Hemocytometer.
9. Inverted Phase-Contrast Microscope.

2.2 PCR Analysis

1. Phire tissue direct PCR Master kit (Thermo Scientific Cat# F-170S).
2. 0.2 ml PCR tubes.
3. Bench centrifuge for 1.5 ml tubes (with adapters for 0.2 ml PCR tubes).
4. PCR thermocycler.
5. Equipment for DNA electrophoresis.

3   Methods

3.1   Parasite Cloning

1. From a 25 cm^2 flask, harvest extracellular tachyzoites or mechanically extrude intracellular parasites by scraping the infected monolayer using a cell scraper and syringing three to four times through a 26-gauge needle. Purify tachyzoites from host cell debris by filtering through a 5 μm filter.

2. Count tachyzoites in a hemocytometer and dilute them in cDMEM to 15 parasites per ml in a total volume of 20 ml (*see* **Note 1**).

3. Remove media from a 96-well plate containing HFF monolayers and add 200 μl (containing ~3 parasites) to each well. Centrifuge the leftover parasites (10 min at 2400 × *g*) to obtain a pellet representing the entire population as PCR control sample. The control pellet may be stored at −20 °C or immediately processed for PCR analysis following the instructions in Subheading 3.2, **step 4** to the end of the protocol (*see* **Note 2**).

4. Incubate the infected 96-well plates in a 37 °C incubator at 5% CO$_2$ for at least 4 days (*see* **Note 3**).

5. Select wells containing single plaques of parasites by carefully inspecting the wells using an inverted phase contrast microscope.

3.2   Parasite Harvesting

1. For wells containing single plaques, gently pipet the media up and down three times to resuspend extracellular parasites without extensively damaging the infected monolayer. Transfer 150 μl from each well to a corresponding 0.2 ml PCR tube (*see* **Note 4**).

2. Spin the samples at 16,000 × *g* for 10 min in a microcentrifuge.

3. Gently remove the supernatant with a pipette (*see* **Note 5**).

4. Resuspend the pellet in 10 μl of a solution composed by 10 μl of Dilution Buffer and 0.25 μl of DNARelease Additive (*see* **Note 6**) by pipetting up and down several times.

5. Incubate the tube for 4 min at RT followed by 2 min at 98 °C (*see* **Note 7**).

6. At this point you can store the tube at −20 °C or proceed with the PCR analysis.

3.3   PCR Reaction

1. Perform PCR in a final volume of 10 μl containing:
   - 2 μl of H$_2$O.
   - 1 μl of 5 μM Forward primer.
   - 1 μl of 5 μM Reverse primer.
   - 5 μl of 2× Phire Tissue Direct PCR Master Mix (*see* **Note 8**).
   - 1 μl of the sample from Subheading 3.2, **step 6** (*see* **Note 9**).

2. Use the following thermal cycles: initial denaturation for 5 min at 98 °C followed by 35 cycles of: 5 s at 98 °C, 5 s at 50–60 °C (*see* **Note 10**) and 20 s ≤ 1 kb or 20 s/kb >1 kb at 72 °C. Perform a single final elongation step for 1 min at 72 °C, then hold at 4 °C.

3. Run the whole PCR reaction on an agarose gel.

4   Notes

1. Usually seeding 3 tachyzoites/well results in 30–40 single plaques per 96-well plate when using a type I *T. gondii* strain such as RH. To obtain a similar number of single plaques per 96-well plate for type II strains, we typically plate 5 tachyzoites/well by creating a suspension of 25 parasites/ml. In either case these densities are set to maximize the number of clones. Wells should be carefully inspected for single plaques. Because it is sometimes not possible to be entirely sure that a well is clonal, additional analyses should be performed to assess clonality after the initial screening.

2. Analyzing the parasite population before screening the ensuing clones might help inform the abundance of parasites carrying the desire genetic modification. If the expected PCR product is barely detectable or completely absent using primers designed to amplify DNA only from the recombinant parasite, this means that it is not very representative among the population and might require analyzing hundreds of clones. If the desired genome manipulation is absent in the population the investigator might opt to retry the transfection.

3. The protocol is highly reproducible and also works well starting from very small plaques, allowing early PCR analysis such as 4 days post-cloning when type I is used. Type II strains, or other slow growing strains, require at least 2 more days post-cloning to obtain plaques of similar size to those of type I strains.

4. If the PCR reaction is analyzed the same day of parasite withdrawal from the 96-well plate, the 50 µl of media left in the wells is sufficient for host cell and parasite survival and more media (typically other 150 µl) can be added to the positive clones identify by the PCR analysis. If the PCR result is not expected the same day, add 150 µl of fresh growth media to all wells being analyzed.

5. The parasite pellet may be poorly visible or invisible if starting from very small plaques. A visible pellet is not required for proceeding further. Pipet carefully the DNARelease Additive several times over the surface where the pellet is expected to be from centrifugation.

6. Prepare a common mix of this solution for all the samples by scaling up the following solutions for 1 sample: mix 10 μl of Dilution Buffer and 0.25 μl of DNARelease Additive.

7. Use a PCR thermocycler for these incubations to avoid sample evaporation during the 2 min at 98 °C.

8. We have failed to obtain PCR amplification from parasites resuspended in the Thermo Scientific DNARelease Additive, that releases the genomic DNA, when commercial DNA polymerases other than that one provided by the Thermo Scientific kit were used.

9. Set also separate PCR reactions containing 1 μl of either the precloning population or parental DNA as positive and negative control template, respectively.

10. The optimal annealing temperature for Phire Hot Start II DNA Polymerase may differ significantly from that of Taq-based polymerases. As a basic rule, for primers >20 nt, anneal for 5 s at a temperature that is 3 °C higher than the T_m of the lower T_m primer. For primers ≤20 nt, use an annealing temperature equal to the T_m of the lower T_m primer.

Acknowledgments

Financial Support: This work was supported by the U.S. National Institutes of Health (V.B.C. and M.D.C., grant number R01AI120607) and DCBB, University of Perugia, Italy, project FRB_2014.

References

1. Di Cristina M, Carruthers VB (2018) New and emerging uses of CRISPR/Cas9 to genetically manipulate apicomplexan parasites. Parasitology 145(9):1119–1126

2. Shen B, Brown K, Long S, Sibley LD (2017) Development of CRISPR/Cas9 for efficient genome editing in *Toxoplasma gondii*. Methods Mol Biol (Clifton, NJ) 1498:79–103

3. Wang JL, Huang SY, Behnke MS, Chen K, Shen B, Zhu XQ (2016a) The past, present, and future of genetic manipulation in *Toxoplasma gondii*. Trends Parasitol 32:542–553

4. Roos DS, Donald RG, Morrissette NS, Moulton AL (1994) Molecular tools for genetic dissection of the protozoan parasite *Toxoplasma gondii*. Methods Cell Biol 45:27–63

5. Roos DS, Sullivan WJ, Striepen B, BohneWand Donald RG (1997) Tagging genes and trapping promoters in *Toxoplasma gondii* by insertional mutagenesis. Methods 13:112–122

6. Soete M, Hettman C, Soldati D (1999) The importance of reverse genetics in determining gene function in apicomplexan parasites. Parasitology 118(suppl):S53–S61

7. Gajria B, Bahl A, Brestelli J, Dommer J, Fischer S, Gao X, Heiges M, Iodice J, Kissinger JC, Mackey AJ, Pinney DF, Roos DS, Stoeckert CJ Jr, Wang H, Brunk BP (2008) ToxoDB: an integrated *Toxoplasma gondii* database resource. Nucleic Acids Res 36(Database issue):D553–D556

8. Fox BA, Ristuccia JG, Gigley JP, Bzik DJ (2009) Efficient gene replacements in *Toxoplasma gondii* strains deficient for nonhomologous end joining. Eukaryot Cell 8(4):520–529

9. Huynh MH, Carruthers VB (2009) Tagging of endogenous genes in a *Toxoplasma gondii* strain lacking Ku80. Eukaryot Cell 8(4):530–539

10. Fox BA, Falla A, Rommereim LM, Tomita T, Gigley JP, Mercier C, Cesbron-Delauw MF, Weiss LM, Bzik DJ (2011) Type II *Toxoplasma gondii* KU80 knockout strains enable functional analysis of genes required for cyst development and latent infection. Eukaryot Cell 10:1193–1206

11. Sidik SM, Hackett CG, Tran F, Westwood NJ, Lourido S (2014) Efficient genome engineering of *Toxoplasma gondii* using CRISPR/Cas9. PLoS One 9(6):e100450

12. Di Cristina M, Dou Z, Lunghi M, Kannan G, Huynh MH, McGovern OL, Schultz TL, Schultz AJ, Miller AJ, Hayes BM, van der Linden W, Emiliani C, Bogyo M, Besteiro S, Coppens I, Carruthers VB (2017) *Toxoplasma* depends on lysosomal consumption of autophagosomes for persistent infection. Nat Microbiol 2:17096

Chapter 7

CRISPR/Cas9-Mediated Generation of Tetracycline Repressor-Based Inducible Knockdown in *Toxoplasma gondii*

Damien Jacot and Dominique Soldati-Favre

Abstract

The phylum Apicomplexa groups numerous pathogenic protozoan parasites including *Plasmodium*, the causative agent of malaria, *Cryptosporidium* which can cause severe gastrointestinal infections, as well as *Babesia*, *Eimeria*, and *Theileria* that account for considerable economic burdens to poultry and cattle industry. *Toxoplasma gondii* is the most ubiquitous and opportunistic member of this phylum able to infect all warm-blooded animals and responsible for severe disease in immunocompromised individuals and unborn fetuses.

Due to its ease of cultivation and genetic tractability *T. gondii* has served as recipient for the transfer and adaptation of multiple genetic tools developed to control gene expression. In these parasites, a collection of tight conditional systems exists to control gene expression at the levels of transcription, RNA degradation or protein stability. The recent implementation of the CRISPR/Cas9 technology considerably reduces time and effort to generate transgenic parasites and at the same time increases to an ultimate level of precision the editing of the parasite genome. Here, we provide a step-by-step protocol for CRISPR/Cas9-mediated generation of tetracycline repressor-based inducible knockdown in *T. gondii*.

Key words *Toxoplasma gondii*, Tetracycline repressor, Tetracycline transactivator, Inducible knockdown, CRISPR/Cas9, gRNA, Homologous recombination

1 Introduction

Studies of essential genes via the generation of inducible knockdown (iKD) strains have been instrumental to investigate the biology of *Toxoplasma gondii*. Over the last two decades, several inducible systems have been successfully established (Fig. 1a) [1–4]. The first to be developed and the most widely used so far is a tetracycline repressor-based system that controls the transcription of the gene of interest (GOI) [5, 6]. This system is based on a transactivator composed of the tetracycline repressor fused to an activating domain isolated from a genetic screen in the parasite and named transactivator trap identified 1 (TATi-1) [6]. By genetic

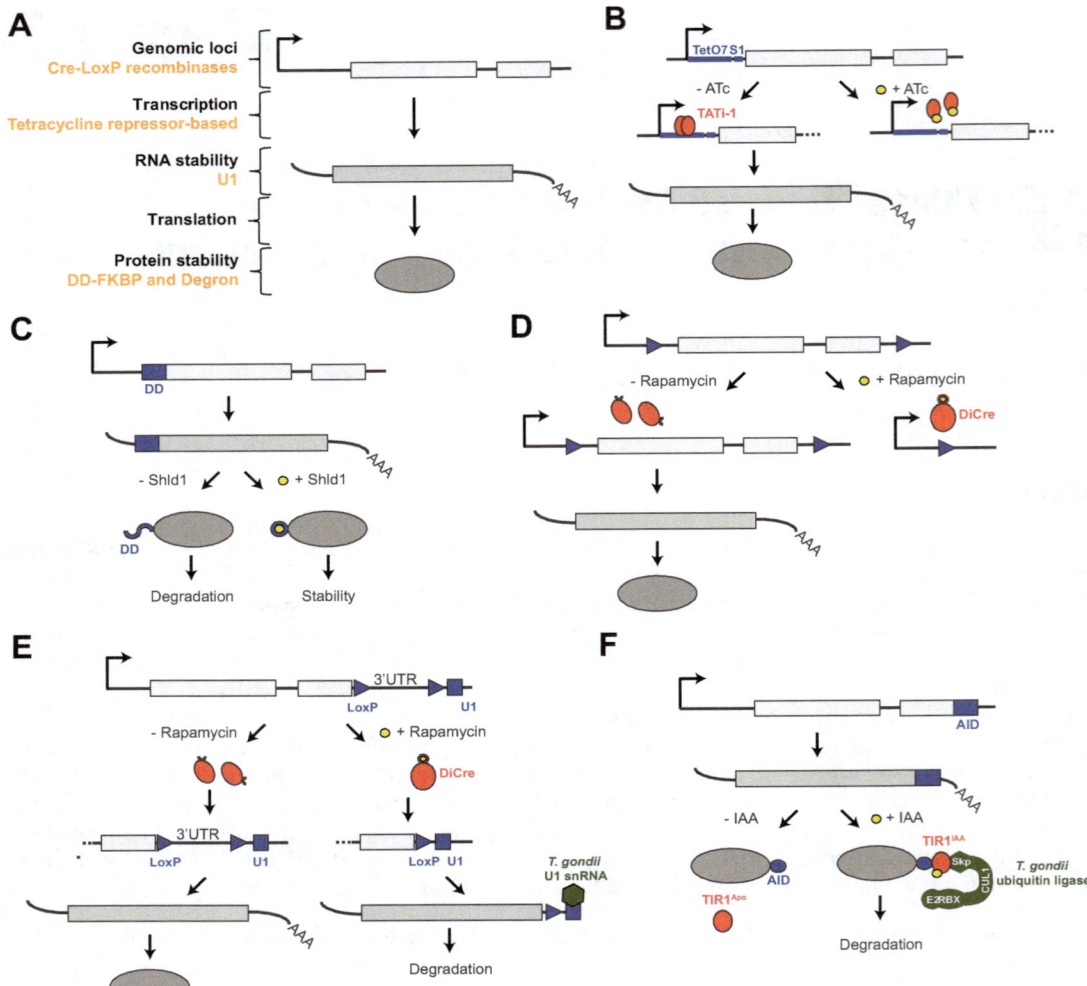

Fig. 1 (**a**) Schematic representation of the various inducible systems developed for *T. gondii*. These systems act at different levels through direct modifications at the genomic level, blocking transcription or affecting RNA stability or protein degradation. (**b**) In the tetracycline repressor-based system, the endogenous promoter is replaced by a tetO regulatable promoter. The transactivator TATi-1 binds to the tetO sequences and drives the transcription of the GOI. The addition of anhydrotetracycline (ATc) results in gene silencing. TATi-1 should be either contained in the inducible plasmid or constitutively expressed in the recipient strain. (**c**) The DD-fused POI is rapidly degraded unless Shld1 is added. Shld1 binds and folds the DD preventing protein degradation. The DD can be placed either in the N-terminus or C-terminus of the protein. Although more complicated to engineer N-terminal tagging appears to regulate better. (**d**) The GOI is flanked by two loxP sites. The addition of rapamycin reconstitutes a functional DiCre recombinase, which subsequently excises the GOI. This system is dependent on a recipient strain constitutively expressing the two inactive fragments of the Cre recombinase. (**e**) The 3′ UTR of the GOI is replaced by the SAG1 3′ UTR flanked by two loxP sites and a 3′ U1 snRNA recognition sequence. The addition of rapamycin leads to U1 transposition immediately after the STOP codon. This results in the recruitment of the *T. gondii* U1 snRNP (small nuclear ribonucleic particles) to the pre-mRNA which inhibits polyadenylation and therefore pre-mRNA maturation. This system is dependent on a recipient strain constitutively expressing the two inactive fragments of the Cre recombinase. (**f**) The auxin-inducible

engineering, the GOI is placed under the control of a regulatable promoter containing 7 tet-Operators (tetO). TATi-1 binds to the tetO sequences and drives the transcription of the GOI. Addition of anhydrotetracycline (ATc) induces a conformational change in TATi-1, resulting in its dissociation from tetO, thereby silencing the gene (Fig. 1b).

Alternative and complementary approaches are available to conditionally control gene expression in *T. gondii*. The ligand-controlled destabilization domain (DD derived from FKBP) confers rapid and reversible protein stabilization (Fig. 1c) [1]. In this system, the DD-fused protein of interest (POI) is rapidly degraded unless the synthetic ligand, called Shield-1 (Shld1) is added to selectively bind and fold DD and stabilize the fusion protein. The controlled assembly of the Cre recombinase by rapamycin has been exploited to control the excision of LoxP flanked genes (Fig. 1d) [2]. Here the DiCre recombinase is split into two inactive fragments fused to either the rapamycin-binding proteins FRB or FKBP. Addition of rapamycin brings FRB and FKBP together and thus reconstitutes a functional enzyme able to excise the loxP-flanked GOI. Based on the same DiCre-mediated strategy, U1 small nuclear ribonucleic particles-mediated gene silencing was also established (Fig. 1e) [3]. Rapamycin-induction resulted in the repositioning of the U1 recognition sites adjacent to the termination codon of the GOI, leading to pre-mRNA degradation and efficient iKD. Importantly, both last methods rely heavily on the efficiency of the rapamycin-dependent reconstitution of a functional Cre recombinase. Finally, an auxin-inducible degron (AID) system was established (Fig. 1f). In a parasite strain constitutively expressing the *Oryza sativa* transport inhibitor response 1 (TIR1), addition of auxin (indole-3-acetic acid, IAA) results in the rapid degradation of the AID-tagged POI [4, 7].

In its first version, the tetracycline repressor-based system required two rounds of transfection and selection before obtaining the final inducible strain [6]. First an inducible second copy of the GOI is integrated in a strain constitutively expressing TATi-1. Then, knockout (KO) of the endogenous GOI resulted in the iKD strain. Although this system was successfully used to generate numerous iKDs, it required laborious cloning steps and the amplification of large homology regions to produce vectors favoring homologous recombination. Indeed, *T. gondii* possesses an efficient non-homologous end joining repair machinery (NHEJ), which limits the use of homology-directed approaches unless

Fig. 1 (continued) degron (AID) sequence is inserted at the C-terminus of the GOI. In the absence of auxin, the plant auxin receptor TIR1 is inactive (Apo state) allowing the POI to be expressed. Upon the addition of auxin (indole-3-acetic acid, IAA), auxin-bound TIR1 assembles into an active ubiquitin ligase complex. This complex now recognizes and polyubiquitinates the AID, targeting the POI to degradation

large homology regions are provided. The isolation of ΔKu80 strains, a key component of the NHEJ [8–10], helped overcome this issue and allowed the efficient generation of transgenic strains using shorter homology regions (500–300 bp). As a consequence, two more streamlined versions of the system were developed. In one, the endogenous promoter of the GOI is directly replaced by the tetO-inducible promoter in a TATi-1 constitutively expressing strain [11–13]. An alternative single-step and self-contained approach consists in a double homologous recombination strategy where a vector expressing TATi-1 under the control of a constitutive tubulin promoter (pTub8) is integrated downstream of the 5′ UTR of the GOI. On the other end, the 3′ recombination region is designed to result in the replacement of the endogenous promoter by the tetO-inducible one. Simultaneously, a Myc tag can be placed at the N-terminus of the GOI [14–17]. The recent implementation of the CRISPR/Cas9 technology in *T. gondii* considerably improved site-targeted homologous recombination, allowing efficient gene targeting using very short homology regions [18–20]. This opened the possibility to generate amplicons by PCR, using primers containing homology regions of around 30 bp and plasmids as template, avoiding laborious cloning of 5′ and 3′ flanking regions. In that context, the AID system was described in combination with the CRISPR/Cas9 system for successful and rapid generation of iKD strains in *T. gondii* [4, 21].

Here, we describe a detailed protocol for the rapid generation of CRISPR/Cas9-mediated tetracycline repressor-based iKD in *Toxoplasma gondii*. This technique is based on the same single-step and self-contained strategy as previously described [15]. The plasmid contains a constitutively expressed TATi-1 cassette, a hypoxanthine-xanthine-guanine phosphoribosyl transferase (HXGPRT) selection cassette, a tetO-inducible promoter and an N-terminal Myc epitope-tag (*see* Fig. 2a). A PCR-generated amplicon with 30 bp 5′ and 3′ flanking homology region to the targeted GOI is used, instead of a plasmid. Double homologous recombination at the locus of interest is triggered by CRISPR/Cas9 genome editing (Fig. 2a). This strategy was well established in the RHΔHXGPRTΔKu80 parasite strain [22–25]. The ΔHXGPRT is required to use HXGPRT as positive selectable marker [26] while ΔKu80 is eliminating random integration and hence indirectly favors the isolation of homologous recombination events. CRISPR/Cas9 mediated integration of KO vectors in wild-type parasites using short homology regions (30 bp) was demonstrated to be successful [18–20] suggesting that wt strains can be used for the generation of tetracycline repressor-based iKDs. Finally, this system is also suitable for in vivo virulence assay [6, 16]. However, it is important to mention that expression of the Tet-transactivator can affect virulence [27]. In conclusion, this self-contained system

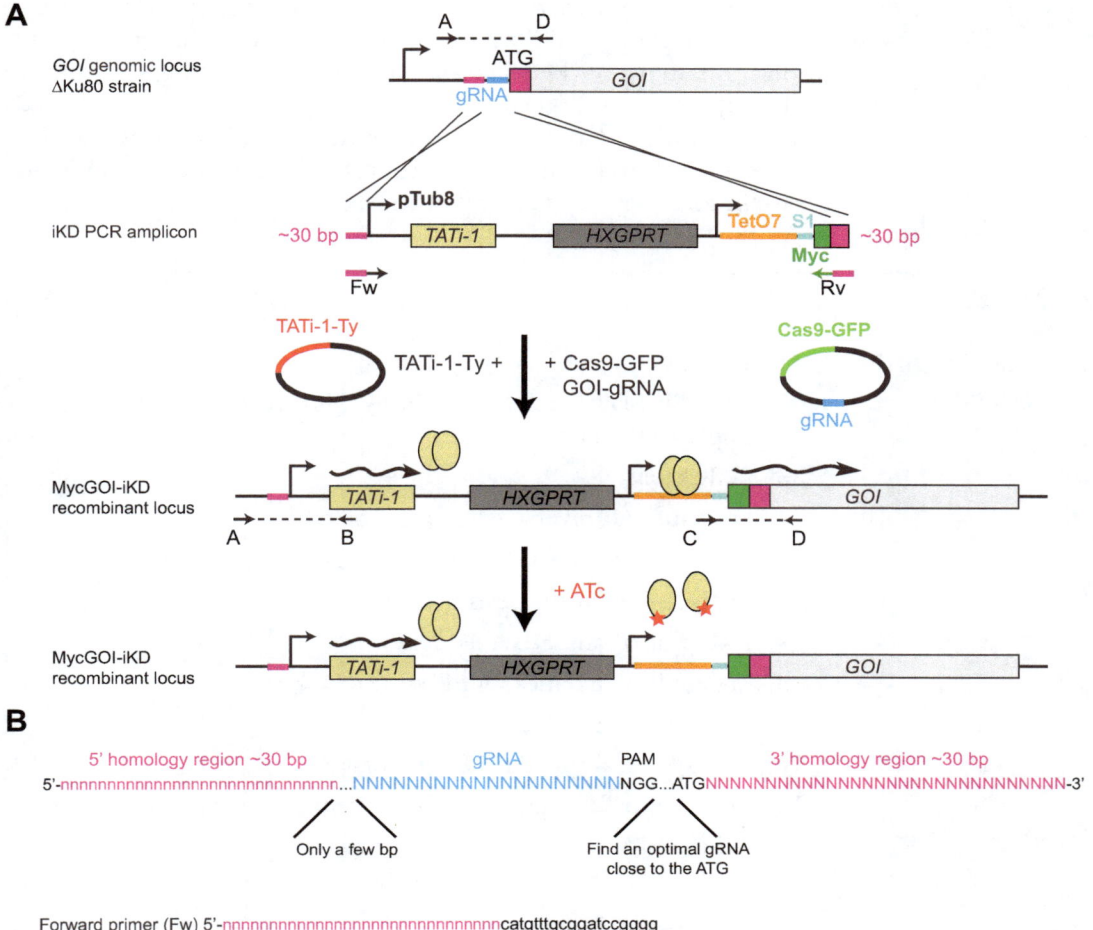

Fig. 2 (**a**) Schematic representation of the tetracycline repressor-based inducible knockdown strategy. The PCR amplicon contains all the elements for transactivation and permits N-terminal tagging of the GOI. A short sequence of the Surface Antigen 1 (SAG1) promoter is used as minimal promoter to ensure transactivation. Double homologous recombination is assisted by CRISPR/Cas9 and initial transactivation facilitated by transient transfection of TATi-1-Ty. Upon successful recombination, the addition of ATc results in gene silencing. (**b**) Schematic representation of the strategy used to design the 5′ and 3′ homology regions as well as the gRNA sequence. Forward and reverse primer sequences for the KOD PCR are presented

offers the potential to rapidly generate robust iKDs of any gene in wild-type background type I strains.

This strategy could also be implemented in cyst-forming strains such as Me49ΔHXGPRTΔKu80, as well as PruΔHXGPRTΔKu80 [8]. Although ATc regulates gene expression within in vitro produced cysts, transactivation and therefore expression of the GOI appears to be reduced even in absence of ATc (Soldati-Favre, unpublished). Furthermore, ATc does not cross the blood–brain barrier, limiting its utilization to investigate the chronic stage of infection in vivo. The blood–brain barrier crossing compound Doxycycline, a well-known alternative to ATc could not be used as this antibiotic targets translation in the apicoplast and is toxic for *T. gondii* [5]. So far, an efficient, robust and stage-specific inducible system for in vivo cysts is still missing.

2   Materials

2.1 Site Directed Mutagenesis

1. Thermocycler.
2. Q5® Site-Directed Mutagenesis Kit Protocol (E0554, New England Biolabs).
3. PCR tubes.
4. Forward and reverse primer (*see* below).
5. pSag1-Cas9-NLS-GFP/pU6-gRNA plasmid [19].
6. Agarose Electrophoresis System.
7. 1 kb plus or any DNA ladder.
8. Restriction enzymes DpnI and SacI.
9. Competent *E. coli* cells.
10. 100 µg/ml ampicillin LB agar plates.
11. Microcentrifuge and benchtop centrifuge with 15 ml tube holders.
12. 100 µg/ml ampicillin LB broth.
13. Plasmid extraction kit.
14. M13 reverse universal primer.

2.2 KOD PCR

1. Thermocycler.
2. PCR tubes.
3. Forward and reverse primer (*see* below).
4. KOD HiFi DNA polymerase (71085-3, Merck Millipore).
5. pTub8TATi1-HXGPRT-tetO7S1myc [15] This plasmid will be available on Addgene.
6. 3 M sodium acetate in H_2O.
7. 100% EtOH and 70% EtOH in H_2O.
8. Agarose Electrophoresis System.
9. Microcentrifuge.

2.3 Parasites Transfection and Selection

Only the specific materials for *T. gondii* transfection are listed here. *T. gondii* general cell culture is not included. Additional protocols can be found in [28].

1. RHΔHXGPRTΔKu80 [10] parasite strain and human foreskin fibroblasts (HFFs).

2. General *T. gondii* cell culture equipment (dish, 96-well plate, pipette. . .).

3. Cytomix: 120 mM KCl, 0.15 mM $CaCl_2$, 10 mM K_2HPO_4/KH_2PO_4 pH 7.6, 25 mM HEPES pH 7.6, 2 mM, EGTA, 5 mM $MgCl_2$ in H_2O. Should be prepared in large batches; filter-sterilized and stored at −20 °C or 4 °C.

4. ATP: 100 mM in H_2O, pH 7.9 with KOH.

5. Glutathione (GSH): 100 mM in H_2O, pH 7.6 with KOH.

6. 4 mm gap electroporation cuvettes (Cell Projects Limited).

7. BTX ECM 630 or Bio-Rad electroporator or Amaxa system.

8. Benchtop centrifuge with 15 ml tube holders.

9. pTub8-TATi-1-Ty plasmid [29].

10. KOD PCR amplicons (*see* below).

11. Xanthine (250× stock solution): 12.5 mg/ml in H_2O, 0.1 N KOH.

12. Mycophenolic acid (MPA, 250× stock solution): 6.25 mg/ml in 100% MetOH.

13. Anhydrotetracycline (ATc): 1 mg/ml stock solution in 100% EtOH.

14. 4% paraformaldehyde (PFA)/0.05% glutaraldehyde (GA) in PBS.

15. 0.1 M glycine in PBS.

16. 2% BSA in PBS.

17. 0.2% Triton X-100 in PBS.

18. C-Myc antibodies (9E10).

19. GAP45 antibodies [30].

20. Alexa Fluor 488 and Alexa Fluor 594 conjugated goat anti-mouse/rabbit secondary antibodies.

21. Fluorescence microscope.

22. SDS-PAGE electrophoresis apparatus and prestained protein ladder.

23. Actin-1 antibodies [31] or any other *T. gondii* loading-control antibodies.

24. Horseradish Peroxidase conjugated goat anti-rabbit/mouse secondary antibodies.

25. Chemiluminescence imaging system.

3   Methods

3.1   Design
of the gRNA

1. Genomic DNA sequences of *T. gondii* can be found on http:// toxodb.org/toxo/. A detailed protocol to extract DNA sequences is described in [21]. Select an optimal gRNA directly 5′ to the start codon (ATG) of the GOI (*see* Fig. 2a, b and **Note 1**). Multiple online tools are available for optimal gRNA design. We recommend using The Eukaryotic Pathogen CRISPR guide RNA/DNA Design Tool http://grna.ctegd. uga.edu/. Be careful to choose the appropriate *T. gondii* strain. Select only a gRNA sequence that has a 3′ NGG protospacer adjacent motif (PAM). The gRNAs can be either on the forward or reverse DNA strand.

3.2   Site Directed
Mutagenesis
for GOI-Specific gRNA
CRISPR/Cas9 Plasmid
Generation

1. The Q5® site-directed mutagenesis kit protocol (E0554) from New England Biolabs is used here but any other equivalent kit can be used to modify the pSag1-Cas9-NLS-GFP/pU6-gRNA plasmid [19].

2. Site-directed mutagenesis PCRs are performed with a reverse universal primer and a forward primer containing the new gRNA.

3. Reverse universal primer: aacttgacatccccatttac.

4. Forward   gRNA   primer: (G)NNNNNNNNNNNNNNNNNNNN gttttagagctagaaatagc.

5. The Ns correspond to the 20 nucleotides of the gRNA sequence and (G) is an optional G at the 5′ end (*see* **Note 1**).

6. Assemble the following reagents in a PCR tube.

Q5 Hot Start High-Fidelity 2× Master Mix	6.25 µl
10 µM forward primer	0.625 µl
10 µM reverse primer	0.625 µl
Template DNA (1–25 ng/µl)	1 µl
Nuclease-free water	4 µl

7. Mix reagents completely, and then transfer to a thermocycler.

8. Perform the following cycling conditions:

98 °C	30 s
98 °C	10 s
57 °C	30 s
72 °C	5 min (repeat **steps 2–4** 25×)
72 °C	5 min
Hold	4 °C

9. Load 1 μl of the PCR reaction on a DNA gel to confirm a successful reaction. The expected band should be around 10 kb.

10. If PCR is positive, assemble the following reagents in an Eppendorf tube:

PCR Product	1 μl
2× KLD reaction buffer	2.5 μl
10× KLD enzyme mix	0.5 μl
Nuclease-free water	1 μl

11. Mix well by pipetting up and down and incubate at room temperature for 5–10 min (*see* **Note 2**).

12. Thaw a tube of chemically competent *E. coli* cells on ice.

13. Add the reaction from **step 11** to the tube of thawed cells.

14. Place the mixture on ice for 10 min.

15. Heat shock at 42 °C for 30 s.

16. Place on ice for 5 min.

17. Plate on Amp LB agar.

18. The next day, pick and grow 3–4 single colonies overnight in 3 ml LB containing ampicillin at 37 °C. Pellet the bacterial cultures and extract the plasmids using a plasmid extraction kit.

19. Perform an analytical restriction digest with appropriate enzymes (such as SacI) to check plasmid integrity. Some plasmids might include the new gRNA but have lost parts of the plasmid during mutagenesis.

20. Confirm appropriate pattern on an agarose gel.

21. If the analytical digest is correct, send plasmids for sequencing using the M13 universal reverse primer.

3.3 KOD PCR

1. Design the 5′ homology region directly 5′ to the gRNA sequence. This region should not include the gRNA sequence to avoid cleavage of the template vector after integration (*see* Fig. 2a, b). Both the 3′ and 5′ homology regions should contain around 30 nucleotides.

2. Design the 3′ homology region following the ATG of the GOI (*see* Fig. 2a, b and **Note 3**).

3. The KOD PCRs (*see* **Note 4**) on the inducible vector pTub8-TATi1-HXGPRT-tetO7S1myc are performed with the following primers:

    Forward primer (Fw): 5′-nnnnnnnnnnnnnnnnnnnnnnnnnnnnnn catgtttgcggatccggggg

Reverse primer (Rv):
5′NNNNNNNNNNNNNNNNNNNNNNNNNNNNNNNNNNCAGGTCCTCCT
CGGAGATGA.

The 5′ and 3′ homology regions are represented with n and N respectively. To design a construct without an N-terminal Myc tag (*see* **Note 5**).

4. The amplicon will include the selectable marker HXGPRT as well as the transactivator TATi-1 driven by a constitutive tubulin (pTub8) promoter (*see* **Note 6**).

5. Assemble the following reagents in a PCR tube. 2 KOD reactions (50 μl each) are usually sufficient to obtain enough DNA for transfection (10–15 μg).

Nuclease-free water	32.6 μl
10× buffer#1 for KOD HiFi DNA polymerase	5 μl
dNTPs (final concentration 0.2 mM)	5 μl
MgCl2 (final concentration 1 mM)	2 μl
Template DNA (1–25 ng/μl)	1 μl
10 μM forward primer	2 μl
10 μM reverse primer	2 μl
KOD HiFi DNA polymerase (2.5 U/μl)	0.4 μl

6. Mix reagents completely, and then transfer to the thermocycler.

7. Perform the following cycling conditions:

98 °C	15 s
98 °C	15 s
58 °C	5 s
72 °C	40 s (repeat **steps 2–4** 25×)
72 °C	2 min
Hold	4 °C

8. Precipitate PCR reactions in microcentrifuge tubes using 10% Sodium acetate 3 M and 2–3× volume of 100% EtOH (*see* **Note 7**).

9. Incubate at −20 °C overnight or minimum for 2 h.

10. Centrifuge at 15,000 × *g* speed for 30 min at 4 °C.

11. Carefully remove and discard the supernatant.

12. Wash the pellet by adding 500 μl 70% cold ethanol. Centrifuge at 15,000 × *g* speed for 10 min at 4 °C, and carefully remove and discard the supernatant.

13. Air-dry the pellet for 20 min and resuspend in 50 μl dH$_2$O.-Combine the two PCRs to obtain a final volume of 100 μl.

14. Check DNA quantity, a least 10–15 μg are required for one transfection. If the concentration is not sufficient, perform an additional KOD PCR, precipitate and resuspend the pellet with the 100 μl from **step 13**.

3.4 Parasite Transfection and Selection

Only a specific protocol for *T. gondii* transfection is presented here. The general procedure for *T. gondii* cell culture is not included. Additional protocols can be found in [28].

1. Harvest *T. gondii* RHΔHXGPRTΔKu80 (*see* **Note 8**) parasites from a 6 cm dish of fully lysed HFFs and pellet by spinning at 1000 rpm for 10 min at RT in a 15 ml falcon tube. A 6 cm dish contains a typical yield of 5–6 × 10^7 parasites which is sufficient for 3–4 transfections.

2. Resuspend the pellet in 3 ml of cytomix. Add 30 μl of ATP (100 mM) and 30 μl of GSH (100 mM) per ml of cytomix used.

3. Combine 650 μl of the resuspended parasites with 100 μl of purified KOD PCR (Subheading 3.3, **step 14**). Add 20 μg of your modified pSag1-Cas9-NLS-GFP/pU6-gRNA vector that will be transfected transiently as circular plasmid. We also recommend to co-transfect 20 μg of circular pTub8-TATi-1-Ty plasmid [29] to improve transactivation during the first parasite cell cycles (*see* **Note 9**). Be careful to not exceed the maximal 800 μl volume of the cuvette.

   In rare cases, one of these last vectors can integrate. Absence of integration can be checked latter (*see* Subheading 3.4, **step 8**).

4. Transfer the transfection mix into a 4 mm gap electroporation cuvette.

5. Electroporate the parasites with two pulses of 2000 V, 50 U, 25 mF using a BTX ECM 630 electroporator or according to electroporator manufacturer's instructions.

6. Transfer the parasite into fresh dishes with confluent HFFs and incubate them at 37 °C, 5% CO$_2$.

7. Twenty-four hours after transfection add 25 μg/ml mycophenolic acid and 50 μg/ml xanthine. MPA/xanthine should kill parasites lacking the selection cassette within 2–3 days.

8. When a drug-resistant population emerges, assess the transfected pool of parasites by indirect immunofluorescence assay (IFAs) using c-Myc and GAP45 antibodies. Regulation of the inducible copy should be tested using 1 μg/ml of ATc. Typically, 24 and 48 h ATc treatment can be investigated (*see* **Note 10**). For IFAs, a 24 h pretreatment before inoculation of the IFA plate is recommended for a 48 h time point.

(a) Inoculate a 24-well plate containing coverslips and HFF monolayer ± ATc.

(b) After 24 h fix with 4% PFA/0.05% glutaraldehyde in PBS for 10 min and quench with 0.1 M glycine/PBS for at least 5 min.

(c) Permeabilize the cells for 20 min using 0.2% Triton X-100/PBS.

(d) Block in 2% BSA/PBS for 20 min.

(e) Proceed with indirect fluorescence microscopy using primary antibodies against c-Myc (mouse) and GAP45 or other (rabbit), and then secondary antibodies Alexa Fluor 488 and 594 against mouse and rabbit. Perform all incubations in 2% BSA/PBS and washes with PBS. Absence of integration of pSag1-Cas9-NLS-GFP/pU6-gRNA and pTub8-TATi-1-Ty vectors can also be assessed at this stage using Ty and GFP markers.

9. Western blot analysis can be performed to confirm Myc tagging of the protein and proper regulation. 24 and 48 h ± ATc treatment is recommended. 10^6 parasites per lane are typically used. Actin antibodies can be used as loading control.

10. Correct integration of the inducible vector should be confirmed by PCR analysis using appropriate primers (*see* Fig. 2a and **Note 11**). Primers A–B and C–D are used to confirm 5′ and 3′ integrations respectively. The presence or absence of the endogenous locus is evaluated with primers A–D (*see* **Note 12**). GoTaq Green Master Mix or any other equivalent polymerase can be used for PCR amplification by following manufacturer's protocol.

11. If **steps 8–10** are successful, clone the parasites by limiting dilution in 96 well plates.

12. After 7 days, pick several single plaques corresponding to individual clones.

13. Screen each clone by IFAs using c-Myc antibodies.

14. Confirm by PCR analyses the 5′ and 3′ integrations with primers A–B and C–D respectively as well as absence of the endogenous locus with primers A–D (*see* Fig. 2a).

15. Assess each positive clone for proper ATc (1 μg/ml) regulation by western blotting and IFAs as previously described.

16. If successful, proceed to full phenotyping.

4   Notes

1. Ideally, the selected gRNA should be close to the start codon ATG (between 0 and 200 bp). It is not necessary to remove the entire endogenous promoter. If the selected gRNA is very distant from the ATG (more than 200 bp), the probability of successful double homologous recombination will be reduced. Due to unpredictable efficiency among different gRNAs, more than one guide could be designed but each gRNA has to be transfected independently. For efficient transcription of gRNAs driven by the U6 promoter, a G should ideally be the first base of the 20 bp guide sequence at the 5′ position. For gRNAs that do not begin with a G, an additional G is recommended at the 5′ of the guide sequence, resulting in a 21 bp sequence (5′-GNNNNNNNNNNNNNNNNNNNN). The addition of a 5′ G does not alter the specificity of the gRNA or affect the efficiency of Cas9 cleavage [32].

2. To improve mutagenesis efficiency, an additional and prolonged DpnI digestion can be performed after the KLD step to remove residual parental vectors. Increase the volume to 50 μl with dH$_2$O, add the appropriate restriction enzyme buffer and 0.5 μl of DpnI. DpnI recognizes and cuts methylated DNA. The PCR product is not methylated in contrast to the template DNA plasmid.

3. The 3′ homology region could include the ATG of the GOI, though this is not necessary. The start codon will be encoded in the Myc tag.

4. KOD HiFi polymerase elongation rate and processivity are respectively five times and 10–15 times higher than Pfu DNA polymerase. This results in high-fidelity and high-yield DNA amplification.

5. This design will introduce a Myc tag at the N-terminal end of the GOI (Fig. 2a, b). If N-terminal tagging with Myc is not possible or desired, the same procedure can be done using a different reverse primer starting before the Myc tag. In that situation the 3′ homology region should contain the first methionine.
   Reverse   primer   (Rv)   without   Myc:
   5′-NNNNNNNNNNNNNNNNNNNNNNNNNNNNNNNCAT tttgatatccctaggaattc.

6. The expression of the trans-activator TATi-1 is driven by a strong constitutive promoter. If the expression of the GOI is cell cycle dependent, the endogenous promoter could be used to drive the expression of the TATi-1. However, gRNA and 5′ homology region design should be designed carefully to include the entire endogenous promoter. Transactivation likely requires a strong promoter to express enough TATi-1 to

sustain the expression of the GOI. Weak endogenous promoters might therefore not be suitable for transactivation. Several iKD of genes displaying a cell cycle dependent profile were made using a pTub8-TATi-1 constitutive promoter suggesting that transcriptional control can be by-passed, at least in some cases.

7. Sodium acetate precipitation and resuspension of the PCR fragments in dH_2O is required to remove the excess of salt present in the PCR mix that interfere with the cytomix composition resulting in low efficiency of parasite transfection.

8. The RHΔHXGPRTΔKu80 strain is preferred for this strategy. ΔHXGPRT is required for proper selection with the HXGPRT selectable marker [26]. ΔKu80 is needed for the success and high efficiency of homologous recombination. If RHΔHXGPRT background is required, the same strategy can be used. However, the 30 bp homology regions might not be sufficient for proper recombination as the NHEJ machinery is active and could result in nonhomologous random integration of the inducible constructs, as well as mutations in the gRNA targeted region before integration of the inducible vector. Integration of KO vectors in RH wild-type parasites using short homology regions was demonstrated to be efficient, suggesting that the 30 bp could be enough for certain cases [18–20]. However, we have not tested that formally using the tetracycline repressor-based inducible system and have used only ΔKu80 parasites for the generation of iKD. Conventional cloning methods can be used to insert larger 5′ and 3′ homology regions in the same inducible vector as described in [15, 16, 22, 23]. This will improve integration efficiency and assure proper targeting of the inducible vector.

9. Establishment of the transactivation process is presumed to be a critical limiting step for the generation of tetracycline repressor-based inducible system. Transient episomal transfection of a plasmid expressing the transactivator TATi-1 (pTub8-TATi-1-Ty) during the first cell cycle could improve the proper establishment of the transactivation.

10. Twenty-four hours of ATc treatment is often enough to detect regulation. Careful analysis by IFAs and western blotting at multiple time points to assess downregulation should be performed before any phenotyping. ATc is stable for at least 1 week in culture. Proper concentration of ATc should be used as high concentration of ATc is toxic [5] and affect apicoplast inheritance [14]. Prolonged treatment with ATc can result with the emergence of parasites that lost ATc regulation of the GOI. The time frame for proper regulation of the GOI is different for every gene. Already produced mRNA and

proteins could have very different stability that will affect the timing of downregulation. Downregulation of the gene is sometime only partial. This strategy is a knockdown and there will always be some residual expression.

11. If N-terminal tagging of the GOI is not possible, PCR analysis is the only method to assess integration of the inducible vector. Generation of specific antibodies or additional tagging in the C-terminal region would be required to assess regulation. We do not recommend qRT-PCR to evaluate proper regulation.

12. Primers A and D should be designed respectively in 5′ and 3′ of the homology regions.
    Primer B: 5′-GAGCGAGTTTCCTTGTCGTCAGGCC.
    Primer C: 5′-CGCTGCACCACTTCATTATTTCTTCTGG.

Acknowledgments

The author would like to thank Nicolò Tosetti, Aarti Krishnan, and Hung Ryan Vuong for careful reading of the manuscript.
This research was supported by the Swiss National Science Foundation 310030B_166678.

References

1. Herm-Gotz A, Agop-Nersesian C, Munter S, Grimley JS, Wandless TJ, Frischknecht F, Meissner M (2007) Rapid control of protein level in the apicomplexan *Toxoplasma gondii*. Nat Methods 4(12):1003–1005. https://doi.org/10.1038/nmeth1134

2. Andenmatten N, Egarter S, Jackson AJ, Jullien N, Herman JP, Meissner M (2013) Conditional genome engineering in *Toxoplasma gondii* uncovers alternative invasion mechanisms. Nat Methods 10(2):125–127. https://doi.org/10.1038/nmeth.2301

3. Pieperhoff MS, Pall GS, Jimenez-Ruiz E, Das S, Melatti C, Gow M, Wong EH, Heng J, Muller S, Blackman MJ, Meissner M (2015) Conditional U1 gene silencing in *Toxoplasma gondii*. PLoS One 10(6):e0130356. https://doi.org/10.1371/journal.pone.0130356

4. Long S, Brown KM, Drewry LL, Anthony B, Phan IQH, Sibley LD (2017) Calmodulin-like proteins localized to the conoid regulate motility and cell invasion by *Toxoplasma gondii*. PLoS Pathog 13(5):e1006379. https://doi.org/10.1371/journal.ppat.1006379

5. Meissner M, Brecht S, Bujard H, Soldati D (2001) Modulation of myosin a expression by a newly established tetracycline repressor-based inducible system in *Toxoplasma gondii*. Nucleic Acids Res 29(22):E115

6. Meissner M, Schluter D, Soldati D (2002) Role of *Toxoplasma gondii* myosin a in powering parasite gliding and host cell invasion. Science 298(5594):837–840. https://doi.org/10.1126/science.1074553

7. Brown KM, Long S, Sibley LD (2017) Plasma membrane association by N-acylation governs pkg function in *Toxoplasma gondii*. MBio 8(3). https://doi.org/10.1128/mBio.00375-17

8. Fox BA, Falla A, Rommereim LM, Tomita T, Gigley JP, Mercier C, Cesbron-Delauw MF, Weiss LM, Bzik DJ (2011) Type II *Toxoplasma gondii* KU80 knockout strains enable functional analysis of genes required for cyst development and latent infection. Eukaryot Cell 10 (9):1193–1206. https://doi.org/10.1128/EC.00297-10

9. Fox BA, Ristuccia JG, Gigley JP, Bzik DJ (2009) Efficient gene replacements in *Toxoplasma gondii* strains deficient for nonhomologous end joining. Eukaryot Cell 8 (4):520–529. https://doi.org/10.1128/EC.00357-08

10. Huynh MH, Carruthers VB (2009) Tagging of endogenous genes in a *Toxoplasma gondii* strain lacking Ku80. Eukaryot Cell 8

(4):530–539. https://doi.org/10.1128/EC.00358-08

11. Sheiner L, Demerly JL, Poulsen N, Beatty WL, Lucas O, Behnke MS, White MW, Striepen B (2011) A systematic screen to discover and analyze apicoplast proteins identifies a conserved and essential protein import factor. PLoS Pathog 7(12):e1002392. https://doi.org/10.1371/journal.ppat.1002392

12. Francia ME, Jordan CN, Patel JD, Sheiner L, Demerly JL, Fellows JD, de Leon JC, Morrissette NS, Dubremetz JF, Striepen B (2012) Cell division in Apicomplexan parasites is organized by a homolog of the striated rootlet fiber of algal flagella. PLoS Biol 10(12):e1001444. https://doi.org/10.1371/journal.pbio.1001444

13. Sampels V, Hartmann A, Dietrich I, Coppens I, Sheiner L, Striepen B, Herrmann A, Lucius R, Gupta N (2012) Conditional mutagenesis of a novel choline kinase demonstrates plasticity of Phosphatidylcholine biogenesis and gene expression in Toxoplasma gondii. J Biol Chem 287(20):16289–16299. https://doi.org/10.1074/jbc.M112.347138

14. Jacot D, Daher W, Soldati-Favre D (2013) Toxoplasma gondii myosin F, an essential motor for centrosomes positioning and apicoplast inheritance. EMBO J. https://doi.org/10.1038/emboj.2013.113

15. Salamun J, Kallio JP, Daher W, Soldati-Favre D, Kursula I (2014) Structure of Toxoplasma gondii coronin, an actin-binding protein that relocalizes to the posterior pole of invasive parasites and contributes to invasion and egress. FASEB J 28(11):4729–4747. https://doi.org/10.1096/fj.14-252569

16. Graindorge A, Frenal K, Jacot D, Salamun J, Marq JB, Soldati-Favre D (2016) The Conoid associated motor MyoH is indispensable for Toxoplasma gondii entry and exit from host cells. PLoS Pathog 12(1):e1005388. https://doi.org/10.1371/journal.ppat.1005388

17. Dogga SK, Mukherjee B, Jacot D, Kockmann T, Molino L, Hammoudi PM, Hartkoorn RC, Hehl AB, Soldati-Favre D (2017) A druggable secretory protein maturase of Toxoplasma essential for invasion and egress. Elife 6. https://doi.org/10.7554/eLife.27480

18. Di Cristina M, Carruthers VB (2018) New and emerging uses of CRISPR/Cas9 to genetically manipulate apicomplexan parasites. Parasitology 145:1119–1126. https://doi.org/10.1017/S003118201800001X

19. Shen B, Brown KM, Lee TD, Sibley LD (2014) Efficient gene disruption in diverse strains of Toxoplasma gondii using CRISPR/CAS9.

MBio 5(3):e01114-14. https://doi.org/10.1128/mBio.01114-14

20. Sidik SM, Hackett CG, Tran F, Westwood NJ, Lourido S (2014) Efficient genome engineering of Toxoplasma gondii using CRISPR/Cas9. PLoS One 9(6):e100450. https://doi.org/10.1371/journal.pone.0100450

21. Brown KM, Long S, Sibley LD (2018) Conditional knockdown of proteins using Auxin-inducible Degron (AID) fusions in Toxoplasma gondii. Bio Protoc 8(4). https://doi.org/10.21769/BioProtoc.2728

22. Frenal K, Jacot D, Hammoudi PM, Graindorge A, Maco B, Soldati-Favre D (2017) Myosin-dependent cell-cell communication controls synchronicity of division in acute and chronic stages of Toxoplasma gondii. Nat Commun 8:15710. https://doi.org/10.1038/ncomms15710

23. Jacot D, Tosetti N, Pires I, Stock J, Graindorge A, Hung YF, Han H, Tewari R, Kursula I, Soldati-Favre D (2016) An Apicomplexan actin-binding protein serves as a connector and lipid sensor to coordinate motility and invasion. Cell Host Microbe 20(6):731–743. https://doi.org/10.1016/j.chom.2016.10.020

24. Jia Y, Marq JB, Bisio H, Jacot D, Mueller C, Yu L, Choudhary J, Brochet M, Soldati-Favre D (2017) Crosstalk between PKA and PKG controls pH-dependent host cell egress of Toxoplasma gondii. EMBO J 36(21):3250–3267. https://doi.org/10.15252/embj.201796794

25. Bullen HE, Jia Y, Yamaryo-Botte Y, Bisio H, Zhang O, Jemelin NK, Marq JB, Carruthers V, Botte CY, Soldati-Favre D (2016) Phosphatidic acid-mediated signaling regulates Microneme secretion in Toxoplasma. Cell Host Microbe 19(3):349–360. https://doi.org/10.1016/j.chom.2016.02.006

26. Donald RG, Carter D, Ullman B, Roos DS (1996) Insertional tagging, cloning, and expression of the Toxoplasma gondii hypoxanthine-xanthine-guanine phosphoribosyltransferase gene. Use as a selectable marker for stable transformation. J Biol Chem 271(24):14010–14019

27. Gras S, Jackson A, Woods S, Pall G, Whitelaw J, Leung JM, Ward GE, Roberts CW, Meissner M (2017) Parasites lacking the micronemal protein MIC2 are deficient in surface attachment and host cell egress, but remain virulent in vivo. Wellcome Open Res 2:32. https://doi.org/10.12688/wellcomeopenres.11594.2

28. Kim K, Weiss LM (2004) Toxoplasma gondii: the model apicomplexan. Int J Parasitol 34

(3):423–432.   https://doi.org/10.1016/j.ijpara.2003.12.009

29. Pino P, Sebastian S, Kim EA, Bush E, Brochet M, Volkmann K, Kozlowski E, Llinas M, Billker O, Soldati-Favre D (2012) A tetracycline-repressible transactivator system to study essential genes in malaria parasites. Cell Host Microbe 12(6):824–834. https://doi.org/10.1016/j.chom.2012.10.016

30. Plattner F, Yarovinsky F, Romero S, Didry D, Carlier MF, Sher A, Soldati-Favre D (2008) *Toxoplasma* profilin is essential for host cell invasion and TLR11-dependent induction of an interleukin-12 response. Cell Host Microbe

3(2):77–87.   https://doi.org/10.1016/j.chom.2008.01.001

31. Herm-Gotz A, Weiss S, Stratmann R, Fujita-Becker S, Ruff C, Meyhofer E, Soldati T, Manstein DJ, Geeves MA, Soldati D (2002) *Toxoplasma gondii* myosin a and its light chain: a fast, single-headed, plus-end-directed motor. EMBO J 21(9):2149–2158. https://doi.org/10.1093/emboj/21.9.2149

32. Ran FA, Hsu PD, Wright J, Agarwala V, Scott DA, Zhang F (2013) Genome engineering using the CRISPR-Cas9 system. Nat Protoc 8 (11):2281–2308. https://doi.org/10.1038/nprot.2013.143

Chapter 8

Assessing Rhoptry Secretion in *T. gondii*

Catherine Suarez, Melissa B. Lodoen, and Maryse Lebrun

Abstract

Rhoptries are key secretory organelles for *Toxoplasma gondii* invasion. Here, we describe how to assess the ability of *T. gondii* tachyzoites to secrete their rhoptry contents in vitro.

Key words Rhoptries, Secretion, Reporter assay, FRET, SeCreET

1   Introduction

The invasive stages of *Toxoplasma gondii* and other apicomplexan parasites are characterized by the presence of an apical complex composed of specialized secretory organelles. These include micronemes and rhoptries, which are sequentially secreted during active invasion of the parasite into its host cell [1]. Rhoptries contain both proteins and membranous material [2], which are directly injected into the host cell cytoplasm in order to invade and hijack crucial host functions necessary to establish and maintain infection [3, 4]. Rhoptry effectors play roles in (1) invasion, (2) nutrient uptake, (3) modification of host cell signaling, and (4) immune escape [5–11]. Therefore, rhoptry exocytosis is an essential step for the lifestyle of these parasites, which is in turn connected to the upstream microneme secretion (*see* Chapter 9) and attachment of the parasite to the host cell.

Upon contact with the host cell, rhoptries release vesicles into the host cell cytosol that associate with the nascent parasitophorous vacuole membrane (PVM) in which the parasite replicates [12]. These vesicles containing rhoptry proteins can be visualized by treating ready-to-invade parasites with cytochalasin D (CytD), an actin-disrupting drug that blocks parasite motility and invasion but does not prevent attachment. The vesicles formed in the presence of CytD, called evacuoles, expand from the site of parasite attachment within the host cell cytosol and can be revealed by immunofluorescence using specific anti-ROP antibodies

Christopher J. Tonkin (ed.), *Toxoplasma gondii: Methods and Protocols*, Methods in Molecular Biology, vol. 2071, https://doi.org/10.1007/978-1-4939-9857-9_8, © Springer Science+Business Media, LLC, part of Springer Nature 2020

[12]. Later, it was discovered that parasite-derived rhoptry bulb proteins, such as phosphatase 2C (PP2C-Hn) and ROP16, are translocated to the host nucleus [9, 13]. ROP16 is a kinase that phosphorylates the host transcriptional factors, STAT3 and STAT6, to negatively regulate the production of IL-12 and Th1 inflammatory responses [9, 14]. Other rhoptry bulb proteins are either diluted in the host cytoplasm [15] or targeted to the cytoplasmic face of the PVM to prevent accumulation of immune-related GTPases at the PVM and disarm the IFN-γ-mediated immune response [16–18]. Finally, it has also been shown that not only are rhoptry bulb proteins injected into the host cell, but a complex of rhoptry neck proteins (RON2/RON4/$RON4_{L1}$/RON5/RON8) is also inserted into the host cell plasma membrane. This complex is used for intimate attachment of the parasite to its host cell and invasion. RON4, $RON4_{L1}$, RON5, and RON8 localize to the cytosolic face of the host membrane, while RON2 is a transmembrane protein containing a short extracellular domain and a large intra-cytoplasmic domain [7, 19–22]. Through multiple specific interaction motifs, RON proteins recruit host adaptor proteins (ALIX, CD2AP, CIN85, TSG101), which have been proposed to stabilize the interaction between the parasite and the host cortical cytoskeleton [23].

Here we describe four methods to assess secretion of this organelle and export of its contents into the host cell for *T. gondii* tachyzoites.

The first method relies on the ability of tachyzoites to secrete rhoptry derived vesicles when invasion is prevented [12, 24] by CytD and evacuoles are formed and quantified (Fig. 1a).

The second method visualizes the phosphorylation of STAT6 induced by ROP16 secretion into the host cell, using phosphorylation-specific antibodies directed against STAT6 (Tyr 641) (Fig. 1b). The last two methods use different reporter systems based on the engineering of transgenic *T. gondii* parasites (Fig. 1c, d). These rely on the expression of a rhoptry fusion protein (toxofilin), which is secreted into the host cell and can be detected by fluorescence microscopy and/or fluorescence-activated cell sorting (FACS).

2 Evacuole Detection Assay

2.1 Materials

1. Human Foreskin Fibroblasts (HFFs): American Type Culture Collection-CRL 1634.

2. Complete *T. gondii* culture medium: Dulbecco's modified essential medium (DMEM) supplemented with 5% fetal calf serum, 2 mM glutamine, and a cocktail of penicillin (10,000 U/mL) and streptomycin (10,000 μg/mL).

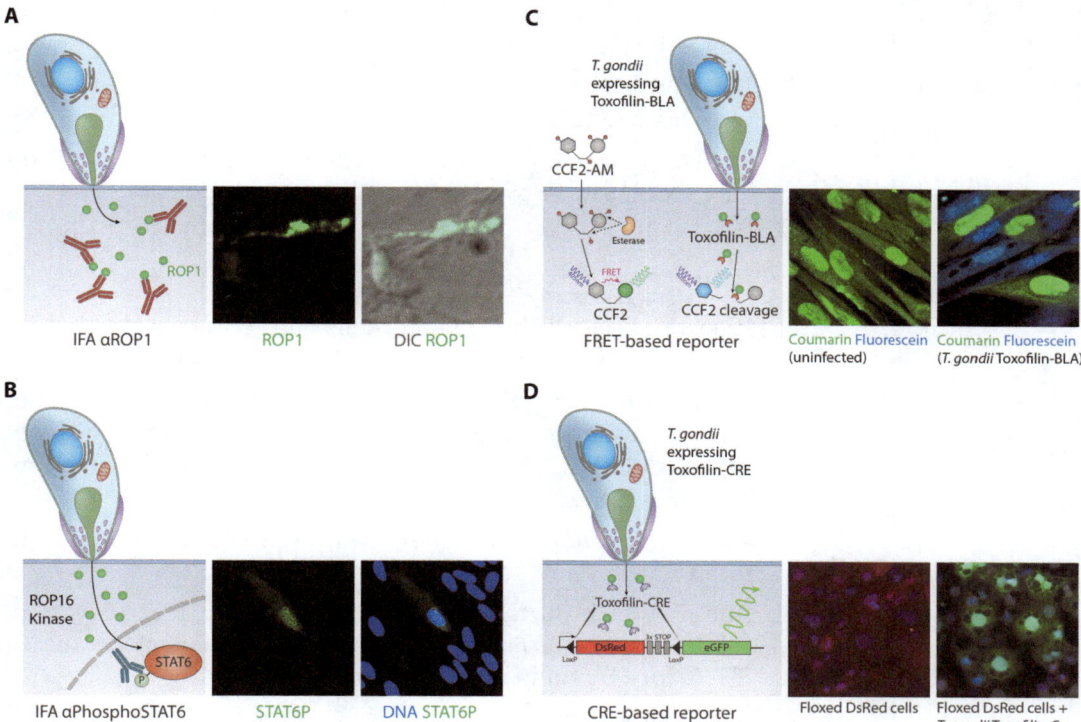

Fig. 1 (**a**) Left, schematic of evacuole detection assay. Right, IFA showing a secretion event. ROP1 staining in green. (**b**) Left, schematic of ROP16 mediated phosphorylation of STAT6 into the host nucleus. Right, STAT6P staining in green, DNA in blue. (**c**) Left, schematic of FRET-Based Secretion Assay. Right, uninfected cells loaded with CCF2 display a green fluorescent signal due to FRET. Disruption of FRET in cells infected by toxofilin-BLA parasites results in a blue fluorescent signal. (**d**) Left, schematic of SeCreEt Reporter Assay. Right, uninfected DsRed cells express DsRed, and cells infected by toxofilin-Cre parasites express eGFP

3. Tissue culture CO_2 incubators maintained at 37 °C and 5% CO_2.

4. Cytochalasin D (CytD): prepared at 1 mM in DMSO (stored at −20 °C) and used at 1 μM final concentration.

5. Glass coverslips: thickness #1.5 and 12 mm diameter (Thermo fisher scientific; cat. 11846933).

6. 24-well cell culture plates to place the coverslips and grow the HFFs onto.

For the immunofluorescence assays (IFA):

1. Quenching solution: 0.1 M glycine in Phosphate-buffered saline (PBS).

2. Blocking solution: 3% Bovine Serum Albumin (BSA) in PBS.

3. Rabbit anti-TgROP1(S2b) [25].

4. Mouse anti-TgSAG1 (T4 1E5) [26].

5. Alexa Fluor® rabbit and mouse conjugated secondary antibodies (Molecular Probes™; rabbit 594 cat. A11012, mouse 488 cat. A11029).

6. Hoechst 33342 dye.

7. Antifading mounting medium (Thermo fisher scientific; Prolong Gold, cat. P36930).

8. Glass slides (Knittel Glass; StarFrost®, cat. VS1137#1FKB.0).

2.2 Methods

Evacuoles detection assay:

1. Prepare HFF cells by seeding them onto coverslips inside the 24-well plate and use them when they reach confluency.

2. The day of the experiment use freshly egressed tachyzoites and prepare a dilution of 200,000 parasites/μL considering you will need 250 μL of this solution per coverslip (each condition requires triplicates).

3. Treat these extracellular parasites with 1 μM CytD for 10 min at room temperature (20 °C to 25 °C).

4. Add 5×10^6 CytD-treated tachyzoites per HFF coverslip (250 μL/coverslip), allow the parasites to settle and invade at 37 °C for 15 min in the incubator.

5. Aspirate the medium out of the wells and fix the coverslips with 4% formaldehyde in PBS for 15 min before proceeding to IFA. *Note*: Coverslips can be stored in PBS at 4 °C or processed for IFA straight away.

IFA to detect ROP1 secretion into the host cell:

1. Incubate fixed coverslips with the quenching solution for 2 min.

2. Remove the quenching solution and add blocking solution for 30 min.

3. Remove the blocking solution and incubate the sample with 0.3% BSA solution (blocking solution diluted 10× in PBS) containing rabbit anti-ROP1 (dilution 1:3000) and mouse anti-SAG1 T4 1E5 (1:2000) for 1 h at RT.

4. Wash coverslips 3× with PBS for 5 min.

5. Incubate samples with PBS 0.3% BSA solution containing the Alexa Fluor® conjugated secondary antibodies (dilution 1:4000) for 45 min.

6. Remove the secondary antibodies and counterstain the nuclei with Hoechst (1 μg/mL) for 5 min.

7. Wash coverslips with PBS 3× for 3 min and mount the coverslips with one drop of mounting medium on a glass slide.

This staining will label the evacuoles (abortive invasions). Counts can be determined by microscopic examination. Routinely, a minimum of 30 fields per coverslip are counted. The fields are chosen randomly.

3 ROP16 Mediated Phosphorylation of STAT6 into the Host Nucleus

3.1 Materials

1. Human Foreskin Fibroblasts (HFFs).

2. Complete *T. gondii* culture medium: Dulbecco's modified essential medium (DMEM) supplemented with 5% fetal calf serum, 2 mM glutamine and a cocktail of penicillin 10,000 U/mL) and streptomycin (10,000 μg/mL).

3. Glass coverslips: thickness #1.5 and 12 mm diameter (Thermo fisher scientific; cat. 11846933).

4. 24-well cell culture plates to place the coverslips and grow the HFFs onto.

For the immunofluorescence assays (IFA):

1. Quenching solution: 0.1 M glycine in PBS.

2. Blocking solution: 3% BSA in PBS.

3. Rabbit anti- STAT6-P ^{Tyr641} (Cell Signaling 56554S).

4. Mouse anti-TgSAG1 (T4 1E5).

5. Alexa Fluor® mouse and rabbit conjugated secondary antibodies (Molecular Probes™, rabbit 594 cat. A11012, mouse 488 cat. A11029).

6. Hoechst 33342 dye.

7. Antifading mounting medium (Thermo fisher scientific; Prolong Gold, cat. P36930).

8. Glass slides (Knittel Glass; StarFrost®, cat. VS1137#1FKB.0).

3.2 Methods

Invasion assay:

1. Prepare HFF cells by seeding them onto coverslips inside the 24-well plate and use them when they reach confluency.

2. The day of the experiment use freshly egressed tachyzoites and prepare a dilution of 2000 parasites/μL in cold complete medium considering you will need 250 μL of this solution per coverslip (each condition requires triplicates).

3. Add 5×10^5 treated tachyzoites per coverslip (250 μL/coverslip) and allow the parasites to settle on ice for 20 min. In the meantime switch on the water bath to 38 °C.

4. Spin the 24-well plate at $250 \times g$ for 1 min.

5. Switch off the water bath and place the plate in it for 20 min (the plate will float and will reach 37 °C quickly).

6. Aspirate the medium out of the well and wash 3× with PBS before fixing the coverslips with ice-cold methanol at −20 °C for 8 min.

7. Aspirate the methanol out of the wells and wash 3× with PBS. Coverslips can be stored in PBS at 4 °C or processed for IFA straight away.

IFA to detect STAT6-P in the host nucleus:

1. Add blocking solution for 1 h.

2. Remove the blocking solution and incubate the sample with 0.3% BSA solution containing rabbit anti-STAT6-P (dilution 1:600) and mouse anti-SAG1 T4 1E5 (1:2000) overnight at 4 °C.

   Next day:

3. Wash coverslips 3× with PBS for 5 min.

4. Incubate samples with PBS 0.3% BSA solution containing the Alexa Fluor® conjugated secondary antibodies (dilution 1:4000) for 45 min.

5. Remove the secondary antibodies and counterstain the nuclei with Hoechst (1 µg/mL) for 5 min.

6. Wash coverslips with PBS 3× for 3 min and mount the coverslips with one drop of mounting medium on a glass slide.

This staining will label the host nuclei and the parasite surface, respectively. STAT6-P-positive host cells containing a parasite vacuole (productive invasions) or not (abortive invasion) can be determined by microscopic examination. Routinely, a minimum of 30 fields per coverslip are counted and normalized to the total number of host cell nuclei. Counts can be automated using imaging software such as ImageJ or ZEN.

3.3 Notes

1. Methanol fixation/permeabilization is necessary to favour accessibility of the anti-PhosphoSTAT6 antibodies into the cell nucleus. This improves the staining when compared to triton permeabilization.

2. It is worth noting that overnight incubation at 4 °C with this antibody greatly improves the signal.

4 FRET-Based Secretion Assay

4.1 Materials

1. Human foreskin fibroblasts (HFFs).

2. *T. gondii* RH strain tachyzoites stably expressing toxofilin-HA-beta lactamase (BLA) [15].

3. Tissue culture CO_2 incubators maintained at 37 °C and 5% CO_2.

4. Complete *T. gondii* culture medium: Dulbecco's modified essential medium (DMEM) supplemented with 10% fetal bovine serum, 2 mM glutamine, penicillin (100 U/mL), and streptomycin (100 μg/mL).

5. Chambered cover glass, such as Nunc Lab-Tek or Lab-Tek II products.

6. Tissue culture-coated 12-well or 6-well plates.

7. Invitrogen LiveBLAzer™ FRET-B/G Loading Kit with CCF2-AM (cat #K1032).

8. Fluorescence microscope equipped with a filter set that can distinguish coumarin and fluorescein.

Example:	Chroma filter set (cat. #19011)
	Excitation filter: AT405/30×
	Dichroic mirror: AT440DC
	Emission filter: AT450lp (long-pass)

9. FACS machine equipped with a 405 nm laser.

4.2 Methods

1. Seed HFFs in chambered cover glass wells or in well plates and culture to confluence at 37 °C. Chambered cover glass products are optimal for live cell microscopy, and well plates are optimal for harvesting the cells and analysis by flow cytometry, as described below.

2. On the day before the assay, add 1 mL of a freshly lysed culture of toxofilin-BLA-expressing *T. gondii* tachyzoites (approximately 2×10^7 parasites) to a T25 flask of confluent HFF and culture for 24 h at 37 °C.

3. On the day of the assay, the T25 flask should have HFFs containing large vacuoles of intracellular tachyzoites.

4. Scrape down the cells in the flask, syringe lyse the infected cell culture to liberate the parasites from the cells, and transfer the culture to a 15 mL conical tube.

5. Add *T. gondii* culture medium to a total volume of 15 mL and pellet by centrifugation at $400 \times g$ for 7 min.

6. Aspirate the supernatant and resuspend the pellet in 15 mL of *T. gondii* culture medium to wash. Pellet the parasites by centrifugation at $400 \times g$ for 7 min.

7. Aspirate the supernatant and resuspend the parasite pellet in 1 mL of *T. gondii* culture medium for counting.

8. Count the parasites and infect the monolayer of HFFs (in either chambered cover glass or in well plates) with toxofilin-BLA-expressing parasites at the desired multiplicity of infection (MOI) in *T. gondii* culture medium. Standard MOIs for

T. gondii infection of HFFs range from 1 to 10; however, higher MOIs can also be used if a high percentage of infected cells is desired.

9. Incubate the chambered cover glass or well plates at 37 °C for the desired time period (*see* Subheading 4.3).

10. Mix the CCF2-AM substrate according to the Invitrogen protocol for Standard Substrate Loading to make a 6× solution.

11. Gently add the CCF2-AM substrate directly to the infected cell monolayer at a 1× final concentration.

12. Incubate the cells at room temperature *in the dark* for 30 min.

13. *Visualize by microscopy:*

    Cells cultured in chambered cover glass wells can be visualized on an inverted microscope with the appropriate filter sets to detect the coumarin and fluorescein fluorescence by live cell microscopy.

    Analyze by flow cytometry:

    Cells cultured in well plates can be gently washed with PBS, trypsinized, and resuspended in PBS with 3% serum. The resuspended cell population can be analyzed by flow cytometry on instruments with a 405 nm laser.

    CCF2 is comprised of a cephalosporin core linking two fluorophores: 7-hydroxycoumarin and fluorescein. The CCF2-AM substrate is cell permeable, and after entering cells, intracellular esterases cleave the acetyl methyl group, trapping CCF2 in the cell cytosol. When the intact CCF2 is excited at 409 nm, the emission from the coumarin at 447 nm excites the nearby fluorescein, resulting in FRET and emission from the fluorescein at 520 nm, producing a green fluorescent signal. In the presence of beta-lactamase (BLA), the cephalosporin core is cleaved, separating the two fluorophores and disrupting FRET, such that excitation of the coumarin at 409 nm results in emission at 447 nm, which is detected as a blue fluorescent signal.

    During *T. gondii* invasion of host cells, the rhoptry protein toxofilin is secreted into the host cell cytosol. In cells infected with the toxofilin-BLA-expressing line of *T. gondii*, BLA is introduced into cells due to its fusion to toxofilin.

    Cells loaded with CCF2-AM produce green fluorescence when excited at 409 nm, due to FRET. During *T. gondii* invasion and rhoptry secretion of toxofilin-BLA, FRET is disrupted, and excitation of cells at 409 nm results in blue fluorescence, which can be used as a highly sensitive read-out for rhoptry secretion.

4.3 Notes

1. After several hours in the substrate solution, HFFs begin to round up and peel off the plate, particularly if they are plated on glass.

2. If the substrate solution is washed off the cells, the signal will diminish within 1–2 h.

3. If analyzing the cells by fluorescence microscopy, note that photobleaching may reduce the fluorescent signal in the field of view relatively quickly.

4. Any extracellular toxofilin-BLA-expressing tachyzoites that have taken up the substrate solution will also turn blue, indicating that the CCF2 substrate is accessible to toxofilin-BLA within the parasites.

5. Although HFF readily take up the substrate solution, phagocytic cells such as macrophages do not take up the substrate solution as efficiently, and the alternative protocol for substrate loading (provided in the Invitrogen LiveBLAzer™ FRET-B/G Loading Kit manual) may be more efficient than the standard protocol.

6. In cells in which rhoptry secretion has occurred and BLA has cleaved CCF2 and separated the coumarin and fluorescein fluorophores, excitation of the cells at 488 nm will still result in emission at 520 nm because this fluorophore is still inside the cells. As a result, when excited at 409 nm or at 488 nm, the cells will fluoresce at 447 nm (blue) or 520 nm (green), respectively.

7. Individual investigators will need to determine the optimal time period of infection, depending on their specific research question. High MOI infections may result in lysis of the HFF sooner than low MOI infections, due to superinfection. As a result, in the case of high MOI infections, it is recommended that the time period of the infection be relatively short (e.g., less than 2 or 3 h). A 1 h infection is sufficient to detect blue cells in the BLA assay.

5   SeCreEt Reporter Assays

5.1   Materials

1. Human foreskin fibroblasts (HFFs).

2. Cre-reporter cells, such as the immortalized mouse fibroblast Cre-reporter line [27] engineered by the lab of Dr. Helen Blau, Stanford University School of Medicine.

3. *T. gondii* RH strain SeCreEt (Secreted Cre, Epitope-tagged) tachyzoites stably expressing toxofilin-Cre [27].

4. Tissue culture CO_2 incubators maintained at 37 °C and 5% CO_2.

5. Complete *T. gondii* culture medium: Dulbecco's modified essential medium (DMEM) supplemented with 10% fetal bovine serum, 2 mM glutamine, penicillin (100 U/mL), and streptomycin (100 µg/mL).

6. High potassium Endo buffer [28]: 44.7 mM K_2SO_4, 10 mM $MgSO_4$, 5 mM glucose, 3.5 mg/mL BSA, 106 mM sucrose, 20 mM Tris-H_2SO_4 (pH 8.2).

7. 24-well plates.

8. Coverslips.

9. Glass slides.

10. Microscope equipped with filters to detect fluorescence from the Cre-reporter cells.

5.2   Methods

1. On the day before the assay, seed Cre-reporter cells on coverslips in 24-well plates at a density of 2×10^4 cells per well.

2. On the same day, add 1 mL of a freshly lysed culture of toxofilin-Cre tachyzoites (approximately 2×10^7 parasites) to a T25 flask of confluent HFF and culture for 24 h at 37 °C.

3. On the day of the assay, the T25 flask should have HFFs containing large vacuoles of intracellular tachyzoites. Remove the medium and replace it with 5 mL of high potassium Endo buffer.

4. Scrape down the cells in the flask, syringe lyse the infected cell culture to liberate the parasites from the cells, and transfer the culture to a 15 mL conical tube.

5. Add Endo buffer to a total volume of 15 mL and pellet by centrifugation at $400 \times g$ for 7 min.

6. Aspirate the supernatant and resuspend the pellet in 15 mL of Endo buffer to wash. Pellet the parasites by centrifugation at $400 \times g$ for 7 min.

7. Aspirate the supernatant and resuspend the parasite pellet in 1 mL of Endo buffer for counting.

8. Wash the Cre-reporter cells with 1 mL of PBS and replace with 300 µL of Endo buffer.

9. Count the parasites and add them in 200 µL Endo buffer to the Cre-reporter cells at the desired MOI (*see* Subheading 5.3 about MOI).

10. Allow the parasites to settle onto the monolayer for 20 min.

11. Gently remove the Endo buffer, wash with 1 mL of prewarmed PBS to remove any unattached parasites, and replace the medium with prewarmed *T. gondii* culture medium to synchronize invasion.

12. Incubate the cells at 37 °C for the desired time period (*see* Subheading 5.3 about time periods of infection and detection of eGFP fluorescence).

13. Fix the coverslips, stain with antibodies if desired, and visualize by microscopy.

The Cre-reporter cells [27] constitutively express DsRed, and in the event of Cre-mediated recombination, the enhanced GFP (eGFP) will be expressed. As a result, rhoptry secretion by the toxofilin-Cre tachyzoites is detected by the expression of eGFP in the cells.

5.3 Notes

1. Cre-reporter cells that are based on the transcription of eGFP and the loss of DsRed expression after Cre-mediated recombination may remain DsRed[+] even after Cre-mediated recombination at the loxP sites, due to residual DsRed protein in the cells. These eGFP[+]DsRed[+] double fluorescent cells are detectable by 4–6 h post-infection (hpi).

2. In the Cre-reporter cells [27], the detection of eGFP signal is maximal at 18–24 hpi.

3. When cells are infected at a low MOI (less than 0.5), there will likely be cells in the culture that express eGFP fluorescence but lack an intracellular parasite. These cells have been studied extensively and may be the result of cells into which the parasites have secreted but not invaded (abortive invasion), cell division events that occurred after the cells expressed eGFP, or in some cell types, cell-intrinsic mechanisms of parasite killing in cells after Cre-mediated recombination [29].

4. One suggested method for analyzing the efficiency of rhoptry secretion and Cre-mediated recombination is to restrict the analysis to eGFP[+] cells with single invasion events and at least two parasites per vacuole, as an indication of productive infection.

Acknowledgments

Our research on rhoptry secretion is supported by the Laboratoire d'Excellence (LabEx) (ParaFrap ANR-11-LABX-0024) and by the Fondation pour la Recherche Médicale (Equipe FRM EQ. 20170336725) to M.L. M.B.L. is supported by NIH R01AI20846. We would like to thank Julien Marcetteau for the graphic design of the figure and Anita Koshy for helpful comments.

References

1. Carruthers VB, Sibley LD (1997) Sequential protein secretion from three distinct organelles of *Toxoplasma gondii* accompanies invasion of human fibroblasts. Eur J Cell Biol 73:114–123

2. Dubremetz JF (2007) Rhoptries are major players in *Toxoplasma gondii* invasion and host cell interaction. Cell Microbiol 9:841–848

3. Besteiro S, Dubremetz JF, Lebrun M (2011) The moving junction of apicomplexan parasites: a key structure for invasion. Cell Microbiol 13:797–805. https://doi.org/10.1111/j.1462-5822.2011.01597.x

4. Boothroyd JC, Dubremetz JF (2008) Kiss and spit: the dual roles of *Toxoplasma* rhoptries. Nat Rev Microbiol 6:79–88

5. Counihan NA et al (2017) Plasmodium falciparum parasites deploy RhopH2 into the host erythrocyte to obtain nutrients, grow and

replicate. Elife 6. https://doi.org/10.7554/eLife.23217

6. Ito D, Schureck MA, Desai SA (2017) An essential dual-function complex mediates erythrocyte invasion and channel-mediated nutrient uptake in malaria parasites. Elife 6. https://doi.org/10.7554/eLife.23485

7. Lamarque M et al (2011) The RON2-AMA1 interaction is a critical step in moving junction-dependent invasion by apicomplexan parasites. PLoS Pathog e1001276:7

8. Saeij JP et al (2006) Polymorphic secreted kinases are key virulence factors in toxoplasmosis. Science 314:1780–1783. https://doi.org/10.1126/science.1133690

9. Saeij JP et al (2007) *Toxoplasma* co-opts host gene expression by injection of a polymorphic kinase homologue. Nature 445:324–327

10. Taylor S et al (2006) A secreted serine-threonine kinase determines virulence in the eukaryotic pathogen *Toxoplasma gondii*. Science 314:1776–1780

11. Tonkin ML et al (2011) Host cell invasion by apicomplexan parasites: insights from the co-structure of AMA1 with a RON2 peptide. Science 333:463–467. https://doi.org/10.1126/science.1204988

12. Hakansson S, Charron AJ, Sibley LD (2001) *Toxoplasma* evacuoles: a two-step process of secretion and fusion forms the parasitophorous vacuole. EMBO J 20:3132–3144

13. Gilbert LA, Ravindran S, Turetzky JM, Boothroyd JC, Bradley PJ (2007) *Toxoplasma gondii* targets a protein phosphatase 2C to the nuclei of infected host cells. Eukaryot Cell 6:73–83

14. Ong YC, Reese ML, Boothroyd JC (2010) *Toxoplasma* rhoptry protein 16 (ROP16) subverts host function by direct tyrosine phosphorylation of STAT6. J Biol Chem 285:28731–28740. https://doi.org/10.1074/jbc.M110.112359. M110.112359 [pii]

15. Lodoen MB, Gerke C, Boothroyd JC (2010) A highly sensitive FRET-based approach reveals secretion of the actin-binding protein toxofilin during *Toxoplasma gondii* infection. Cell Microbiol 12:55–66. https://doi.org/10.1111/j.1462-5822.2009.01378.x. CMI1378 [pii]

16. Fentress SJ et al (2010) Phosphorylation of immunity-related GTPases by a *Toxoplasma gondii*-secreted kinase promotes macrophage survival and virulence. Cell Host Microbe 8:484–495. https://doi.org/10.1016/j.chom.2010.11.005

17. Steinfeldt T et al (2010) Phosphorylation of mouse immunity-related GTPase (IRG) resistance proteins is an evasion strategy for virulent *Toxoplasma gondii*. PLoS Biol 8:e1000576. https://doi.org/10.1371/journal.pbio.1000576

18. Zhao YO, Khaminets A, Hunn JP, Howard JC (2009) Disruption of the *Toxoplasma gondii* parasitophorous vacuole by IFNgamma-inducible immunity-related GTPases (IRG proteins) triggers necrotic cell death. PLoS Pathog 5:e1000288

19. Besteiro S, Michelin A, Poncet J, Dubremetz JF, Lebrun M (2009) Export of a *Toxoplasma gondii* rhoptry neck protein complex at the host cell membrane to form the moving junction during invasion. PLoS Pathog 5:e1000309

20. Guerin A, El Hajj H, Penarete-Vargas D, Besteiro S, Lebrun M (2017) RON4L1 is a new member of the moving junction complex in *Toxoplasma gondii*. Sci Rep 7:17907. doi:https://doi.org/10.1038/s41598-017-18010-9

21. Straub KW, Cheng SJ, Sohn CS, Bradley PJ (2009) Novel components of the Apicomplexan moving junction reveal conserved and coccidia-restricted elements. Cell Microbiol 11:590–603. https://doi.org/10.1111/j.1462-5822.2008.01276.x. CMI1276 [pii]

22. Tyler JS, Boothroyd JC (2011) The C-terminus of *Toxoplasma* RON2 provides the crucial link between AMA1 and the host-associated invasion complex. PLoS Pathog 7:e1001282. https://doi.org/10.1371/journal.ppat.1001282

23. Guerin A et al (2017) Efficient invasion by *Toxoplasma* depends on the subversion of host protein networks. Nat Microbiol 2:1358–1366. https://doi.org/10.1038/s41564-017-0018-1

24. Miller LH, Aikawa M, Johnson JG, Shiroishi T (1979) Interaction between cytochalasin B-treated malarial parasites and erythrocytes. Attachment and junction formation. J Exp Med 149:172–184

25. Lamarque MH et al (2014) Plasticity and redundancy among AMA-RON pairs ensure host cell entry of *Toxoplasma* parasites. Nat Commun 5:4098. https://doi.org/10.1038/ncomms5098

26. Couvreur G, Sadak A, Fortier B, Dubremetz JF (1988) Surface antigens of *Toxoplasma gondii*. Parasitology 97(Pt 1):1–10

27. Koshy AA et al (2010) *Toxoplasma* secreting Cre recombinase for analysis of host-parasite interactions. Nat Methods 7:307–309. https://doi.org/10.1038/nmeth.1438. nmeth.1438 [pii]

28. Endo T, Tokuda H, Yagita K, Koyama T (1987) Effects of extracellular potassium on acid release and motility initiation in *Toxoplasma gondii*. J Protozool 34:291–295

29. Koshy AA et al (2012) *Toxoplasma* co-opts host cells it does not invade. PLoS Pathog 8: e1002825. https://doi.org/10.1371/journal. ppat.1002825. PPATHOGENS-D-11-02798 [pii]

Chapter 9

High-Throughput Measurement of Microneme Secretion in *Toxoplasma gondii*

Kevin M. Brown, L. David Sibley, and Sebastian Lourido

Abstract

Micronemes are specialized secretory organelles present in all motile forms of apicomplexan parasites. Microneme vesicles hold adhesins and other proteins that are secreted to facilitate parasite attachment, invasion of host cells, and egress following replication—all processes indispensable for cell-to-cell transmission of these obligate intracellular parasites. Defining the signaling pathways that lead to microneme secretion is an important part of understanding the infectious cycle of apicomplexan parasites. However, the classical method of measuring microneme secretion by immunoblotting for microneme proteins in parasite excreted/secreted antigen (ESA) preparations is low-throughput and only semiquantitative. We recently reported a new luciferase-based method for measuring microneme secretion in a 96-well format with high sensitivity in the model apicomplexan *Toxoplasma gondii*. Here, we aim to elaborate on this detection method and review current practices for stimulating microneme secretion in vitro.

Key words Microneme secretion, Luciferase, Reporter, *Toxoplasma gondii*

1 Introduction

Apicomplexan parasites have dedicated part of their secretory pathway to generate the specialized organelles that mediate migration through tissues, alternatively invading and egressing from host cells as part of the lytic cycle. Micronemes, one of these specialized organelles, are small elongated secretory vesicles that develop from the Golgi-endosomal network and accumulate at the apical end of apicomplexan zoites (*see* review [1]). The number of micronemes in a given parasite varies widely among apicomplexans depending on the species and life stage [1]. Zoites that display extensive gliding motility, migration, and active invasion and egress (e.g., *Toxoplasma gondii* tachyzoites), carry abundant micronemes (Fig. 1a). The functional link between micronemes and motility lies in the microneme cargo: adhesive proteins for parasite attachment and substrate-based motility (modular microneme (MIC) adhesins), structural proteins for moving junction formation and

Christopher J. Tonkin (ed.), *Toxoplasma gondii: Methods and Protocols*, Methods in Molecular Biology, vol. 2071,
https://doi.org/10.1007/978-1-4939-9857-9_9, © Springer Science+Business Media, LLC, part of Springer Nature 2020

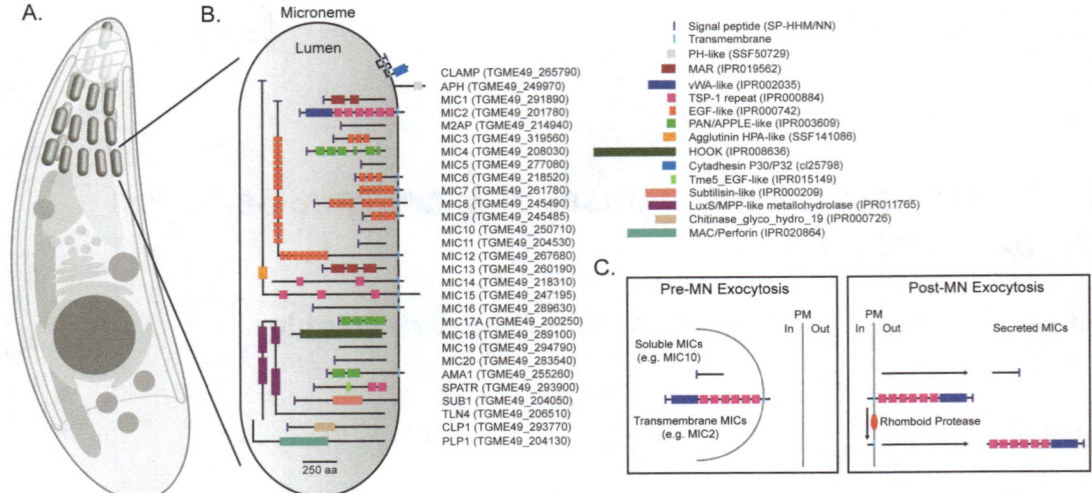

Fig. 1 Microneme Secretion in *Toxoplasma gondii*. (**a**) Diagram of a *T. gondii* tachyzoite illustrating the location of the micronemes at the apical end of the cell. (**b**) Domain structure of known microneme proteins. Full-length proteins are drawn, although many are known to undergo proteolytic processing during trafficking and secretion, such as removal of the signal peptide. (**c**) Predicted topology of microneme proteins before and after microneme (MN) exocytosis. Membrane-tethered adhesins are released from the surface of the parasite by their intra-membrane cleavage by rhomboid proteases. *PM* plasma membrane

invasion (AMA1, CLAMP), and a pore-forming perforin for egress (PLP1). Figure 1b lists the known *T. gondii* microneme proteins and summarizes their domains, which function following secretion.

A variety of signaling pathways have been shown to contribute to microneme secretion in *T. gondii*. Increasing cytosolic Ca^{2+} concentrations through the release of intracellular stores [2–4] or entry from the extracellular environment [5] have been associated with microneme secretion through the activation of calcium-dependent protein kinases [6] and vesicular trafficking [7]. Activation of cGMP signaling through the action of cGMP-dependent protein kinase (PKG) has also been show to stimulate microneme secretion, in part through the release of intracellular Ca^{2+} stores [8–12]. More recently, microneme secretion has been linked to an increased production of phosphatidic acid (PA) at the parasite membrane, which enhances trafficking of micronemes to the plasma membrane [13]. Isolated extracellular parasites can be treated with various compounds to stimulate microneme secretion. A list of commonly used the so-called secretagogues is provided in Table 1, along with their presumed mechanism of action. The action of several secretagogues is enhanced by the presence of bovine serum albumin (BSA), which is thought to stimulate the guanylate cyclase that produces cGMP [8].

Adhesive MICs are anchored to the plasma membrane of the parasite by transmembrane domains (TMs) after exocytosis. Many

Table 1
Commonly used microneme secretagogues in _T. gondii_

Secretagogue	Concentration	Mode of action	Relative strength	References
A23187	1–5 µM	Elevated cytosolic Ca^{2+}	+	[2]
Ethanol	1% (v/v)	Activation of PI-PLC-dependent PIP_2 hydrolysis; elevated IP_3 (Ca^{2+} release) and PA	+	[3, 4, 13]
Propranolol	500 µM	Inhibition of PA phosphatase; elevated PA	+++	[13]
zaprinast	500 µM	Inhibition of cGMP PDEs; elevated cGMP; elevated cytosolic Ca^{2+}	++	[8, 28]
BSA	1% (w/v)	Elevated cGMP	++	[8]
BSA and ethanol	1% (w/v) BSA, 1% (v/v) ethanol	_See_ above	+++	[8, 10]
BSA and zaprinast	1% (w/v) BSA, 500 µM zaprinast	_See_ above	++++	[8]

of these proteins are type I transmembrane proteins with a C-terminal TM and short cytoplasmic tails (e.g., MICs 2, 6, 7, 8, 9, 12, 14, 15, 16, and AMA1). These membrane-bound MICs can also serve as anchors for their binding partners (e.g., MIC1/4 tethering to MIC6, M2AP tethering to MIC2, and MIC3 tethering to MIC8). The ectodomains of these adhesins have diverse motifs for substrate binding (Fig. 1c), often in tandem arrays. Although their ligands are largely unknown, these adhesins are thought to bind proteins (e.g., MIC2 binding of ICAM1 [14]) and glycans in the matrix or host-cell membrane (e.g., MIC1 binding of lactose [15]; MIC4 binding of galactose [16]) to provide traction for motility. The cytoplasmic tails of MIC2, and several other microneme proteins, is proposed to interact with actin filaments through a conserved apicomplexan protein, which links the adhesins to fixed myosin motors that provide the force for gliding motility and invasion [17, 18].

Micronemal adhesins are efficiently shed from the surface of the parasite by the action of rhomboid proteases—although other proteases can contribute to shedding [19]. Shedding can be influenced by substrate binding [20]; however, the turnover of microneme adhesins occurs too rapidly to quantify secretion by surface staining. Therefore, measuring secreted and shed micronemal proteins collected from the supernatants of parasite suspensions has been the most common method for assessing microneme secretion [2, 3]. Using this method, the secretion of several microneme

proteins has been quantified by immunoblot. Because of the availability of a reliable hybridoma against MIC2 (6D10, [21]), most
reported measurements of microneme secretion have been based
on this marker and, when evaluated, other microneme proteins
follow the same pattern of secretion [4, 22]. Therefore, although
different populations of micronemes have been observed in
T. gondii tachyzoites [23], they appear to be secreted to the same
extent in response to similar signaling pathways.

The most significant limitations of measuring microneme
secretion by immunoblot are relatively large numbers of parasites
needed to achieve a detectable signal, the low throughput of the
approach, and its variability. To address these challenges, we developed a microneme secretion assay based on the expression of an
engineered allele of MIC2 that carries *Gaussia* luciferase as part of
its ectodomain (MIC2-GLuc, Fig. 2). In the copepod from where it
originates, *Gaussia* luciferase is secreted from the cells that produce
it, and it has been similarly used as a naturally secreted reporter in
mammalian cells [24]. MIC2-GLuc appropriately localizes to the
micronemes, and retains its luciferase activity in both parasite
lysates and secreted fractions [8]. The amount of secreted fusion
protein can be quantitatively estimated by measuring luciferase
activity, and results in a 10,000-fold increase in sensitivity over
immunoblot detection of secreted MIC2 (Table 2). The ease of
sample preparation and the decreased numbers of parasites required
for each condition, makes this luciferase-based assay a versatile and
high-throughput approach to study the signaling pathways and
conditions that govern microneme secretion.

2 Materials

2.1 Parasite Transfection

1. Human foreskin fibroblasts (HFF) cells (ATCC, cat. no. SCRC-1041).

2. D10 medium: For 1 l, combine 1 package Dulbecco's Modified Eagle's Medium (DMEM) powder (Thermo Fisher,
   Gibco cat. no. 12100046), 3.7 g $NaHCO_3$, 100 ml FBS,
   10 ml of 200 mM L-glutamine, 1 ml of 10 mg/ml gentamycin,
   and dH_2O to 1 l. Sterilize by 0.45 μm filtration.

3. Tissue-culture supplies such as 25 cm^2 cell culture flask (T-25),
   96-well plates, 24-well plates, and cell scrapers.

4. 37 °C, 5% CO_2 incubator and biosafety cabinet.

5. 1× PBS, tissue-culture grade.

6. 0.05% trypsin, 0.02% EDTA solution (w/v).

7. Parasite strains: commonly used *T. gondii* strains (type I RH or
   GT1 strains, type II ME49 or PRU strains), available from
   ATCC (www.atcc.org). Strains with *KU80* deleted are well-

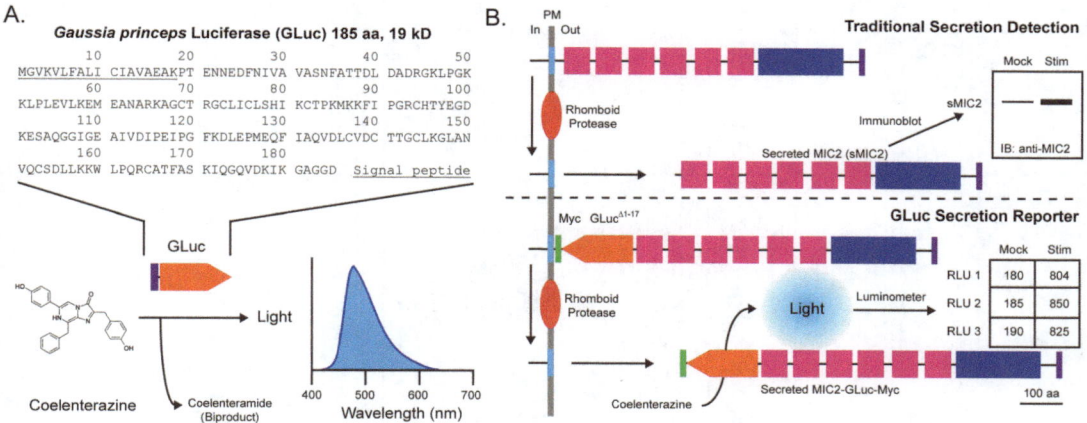

Fig. 2 Luciferase-based detection of microneme secretion. (**a**) *Gaussia* luciferase (GLuc) sequence, and illustration of the luciferase reaction highlighting the spectrum of light produced during oxidation of the substrate coelenterazine. (**b**) Diagram of MIC2 secretion in traditional and GLuc assay, including simulated data

suited for gene editing using a repair template as they have impaired nonhomologous end-joining. Strains with *HXGPRT* deleted provide the proper genetic background for positive selection of plasmids bearing this marker, like pMIC2-GLuc-Myc, HXGPRT [8]. When introducing the MIC2-GLuc reporter, we recommend starting with RHΔ*hxgprt* or RHΔ*hxgprt*Δ*ku80* [25]. Alternatively, RH MIC2-GLuc-Myc [8] has recently been submitted to BEI Resources (www.beiresources.org) for distribution.

8. Plasmid: pMIC2-GLuc-Myc, HXGPRT [8]; available from upon request.

9. Blunt-end needles (25 gauge) and 10 ml syringes.

10. Filter holder (Whatman, cat. no. 420200) and polycarbonate filter membranes (3 μm pore) (Whatman, cat. no. 110612).

11. Centrifuge capable holding 15 or 50 ml conical vials that can spin at $400 \times g$.

12. Cytomix transfection buffer: 120 mM KCl, 0.15 mM $CaCl_2$, 10 mM K_2HPO_4/KH_2PO_4, 25 mM HEPES, 2 mM EDTA, 5 mM $MgCl_2$, pH 7.6, sterilized by 0.45 μm filtration.

13. $100\times$ ATP (0.2 M).

14. $100\times$ Glutathione (0.5 M).

15. Electroporation cuvettes: BTX640 (BTX Harvard Apparatus).

16. Square-wave electroporation system ECM-830 (BTX Harvard Apparatus).

Table 2
Comparison of traditional and GLuc microneme secretion assays

Detection method	Transgenic reporter	Sample format	Detection equipment	Key reagents	Assay time	Sample limit	Detection limit[a]
Immunoblotting	None	ESA samples resolved by SDS-PAGE and blotted onto nitrocellulose membrane	Standard immunoblotting equipment	MIC protein antisera	1–2 days	10–20[b]	10^7 parasites/ml
GLuc assay	pMIC2-GLuc-Myc-HXGPRT	ESA samples arrayed in 96-well plates	96-well plate luminometer with optional plate stacker	BioLux® *Gaussia* luciferase kit (NEB)	30 min	96 × number of plates	10^3 parasites/ml

[a]Concentration of parasites needed to detect MIC2-GLuc-Myc in 10 µl stimulated ESA by immunoblotting (mouse anti-Myc monoclonal at 1:2000 dilution, detected with an IRDye-conjugated goat anti-mouse secondary at 1:2000 dilution, imaged on a Licor Odyssey scanner) or GLuc assay (BioLux® *Gaussia* luciferase assay kit detected with a Cytation 3 plate-reader) [8]

[b]Confined to number of lanes of standard SDS-PAGE gel

17. Mycophenolic acid (10 mg/ml in 100% EtOH) and xanthine (20 mg/ml in 1N NaOH) to select for pMIC2-GLuc-Myc, HXGPRT.

18. HHE: 1× Hank's Balanced Salt Solution, 10 mM HEPES, 1 mM EGTA, sterilized by 0.45 µm filtration.

2.2 Stimulating Microneme Secretion and Collecting ESA in 96-Well Plate Format

1. *T. gondii* line expressing MIC2-GLuc-Myc grown in HFF monolayers.

2. Blunt-end needles (25 gauge) and 10 ml syringes.

3. 50 ml polystyrene conical vials.

4. 18 °C water bath (an ice-bucket with ice water and thermometer will suffice).

5. Filter holder (Whatman, cat. no. 420200) and polycarbonate filter membranes (3 µm pore) (Whatman, cat. no. 110612).

6. Extracellular (EC) buffer: 5 mM KCl, 142 mM NaCl, 1 mM $MgCl_2$, 1.8 mM $CaCl_2$, 5.6 mM D-glucose, 25 mM HEPES pH 7.4, sterilized by 0.45 µm filtration.

7. Intracellular (IC) buffer: 142 mM KCl, 5 mM NaCl, 1 mM $MgCl_2$, 5.6 mM D-glucose, 2 mM EGTA, 25 mM HEPES pH 7.4, sterilized by 0.45 µm filtration.

8. Hemocytometer.

9. Refrigerated centrifuge with buckets for conical vials and swings for 96-well plates capable of spinning at 2000 × *g*.

10. Secretagogue preparation (*see* Table 1): DMSO can be used for preparing stocks of 10 mM A23187, 50 mM propranolol, and 100 mM zaprinast. 2× stimulation buffer can be prepared in IC or EC secretion buffers: 2–10 µM A23187 ([vehicle] = 0.02–0.1% DMSO in secretion buffer), 1 mM propranolol ([vehicle] = 2% DMSO in secretion buffer), 1 mM zaprinast ([vehicle] = 2% DMSO in secretion buffer), 2% ethanol (v/v) (use secretion buffer as the untreated control), 2% (w/v) BSA (use secretion buffer as the untreated control).

11. 96-Well polystyrene V-bottom plates.

12. 200 µl multichannel pipette.

13. 37 °C water bath.

14. Timer.

15. Ice for halting microneme secretion.

16. 96-Well PCR plate for cell-free ESA.

2.3 Measuring Secreted MIC2-GLuc-Myc in ESA in 96-Well Plates

1. 96-Well half-area white opaque assay plates.

2. BioLux® *Gaussia* luciferase assay kit (New England Biolabs, *see* Note 1).

3. 20 and 200 µl multichannel pipettes.

4. 50 ml reagent reservoirs.

5. Plate-reading luminometer.

3   Protocols

3.1   Parasite Transfection

T. gondii can be propagated using previously described protocols in a variety of mammalian cell lines [26]. Here we describe propagation in HFFs using aseptic technique throughout.

1. Infect confluent HFFs cells grown in a T-25 flask with sufficient *T. gondii* parasites (RHΔ*hxgprt*Δ*ku80* [25] or other Δ*hxgprt* line) to achieve ~75% host-cell lysis 2 days postinfection. The exact number of parasites should be determined empirically; however, one tenth the volume of a freshly lysed T-25 is usually sufficient.

2. After 2 days of growth, scrape the monolayer, collect the media containing extracellular parasites and resuspended host cells in a 50 ml conical vial, and pass them through a 25 gauge needle three to five times to disrupt the remaining host cells. Filter the parasites using 3 μm polycarbonate membranes to remove host-cell debris.

3. Centrifuge the filtered culture at $400 \times g$ for 10 min at 18 °C, resuspend the pellets in 10 ml HHE.

4. Count 10 μl of the 10 ml parasite suspension using a hemocytometer.

5. Centrifuge the 10 ml parasite suspension again at $400 \times g$ for 10 min at 18 °C.

6. Resuspend the parasite cell pellet in Cytomix to achieve a parasite density of 4×10^7/ml.

7. Prepare the transfection mix. In an electroporation cuvette, combine the following:

Parasites suspension in Cytomix:	250 μl
pMIC2-GLuc-Myc, HXGPRT:	10 μg
100× ATP	3 μl
100× glutathione	3 μl
Cytomix	to 300 μl

8. Mix the components in the cuvette and electroporate in the ECM-830 with 1.7 kV, 176 μs pulse length, and 2 pulses with 100 ms interval. Following electroporation, transfer the parasites into T-25 flasks with confluent HFFs and grow them at 37 °C, 5% CO_2.

3.2 Drug Selection and Cloning

1. 24 h after electroporation and recovery, select for stable trans-formants harboring the pMIC2-GLuc-Myc, HXGPRT plasmid using D10 containing MPA/xanthine (25 µg/ml each). Sub-culture the parasites as needed until the drug-resistant pool becomes stable (3–5 passages).

2. When the drug-resistant pool becomes stable, harvest and count the extracellular parasites with a hemocytometer (as described in Subheading 3.1, **steps 2–4**).

3. Dilute to ~20 parasites/ml in D10 (without drug). Subse-quently, aliquot 150 µl/well of the parasite suspension into 96-well plates seeded with confluent HFFs and return to 37 °C, 5% CO_2. Two 96-well plates should yield sufficient clones to identify a strain carrying the reporter. Do not move the plates during this time to ensure proper plaque formation.

4. After 7–10 days, inspect each well of the 96-well plates under an inverted phase-contrast microscope (e.g., Nikon TS100) to identify wells that contain a single plaque. Transfer parasites from single-plaque wells into 24-well plates containing conflu-ent HFFs. Propagate in this format until a single clone is confirmed.

5. To check single clones for MIC2-GLuc-Myc expression, per-form an indirect immunofluorescence assay on 5–10 clones using mouse-anti-Myc (Biolegend) antisera as described previ-ously [8] using the parental line as a negative control. The staining pattern for MIC2-GLuc-Myc should resemble that of endogenous MIC2 (i.e., localized to the apical third of the parasite).

6. Once positive clones are identified, they should be transferred into T-25 flasks and cryopreserve for future use.

3.3 Stimulating Microneme Secretion and Collecting ESA in 96-Well Plate Format

1. Infect confluent HFFs cells grown in T-25 flasks with sufficient *T. gondii* parasites to achieve ~25% host cell lysis 2 days postin-fection (*see* **Note 2**).

2. After 2 days of growth, scrape the semilysed monolayers, col-lect the media containing extracellular parasites and resus-pended host cells in a 50 ml conical vial, shift the parasites to an 18 °C water bath (an ice bucket filled to 5 cm with ice water and thermometer works well for this) to prevent premature microneme secretion, and pass them through a 25 gauge nee-dle three to five times to disrupt host cells and release all the parasites. Filter the parasites using 3 µm polycarbonate mem-branes to remove host-cell debris. Centrifuge the filtered cul-ture at $400 \times g$ for 10 min at 18 °C, resuspend the pellets in 10 ml HHE (at 18 °C) and count the parasites. Centrifuge again and resuspend the parasite cell pellet in EC buffer (18 °C) at a concentration of 2×10^7/ml.

3. Add 1×10^6 parasites in 50 µl EC buffer or EC buffer alone in triplicate to wells of a 96-well V-bottom plate.

4. Add 50 µl of $2\times$ stimulation buffer (EC buffer, secretagogue at $2\times$ the final desired concentration), and 50 µl mock stimulation buffer (vehicle control stimulation buffer) to the appropriate wells.

5. Immediately shift the parasite plate to a 37 °C water bath with 1 cm height water and incubate for 10 min to induce microneme secretion.

6. After stimulating secretion, stop secretion by shifting the plate to ice for 5 min.

7. Centrifuge at $1200 \times g$ at 4 °C for 10 min. Remove the top 50 µl cell-free supernatant from each well without disturbing the pellet and transfer to a PCR plate. This supernatant contains the ESA that will be assayed for microneme content. Perform the GLuc assay step immediately or freeze the ESA samples at −20 °C for analysis at a later date.

3.4 Measuring Secreted MIC2-GLuc-Myc in ESA in 96-Well Plate Format

1. The BioLux *Gaussia* Flex luciferase assay kit (NEB) includes three components: substrate, stabilizer, and buffer. Prepare the Gluc stabilized assay solution. To prepare sufficient assay reagent for a full plate (96 tests), add 50 µl of BioLux Gluc Substrate and 0.8 ml BioLux Flex stabilizer to 5 ml of BioLux Gluc Assay Buffer immediately before performing the assay. Maintain this reagent ratio if fewer tests are needed. Mix well by inverting the tube several times (do not vortex). Incubate reagent for 25 min protected from light.

2. Set the luminometer to read the proper wells of a 96-well plate (open lum configuration, no filter range needed, 1 s integration).

3. Add 10 µl of sample from Subheading 3.3, **step 7** per well in white, opaque, half-area 96-well plates.

4. Using a multichannel pipet, quickly add 50 µl of the Gluc stabilized assay solution to each well. The signal will reach maximum at approximately 1 min postaddition and remain relatively stable for 20 min.

5. Read the plate on the luminometer.

6. Subtract the buffer-only values from their corresponding ESA values to correct for background luminescence (*see* **Note 3**).

4 Notes

1. *BioLux Gaussia Flex kit.*

   The BioLux Gaussia Flex kit (NEB) was discontinued during the publication of this manuscript. The Pierce Gaussia Luciferase Glow Assay Kit may be used in its place (Thermo Fisher Scientific, cat. no. 16160).

2. *Estimating parasite numbers for microneme secretion assays.*

   For the RH strain of *T. gondii*, a single T-25 of HFFs should yield approximately 5×10^7 parasites after the final round of egress. The yield from other strains should be determined empirically and the cultures scaled appropriately. In general, 3×10^6 parasites will be needed for each treatment condition performed in triplicate. Therefore, for RH one T-25 should be sufficient for 16 tests in triplicate (48 tests total) so plan to use 2–3 T-25s per 96-well plate. A basic experiment will include triplicate wells for the following: mock stimulation buffer only, stimulation buffer only, parasites with mock-stimulation buffer, and parasites with stimulation buffer. The buffer only controls are important for subtracting background luminescence values from the MIC2-GLuc-Myc values.

3. *Replicates and data analysis.*

   For robust analysis of microneme secretion, experiments should be performed three times ($N = 3$ biological replicates) using three replicates per treatment ($n = 3$ technical replicates). Following data collection, correct the relative luminescence unit (RLU) values by subtracting the mean background RLU value (i.e., buffer-only control) from the corresponding ESA RLU values. The mean corrected RLU values for each treatment ($n = 3$) should be averaged from three experiments ($N = 3$). Graph mean RLU values vs. treatment $\pm$ SEM as previously reported [8, 27]. Statistical differences between two treatments (e.g., mock stimulation vs. stimulation) can be determined using a Student's unpaired t-test with a significance probability threshold of $P < 0.05$. When making several comparisons (e.g., mock stimulation vs. stimulation A vs. stimulation B), a two-way analysis of variance (ANOVA) can be performed using Tukey's multiple comparison test with a significance threshold of $P < 0.05$.

Acknowledgments

Work in the authors' labs was supported by an AHA grant 15POST22130001 to KMB, NIH grants AI118426 and AI034036 to LDS, and 1DP5OD017892 and 1R21AI123746 to SL.

References

1. Carruthers VB, Tomley FM (2008) Microneme proteins in apicomplexans. Subcell Biochem 47:33–45

2. Carruthers VB, Sibley LD (1999) Mobilization of intracellular calcium stimulates microneme discharge in *Toxoplasma gondii*. Mol Microbiol 31:421–428

3. Carruthers VB, Moreno SNJ, Sibley LD (1999) Ethanol and acetaldehyde elevate intracellular $[Ca^{2+}]$ calcium and stimulate microneme discharge in *Toxoplasma gondii*. Biochem J 342:379–386

4. Lovett JL, Marchesini N, Moreno SN, Sibley LD (2002) *Toxoplasma gondii* microneme secretion involves intracellular Ca^{2+} release from IP_3/ryanodine sensitive stores. J Biol Chem 277(29):25870–25876

5. Pace DA, McKnight CA, Liu J, Jimenez V, Moreno SN (2014) Calcium entry in *Toxoplasma gondii* and its enhancing effect of invasion-linked traits. J Biol Chem 289(28):19637–19647. https://doi.org/10.1074/jbc.M114.565390

6. Lourido S, Shuman J, Zhang C, Shokat KM, Hui R, Sibley LD (2010) Calcium-dependent protein kinase 1 is an essential regulator of exocytosis in *Toxoplasma*. Nature 465:359–362

7. Farrell A, Thirugnanam S, Lorestani A, Dvorin JD, Eidell KP, Ferguson DJ, Anderson-White BR, Duraisingh MT, Marth GT, Gubbels MJ (2012) A DOC2 protein identified by mutational profiling is essential for apicomplexan parasite exocytosis. Science 335((6065)):218–221. https://doi.org/10.1126/science.1210829

8. Brown KM, Lourido S, Sibley LD (2016) Serum albumin stimulates protein kinase G-dependent microneme secretion in *Toxoplasma gondii*. J Biol Chem 291(18):9554–9565. https://doi.org/10.1074/jbc.M115.700518

9. Sidik SM, Hortua Triana MA, Paul AS, El Bakkouri M, Hackett CG, Tran F, Westwood NJ, Hui R, Zuercher WJ, Duraisingh MT, Moreno SN, Lourido S (2016) Using a genetically encoded sensor to identify inhibitors of *Toxoplasma gondii* Ca^{2+} signaling. J Biol Chem 291(18):9566–9580. https://doi.org/10.1074/jbc.M115.703546

10. Brown KM, Long S, Sibley LD (2017) Plasma membrane association by N-acylation governs PKG function in *Toxoplasma gondii*. MBio 8(3). https://doi.org/10.1128/mBio.00375-17

11. Howard BL, Harvey KL, Stewart RJ, Azevedo MF, Crabb BS, Jennings IG, Sanders PR, Manallack DT, Thompson PE, Tonkin CJ, Gilson PR (2015) Identification of potent phosphodiesterase inhibitors that demonstrate cyclic nucleotide-dependent functions in apicomplexan parasites. ACS Chem Biol 10(4):1145–1154. https://doi.org/10.1021/cb501004q

12. Stewart RJ, Whitehead L, Nijagal B, Sleebs BE, Lessene G, McConville MJ, Rogers KL, Tonkin CJ (2017) Analysis of Ca(2)(+) mediated signaling regulating *Toxoplasma* infectivity reveals complex relationships between key molecules. Cell Microbiol 19(4). https://doi.org/10.1111/cmi.12685

13. Bullen HE, Jia Y, Yamaryo-Botte Y, Bisio H, Zhang O, Jemelin NK, Marq JB, Carruthers V, Botte CY, Soldati-Favre D (2016) Phosphatidic acid-mediated signaling regulates microneme secretion in *Toxoplasma*. Cell Host Microbe 19(3):349–360. https://doi.org/10.1016/j.chom.2016.02.006

14. Barragan A, Brossier F, Sibley LD (2005) Transepithelial migration of *Toxoplasma gondii* involves an interaction of intercellular adhesion molecule 1 (ICAM-1) with the parasite adhesin MIC2. Cell Microbiol 7(4):561–568. https://doi.org/10.1111/j.1462-5822.2005.00486.x

15. Lourenco EV, Pereira SR, Faca VM, Coelho-Castelo AA, Mineo JR, Roque-Barreira MC, Greene LJ, Panunto-Castelo A (2001) *Toxoplasma gondii* micronemal protein MIC1 is a lactose-binding lectin. Glycobiology 11(7):541–547

16. Marchant J, Cowper B, Liu Y, Lai L, Pinzan C, Marq JB, Friedrich N, Sawmynaden K, Liew L, Chai W, Childs RA, Saouros S, Simpson P, Roque Barreira MC, Feizi T, Soldati-Favre D, Matthews S (2012) Galactose recognition by the apicomplexan parasite *Toxoplasma gondii*. J

Biol Chem 287(20):16720–16733. https://doi.org/10.1074/jbc.M111.325928

17. Jacot D, Tosetti N, Pires I, Stock J, Graindorge A, Hung YF, Han H, Tewari R, Kursula I, Soldati-Favre D (2016) An apicomplexan actin-binding protein serves as a connector and lipid sensor to coordinate motility and invasion. Cell Host Microbe 20 (6):731–743. https://doi.org/10.1016/j.chom.2016.10.020

18. Frenal K, Dubremetz JF, Lebrun M, Soldati-Favre D (2017) Gliding motility powers invasion and egress in Apicomplexa. Nat Rev Microbiol 15(11):645–660. https://doi.org/10.1038/nrmicro.2017.86

19. Shen B, Brown K, Long S, Sibley LD (2017) Development of CRISPR/Cas9 for efficient genome editing in Toxoplasma gondii. Methods Mol Biol 1498:79–103. https://doi.org/10.1007/978-1-4939-6472-7_6

20. Krishnamurthy S, Deng B, Del Rio R, Buchholz KR, Treeck M, Urban S, Boothroyd J, Lam YW, Ward GE (2016) Not a simple tether: binding of Toxoplasma gondii AMA1 to RON2 during invasion protects ama1 from rhomboid-mediated cleavage and leads to dephosphorylation of its cytosolic tail. MBio 7(5). https://doi.org/10.1128/mBio.00754-16

21. Wan KL, Carruthers VB, Sibley LD, Ajioka JW (1997) Molecular characterisation of an expressed sequence tag locus of Toxoplasma gondii encoding the micronemal protein MIC2. Mol Biochem Parasitol 84(2):203–214

22. Kafsack BF, Pena JD, Coppens I, Ravindran S, Boothroyd JC, Carruthers VB (2009) Rapid membrane disruption by a perforin-like protein facilitates parasite exit from host cells. Science 323(5913):530–533. https://doi.org/10.1126/science.1165740

23. Kremer K, Kamin D, Rittweger E, Wilkes J, Flammer H, Mahler S, Heng J, Tonkin CJ, Langsley G, Hell SW, Carruthers VB, Ferguson DJ, Meissner M (2013) An overexpression screen of Toxoplasma gondii Rab-GTPases reveals distinct transport routes to the micronemes. PLoS Pathog 9(3):e1003213. https://doi.org/10.1371/journal.ppat.1003213

24. Tannous BA, Kim DE, Fernandez JL, Weissleder R, Breakefield XO (2005) Codon-optimized Gaussia luciferase cDNA for mammalian gene expression in culture and in vivo. Mol Ther 11(3):435–443. https://doi.org/10.1016/j.ymthe.2004.10.016

25. Huynh MH, Carruthers VB (2009) Tagging of endogenous genes in a Toxoplasma gondii strain lacking Ku80. Eukaryot Cell 8 (4):530–539

26. Roos DS, Donald RGK, Morrissette NS, Moulton AL (1994) Molecular tools for genetic dissection of the protozoan parasite Toxoplasma gondii. Methods Cell Biol 45:28–61

27. Long S, Brown KM, Drewry LL, Anthony B, Phan IQH, Sibley LD (2017) Calmodulin-like proteins localized to the conoid regulate motility and cell invasion by Toxoplasma gondii. PLoS Pathog 13(5):e1006379. https://doi.org/10.1371/journal.ppat.1006379

28. Lourido S, Moreno SN (2015) The calcium signaling toolkit of the Apicomplexan parasites Toxoplasma gondii and Plasmodium spp. Cell Calcium 57(3):186–193. https://doi.org/10.1016/j.ceca.2014.12.010

Chapter 10

Plate-Based Quantification of Stimulated *Toxoplasma* Egress

Emily Shortt and Sebastian Lourido

Abstract

Apicomplexans are obligate parasites that replicate inside host cells, within a subcellular compartment called the parasitophorous vacuole. Egress is the process by which apicomplexan parasites like *Toxoplasma gondii* exit from host cells, rupturing the parasitophorous vacuole and host-cell plasma membranes in the process. *T. gondii* retains the ability to egress throughout most of its intracellular replicative cycle, and this process has been associated with parasite signaling pathways that include the modulation of intracellular calcium, cyclic nucleotides, phosphatidic acid, and pH, which can be manipulated genetically or pharmacologically. Here we describe two methods of assessing stimulated parasite egress from host cells by measuring the permeabilization of host-cell membranes that occurs during this process. The first method measures the release of lactate dehydrogenase (LDH) from host cells, which is quantified in a colorimetric assay that detects LDH by the enzymatic generation of red formazan. The second method measures entry of the cell-impermeant 4′,6-diamidino-2-phenylindole (DAPI) DNA dye, which stains host-cell nuclei (HCN) as parasites egress. Both described methods complement, with higher throughput, video-microscopy approaches that are well suited to examine the dissociation of parasite vacuoles that follows host-cell permeabilization.

Key words *Toxoplasma gondii*, Egress, Host-cell lysis, Membrane rupture

1 Introduction

The asexual portion of the apicomplexan life cycle is based on repeated rounds of replication within host cells. Following invasion, parasites typically undergo several mitotic divisions within a parasitophorous vacuole before emerging to reinvade and repeat the cycle in adjacent host cells. This lytic cycle is responsible for most of the pathogenesis associated with apicomplexan infections [1]. Egress is the active process through which apicomplexans exit from the infected host cells. This process lyses the parasitophorous vacuole and host-cell membranes, resulting in cell death [2]. Some apicomplexans, like *Toxoplasma gondii*, retain the ability to egress throughout most of the intracellular replicative cycle, while others, like *Plasmodium* spp., only form the necessary cellular structures

Christopher J. Tonkin (ed.), *Toxoplasma gondii: Methods and Protocols*, Methods in Molecular Biology, vol. 2071, https://doi.org/10.1007/978-1-4939-9857-9_10, © Springer Science+Business Media, LLC, part of Springer Nature 2020

immediately prior to egress, during their final cell cycle [3]. For that reason, *T. gondii* has become a useful model to investigate the parasite signaling pathways that regulate egress, which include the modulation of intracellular Ca^{2+} [4], cyclic nucleotides [5], phosphatidic acid [6], and pH [7, 8].

Stimulated *T. gondii* egress was first observed in response to the Ca^{2+} ionophore A23187 [9]. Since then egress has been shown to occur in response to a variety of stimuli ranging from phosphodiesterase inhibitors [5] to host-cell rupture [10]. These studies have mainly relied on the static examination of infected monolayers or time-lapse video microscopy following stimulation with a given agonist. Genetic and pharmacological studies of this type have revealed the involvement of microneme secretion and parasite motility in *T. gondii* egress and cell spread [11–13]. However, standard microscopy lacks the throughput and ease of quantification needed to explore a broad range of agonists and inhibitors at varying concentrations.

To achieve a higher-throughput and a more quantitative measure of egress, we describe two plate-based assays that rely on host-cell permeabilization during egress. The first assay is a colorimetric endpoint assay that measures lactate dehydrogenase (LDH) release from host cells (Fig. 1a). LDH is an abundant cytosolic enzyme that is released into the culture supernatant when parasites lyse the host-cell membrane during egress. LDH activity can be measured indirectly by a coupled assay in which the lactate-dependent generation of NADH results in the conversion of a tetrazolium salt to a red formazan product by diaphorase. Red formazan generation is detected by absorbance at 490 nm and is proportional to the amount of LDH released. This is an endpoint assay in that it measures the total amount of egress that has occurred in a given amount of time—5 min in the described protocol. In contrast, the second method is a time-lapse video microscopy assay optimized for a high-content imager (Fig. 1b). The egress agonist and cell-impermeant DNA dye 4′,6-diamidino-2-phenylindole (DAPI) are added together to infected cell monolayers. Within seconds of parasites egress, DAPI enters the host cells and stains their nuclei, causing them to fluoresce blue. After the egress period—9 min, for the purpose of this description—a solution of Triton X-100 is added to each well, lysing the remaining host cells and allowing for the enumeration of the total number of host cells in the monolayer. The stained host nuclei are amenable to automated counting due to their homogenous size and staining intensity, and we use the number of stained nuclei as a proxy for the extent of parasite egress in a monolayer. Stained host nuclei are counted every 10 s during a 9 min incubation with the agonist, producing a kinetic trace of egress over time (*see* **Note 1**).

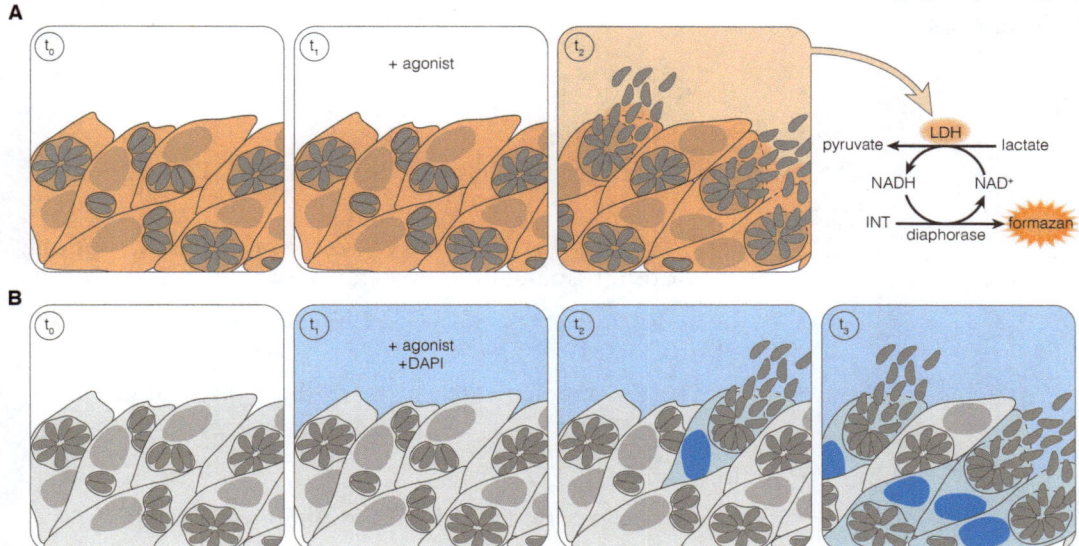

Fig. 1 Schematic of the two different egress assays presented in the protocol. (**a**) The LDH release assay monitors the release of LDH from infected host cells following stimulated parasite egress. LDH in the supernatant is quantified using a colorimetric assay that reads out its catalysis of a tetrazolium salt (INT) into red formazan. (**b**) The DAPI entry assay monitors permeabilization of host cells dynamically by visualizing the number of fluorescent host cell nuclei following the addition of an egress agonist

In addition to determining the consequences of genetic manipulations on *T. gondii* egress, these methods can be used to identify compounds that inhibit or stimulate egress. For the purposes of this protocol, we will use the pyrazolopyrimidine derivative 3-MB-PP1, which inhibits egress of wildtype *T. gondii* through the inhibition of CDPK1 [14]. Other inhibitors and agonists or genetic manipulations may be substituted to study different aspects of the pathways that govern egress.

The methods presented focus on the permeabilization of the host-cell membrane to measure egress. Other assays, which measure egress by the number of intact vacuoles present after stimulation, may additionally take into account the initiation of parasite motility. This distinction should be kept in mind when comparing different studies and interpreting results. In addition to a kinetic trace, the DAPI method provides low magnification time-lapse video microscopy suitable for inspection of the monolayers to examine the motility of parasites immediately before and during egress, and this visualization can be enhanced if fluorescent parasites lines are used. Ideally the presented methods complement finer imaging of egress, by helping investigators identify the most informative conditions to analyze in greater detail.

2   Materials

- CO_2 incubator.
- Inverted microscope.
- Tissue culture treated 96-well plates, such as TPP low evaporation plates (cat. no. 92096).
- Cytation plates: PerkinElmer cell-carrier 96, black, optically clear bottom, tissue-culture treated (cat. no. 6005550).
- Human foreskin fibroblast (HFF) cells, such as ATCC cat. no. SCRC-1041.
- D10: DMEM supplemented with 10% heat-inactivated FBS.
- PBS.
- 0.05% trypsin–EDTA.
- Multichannel pipette for volumes from 50 to 200 µl.
- Reagent reservoirs.
- Micropipettes for volumes from 0.5 to 1000 µl.
- Pipet aid.
- Serological pipettes: 5 ml, 10 ml.
- Multichannel aspirator.
- *T. gondii* cell lines.
- HHE: Hank's Balanced Salts (Sigma cat. no. H2387) prepared in dH_2O and supplemented with 0.1 mM EGTA and 10 mM HEPES. Adjust pH to 7.4 using NaOH and sterile filter. Store protected from light.
- 3 µm filters: 3 µm pore polycarbonate membrane (GVS Life Sciences cat. no. 1215036) in a Whatman filter support (GE Healthcare/Whatman cat. no. 420400).
- 5 ml luer-lock syringes.
- 15 ml conical tubes.
- 1.5 ml microcentrifuge tubes.
- Hemocytometer.
- Refrigerated clinical centrifuge and rotors (including multiwell plate rotor bucket).
- Methanol.
- Small water bath prepared by filling a shallow dish with 0.5 cm sterile 37 °C water and placing it in the incubator.
- Ringer's Solution: 155 mM NaCl, 3 mM KCl, 2 mM $CaCl_2$, 1 mM $MgCl_2$, 3 mM NaH_2PO_4, 10 mM HEPES pH 7.4, 10 mM glucose, 1% heat-inactivated FBS.

- A23187 (Calbiochem cat. no. 100105) resuspended in DMSO to 2 mM.

- 3-MB-PP1 (EMD Millipore cat. no. 529582) resuspended in DMSO to 10 mM.

- Cytotox 96 nonradioactive cytotoxicity assay kit (Promega cat. no. G1780).

- Plate reader, such as Biotek epoch microplate spectrophotometer.

- Fluorobrite D10: Fluorobrite DMEM (Life Technologies cat. no. A1896701) supplemented with 10% heat-inactivated FBS.

- Triton X-100.

- DAPI (Molecular Probes cat. no. D1306), resuspended in dH_2O to 14.3 mM.

- Biotek Cytation 3 imaging multimode reader with CO_2 control, dual reagent injector module, equipped with laser autofocus, operated with the Gen5 software package; or a comparable high-content imager and software.

- 70% ethanol.

- MilliQ H_2O.

- Microsoft Excel.

- Graphing software, such as GraphPad Prism.

- Immunofluorescence blocking solution: 5% normal goat serum, 5% heat-inactivated FBS in PBS.

- Rabbit anti-aldolase antibody [15] (or another general anti-*Toxoplasma* antibody).

- Alexa 594-conjugated goat anti-rabbit antibody.

- Hoescht-33258 (Santa Cruz Biotechnology cat. no. sc-394039).

- Imaging software, such as FIJI [16, 17], with Cell Counter plug-in.

3   Methods

3.1   Preparing HFFs

Three to four days prior to the experiment, seed 96-well plates with HFF cells; one plate will be the assay plate and one plate will be for the immunofluorescence assay (IFA) (*see* **Note 2**).

1. Aspirate the growth medium from a confluent 12.5 cm^2 flask of HFFs, wash the monolayer twice with 5 ml of PBS, and aspirate the PBS. Add 300 μl of 0.05% trypsin–EDTA and return the flask to the incubator for 2 min; tap the flask to dislodge the cells and check using an inverted light microscope that the cells are detached from the flask (*see* **Note 3**).

2. Add enough D10 medium to the flask of trypsinized HFFs to total 200 μl of HFF suspension per assay well (*see* **Note 4**). Gently pipette up and down to wash the cells off the sides of the flask.

3. Pipette the cell suspension into a sterile reagent reservoir and use a multichannel pipette to dispense 200 μl of cell suspension into each well of the appropriate tissue culture treated 96-well plates (*see* **Note 5**). Place the 96-well plates in the 5% CO_2 incubator at 37 °C.

3.2 Infecting the Monolayers

One day prior to the experiment, infect the confluent HFF monolayer in the prepared 96-well plate with *Toxoplasma*. Also infect the monolayer in the accompanying 96-well Cytation plate for an IFA.

1. Harvest parasites from a freshly lysed flask. For each strain, place a 3 μm filter with attached 5 ml syringe over a 15 ml conical tube and prewet the membrane with 5 ml of HHE. Place the parasite suspension in the syringe and allow it to enter the filter by gravity, then wash the syringe and filter with 5 ml of HHE. Centrifuge the parasites in a clinical centrifuge for 10 min at $400 \times g$ at 4 °C.

2. Aspirate the supernatant and resuspend the parasite pellet in 5 ml of HHE. Count a 1:10 dilution of the parasite suspension using a hemocytometer (*see* **Note 6**).

3. Dilute parasites to 2.5×10^5 parasites per ml in D10 in a volume sufficient to infect the wells to be tested; each well will require 200 μl of parasite suspension (*see* **Note 7**).

4. Aspirate the growth medium from the HFF monolayers using a multichannel aspirator and use a multichannel pipette to add 200 μl of parasite suspension to each well. Add 200 μl of fresh D10 to wells that will remain uninfected.

5. Centrifuge the infected plates in a clinical centrifuge for 5 min at $290 \times g$, 4 °C, to spin the parasites onto the monolayer, and return the plates to the 5% CO_2 incubator at 37 °C for 24 h.

6. At this point the infected plates will be treated according to the assay that will be performed. Continue with Subheading 3.3 for IFA, Subheading 3.4 for LDH release assay, and Subheading 3.6 for DAPI entry assay.

3.3 Preparation of Infected Plate for IFA

1. Aspirate the growth medium from the plate infected for IFA using a multichannel aspirator and use a multichannel pipette to gently wash three times with 200 μl Ringer's Solution.

2. Add 200 μl ice-cold 100% methanol to each well and place the plate on ice for 2 min to allow fixation and permeabilization to proceed (*see* **Note 8**).

3. Aspirate the methanol and wash the fixed and permeabilized monolayer gently three times with 200 μl PBS, then add 200 μl PBS to each well and keep the plate at 4 °C until processing for IFA (continued in Subheading 3.11).

3.4 Stimulation of Parasite Egress for LDH Release Assay

1. Several hours prior to the experiment, fill a small dish with about 0.5 cm sterile water and place it in the incubator at 37 °C to create a shallow water bath.

2. Prepare dilutions of 3-MB-PP1 in Ringer's Solution containing the same amount of DMSO as the lowest dilution tested (0.2% in this example). First prepare the Ringer's Solution with 0.2% DMSO by mixing 20 μl of DMSO into 10 ml of Ringer's Solution. Next prepare the 3-MB-PP1, first by diluting the 10 mM stock solution to a new 20 μM stock by mixing 4 μl of 10 mM 3-MB-PP1 into 2 ml of Ringer's Solution, then by preparing the following dilution series: 10 μM, 2 μM, 1 μM, 0.5 μM, 0.25 μM, 0.125 μM using the 0.2% DMSO in Ringer's Solution as the solute for each (*see* **Notes 9** and **10**).

3. Prepare A23187 at 4 μM in Ringer's Solution by mixing 4 μl of A23187 stock (2 mM) with 1996 μl Ringer's Solution; this is four times the desired final concentration of 1 μM. Prepare an equal dilution of DMSO (4 μl into 2 ml total Ringer's Solution) to assess the effect of the inhibitor on LDH release without stimulation (*see* **Notes 9** and **11**).

4. In an empty 96-well plate, arrange the 3-MB-PP1 dilutions in the same order as they will be added to the infected cells. Prepare one set for pretreatment and one set for use during stimulation, with a maximum volume 150 μl of 3-MB-PP1 per well. For this example, you will need two sets of 150 μl pretreatment wells and two sets of 150 μl stimulation wells, which is enough for triplicate wells of each condition for one strain.

5. Dilute the pretreatment inhibitor dilution series with 150 μl of Ringer's Solution to bring the inhibitor concentration to the desired final concentration.

6. Remove growth medium from infected wells using a multichannel aspirator and use a multichannel pipette to wash once with 200 μl Ringer's Solution, then aspirate the Ringer's Solution.

7. Add 50 μl of the pretreatment condition to the appropriate wells using a multichannel pipette. Place the plate in the prepared 37 °C water bath and incubate 20 min.

8. Add 150 μl of the 4× A23187 agonist solution to one of the remaining inhibitor dilution series and add 150 μl Ringer's Solution plus DMSO from **step 3** to the other remaining inhibitor dilution series (*see* **Note 12**). Add 50 μl of each stimulation condition to the appropriate wells using a

multichannel pipette. Place the plate in the prepared 37 °C water bath and allow egress to proceed for 5 min (*see* **Note 13**).

9. Centrifuge the plate in a clinical centrifuge for 5 min at $400 \times g$, 4 °C, to pellet the egressed parasites and cell debris.

10. Carefully transfer 50 μl of the supernatant from each well to a new 96-well plate. Take care not to disturb the monolayer.

11. Lyse the uninfected well designated as the total lysis control by adding 10 μl of lysis solution provided with the Cytotox Assay kit, scraping the monolayer with a pipette tip, and pipetting up and down to resuspend the cells (*see* **Note 14**). Transfer 50 μl of cell lysate to the 96-well plate. The assay plate can be discarded at this point.

12. Supernatants may be held at 4 °C for 2–3 h before continuing to develop the assay in Subheading 3.5.

3.5 Quantification of Host-Cell Lysis Using the Cytotox Assay Kit

1. Prepare substrate mixture by adding 12 ml of Assay Buffer to 1 vial of Substrate. You will use 6 ml of prepared substrate per 96-well plate (*see* **Note 15**).

2. Use a multichannel pipette to add 50 μl of prepared substrate to each well containing experiment supernatants.

3. Incubate in the dark for 30 min at room temperature.

4. Use a multichannel pipette to add 50 μl of stop buffer to each well (*see* **Note 16**). Air bubbles can affect the absorbance reading and should be popped with a pipette tip or needle.

5. Use a plate reader to measure the absorbance at 490 nm. Complete the readings within 1 h of adding stop buffer, as the formazan product will precipitate over time.

6. Calculate the relative amount of egress:

$$\%\text{Egress} = (\text{Sample} - \text{Uninfected})/(\text{Total lysis} - \text{Uninfected})$$

3.6 Solutions for DAPI Entry Assay

1. Prepare the egress agonist solution of A23187 at 12 μM plus 1.5% (v/v) DMSO in Fluorobrite D10 with 5 μg/ml DAPI, which is three times the desired effective concentration of 4 μM A23187 in Fluorobrite D10 with 0.5% (v/v) DMSO. Prepare enough for 100 μl per well of the assay plus 1.4 ml for priming the injector (*see* **Notes 17–19**).

2. Prepare the 3-MB-PP1 inhibitor solution at 6 μM, by diluting the 10 mM stock first to 100 μM and then by mixing 30 μl of the 100 μM solution per 500 μl of Fluorobrite D10 (*see* **Note 18**). Also prepare the corresponding vehicle control of DMSO in Fluorobrite D10. You will need 25 μl per well of inhibitor or vehicle control.

3. Prepare the 1% Triton X-100 solution in Fluorobrite D10. Prepare enough for 50 μl per well of the assay plus 1.4 ml for priming the injector.

4. Prepare 500 μl Fluorobrite D10 containing 5 μg/ml DAPI.

3.7 Preparation of Infected Plates for DAPI Entry Assay

1. Several hours prior to the experiment, fill a small dish with about 0.5 cm sterile water and place it in the incubator at 37 °C to create a shallow water bath.

2. Aspirate the growth medium from the wells using a multichannel aspirator and use a multichannel pipette to gently wash the infected monolayers three times with 200 μl Ringer's Solution and aspirate the Ringer's Solution.

3. Add 25 μl Fluorobrite D10 to each well, then add 25 μl of 3-MB-PP1 or vehicle control to the appropriate wells (*see* **Note 20**). Incubate the plate at 37 °C for 20 min.

4. To the uninfected well that will be used for focusing, add 25 μl 1% Triton X-100 and 25 μl of 5 μg/ml DAPI.

3.8 Preparation of Cytation 3 High-Content Plate Reader

1. Set up the protocol in the Gen5 software, using a PE Cell Carrier 96 plate without the lid. Choose to select wells "at runtime."

2. Set the temperature for the assay to 37 °C and select the option to "preheat before continuing with next step."

3. Set up the prestimulation imaging loop in Well Mode. In a kinetic step, set the run time as 1 s (0:01.00) and interval as 1 s (0:01.00) and set up the read for endpoint imaging with filters using the 4× objective. The microscopy channels you will use for imaging are bright field (BF) and DAPI (377 excitation, 477 emission) with one image per well. Select the option to use the focal height of the first read for all reads in well mode block. For both channels, deselect the "auto" option; for BF choose Laser Auto Focus as the focus method (Fig. 2).

4. Set up the first injection, which will be 100 μl of A23187 and DAPI solution. For dispenser 1 set the volume to 100 μl and the rate to 225 μl per second; no priming is necessary.

5. Set up the post-stimulation imaging loop by repeating **step 3** except set the run time as 9 min (9:00.00) and the interval as 10 s (0:10.00). Append the reads to the previous kinetic data to carry the read parameters from the previous step.

6. Set up the second injection, which will be 50 μl of the 1% Triton X-100 solution. Repeat **step 4**, except choose dispenser 2 and set the volume to 50 μl.

7. Set up the 100% lysis imaging loop by repeating **step 5**, except set the run time as 20 s (0:20.00) and the interval as 5 s

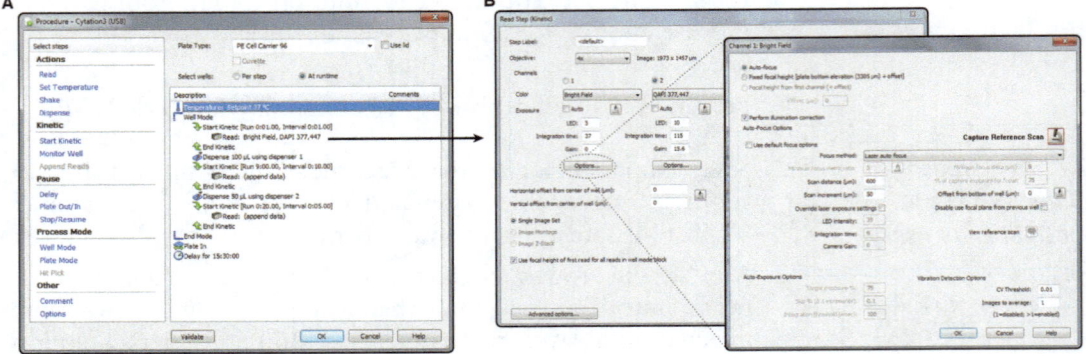

Fig. 2 Configuration of the Cytation 3 for the DAPI entry assay. (**a**) Snapshot of the procedure setup window indicating the order of reads and dispenser injections. (**b**) Imaging configuration and focus options

(0:05.00). This concludes the kinetic step as well as the well mode (*see* **Note 21**).

8. At least 30 min prior to the experiment, set the Cytation 3 to incubate at 37 °C. Also turn on the CO_2 regulator to 5%. At this point it is important to make sure the plate tray is kept in so that the chamber can heat up and the gases can equilibrate.

9. Prime each of the injectors with 1.4 ml of A23187 solution or Triton X-100 solution; in this protocol, the agonist solution is assigned to injector 1 and the Triton X-100 solution to injector 2. It is critical to place the priming plate on the plate carrier before performing the priming step.

10. Focus the imaging plate reader and set the exposure for each channel (*see* **Note 22**). To focus the bright field, use an infected well (with 50 µl Fluorobrite in the well). Bright field is also used for the laser auto focus reference scan, so use this well to capture the reference scan. To focus the DAPI channel, use the uninfected well of HFFs to which you have added Triton X-100 and 5 µg/ml DAPI, which will allow you to visualize the HCN.

3.9 Kinetic Analysis of Parasite Egress

1. Starting with a plate of infected HFFs with 50 µl of medium per well, (from Subheading 3.7, **step 3**), start a new experiment in the Gen5 software and choose the protocol created in Subheading 3.8.

2. Click the "Read Now" button (green arrow) and select the wells to be assayed, then click "OK."

3. Place the plate in the plate carrier of the Cytation 3 and remove the lid, then click OK on the popup menu. The temperature will equilibrate to 37 °C, if necessary, and the protocol will begin (*see* **Note 23**).

4. When the assay is finished, clean the injectors by priming each with 2.5 ml of 70% ethanol and 5 ml of milliQ water. It is critical to place the priming plate on the plate carrier before proceeding with priming; rinse and dry the priming plate when finished.

3.10 Data Transformation and Graphing

1. To set up the cell counting analysis, click on an image in the plate view to open it and navigate to a time point with substantial numbers of stained HCN. Click "Analyze" and set up a new image analysis data reduction step for cell counting in the DAPI channel. Select "bright object on dark background" and "split touching objects." Choose a threshold value, as well as minimum and maximum object sizes; a threshold of 5600 and size range of 11–30 μm should be appropriate. To check how well your settings are working, select "highlight objects" and click "Start;" this will allow the cell counting analysis to run and will highlight the objects that have been counted. Adjust the threshold and size range parameters as needed to maximize the number of HCN being counted while minimizing incorrect calls (e.g., splitting large objects into smaller ones or counting objects that are too small). It will take several minutes for the cell counting analysis to iterate over the entire data set.

2. Set up the data transformations to convert from raw number of HCN to a scale of 0–100% egress. Click the data reduction icon, where you will see cell counting already listed. Under transformations, click "Custom" and choose "select multiple data sets," then assign the data sets as follows:

Data sets	Plate	Data in	Read(s)
DS1	Current plate	HCN	All
DS2	Current plate	HCN	1
DS3	Current plate	HCN	62[a]

[a]This is the last read

Give the new data set a name—egress_score. Select "single formula for all wells" and set the plate formula as (DS1–DS2)/(DS3–DS2) then click "OK" to record the transformation. Set up another custom transformation for which the "data in" is "egress_score" reads: "all." Select "single formula for all wells" and set the plate formula as $DS1*100$. Give the new data set a name (% egress), then click OK to record the transformation. It may take several minutes for the data transformations to iterate over the entire data set.

3. To export the data, select the desired data (% egress) from the drop-down menu in the plate view. Double click on a well, then

select the data radio button (instead of graph). Click select wells and choose the wells you assayed; the data for these wells will populate a table. Click the "export to Excel" button (green x next to "edit table"). This process will need to be repeated for each plate of data and for each data type (if you want to export raw HCN, egress_score, % egress).

4. Open the exported data in Microsoft Excel. Convert the Time column from its current format (mm:ss) to seconds. Any additional labeling of data columns is optional.

5. Plot the data in GraphPad Prism. Choose an XY graph and for Y enter 3 replicate values in side-by-side columns. Label the columns by strain name and treatment condition, if applicable. For the X column, insert the time values in seconds. Copy and paste the Y values from Microsoft Excel into the correct column. Select the rows for the last five time points and exclude them (*see* **Note 24**). New data are automatically plotted, and graphs can be found under the Graphs section.

3.11 Assessment of MOI by IFA

1. Starting with a Cytation plate with fixed and permeabilized infected cells, stored in PBS at 4 °C (from Subheading 3.3), remove the PBS and add 100 μl per well of immunofluorescence blocking solution. Incubate 15 min.

2. Remove the blocking solution and add 50 μl per well of primary antibody solution (1:2500 dilution of rabbit anti-aldolase or another anti-*Toxoplasma* antibody at the appropriate dilution). Incubate 30–45 min at room temperature.

3. Remove the primary antibody and wash gently three times with 200 μl PBS. Add 100 μl per well immunofluorescence blocking solution and incubate 5 min.

4. Remove the blocking solution and add 50 μl per well of secondary antibody solution (1:1000 dilution of Alexa 594-conjugated goat anti-rabbit) containing 10 μM Hoechst. Incubate in the dark 30–45 min at room temperature.

5. Remove the secondary antibody and wash gently three times with 200 μl PBS. Add 200 μl per well PBS for imaging, and store plate in the dark at 4 °C until ready to image.

6. Set up the IFA imaging protocol in the Gen5 software, using a PE Cell Carrier 96 plate with the lid. Choose to select wells "at runtime." Set up the read for endpoint imaging with filters using the 20× objective. The microscopy channels you will use for imaging are DAPI (377 excitation, 477 emission) and Texas Red (586 excitation, 647 emission) with a 2 by 2 montage of images in each well without stitching.

7. For both channels, deselect the "auto" option then focus the imaging plate reader and set the exposure for each channel (*see* **Note 22**).

8. In the Gen5 software, start a new experiment and choose the protocol that you set up in **steps 6** and **7**.

9. Click the "Read Now" button (green arrow) and select the wells you want to image, then click "OK."

10. Place the plate in the plate carrier of the Cytation 3 with the lid on, then click "OK" on the popup menu to begin the protocol.

11. Images are saved as individual TIFs (1 per imaging channel, so 8 files per imaged well). Open FIJI [16, 17] and open the corresponding images (BF and Texas Red) for one quadrant of the montage in the desired well. If necessary, adjust the brightness and contrast of the individual images. When you are satisfied with the brightness and contrast, merge the images into a two-color composite by assigning DAPI to the blue channel and Texas Red to the red channel. Start the Cell Counter plug-in and initialize the image, then select the cell counter type. Count the HCN (excluding those at the frame edge) and then switch to another cell counter type and count the parasite vacuoles (excluding those at the frame edge). Record the values for each counter type (*see* **Note 25**).

12. Calculate the ratio of parasite vacuoles per HCN for each image and plot the values using GraphPad Prism. At least two images should be counted for each condition (strain or treatment condition).

4 Notes

1. This assay can also be performed in an endpoint fashion. Instead of imaging every 10 s during the egress period to generate a kinetic trace, the agonist and DAPI can be added and incubated with the infected monolayer at 37 °C for the desired egress period, followed by a single image of the well and the addition of Triton X- 100 to estimate total cell numbers.

2. When interpreting the data from plate-based egress assays, it is important that all wells be infected to the same extent. To determine whether this is the case, a second 96-well plate can be set up in parallel and used to perform an in-plate IFA using a general parasite antibody and a Hoechst DNA stain. Then count parasite vacuoles and HCN and calculate a multiplicity of infection (parasite vacuoles per host cell nucleus). If fluorescent *Toxoplasma* strains are used, live microscopy may be substituted for the IFA to compare multiplicity of infection between wells.

3. Allot one 12.5 cm^2 flask of confluent HFF cells per half plate (48 wells) to be seeded at this time point.

4. For LDH release assay, seed 48 wells of HFFs per *Toxoplasma* strain being assayed with a 5-concentration 3-MB-PP1 dilution series, plus a row of vehicle control and uninfected wells, as

described in this protocol. The uninfected wells are reserved to test the effect of drugs on host cell lysis and for a total lysis control. For the DAPI entry assay, seed 7 wells, which is 3 wells of HFFs per *Toxoplasma* strain per condition being assayed plus one uninfected well, which is reserved for focusing the imager. For IFAs, seed one well of HFFs per *Toxoplasma* strain per condition being assayed.

5. For LDH release assay, it is not necessary to use optically clear, black 96-well plates; any tissue-culture treated 96-well plate will suffice. For the DAPI entry assay and for IFA, which rely on imaging, use optically clear, black 96-well plates as described in the materials as Cytation plates.

6. The expected parasite yield from a lysed 12.5 cm^2 flask is 1–3×10^7.

7. This concentration will need to be empirically determined for each *Toxoplasma* strain used, with the goal of a multiplicity of infection equal to 1. We have successfully used a range of concentrations between 2.5–5 and 10^5 parasites per ml.

8. Use a different fixation method if required for the *Toxoplasma* antibody of choice.

9. The Ringer's Solution with 0.2% DMSO serves as a vehicle control, because 3-MB-PP1 is resuspended in DMSO. The percentage of DMSO included in this solution will vary based on the lowest concentration of 3-MB-PP1 used in the assay, to measure any background lysis from the maximum concentration of vehicle.

10. These concentrations of inhibitor are twice the final desired concentration that the parasites will experience in this example.

11. A23187 is prepared at 4× the desired final concentration. Zaprinast is an alternative agonist that may be used. Prepare it at 2 mM in Ringer's Solution, which is four times the desired effective concentration of 500 μM.

12. Mixing the agonist solution (or vehicle control) with the inhibitor dilution series before using it to stimulate egress ensures that the inhibitor concentration remains the same during stimulation of egress. This is particularly important when using reversible inhibitors like 3-MB-PP1, which could be washed out during the stimulation period. This addition also dilutes the agonist and inhibitor from 4× and 2×, respectively, to the desired final concentration.

13. It is possible to use shorter incubation times for the egress stimulation step, but in our hands, these show greater variability. Additionally, it is possible to increase the incubation time up to 30 min, but this may cause increased background lysis.

14. It is possible to prepare your own lysis solution. The composition is 9% (v/v) Triton X-100.

15. The remaining reconstituted substrate mixture can be stored at −20 °C for several months.

16. It is possible to prepare your own stop buffer. The composition is 1 M acetic acid in water.

17. Zaprinast is an alternative agonist that may be used. Prepare it at 1.5 mM in Fluorobrite D10 with 5 μg/ml DAPI, which is three times the desired effective concentration of 500 μM zaprinast.

18. The egress agonist is prepared at three times the desired effective concentration because it will be diluted over the course of the experiment to a final concentration of 1× (by combining 100 μl of agonist solution with the 25 μl of inhibitor or vehicle solution and 25 μl of Fluorobrite D10 already in the well upon injection, for a final volume of 150 μl). The 3-MB-PP1 inhibitor solution is prepared at twice the desired effective concentration because it will be diluted to 1× upon application to the parasites which already have an equal volume of Fluorobrite D10 in each well.

19. Some agonists may be absorbed by the injector tubing. To compensate for this, we have increased the concentration of agonist used and added a small percentage of DMSO to the solute (0.5% final concentration).

20. The volume of Fluorobrite D10 added at this step will vary with experimental set up. If no inhibitor pretreatment is used, add 50 μl of Fluorobrite D10. The agonist concentration in this example depends on 50 μl total in the wells prior to stimulation.

21. You may wish to program in a step to take the plate back into the carrier and a delay step to hold the plate in the carrier. To do this, choose "Plate Out/In" from the Pause menu and select "move plate in." To program the delay step, choose "Delay" from the "Pause" menu and set the desired delay time (HH:MM:SS format). The procedure shown in Fig. 2 includes the delay step.

22. It is necessary to focus the imager for each new plate, as there can be variation in the focus metrics between plates. You will be asked to "Update" the protocol when you make these changes.

23. If you need to change plates during the protocol, click abort read (to end the programmed delay), then click Read Now. You will be asked to choose between deleting the data in Plate 1 and creating a new Plate 2 for new data. Choose to create a new plate for new read data, then select the wells you want to read.

24. These values in the last 5 rows can be included in the plots, but we have chosen to exclude them because they do not represent egress. Rather, these are the time points taken after 1% Triton

X-100 is added to the wells, and the images are used for scaling the egress from 0 to 100%.

25. It may be possible to automate the counting process through a macro; however, it will be important to ensure that parasite vacuoles can be identified accurately regardless of size, or that single parasites can be counted instead of vacuoles, which would result in a metric of parasites per HCN instead of vacuoles per HCN.

Acknowledgments

This work was supported by the NIH Director's Early Independence Award (1DP5OD017892) and an NIH Exploratory R21 grant (1R21AI123746) to S.L.

References

1. Blader IJ, Coleman BI, Chen C-T, Gubbels M-J (2015) Lytic cycle of *Toxoplasma gondii*: 15 years later. Annu Rev Microbiol 69:463–485

2. Blackman MJ, Carruthers VB (2013) Recent insights into apicomplexan parasite egress provide new views to a kill. Curr Opin Microbiol 16:459–464

3. Striepen B, Jordan CN, Reiff S, van Dooren GG (2007) Building the perfect parasite: cell division in apicomplexa. PLoS Pathog e78:3

4. Lourido S, Moreno SNJ (2015) The calcium signaling toolkit of the Apicomplexan parasites *Toxoplasma gondii* and Plasmodium spp. Cell Calcium 57:186–193

5. Lourido S, Tang K, Sibley LD (2012) Distinct signalling pathways control *Toxoplasma* egress and host-cell invasion. EMBO J 31:4524–4534

6. Bullen HE et al (2016) Phosphatidic acid-mediated signaling regulates microneme secretion in *Toxoplasma*. Cell Host Microbe 19:349–360

7. Roiko MS, Svezhova N, Carruthers VB (2014) Acidification activates *Toxoplasma gondii* motility and egress by enhancing protein secretion and cytolytic activity. PLoS Pathog 10: e1004488

8. Jia Y et al (2017) Crosstalk between PKA and PKG controls pH-dependent host cell egress of *Toxoplasma gondii*. EMBO J 36:3250–3267

9. Endo T, Sethi KK, Piekarski G (1982) *Toxoplasma gondii*: calcium ionophore A23187-mediated exit of trophozoites from infected murine macrophages. Exp Parasitol 53:179–188

10. Moudy R, Manning TJ, Beckers CJ (2001) The loss of cytoplasmic potassium upon host cell breakdown triggers egress of *Toxoplasma gondii*. J Biol Chem 276:41492–41501

11. Black MW, Arrizabalaga G, Boothroyd JC (2000) Ionophore-resistant mutants of *Toxoplasma gondii* reveal host cell permeabilization as an early event in egress. Mol Cell Biol 20:9399–9408

12. Kafsack BFC et al (2009) Rapid membrane disruption by a perforin-like protein facilitates parasite exit from host cells. Science 323:530–533

13. Lavine M, Arrizabalaga G (2007) Invasion and egress by the obligate intracellular parasite *Toxoplasma gondii*: potential targets for the development of new antiparasitic drugs. Curr Pharm Des 13:641–651

14. Lourido S et al (2010) Calcium-dependent protein kinase 1 is an essential regulator of exocytosis in *Toxoplasma*. Nature 465:359–362

15. Starnes GL, Jewett TJ, Carruthers VB, Sibley LD (2006) Two separate, conserved acidic amino acid domains within the *Toxoplasma gondii* MIC2 cytoplasmic tail are required for parasite survival. J Biol Chem 281:30745–30754

16. Schindelin J et al (2012) Fiji: an open-source platform for biological-image analysis. Nat Methods 9:676–682

17. Schneider CA, Rasband WS, Eliceiri KW (2012) NIH Image to ImageJ: 25 years of image analysis. Nat Methods 9:671–675

Chapter 11

Genetic Indicators for Calcium Signaling Studies in *Toxoplasma gondii*

Stephen A. Vella, Abigail Calixto, Beejan Asady, Zhu-Hong Li, and Silvia N. J. Moreno

Abstract

Fluctuations of the cytosolic calcium ion (Ca^{2+}) concentration regulate a variety of cellular functions in all eukaryotes. Cells express a sophisticated set of mechanisms to balance the cytosolic Ca^{2+} levels and the signals that elevate Ca^{2+} in the cytosol are compensated by mechanisms that reduce it. Alterations in Ca^{2+}-dependent homeostatic mechanisms are the cause of many prominent diseases in humans, such as heart failure or neuronal death.

The genetic tractability of *Toxoplasma gondii* and the availability of genetic tools enabled the use of Genetically Encoded Calcium Indicators (GECIs) expressed in the cytoplasm, which started a new era in the studies of *Toxoplasma* calcium signaling. It was finally possible to see Ca^{2+} oscillations prior to exit of the parasite from host cells. Years after Endo et al showed that ionophores triggered egress, the assumption that oscillations occur prior to egress from host cells has been validated by experiments using GECIs. GECIs allowed the visualization of specific Ca^{2+} signals in live intracellular parasites and to distinguish these signals from host cell calcium fluctuations. In this chapter we present an overview describing "tried and true" methods of our lab who pioneered the first use of GECI's in *Toxoplasma*, including GECI choice, methodology for transfection and selection of ideal clones, their characterization, and the use of GECI-expressing parasites for fluorometric and microscopic analysis.

Key words *Toxoplasma*, Calcium signaling, Genetic indicators, GCaMPs, GECOs, Egress, Time lapse, Fura2 measurements

1 Introduction

Ca^{2+} is a universal signaling molecule that regulates essential cellular functions. Ca^{2+} is controlled spatiotemporally, and intracellular organelles balance Ca^{2+} influx and efflux during Ca^{2+} signaling events [1]. Fluorescence Ca^{2+} indicators, whose brightness is sensitive to Ca^{2+} concentration, have been extensively utilized for decades in order to visualize Ca^{2+} dynamics [2]. Ca^{2+} indicators

---

Stephen A. Vella, Abigail Calixto, and Beejan Asady contributed equally to this work.

Christopher J. Tonkin (ed.), *Toxoplasma gondii: Methods and Protocols*, Methods in Molecular Biology, vol. 2071, https://doi.org/10.1007/978-1-4939-9857-9_11, © Springer Science+Business Media, LLC, part of Springer Nature 2020

designed as organic synthetic dyes have improved over the years and exhibit excellent dynamic range and favorable kinetics. Genetically encoded calcium indicators (GECIs) have become powerful tools for the study of calcium signaling and current efforts in protein engineering have significantly increased their performance to match those of organic dyes [3–7]. GECIs have the advantage of enabling noninvasive imaging of defined cells and compartments, whereas organic dyes are prone to organellar compartmentalization and leakage from the cytosol. Targeting of GECIs to various subcellular compartments, using targeting sequences, together with high-resolution microscopy have opened the possibility of selectively monitoring the dynamics of Ca^{2+} with unprecedented spatial resolution. State-of-the-art GECIs include the single-wavelength intensiometric (the intensity of the fluorescence increases proportionally to Ca^{2+} increase) GCaMP's, which are based on circularly permuted green fluorescent protein (cpGFP), calmodulin (CaM), and the Ca^{2+}/CaM-binding "M13" peptide (M13pep) and FRET based indicators, which are ratiometric and require dual-channel recording [5, 8]. Single-wavelength intensiometric GECI's have a larger dynamic range; and thus, tend to be preferred over FRET based indicators. In mammalian cells a large number of probes have been produced for a variety of uses, including targeting to the endoplasmic reticulum, nucleus, mitochondria, Golgi, and endosome/peroxisomes [8]. The GCaMP6 series are highly sensitive probes with three variants available that differ in their kinetics [9] (Table 1). GCaMP6*s* has the slowest kinetics, GCaMP6*m* is faster while maintaining a high response, and GCaMP6*f* is the fastest variant [9].

The specific characteristics of these indicators have been recently reviewed [10]. Multicolor GECI's are also available like the red shifted variants jRGECO1a, jRCaMP1a/b, RCaMP, R-GECO, O-GECO, and CAR-GECO and the blue-shifted variants like B-GECO and GEM-GECO [6, 7]. Red indicators are of particular interest because red fluorescence is absorbed much less than green fluorescence, especially in mammalian cells, and the recently developed jGECO1a has acquired favorable kinetics to match GCaMP6s, giving red fluorophores a competitive advantage for in vivo imaging [11]. GECIs have been applied in a number of studies including neuronal physiology, *Drosophila*, mice, plants, primates, and parasites [12, 13].

The role of Ca^{2+} signaling in the lytic cycle—egress, extracellular motility, invasion, and replication—of *Toxoplasma* has been very well documented. In *Toxoplasma*, Ca^{2+} signaling results in the stimulation of gliding motility, microneme secretion, conoid extrusion, invasion and egress [14]. Many studies of Ca^{2+} signaling during the lytic cycle of *Toxoplasma gondii* were done indirectly by loading extracellular parasites with fluorescent dyes to follow Ca^{2+} changes during their gliding motility; through using Ca^{2+}

Table 1
Genetically encoded calcium indicators that have been used in *Toxoplasma gondii*

GECIs	K_d for Ca^{2+}	Dynamic range (F_{max}/F_{min})	References	Comments
GCaMP3	542 nM	13.5	Tian et al. [5] Borges et al. [13]	Improved dynamic range over first generation
GCaMP5g	460 nM	32.7	Akerboom et al. [45] Sidik et al. [16]	Improved dynamic range over GCaMP3
R-GECO	482 nM	16.0	Campbell et al. [6] Borges et al. [13]	First generation red GECI
B-GECO	164 nM	7	Campbell et al. [6] Borges et al. [13]	First generation blue GECI
GCaMP6f	375 nM	51.8	Kim et al. [9] Borges et al. [13] Brown et al. [20]	Fast on/off kinetics
GCaMP6s	144 nM	63.2	Kim et al. [9] Stewart et al. [21] Kuchipudi et al. [46]	Slow on/off kinetics
LAR-GECO1	24 μM	10	Campbell et al. [23]	Low affinity, endoplasmic reticulum targeted
LAR-GECO1.2	12 μM	8.7	Campbell et al. [23]	Low affinity, mitochondria targeted
jRGECO1a	148 nM	11.6	Kim et al. [11]	Second generation variant of R-GECO
jRCaMP1a	214 nM	3.2	Kim et al. [11]	Second generation red GECI
jRCaMP1b	712 nM	7.2	Kim et al. [11]	Second generation red GECI

ionophores [15], and other exogenous agents to elevate Ca^{2+} and stimulate conoid extrusion or microneme secretion; or using intracellular or extracellular Ca^{2+} chelators to prevent host-cell invasion or egress. The potential use of GECIs across a wide diversity of applications is still beginning to emerge and some pioneer studies have utilized GECIs in high-throughput screens of compounds that disrupt Ca^{2+} signaling in both mammalian cells and parasites [12, 16]. In this chapter we describe the methods used for the creation of *Toxoplasma* tachyzoites expressing GECIs and their validation and use.

2 Instruments and Materials

Hitachi fluorescence spectrophotometer models F-4500 and F-7000 (Hitachi High Technologies Corporation).

BioTek Synergy H1 hybrid multimode reader (BioTek).

Deltavision Elite or similar system for time-lapse experiments.

Hamilton microliter syringes with fixed needles, 5, 10, 25, and 50 μl sizes (Fisher catalog, 80075, 1482453A, 148247, 148245).

Toxoplasma gondii tachyzoites wild type, RH strain.

Human fibroblasts (immortalized via overexpression of the human telomerase reverse transcriptase gene (hTERT)) were originally from BD Biosciences.

Human epithelial HeLa cells (ATCC CCL-2™).

Tissue culture supplies.

GECI plasmids: GCaMP6f (Addgene 40755), GCaMP6m (Addgene 40754), GCaMP6s (Addgene 40753), R-GECO (Addgene 32462), B-GECO (Addgene 32448), jRGECO1a (Addgene 61563), jRCaMP1a (Addgene 61562), jRCaMP1b (Addgene 63136), ER-LAR-GECO1 (Addgene 32444), mito-LAR-GECO1.2 (Addgene 32461).

Toxoplasma plasmids: pCTH3 [17], pDT7S4H3 (a gift from Boris Striepen) [18], pTH3 (modified variant of pCTH3 in which the chloramphenicol cassette has been removed), [13], and pTUBSAG1-IEα_Dsred_DHFR_sag1CATsag1 (a gift from Vern Carruthers) [13, 19] and for UPRT locus: pUPRT::DHFR-GCaMP6(f/s) [20, 21].

Extracellular (Ringer's) buffer: 155 mM NaCl, 3 mM KCl, 2 mM $CaCl_2$, 1 mM $MgCl_2$, 3 mM NaH_2PO_4, 10 mM Hepes, pH 7.3, and 10 mM glucose.

Intracellular buffer: 140 mM potassium gluconate, 10 mM NaCl, 2.7 mM $MgSO_4$, 2 mM ATP (sodium salt), 1 mM glucose, 200 μM EGTA, 65 μM $CaCl_2$ (90 nM free Ca^{2+}), and 10 mM Tris/Hepes, pH 7.3.

Buffer A plus glucose: 116 mM NaCl, 5.4 mM KCl, 0.8 mM $MgSO_4$, 5.5 mM D-glucose, and 50 mM Hepes, pH 7.2.

PolyJet (SignaGen Laboratories, SL100688).

Fura2-AM (ThermoFisher F1221).

Ionomycin (Santa Cruz Biotechnology sc-3592).

Thapsigargin (Abcam ab120286).

Saponin (Sigma S-7900-25g)

Zaprinast (Sigma 684500-25MG).

35 mm glass bottom cover dishes (MatTek Corp P35G-1.5-20-C).

Tissue Culture Cloning Cylinders (Bel-Art 978470100).

3   Methods

3.1   *Plasmid Construction*

It is ideal and possible to generate *T. gondii* tachyzoites stably expressing GECIs. This can be done by stable integration of GECI genes into the genome of *T. gondii*. This has been achieved either through nonhomologous, random integration into the genome [13] or by integration of the GECI genes into a specific locus of the genome like the UPRT (uracil phosphoribosyltransferase) locus, which is not essential for parasite survival in vitro [21]. GECI genes that are introduced at the genomic locus of the UPRT gene are expressed uniformly because they are under the control of the same cis-element across different clones (*see* **Note 1**). Plasmids for nonhomologous/random integration include pCTH3, pTH3, and pDT7S4H3, while plasmids for integration into the UPRT locus using homologous recombination include pUPRT::DHFR-GCaMP6(f/s) [20, 21].

Without a targeting sequence, GECI genes are expressed in the cytosol. The addition of the superoxide dismutase (SOD2) targeting sequence at the 5′-end of the *GECI gene* confers localization to the mitochondria [22]. In our lab we have successfully constructed stable strains expressing GCaMP6f and LAR-GECO1.2 (low affinity red GECI) [23] targeted to the mitochondria (Fig. 1). In order

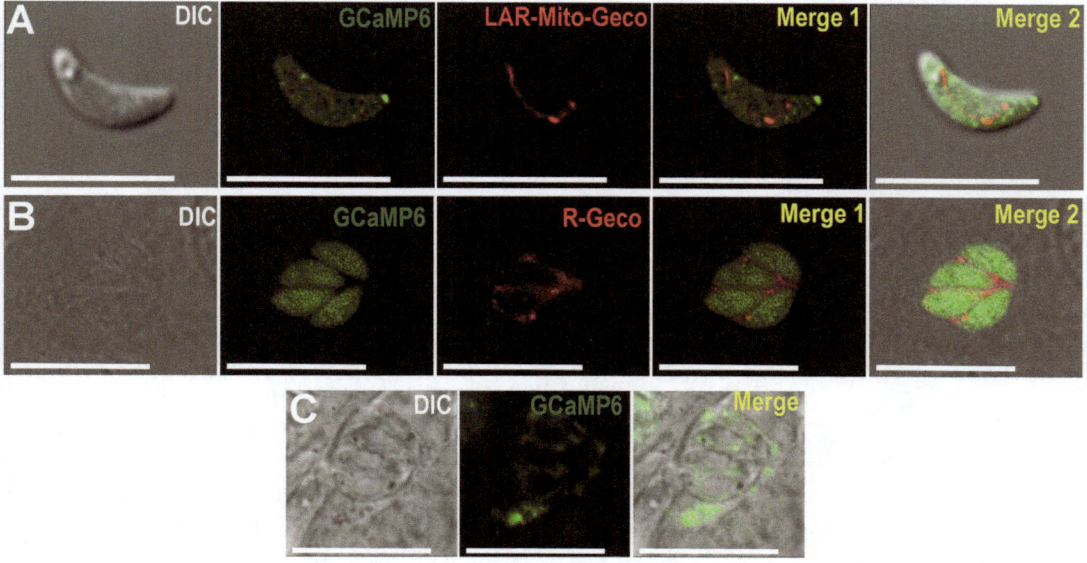

Fig. 1 Images of *Toxoplasma gondii* parasites expressing GCaMP6f in the cytoplasm, mitochondria and parasitophorous vacuole. (**a**) Live cell imaging of extracellular tachyzoites of the RH strain expressing GCaMP6f (pTUBGCaMP6f) (green) in the cytosol and LAR-Geco (pDT7S4H3-SOD2-Mito-LAR-Geco) in the mitochondria (red). (**b**) Live cell imaging of intracellular parasites expressing GCaMP6f (pTUBGCaMP6f) in the cytosol (green) and R-GECO (ptub_SAG1-IEα-R-GECO_dhfr_sag1CATsag1) in the PV (red). (**c**) Live cell imaging of intracellular RH parasites expressing GCaMP6f (pDT7S4H3-P30-GCaMP6f) in PV

to target a GECI to the endoplasmic reticulum the coding sequence of the *P30 gene* (major Surface Antigen 1 of *Toxoplasma*) is fused to its *5′-end* and the ER retention signal HDEL to its 3′ end [17]. We suggest using LAR-GECO1.0, a red GECI whose kinetics favor expression within the endoplasmic reticulum [23]. We have observed expression of GECIs in the ER only transiently (unpublished). Parasites do not appear to tolerate the expression of these indicators in the ER and we have not been able to isolate clones. The addition of the ferredoxin $NADP^+$ reductase (FNR) targeting sequence at the *5′-end* will confer localization to the apicoplast, and we have successfully constructed a stable strain expressing GCaMP6f localized to the apicoplast [24] (unpublished). For expression of GECIs in the parasitophorous vacuole (PV) the vector ptub_SAG1-IE_ DsRed_dhfr_sag1CATsag1 can be used and the GECI of interest like GCaMPs or GECOs can be cloned at the SmaI (5′)/SnaBI (3′) restriction sites, substituting the DsRed gene. Selection can be done using antibiotic resistance or alternatively through enrichment and subclone of a population previously sorted by Fluorescence Activated Cell Sorting (FACS) [17, 24]. We have modified the plasmid pCTH3 [25] by removing the chloramphenicol cassette to generate pTH3. This plasmid has successfully been used to generate stable cell lines expressing GCaMP6f/s alone or in tandem with a (P)2A cleavage site (*see* below **Note 8**) preceding a red fluorescence protein for ratiometric measurements [26]. 2A peptides (P2A, T2A, F2A, and E2A) are highly conserved peptides sequences that fail to form a peptide bond between a glycine and a proline residue at the carboxy terminus of a consensus sequence, through a mechanism termed ribosomal skipping. Translation of the proline and downstream gene continues resulting in two, separate peptide products originating from a single mRNA [27].

3.2 Transfection, Selection and Subcloning

Transfection of *T. gondii* tachyzoites with GECI plasmids is performed using a published protocol [28]. The DNA used for transfection is resuspended in 100 µl of cytomix solution (120 mM KCl, 0.15 mM $CaCl_2$ 10 mM K_2HPO_4/KH_2PO_4, 25 mM HEPES pH 7.6, 2 mM EGTA, 5 mM $MgCl_2$). Freshly isolated and purified parasites are resuspended in the same solution at a concentration of 3.3×10^7/ml. 300 µl of cell suspension and 100 µl of DNA (20–100 µg) is mixed in a 0.4 cm electroporation cuvette. We use a BioRad electroporator with an exponential decay protocol set at 1.5 kV, 25 µF. Pulse time is usually between 0.4 and 0.6 ms.

With the aim of isolating a clonal population, GECI expressing parasites are first selected with drugs if they were transfected with plasmids containing known selectable marker genes like dihydrofolate reductase (DHFR) for pyrimethamine selection and chloramphenicol acetyl transferase for chloramphenicol selection. For GECI genes introduced into the UPRT locus, the pro-drug 5′-fluo-2′-deoxyuridine (FUDR) is used for selection. After selection, drug resistant parasites are serially diluted in 96-well plates and allowed to grow for 6–7 days. Wells with one small plaque are selected for further analysis. When using plasmids devoid of selectable markers, parasites are sorted and enriched by FACS. In this case, parasites can be FACS sorted two independent times to obtain single clones of GECI expressing parasites. Following electroporation, parasites are dispensed into a small T25 flask previously prepared with confluent fibroblasts and allowed to grow until they lyse out. The first FACS sorting can be done with the parasites released from this culture, producing approximately 500–5000 parasites likely expressing the *GECI gene*. This enriched population is dispensed into a new T25 flask and allowed to grow until parasites egress naturally. These parasites can be subjected to a second (and third) round of FACS sorting. In the second sorting, parasites are categorized in weak, medium or strong expression of the *GECI gene*. We typically use parasites with a medium level of GECI expression, because highly fluorescent parasites will likely have higher fluorescence background resulting in a lower functional dynamic range of the GECI fluorescence. After this final FACS sorting, the desired enriched population is diluted into a 96 well plate at 1 parasite/well in order to obtain single clones.

It is possible to express GECIs (GCaMPs or GECOs) at specific compartments like the cytosol (Fig. 1a), mitochondria (Fig. 1a), apicoplast (not shown) or the parasitophorous vacuole (Fig. 1b, c) by using specific targeting signals like the mitochondrial targeting signal of the superoxide dismutase [22], the apicoplast targeting signal of the ferredoxin oxidoreductase [29, 30] and the vector ptub_SAG1-IE_ GECI_dhfr_sag1CATsag1 for PV labeling [19]. Transfection, selection and subcloning is done as described above and these clones expressing rGECO or GCaMP6 in the PV (Fig. 1b, c) are further characterized for their egress phenotype as described below.

3.3 Selecting an Isolate with Ideal Fluorescence Properties (See Note 2)

We usually analyze 10–12 clones for their responses to ionophores, inhibitors and extracellular calcium. Figure 2a, b shows the characterization of 2 clones transfected with GCaMP6f and Fig. 2c, d shows the characterization of two clones expressing GCaMP6s (*see* Table 1 for the characteristics of each indicator). GCaMP6s-expressing parasites show larger fluorescence increase in response to agonists and we attribute this to the slower Ca^{2+} dissociation kinetics of the indicator (compare the response of GCaMP6f to the response of clones 7 and 9 that express GCaMP6s in Fig. 2b).

The procedure to select the fittest clone with maximum response is described:

1. Clonal lines are grown in flasks with confluent hTERT fibroblasts to yield approximately 5×10^8 parasites. Tachyzoites are collected 48 h after infection and when the culture shows

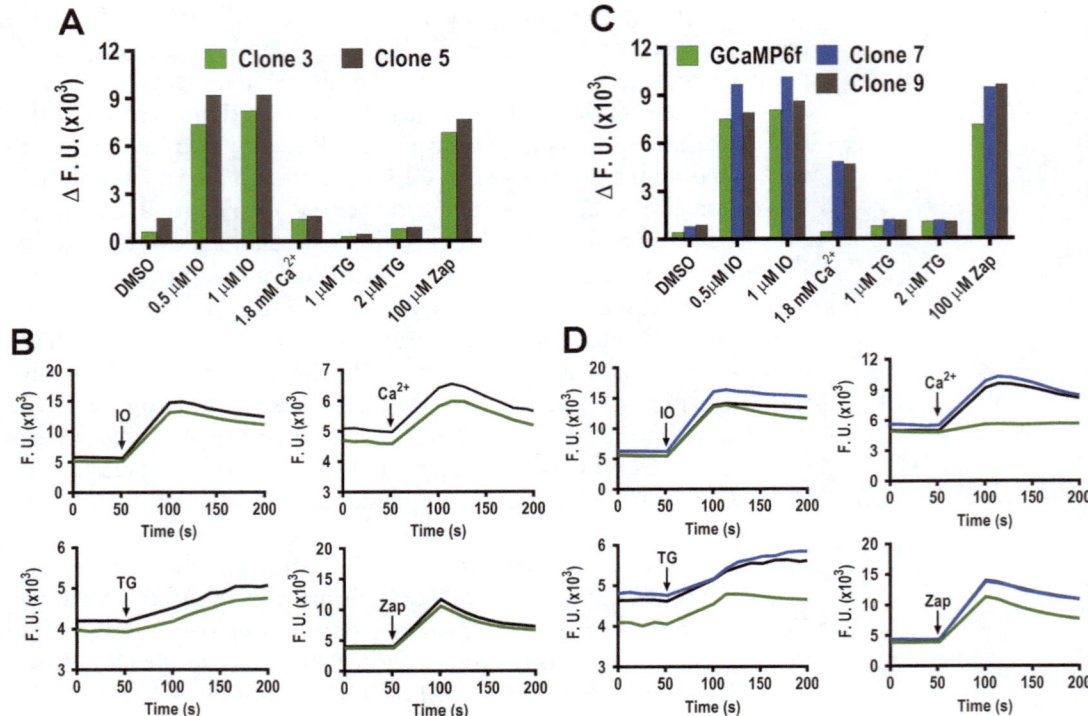

Fig. 2 Characterization of clones in a plate reader. A suspension of 5×10^6 tachyzoites/ml in Ringer's buffer with 100 µM of EGTA is dispensed into each well of a 96 well plate after shaking for 3 min the fluorescence is measured. Reagents are added at 60 s (Subheading 3.3). (**a**) Fluorescence changes before and after the addition of the indicated reagents with two *Toxoplasma* clones (3 and 5). DMSO is used as a control. (**b**) Kinetic measurements for clones 3 and 5 showing changes in the fluorescence of GCaMP6f in function of time. *IO* Ionomycin, *TG* Thapsigargin, *Zap* Zaprinast, Ca^{2+} Extracellular Ca^{2+}, 1.8 mM. (**c**) Same experiment to the one presented in A with clones 7 and 9 that express GCaMP6s and compare with the reference cell line expressing GCamp6f. (**d**) Kinetic measurements with clones 7 and 9. Same conditions as (**b**)

70–80% host cell lysis. Parasites are gently scraped off, purified by filtration through an 8 µM nucleopore membrane and centrifuged at $706 \times g$ for 10 min. The parasites are washed twice and resuspended to a final concentration of 6×10^7 parasites/ ml in extracellular buffer: 155 mM NaCl, 3 mM KCl, 2 mM $CaCl_2$, 1 mM $MgCl_2$, 3 mM NaH_2PO_4, 10 mM Hepes, pH 7.3, and 10 mM glucose.

2. 100 µl of the parasite suspension prepared in 1 is dispensed into each well of a 96 well and 100 µM EGTA is added to each well to chelate extracellular Ca^{2+} (*see* **Note 3**).

3. The plate reader is set to record Green and Red Fluorescence changes using monochromators set to the respective channels: GCaMP6f/s 487 excitation and 508 emission and mScarletI (for ratiometric measurements) 569 excitation and 593 emission. We use a BioTek Synergy H4 Plate Reader with a tungsten halogen and xenon flash as the light source.

4. Fluorescence changes in response to the addition of: DMSO as control for solvent (0.4%), thapsigargin (TG) (0.5 and 1 µM), ionomycin (IO) (0.5 and 1 µM), zaprinast (Zap) (100 µM) and Ca^{2+} (1.8 mM) are measured (Fig. 2).

5. In a standard measurement, 3 min are allowed to establish a baseline followed by the addition of the ionophore or inhibitor. The concentration of the solution of the reagent is adjusted so the volume added is 20 µl per well. Fluorescence is measured for 4 min after addition of the reagent. Representative tracings are shown in Fig. 2b, d.

6. The average fluorescence prior to addition of the reagent is subtracted from the maximum peak fluorescence attained after addition of the reagent to calculate the ΔF shown in Fig. 2a, c of 3 replicative wells for each condition. We select two clones that show largest ΔF indicating larger response to cytosolic Ca^{2+} (Fig. 2).

3.4 Characterization of Isolates: Ensuring Isolate Retains WT Calcium Signaling Properties

These control experiments will measure cytosolic calcium of the GECI expressing mutants, by loading the GECI-expressing tachyzoites with the membrane permeable chemical fluorescent calcium indicator, Fura2-AM, and measuring fluorescence changes from both indicators using a high sensitivity, fast switching, fluorescence spectrophotometer (*see* **Notes 3** and **4**). In addition, if cells express the ratiometric version of GCaMP6 (GCaMP6-mScarlett for example) both the fluorescence of GCaMP and the fluorescence of the reference protein can be recorded for calculation of the fluorescence ratio.

The loading of the chemical indicator to carry out these controls can be performed as follows:

1. *Host cell preparation (see **Note 5**).*

    Confluent T75 flasks of hTERT cells (the surface area of the flask is completely covered by the cell monolayer) are detached and resuspended to a concentration of 5×10^7 host cells/ml in DMEM-HG media with 10% calf serum and aliquoted into 3–5 T75 flasks. These cells should be allowed to grow to complete confluency (typically 5–7 days).

2. *Toxoplasma infection (see **Note 6**).*

    Prior to parasite infection the media of the hTERT flasks (T75s) is replaced with fresh DMEM-HG media containing 1% calf serum prewarmed at 37 °C. 4–6 T75 flasks should be infected with $1.5–2.5 \times 10^7$ parasites per flask 48 h prior to the desired time of collection. The media of these flasks is replaced with the same media 12–24 h after infection to remove any dead parasites and host cell debris.

3. *Collecting parasites.*

    Parasites are collected ~48 h after infection. Ideally, at the time of collection, flasks should contain approximately 50% of host cells lysed and 50% heavily infected. A cell scraper is utilized to detach the entire monolayer, as it should only be partially lysed. This parasite/host cell solution should be transferred and filtered through a vacuum filter holder with receiver, housing a 47 mm, 8.0 μM Nuclepore Track-Etch Membrane. This filtered suspension is then transferred to a 50 ml conical tube and centrifuged at RT for 10 min at 705 × g. The pellet is gently resuspended in 10 ml of Ringer's buffer and a small aliquot diluted for counting. The suspension is centrifuged again at 705 × g for 10 min. The resulting pellet is resuspended at 1 × 10^9 tachyzoites/ml in Ringer's buffers with 1.5% sucrose (loading buffer) for Fura2-AM loading.

4. *Loading of Fura2-AM.*

   Fura2-AM is added to this cell suspension (or to the loading buffer) to a final concentration of 5.15 μM and is allowed to incubate at 26 °C for 27 min, protected from light (*see* **Note 7**). Parasites are then centrifuged at 875 × g for 2 min and washed twice in 1 ml of Ringer's buffer and resuspended at 1 × 10^9 tachyzoites/ml. Parasites are viable for fluorometric experiments for approximately 2–3 h if kept on ice and covered from light.

5. *Fluorometric analysis (Fig. 3).*

   Fluorescence measurements are carried out in a cuvette containing 5 × 10^7 tachyzoites in suspension in 2.5 ml of the appropriate reaction buffer. The parasites have been previously loaded with a fluorescent indicator or are expressing a genetic calcium indicator. The cuvette is placed in a Hitachi F-7000 or F-4500 fluorescence spectrophotometer, which allows kinetic measurements. These experiments are typically performed in extracellular buffer with 100 μM EGTA to chelate contaminating Ca^{2+}. GCaMP6f excitation is 488 nm with emission at 510 nm. If two fluorescent proteins are expressed, such as GCaMP6 and mScarlet, an RFP, red fluorescence can also be measured. mScarlet excitation is 569 nm with emission at 594 nm [31]. Fura2-AM has excitations of 380 nm for its Ca^{2+} un-bound state, and 340 nm for its Ca^{2+}-bound state with emission at 510 nm. The instrument's parameters need to be adjusted to accommodate the consecutive measurements of two reagents (Fura2-AM and GCaMP6f) with appropriate excitation and emission wavelengths selected. The shortest cycle time allowable on the instrument should be selected.

   The cycle time parameter will determine how fast the instrument switches from excitation and emissions from the first reagent to the second. Drugs and reagents are added via an appropriately sized Hamilton syringe during fluorometric readings, whereby changes in fluorescence of the indicators are detected in real time.

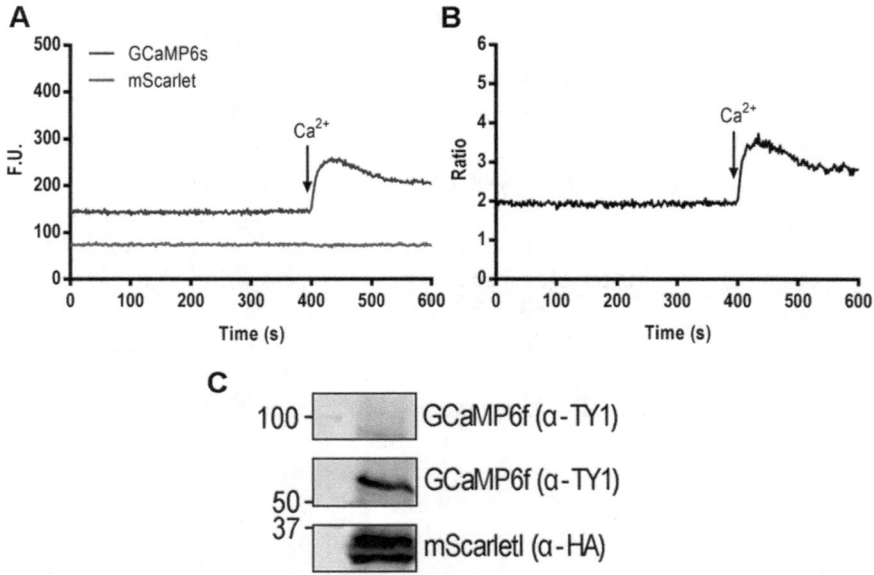

Fig. 3 Ratiometric measurements with a clone expressing GCaMP6s-mScarlet. (**a**) GCaMP and mScarlet fluorescence changes in function of time measured in the F-7000 fluorescence spectrophotometer. (**a**) Parasites at a concentration of 2×10^7 tachyzoites/ml were resuspended in Ringer's buffer with 100 μM of EGTA at a final volume of 2.5 ml. 1.8 mM of Ca^{2+} is added at 400 s. (**b**) Ratio calculation of the fluorescence tracings shown in (**a**). (**c**) Western blots showing the expression of GCaMP6f-Ty1 and mScarletl-3xHA. Antibodies: Mouse α-Ty1 1:2000 (a generous gift from Dr. Etheridge) and Rat α-HA 1:200 (Roche). Secondary: goat α-mouse IRDye 800 (LI-COR) and goat α-rat IRDye 680 (LI-COR)

3.5 Time Lapse Microscopy of GCaMP6f-Expressing Parasites (See Notes 8 and 9)

After successful characterization and isolation of the ideal clone, the clonal line can be used to study cytosolic Ca^{2+} oscillations across the lytic cycle. The methodologies described below are for egress and extracellular motility. These protocols represent a general template and can be tailored (for example, host cell choice, imaging dish, laser exposure, and laser intensity) to match the needs/equipment of the user:

1. *Plating HeLa cells for microscopy.*

    A confluent T25 flask of HeLa cells is split and plated onto 6–8 35 mm glass bottom MatTek dishes and grown overnight using DMEM-HG with 10% FBS. Ideally, the cells should be 60–70% confluent by the next day.

2. *Transient transfection of host cells.*

    For transient transfection of HeLa cells we typically use 3 μL of PolyJet in Vitro DNA transfection Reagent to 1 μg of DNA, as per the manufacturer's instructions.

3. *Infecting for microscopy.*

    From a lysed culture of tachyzoites expressing GCaMP6f we infect with 1×10^6 parasites per MatTek dish of HeLa cells and let them grow overnight. We image these dishes 24 h after the infection and we select parasitophorous vacuoles (PVs) with 2–4 tachyzoites because those are the ones that will allow us to analyze single cell fluctuations without interference of the fluorescence of the neighboring parasite. Parasites in PVs with 8 or more parasites are difficult to single out.

4. *Time lapse for Ca^{2+} oscillations in intracellular parasites.*

We image cells at 37 °C using a Deltavision Elite system. First, the DMEM-HG is replaced with extracellular (Ringer's) buffer. Because this buffer is more defined and does not contain phenol red, which quenches fluorescence, making it the preferred buffer to use for egress experiments. As per settings, we generally use 32% or 10% laser intensity for the FITC (Fluorescein Isothiocyanate), 32% for DIC (Differential Interference Contrast), and 10% laser intensity for TRITC (Tetramethylrhodamine) filter sets with an acquisition rate of 1 frame per second per each channel with approximately 0.150 ms or lower exposure. A typical movie observing Ca^{2+} oscillations and egress lasts about 10–20 min including 1 min of baseline prior to Ca^{2+} or other pharmacological drug addition; the remaining 9–19 min are used to record the response and recovery from the stimuli. The final drug concentrations that can be used are ionomycin (0.1–1 μM), histamine (5 and 100 μM), thapsigargin (1 μM), DTT (5 mM) saponin (0.01%), and nifedipine (10 μM). For Ca^{2+} free experiments, we use Ringer's buffer supplemented with 100 μM or 1 mM EGTA or 1 mM BAPTA. An example of a typical egress video with Thapsigargin stimulation in which the host cells are transiently transfected with R-GECO and infected with GCaMP6f expressing parasites can be seen in Fig. 4. Egress videos are quantified using the FIJI ImageJ plugin suite [32].

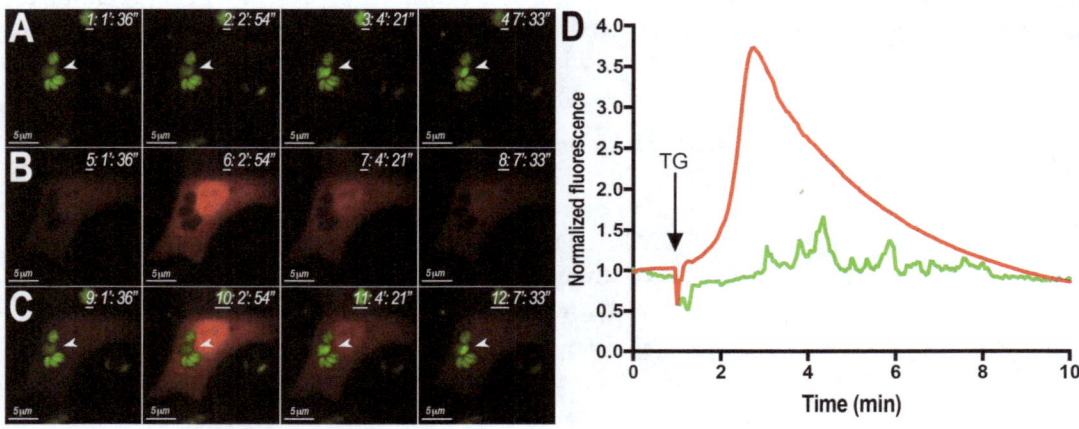

Fig. 4 In Vivo Dual Imaging of Host Cells Infected with GCaMP6f Expressing Parasites. (**a, b**) Still-images obtained from videos showing changes of GCaMP (tachyzoites) and GECO (Hela cells) fluorescence after exposure to 2 μM thapsigargin (TG). (**c**) Overlay of (**a, b**). (**d**) Fluorescence Tracings of Host Cells (red) and Parasites (green) after exposure to thapsigargin (TG). Video taken by Christina Moore

5. *Long term time-lapse microscopy.*

For long-term time-lapse experiments, we typically use Ibidi 35 mm μ-Dish. These are designed with a lid that locks into place in order to minimize evaporation. The main concern when performing a long-term time-lapse experiment is photobleaching and phototoxicity from continual laser exposure. While new microscopes are becoming available that help mitigate these two issues, such as light-sheet microscopy, we adjust our exposure settings on the Deltavision to image each channel every 2 min [33].

6. *Motility experiments.*

For extracellular motility experiments, we use 35 mm glass bottom coverslip dishes (MatTek) that are treated overnight with 2 ml of a 10% FBS solution in a phosphate-buffered saline solution (PBS) at 4 °C. The dishes are washed once with PBS prior to use. Freshly egressed tachyzoites expressing GCaMP6f are collected, purified, and resuspended in 1 ml of Ringer's buffer supplemented with 100 μM EGTA. We usually load ~2.5 × 10^7 parasites divided evenly among 6–8 dishes and incubate the dishes on ice for ~15 min to allow for the parasites to adhere. We use a small tissue culture cloning cylinders (Bel-Art, Cat # 378470100) to keep parasites concentrated in the middle of the dish to increase the efficiency of imaging. After removing the cell cylinder, we wash very gently with 1 ml of Ringer's Buffer and bring the final volume back up to 2 ml with the same buffer supplemented with 100 μM EGTA. We image using a Zeiss LSM 710 confocal microscope set at 37 °C. Prior to imaging, we allow for cells to warm up for ~5 min at 37 °C. After establishment of a 1.5–2 min baseline for imaging, we stimulate gliding motility using pharmacological agents (*see* Time Lapse Egress Protocol for drug concentrations), and approximately an additional 900 frames are recorded. MTrackJ is a FIJI/ImageJ plugin that can manually track objects within a given movie (https://imagescience.org/meijering/software/mtrackj/). MTrackJ interface is simple and user friendly and has successfully been used to track parasites [34]. Typically, our lab uses a custom-made motility algorithm to track calcium oscillations in extracellular parasites and we have successfully applied the algorithm to track egressing parasites [35, 36]. This algorithm uses optical flow and fluorescence intensities to robustly track Ca^{2+} oscillations in extracellular parasites. For this algorithm, images must be input in dimensions of 400 × 400 at a frame rate of 20 fps.

4   Notes

Plasmid Construction

1. The disadvantage of random integration of the GECI gene in an unspecified location of the genome, is that it could result in additional effects on the fitness of the parasites. The expression level of the GECI gene varies within different clones because it depends where it is inserted in the genome. Since calcium levels are tightly regulated in cells, and the GECIs can bind Ca^{2+} to affect the free calcium level, we reasoned that different expression level of the GECIs may have different effect on Ca^{2+} homeostasis. Random integration allows us to select clones with different expression level of the GECIs for different experiments.

Characterization of Isolates

2. GECIs are useful tools to study Ca^{2+} content of organelles and potential microdomains in *Toxoplasma*. GCaMPs have been designed to detect Ca^{2+} via a Ca^{2+} binding protein, calmodulin (CaM). Calmodulins are Ca^{2+} binding proteins expressed in all eukaryotic cells that participate in a number of signaling pathways that control important cellular functions [37]. Introducing extra copies of CaM, by way of a GECI, can potentially alter the Ca^{2+} dynamic in the cell [38]. It is highly recommended to perform control experiments with all GECI-expressing cell lines to determine if the transgenic line still retains the calcium signaling properties of a non-GECI expressing parasite (WT). We usually perform growth assays or plaque assays (Fig. 5a), egress experiments of intracellular parasites (Fig. 5b), response to extracellular Ca^{2+} (Fig. 5c) and test cytosolic Ca^{2+} responses with Fura2-AM loaded parasites (Fig. 5d, e). We check if changes in GECI's fluorescence are concurrent with the changes observed with chemical indicators. The experiment shown in Fig. 5d, e compare the Ca^{2+} response between RH and a clonal line expressing GCaMP6s (compare black and blue tracings). It is evident that the responses are diminished in the GECI expressing parasites and we attribute this to the Ca^{2+}-binding effect of the genetic indicator. It is very likely that the expression of an exogenous copy of GCaMP6 would alter the Ca^{2+} dynamics.

3. For plate reader measurements, we test several concentrations of parasites per well. The number of parasites needs to be adjusted because of the lower sensitivity of the plate reader compared to the fluorescence spectrophotometer. Too few parasites may not be sufficient to produce a response for thapsigargin or Ca^{2+}. These two triggers usually lead to an increase

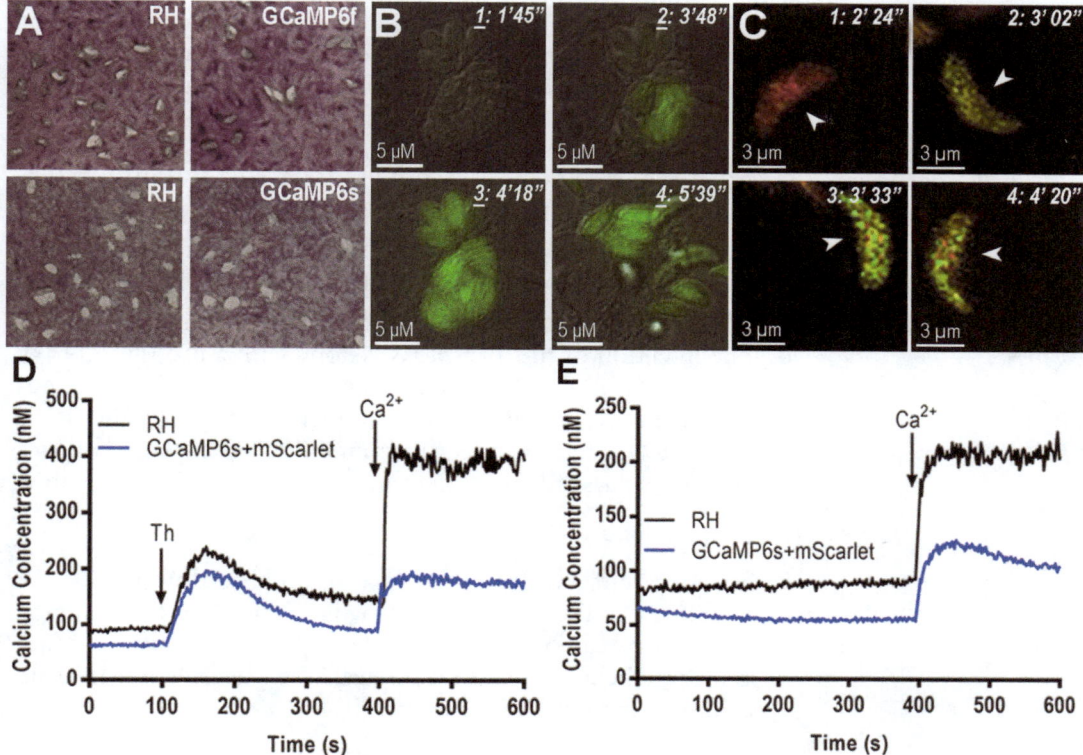

Fig. 5 Physiological characteristics of tachyzoites expressing GECIs. (**a**) Plaques formed after 7 days of growth of 200 freshly isolated and purified tachyzoites per well. The host cells are hTERT previously grown to confluency in 6 well plates. Infected host cell monolayer was fixed with 70% EtOH and stained with crystal violet. Plaque sizes were measured using FIJI. The plaques formed by tachyzoites expressing GCaMPf and GCaMPs were similar to the ones formed by tachyzoites of the RH strain (WT). (**b**) egress experiments of tachyzoites expressing GCaMP6f. Hela cells were grown in MatTek dishes for 24 h and infected with 1 x 10^6 tachyzoites. Egress was stimulated with 100 μM of Zaprinast which was added 1 min after the start of the recording. (**c**) GCaMP6f-Ty1-P2A-mScarletl expressing parasites were loaded in media supplemented with 100 μM EGTA. 1.8 mM Ca^{2+} was added (at ~3 min) leading to an increase in the GCaMP6f fluorescence signal. The signal from the mScarletl is Ca^{2+} insensitive thus allowing for ratiometric analysis. (**d**) tachyzoites expressing GCaMP6s and mScarlet were loaded with FURA2-AM (*see* Subheading 3.4) to measure cytosolic calcium in response to 1 μM thapsigargin, which was added at 100 s and 1.8 mM calcium, added at 400 s. (**e**) Same as (**c**) but only 1.8 mM of calcium was added at 400 s. Cytosolic calcium responses were compared between RH strain (*black tracing*) and the GCaMP6s expressing parasites (*blue tracing*)

of cytosolic Ca^{2+} of 200–300 nM and it is possible that this change could be unnoticed if the number of parasites is too low. If the number of parasites is too high it can oversaturate the reading. We found that 6×10^7 is the ideal number for these experiments.

4. Clones with high background fluorescence are not ideal because they could potentially be unfit. We select clones with the largest range in response to ionophores and inhibitor additions and in general these clones show low background fluorescence.

Parasite Growth, Purification, and Loading

5. Flasks with 75 cm^2 of growth area (T75) produce the highest yield of *Toxoplasma* tachyzoites within a reliable timeframe as long as they are infected with a specific number of parasites per flask (*see* **Note 6**) and the media is changed 8–24 h after the initial infection. Larger flasks, like 175 cm^2 provide a larger surface but the total yield of parasites per flask is not correlative to the size and volume used. We find that the progression of the infection tends to be uneven in larger flasks and the collected time and number of parasites is unpredictable.

6. The infection of the T75 flasks is done with a fixed number of parasites (1–2.5×10^7 total parasites). This number depends on the fitness of the parasites used for infection. Usually, a completely lysed culture will contain a larger proportion of unhealthy parasites and will require a higher infection number.

Fluorometric Experimentation with GECI Cell Lines

7. For more efficient loading it is a better procedure to add the Fura2-AM to the loading buffer, which is used to resuspend the parasites instead of adding it to the suspension. Parasite loading is more efficient and result in healthier parasites when using volumes larger than 300 µl.

Imaging/Microscopy

8. Ca^{2+} dynamics in *T. gondii* parasites expressing GECIs can be studied by video microscopy along its lytic cycle (Fig. 4). In *Toxoplasma* GECI's have been successfully used to visualize Ca^{2+} fluctuations during invasion, egress and gliding [14]. GECI expressing parasites were also used for genetic screens to identify regulators of Ca^{2+} signaling, and probe how pharmacological stimulation induces increases in cytosolic Ca^{2+} levels [16]. Recent work combining Hela cells expressing cytosolic R-GECO infected with parasites expressing GCaMP6f demonstrated that an increase in host cytosolic Ca^{2+} preceded Ca^{2+} oscillations in the parasite [13]. Expression of the B-GECO indicator in the cytosol of Hela and their infection with tachyzoites expressing cytosolic GCaMP3 or GCaMP6 and R-GECO in their PV, allowed to follow simultaneously Ca^{2+} fluctuations in the host cytosol (blue), the PV (red) and the parasite cytosol (green) [13]. This was only possible because of specific expression of genetic indicators in the host cytoplasm, the parasitophorous vacuole and the *Toxoplasma* cytosol. Additionally, GECI's have been applied to extracellular parasites as well in which parasites clones expressing GCaMP6f/s were used to track Ca^{2+} oscillations in motile parasites and link them to motility patterns [13, 35, 36, 39]. GCaMPs are single-wavelength and prone to artifacts such as loss of focus, bleaching, and imprecise initial detection due to low baseline.

A partial solution to this problem is the simultaneous expression of a "reference" indicator insensitive to calcium that will help correct for these issues. Ratiometric studies in *T. gondii* using parasites expressing GCaMP6s and mCherry, both driven by separate promoters, but in the same genomic location has been employed by Stewart et al. [21]. An alternative mechanism to produce two separate proteins is to use the well-characterized 2A system. In this strategy, a short peptide is introduced between the transcripts corresponding to two proteins in the same mRNA. During translation, the ribosome fails to form a peptide bond between a conserved glycine and proline residue. This system has been successfully utilized in *Plasmodium* and *Toxoplasma* [26, 40]. Additionally, our lab has successfully constructed ratiometric strains expressing GCaMP6f-(P)2A-mScarletI [30], and the expression validated by Western Blots (Figs. 3 and 5c), which show that the 2A functions correctly to produce two separate proteins. Fluorometric analysis confirms mScarlet's insensitivity to calcium. In frame fusion of a Ca^{2+} insensitive reference fluorescence protein is not advised due to the potential risk for FRET interaction [41]. These ratiometric strategies enable calibration of the GECI using digitonin or ionomycin, though these studies have been performed in mammalian cells and not in parasites [42]. As GECI's are fluorescent proteins, they are prone to intrinsic factors that should be taken into consideration. GECI performance is susceptible to brightness (extinction coefficient $\times$ quantum yield), pH, folding/stability, and photobleaching, and these factors should be considered when imaging with GECI's [5].

9. GECI's enable for long-term imaging, but care must be taken to avoid phototoxicity. As a general rule, we prefer to use approximately one frame per second for egress experiments and approximately two frames per second for extracellular motility. We also prefer to use GCaMP-expressing parasites over R-GECO and jRGECO1a expressing parasites. GCaMP's are further developed and exhibit a larger dynamic range and less photobleaching [11, 43]. A relatively universal standard for comparing GECI performance is the signal-to-noise ratio (SNR). The SNR is defined as the ratio of the fluorescence signal change ($\Delta F = F_{obs} - F_0$, where F_{obs} is sensor fluorescence at peak [Ca^{2+}] and F_0 is sensor fluorescence at baseline [Ca^{2+}]) to the baseline fluorescence ($F_0\ N^{-1/2}$, where N is the number of photons detected by the sensor) [44]. For extracellular motility experiments, we prefer to use a Zeiss LSM 710 confocal microscope. Confocal microscopy offers enhanced Z-resolution and appears to offer improved sensitivity in detecting Ca^{2+} oscillations in motile parasites.

Additionally, since the light is more focused in a confocal microscope (and coupled to the small size of a *T. gondii* cell (~5 μm)), our cells seem to require less excitation; and thus, we see less phototoxicity versus our widefield microscope. On the contrary, when working with intracellular parasite and egress experiments we prefer to use the Deltavision Elite widefield microscope. Though sacrificing *Z*-resolution versus confocal microscopy, widefield microscopy offers improved area of focus through imaging larger surface area. While imaging both fluorescent host cells as well as parasites, this feature enables for a broader image that encompasses both the entire host cell as well as the parasite to provide for a sharper image in comparison to the LSM710. Though improvements have been made to red GECI's their brightness and photostability are not comparable with the GCaMP series, thus brightness is an important consideration. Because widefield microscope does not attenuate the signal through a pinhole, signal strength is stronger and requires less excitation for visualization. Additionally, the Deltavision also has a "Fast Acquisition" mode that rapidly switches between channels and can be ideal for fast, sensitive multicolor Ca^{2+} imaging experiments to detect Ca^{2+} oscillation, though it should be noted that a confocal is capable of capturing the signaling from 2–4 fluorophores but at a slow speed. If a phase-contrast image is desired, we prefer to use the Deltavision's differential interference contrast. While DIC is possible on the LSM710, it is possible that the Deltavision's use of a more efficient charge-coupled device (CCD) versus a photomultiplier tube (PMT) on the confocal provides for a sharper, crisper image, as a CCD, generally speaking, has a higher quantum yield over a PMT.

Acknowledgments

This work was partially funded by NIH grants AI096836, AI128356, and AI110027 to S.N.J.M.
A.C. was supported by an NIH diversity supplement to AI128356. S.V. was partially supported by a fellowship of the Office of the Vice-President for Research, UGA. We would also like to thank Dr. Muthugapatti Kandasamy from the Biomedical Microscopy Core and Julie Nelson from the Cytometry Shared Resource Laboratory of the University of Georgia.
Eric Dykes helped performed the westerns of the cells expressing GCAMP-mScarlet and Christina Moore made the videos used for Fig. 4.

References

1. Berridge MJ, Bootman MD, Roderick HL (2003) Calcium signalling: dynamics, homeostasis and remodelling. Nat Rev Mol Cell Biol 4 (7):517–529

2. Grynkiewicz G, Poenie M, Tsien RY (1985) A new generation of Ca^{2+} indicators with greatly improved fluorescence properties. J Biol Chem 260(6):3440–3450

3. McCombs JE, Palmer AE (2008) Measuring calcium dynamics in living cells with genetically encodable calcium indicators. Methods 46 (3):152–159

4. Tian L, Hires SA, Mao T, Huber D, Chiappe ME, Chalasani SH, Petreanu L, Akerboom J, McKinney SA, Schreiter ER, Bargmann CI, Jayaraman V, Svoboda K, Looger LL (2009) Imaging neural activity in worms, flies and mice with improved GCaMP calcium indicators. Nat Methods 6(12):875–881

5. Tian L, Hires SA, Looger LL (2012) Imaging neuronal activity with genetically encoded calcium indicators. Cold Spring Harb Protoc 2012(6):647–656

6. Zhao Y, Araki S, Wu J, Teramoto T, Chang YF, Nakano M, Abdelfattah AS, Fujiwara M, Ishihara T, Nagai T, Campbell RE (2011) An expanded palette of genetically encoded Ca(2)(+) indicators. Science 333(6051):1888–1891

7. Akerboom J, Carreras Calderon N, Tian L, Wabnig S, Prigge M, Tolo J, Gordus A, Orger MB, Severi KE, Macklin JJ, Patel R, Pulver SR, Wardill TJ, Fischer E, Schuler C, Chen TW, Sarkisyan KS, Marvin JS, Bargmann CI, Kim DS, Kugler S, Lagnado L, Hegemann P, Gottschalk A, Schreiter ER, Looger LL (2013) Genetically encoded calcium indicators for multi-color neural activity imaging and combination with optogenetics. Front Mol Neurosci 6:2

8. Suzuki J, Kanemaru K, Iino M (2016) Genetically encoded fluorescent indicators for organellar calcium imaging. Biophys J 111 (6):1119–1131

9. Chen TW, Wardill TJ, Sun Y, Pulver SR, Renninger SL, Baohan A, Schreiter ER, Kerr RA, Orger MB, Jayaraman V, Looger LL, Svoboda K, Kim DS (2013) Ultrasensitive fluorescent proteins for imaging neuronal activity. Nature 499(7458):295–300

10. Deo C, Lavis LD (2018) Synthetic and genetically encoded fluorescent neural activity indicators. Curr Opin Neurobiol 50:101–108

11. Dana H, Mohar B, Sun Y, Narayan S, Gordus A, Hasseman JP, Tsegaye G, Holt GT, Hu A, Walpita D, Patel R, Macklin JJ, Bargmann CI, Ahrens MB, Schreiter ER, Jayaraman V, Looger LL, Svoboda K, Kim DS (2016) Sensitive red protein calcium indicators for imaging neural activity. Elife 5:e12727

12. Bassett JJ, Monteith GR (2017) Genetically encoded calcium indicators as probes to assess the role of calcium channels in disease and for high-throughput drug discovery. Adv Pharmacol 79:141–171

13. Borges-Pereira L, Budu A, McKnight CA, Moore CA, Vella SA, Hortua Triana MA, Liu J, Garcia CR, Pace DA, Moreno SN (2015) Calcium signaling throughout the *Toxoplasma gondii* lytic cycle: a study using genetically encoded calcium indicators. J Biol Chem 290(45):26914–26926

14. Hortua Triana MA, Márquez-Nogueras KM, Vella SA, Moreno SN, (2018) Calcium signaling and the lytic cycle of the Apicomplexan parasite *Toxoplasma gondii*. Biochimica et Biophysica Acta (BBA) - Molecular Cell Research 1865 (11):1846–1856

15. Endo T, Sethi KK, Piekarski G (1982) *Toxoplasma gondii*: calcium ionophore A23187-mediated exit of trophozoites from infected murine macrophages. Exp Parasitol 53 (2):179–188.

16. Sidik SM, Hortua Triana MA, Paul AS, El Bakkouri M, Hackett CG, Tran F, Westwood NJ, Hui R, Zuercher WJ, Duraisingh MT, Moreno SN, Lourido S (2016) Using a genetically encoded sensor to identify inhibitors of *Toxoplasma gondii* Ca^{2+} signaling. J Biol Chem 291(18):9566–9580

17. Striepen B, He CY, Matrajt M, Soldati D, Roos DS (1998) Expression, selection, and organellar targeting of the green fluorescent protein in *Toxoplasma gondii*. Mol Biochem Parasitol 92 (2):325–338

18. Brooks CF, Johnsen H, van Dooren GG, Muthalagi M, Lin SS, Bohne W, Fischer K, Striepen B (2010) The *Toxoplasma* apicoplast phosphate translocator links cytosolic and apicoplast metabolism and is essential for parasite survival. Cell Host Microbe 7(1):62–73

19. Kafsack BF, Pena JD, Coppens I, Ravindran S, Boothroyd JC, Carruthers VB (2009) Rapid membrane disruption by a perforin-like protein facilitates parasite exit from host cells. Science 323(5913):530–533

20. Brown KM, Lourido S, Sibley LD (2016) Serum albumin stimulates protein kinase G-dependent Microneme secretion in *Toxoplasma gondii*. J Biol Chem 291 (18):9554–9565

21. Stewart RJ, Whitehead L, Nijagal B, Sleebs BE, Lessene G, McConville MJ, Rogers KL, Tonkin CJ (2017) Analysis of Ca(2)(+) mediated signaling regulating *Toxoplasma* infectivity reveals complex relationships between key molecules. Cell Microbiol 19(4)

22. Brydges SD, Carruthers VB (2003) Mutation of an unusual mitochondrial targeting sequence of SODB2 produces multiple targeting fates in *Toxoplasma gondii*. J Cell Sci 116 (Pt 22):4675–4685

23. Wu J, Prole DL, Shen Y, Lin Z, Gnanasekaran A, Liu Y, Chen L, Zhou H, Chen SR, Usachev YM, Taylor CW, Campbell RE (2014) Red fluorescent genetically encoded Ca^{2+} indicators for use in mitochondria and endoplasmic reticulum. Biochem J 464 (1):13–22

24. Pino P, Foth BJ, Kwok LY, Sheiner L, Schepers R, Soldati T, Soldati-Favre D (2007) Dual targeting of antioxidant and metabolic enzymes to the mitochondrion and the apicoplast of *Toxoplasma gondii*. PLoS Pathog 3(8): e115

25. van Dooren GG, Tomova C, Agrawal S, Humbel BM, Striepen B (2008) *Toxoplasma gondii* Tic20 is essential for apicoplast protein import. Proc Natl Acad Sci U S A 105 (36):13574–13579

26. Wagner JC, Goldfless SJ, Ganesan SM, Lee MC, Fidock DA, Niles JC (2013) An integrated strategy for efficient vector construction and multi-gene expression in *Plasmodium falciparum*. Malar J 12(1):373

27. Szymczak-Workman AL, Vignali KM, Vignali DA (2012) Design and construction of 2A peptide-linked multicistronic vectors. Cold Spring Harb Protoc 2012(2):199–204

28. Jakot D, Meisner M, Sheiner L, Soldati-Favre-D, Striepen B (2014) Genetic manipulation of *Toxoplasma gondii*, 2nd edn. Academic Press, Elsevier

29. Waller RF, Keeling PJ, Donald RG, Striepen B, Handman E, Lang-Unnasch N, Cowman AF, Besra GS, Roos DS, McFadden GI (1998) Nuclear-encoded proteins target to the plastid in *Toxoplasma gondii* and *Plasmodium falciparum*. Proc Natl Acad Sci U S A 95 (21):12352–12357

30. Harb OS, Chatterjee B, Fraunholz MJ, Crawford MJ, Nishi M, Roos DS (2004) Multiple functionally redundant signals mediate targeting to the apicoplast in the apicomplexan parasite *Toxoplasma gondii*. Eukaryot Cell 3 (3):663–674

31. Bindels DS, Haarbosch L, van Weeren L, Postma M, Wiese KE, Mastop M, Aumonier S, Gotthard G, Royant A, Hink MA, Gadella TW Jr (2017) mScarlet: a bright monomeric red fluorescent protein for cellular imaging. Nat Methods 14(1):53–56

32. Schindelin J, Arganda-Carreras I, Frise E, Kaynig V, Longair M, Pietzsch T, Preibisch S, Rueden C, Saalfeld S, Schmid B, Tinevez JY, White DJ, Hartenstein V, Eliceiri K, Tomancak P, Cardona A (2012) Fiji: an open-source platform for biological-image analysis. Nat Methods 9(7):676–682

33. Santi PA (2011) Light sheet fluorescence microscopy: a review. J Histochem Cytochem 59(2):129–138

34. Williams MJ, Alonso H, Enciso M, Egarter S, Sheiner L, Meissner M, Striepen B, Smith BJ, Tonkin CJ (2015) Two essential light chains regulate the MyoA lever arm to promote *Toxoplasma* gliding motility. MBio 6(5): e00845–e00815

35. Fazli MS, Vella SA, Moreno SN, Quinn S (2017) Computational motility tracking of calcium dynamics in *Toxoplasma gondii*. arXiv preprint arXiv:1708.01871

36. Fazli MS, Vella SA, Moreno SN, Quinn S (2018). Unsupervised Discovery of *Toxoplasma gondii* Motility Phenotypes. arXiv preprint arXiv:1801.02591

37. Chin D, Means AR (2000) Calmodulin: a prototypical calcium sensor. Trends Cell Biol 10 (8):322–328

38. Yang Y, Liu N, He Y, Liu Y, Ge L, Zou L, Song S, Xiong W, Liu X (2018) Improved calcium sensor GCaMP-X overcomes the calcium channel perturbations induced by the calmodulin in GCaMP. Nat Commun 9(1):1504

39. Nebl T, Prieto JH, Kapp E, Smith BJ, Williams MJ, Yates JR 3rd, Cowman AF, Tonkin CJ (2011) Quantitative in vivo analyses reveal calcium-dependent phosphorylation sites and identifies a novel component of the *Toxoplasma* invasion motor complex. PLoS Pathog 7(9): e1002222

40. Sidik SM, Huet D, Ganesan SM, Huynh MH, Wang T, Nasamu AS, Thiru P, Saeij JPJ, Carruthers VB, Niles JC, Lourido S (2016) A genome-wide CRISPR screen in *Toxoplasma* identifies essential Apicomplexan genes. Cell 166(6):1423–1435. e12

41. Cho JH, Swanson CJ, Chen J, Li A, Lippert LG, Boye SE, Rose K, Sivaramakrishnan S, Chuong CM, Chow RH (2017) The GCaMP-R family of genetically encoded Ratiometric calcium indicators. ACS Chem Biol 12 (4):1066–1074

42. Park JG, Palmer AE (2015) Measuring the in situ Kd of a genetically encoded Ca^{2+} sensor.

Cold Spring Harb Protoc 2015(1):pdb prot076554

43. Lin MZ, Schnitzer MJ (2016) Genetically encoded indicators of neuronal activity. Nat Neurosci 19(9):1142–1153

44. Yasuda R, Nimchinsky EA, Scheuss V, Pologruto TA, Oertner TG, Sabatini BL, Svoboda K (2004) Imaging calcium concentration dynamics in small neuronal compartments. Sci STKE 2004(219):pl5

45. Akerboom J, Chen TW, Wardill TJ, Tian L, Marvin JS, Mutlu S, Calderon NC, Esposti F, Borghuis BG, Sun XR, Gordus A, Orger MB, Portugues R, Engert F, Macklin JJ, Filosa A, Aggarwal A, Kerr RA, Takagi R, Kracun S, Shigetomi E, Khakh BS, Baier H, Lagnado L, Wang SS, Bargmann CI, Kimmel BE, Jayaraman V, Svoboda K, Kim DS, Schreiter ER, Looger LL (2012) Optimization of a GCaMP calcium indicator for neural activity imaging. J Neurosci 32(40):13819–13840

46. Kuchipudi A, Arroyo-Olarte RD, Hoffmann F, Brinkmann V, Gupta N (2016) Optogenetic monitoring identifies phosphatidylthreonine-regulated calcium homeostasis in *Toxoplasma gondii*. Microb Cell 3(5):215–223

Chapter 12

Phenotyping *Toxoplasma* Invasive Skills by Fast Live Cell Imaging

Georgios Pavlou and Isabelle Tardieux

Abstract

Host cell invasion by *Toxoplasma gondii/T. gondii* tachyzoites is an obligate but complex multistep process occurring in second-scale. To capture the dynamic nature of the whole entry process requires fast and high-resolution live cell imaging. Recent advances in *T. gondii*/host cell genome editing and in quantitative live cell imaging—image acquisition and processing included—provide a systematic way to accurately phenotype *T. gondii* tachyzoite invasive behaviour and to highlight any variation or default from a standard scenario. Therefore, applying these combined strategies allows gaining deeper insights into the complex mechanisms underlying host cell invasion.

Key words *T. gondii* tachyzoite, Host cell invasion, Live cell microscopy, Image processing

1 Introduction

Once it reaches warm-blooded metazoan tissues, the tachyzoite developmental stage of *Toxoplasma gondii/T. gondii* strictly depends on nutrients supplied by hosting cells where to either expand a replicating-prone progeny or where to differentiate as slow replicating bradyzoite developmental stage. This condition imposes to first achieve entry of the target cell by a mechanism that allows rapid biogenesis of an intracellular niche in which the tachyzoite further multiplies. Once the mature progeny fills up the hosting cell, it actively moves out to undergo a transient extracellular phase prior to new successive phases of cell invasion and intracellular multiplication. In this context, the invasive skills of *T. gondii* determine to which extent the parasite population expands, and accordingly the amount of tissue damages which impacts on clinical outcomes. Therefore, a comprehensive and molecular understanding of how tachyzoites access the intracellular niche remains actively investigated with the perspective of designing anti-invasive strategies to combat or prevent the disease.

Christopher J. Tonkin (ed.), *Toxoplasma gondii: Methods and Protocols*, Methods in Molecular Biology, vol. 2071, https://doi.org/10.1007/978-1-4939-9857-9_12, © Springer Science+Business Media, LLC, part of Springer Nature 2020

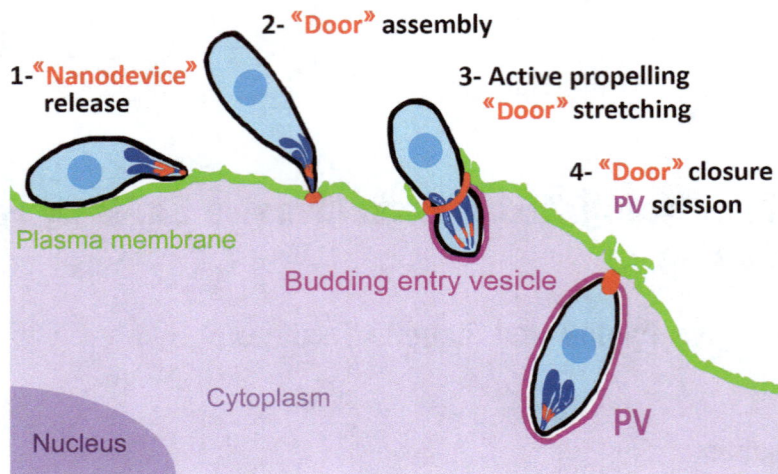

Fig. 1 Schematic depicting the four main steps of the invasion process defined by the RON complex fate. RON stands for *T. gondii* RhOptry Neck complex

Since decades, such **productive invasion** event is described as a short lasting but also as a well-coordinated multistep sequence (Fig. 1) [1]. Despite recent advances in the identification of key molecules of both *T. gondii*—a single-celled eukaryotic parasite—and the metazoan host cell, the whole set of players and the mechanisms that control the transition from an extracellular motile to an no more motile intracellular immotile/replicative tachyzoite, remain unresolved in large part. A major limitation clearly relates to the second-scale dynamic of the entry process, hence difficult to capture and accurately characterize. Indeed, although recent advances in molecular genetics have provided unprecedented tools with the design of genetic screens from which have been generated—and will continue to be—several *T. gondii* mutants potentially disabled in invasive skills [2, 3], the optimal assessment of these is still difficult. However conclusive evidence for any invasion-defective trait that would translate into a specific phenotype can greatly benefit from **fast live microscopy settings** in particular when combined with multiple markers for the *T. gondii* tachyzoite or/and the targeted cell.

Here we provide basic guidelines to set up an optimized experimental framework enabling to collect high-content image datasets from which accurate information can be retrieved using commercial and open source software. By tracking defined objects of interest in time and space, key parameters of the invasion process have been/ can be identified and quantified, and have proven/prove to bring informative mechanistic insights. Importantly, as exemplified below, introducing new variables and upgrading the settings allow automatic analysis of successive steps of the whole invasion event and provide unbiased high-resolution analysis of the invasive capabilities of tachyzoites. Accordingly, any differences with a **standard entry process** including when associated with entry failure can be reliably **qualitatively and quantitatively** assessed and in turn provide information towards a comprehensive mechanistic model of cell invasion.

Recent imaging studies have allowed clarifying or uncovering key events that define successful invasion and can therefore serve as **reference features** for analysing the invasive skills of tachyzoites. They first execute a specific short movement we have described as "impulse" [4], which in association or not with movement production—circular or helical gliding—is characterized by the extrusion of the tubulin-based appendage termed conoid [5]. Conoid extrusion and zoite motility are both controlled by calcium signalling [6–8], but their functional link has been pharmacologically invalidated [9]. Interestingly, entry into the host cell is systematically initiated by zoites with extruded conoids but whether and why this is essential for the process to start has not been solved yet. Cell penetration per se proceeds with the regulated secretion of cargoes prestored in the apical pear-shaped secretory organelles called rhoptries. The identity of molecular triggers for early cargo release is earnestly investigated and these might operate only when conoid is elongated. Several cargoes have been identified and include compounds with distinct final destination such as the host cell (a) Plasma Membrane (hPM) (b) CytoPlasm (hCP), (c) nucleus [10], yet how these are routed and delivered is not known. Delivery of cargoes has indeed rarely been monitored in real time but the visualization of the RhOptry Neck complex—the RON complex—that travels in the rhoptry canal to the tip of the conoidal channel, allowing invasion to begin, appears as **a key early reference feature**. Once the RON material contacts the hPM, it assembles a tight circular interface called a Tight Junction (TJ) between the zoite and the metazoan cell. At this early stage of invasion, local changes in hPM curvature can already be detected with a tightly curved fold surrounding the apex of the tachyzoite while discrete outward projections emerge at the TJ site lining the extracellular part of the *T. gondii* tachyzoite body. Forward progression of the tachyzoite occurs owing to the zoite traction force applied on the TJ with the actin-myosin H activity [11], which is then rapidly relayed by the actin-myosin A motor [4]. Traction force concurs with the stretching of the TJ and the enlargement of the intracellular curved fold that shapes a unique type of entry vesicle. Although deriving from the hPM, the budding entry vesicle selectively incorporates components by virtue of the TJ-associated sieving properties [12, 13]. Invasion is achieved when the hPM-derived bud ultimately pinches off of the hPM [14] leading to a tachyzoite-loaded free vesicle. Rapid and sustained remodelling of this vesicle defined as a bona fide parasite-protective niche named the Parasitophorous Vacuole (PV) allows the tachyzoite to shift to an

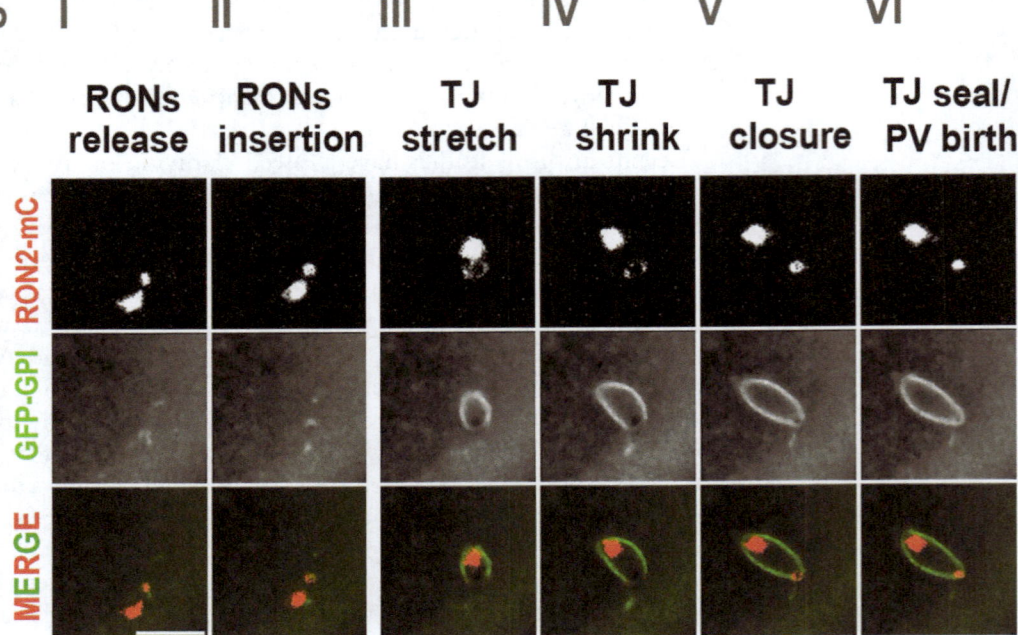

Fig. 2 Host cell invasion is a multistep process that can be decomposed in six steps (I–VI) using key markers from the invading parasite (RON2-mC, red) and the host cell plasma membrane (GFP-GPI, green). Scale bar: 5 μm

intracellular lifestyle [15]. Each of these events—that is, (1) **conoid extrusion/RON secretion**, (2) **RON insertion/TJ assembly** into the hPM, (3) **TJ stretching**, (4) **TJ shrinking**, (5) **TJ closure, and** (6) **PV biogenesis**—constitute six steps that can now serve as **reference features** for scoring tachyzoite invasive skills in the context of any mutation or drug effect under study (Fig. 2).

2   Material

2.1   *T. gondii Cells*

The parasite lines ideally carry one or more fluorescent markers that could include a RON TJ marker to accurately assess the dynamics of invasion and/or any other marker of interest (http://toxodb.org/toxo/). Multiple genetic endogenous tagging can now be easily obtained in both type I and II *T. gondii* strains engineered to lack the gene encoding the *DNA* double-strand break *repair* Ku80 protein hence showing drastic increase in the rate of homologous recombination [16, 17]. In conjunction with these breakthroughs in molecular genetics, LIC-mediated and CRISPR/Cas9 knock-in strategies [2, 3] have undoubtedly eased the introduction of a variety of fluorescent markers thus allowing any laboratory members to image parasites for specific investigation. While care must then be taken to verify expression and functionality of the fusion constructs, a number of these have allowed precise description of preinvasive and invasive *T. gondii* tachyzoite behaviors. As such, we have generated RH (i.e., type 1) Δ*Ku80 T. gondii* strains that express a functional chimeric fluorescent version of the rhoptry-stored RON2 protein which enable visualizing in real time the whole multistep invasion event from the early RON complex release to the TJ closure and the subsequent birth of the PV [4]. Of note the CRISPR/Cas9 knock-in procedure has proved useful for genome editing—gene deletion and point mutations [18, 19]—while conditional silencing systems have allowed analysing loss of function mutants for the so-called "essential" genes [20] and the impact of all those modifications for *T. gondii* invasion-related gene candidates can now be accurately examined in the RON2-mC-expressing tachyzoite lines. Indeed, dynamic imaging of mutants deleted for the *MyoA* gene revealed an alternative mode of entry into host cells that relies on hPM actin-rich protrusions forcing the parasite into a hPM-derived bud [21].

2.2 Metazoan Cells

The human foreskin fibroblasts (HFF-1, ATCC no. SCRC-1041, certified mycoplasma free) have been used to propagate the *T. gondii* tachyzoites in vitro by serial passages in high glucose Dulbecco's Modified Eagle's Medium GlutaMAX (DMEM) supplemented with 10% fetal bovine serum (FBS), 100 units/ml penicillin, and 100 mg/ml streptomycin (i.e., complete medium) at 37 °C with 95% air and 5% CO_2.

The host cell lines used for analyzing invasive skills are diverse due to the particularly broad spectrum of warm-blooded metazoan adherent cells permissive to *T. gondii* tachyzoites. We recommend choosing cells that are easy to transfect for transient or stable transgene expression and that preferentially spread thin and large lamellipodium/lamella area to ease the recording. However invasion of polarized epithelial or endothelial cell monolayers—which display rather columnar architectures—can also be used. In our hands the human U2OS sarcoma cell line (ATCC, Cat#HTB-96; RRID: CVCL_0042) has been convenient for assessing—therefore comparing—invasive behaviors. We can derive from the U2OS cell line a large number of transgenic sublines expressing GFP, mCherry, or any other fluorescent tags in fusion with a variety of constructs targeting the hcPM [4] (i.e., using a transmembrane domain of PM-exposed receptors such as the PDGF receptor or a lipid covalent anchor/tether such as glycosyl-phosphatidylinositol, myristate, and palmitate) or/and the hc cortical cytoskeleton (using lifactin, etc.) (For details, *see* [4]) [15, 21, 22]. During the procedure to obtain the U2OS (or other) cell line of interest, we usually select clones that express low amounts of the fusion construct to limit the risk of mis-localisation or physiological impairment due to transgene overexpression.

2.3 Microscope Platform

We are working with a spinning disk (Yokogawa CSU-X) laser confocal microscope (Nikon Eclipse), a platform that fulfills the speed, sensitivity and resolution requirements for imaging (1) release of the RON material, (2) TJ assembly and function along with (3) parasite penetration. To achieve efficient resolution, we also use the X63 oil objective with a numerical aperture of 1.4. Because of the need to capture emitted signals from distinct fluorophores—exited with distinct laser beams—within only few seconds, fast frame rate video-recording is compulsory. In addition because we also want to capture as many events as possible in the same session to further perform quantitative analysis and apply statistics (i.e., on the same field of view for the appropriate objective), we usually extend the recording periods over two tens of minutes. Therefore, particular care must be taken to limit (1) phototoxicity due to ROS generated from high/long excitation of the fluorophore and (2) photobleaching (*see* **Note 1**). Although phototoxicity might not be apparent for short-imaging time windows as during invasion assay, and clearly depends on the fluorophore and the subcellular localization of the marker of interest. For each marker we therefore optimize the emission filter for a maximal signal and test the best illumination conditions aiming to limit excitation to the level that provides both satisfying signal to noise ratio and spatiotemporal resolution.

Several alternatives to counteract both the phototoxicity and photobleaching exist, including the use of other illumination techniques (Total internal reflection fluorescence—TIRF—light sheet illumination), but increasing the quantum efficiency of the emitted light detector—that is, improving the sensitivity of the camera—is certainly a good start. With these concerns, we use either the EM-CCD (Photometrics CoolSNAP HQ2, Andor iXon) or the sCMOS (Photometrics Prism BSI) cameras having a preference for the second one.

2.4 Additional Microscope Settings

To keep the physiological conditions required for long term live imaging of the *T. gondii* invasion in metazoan cells, a 37 °C temperature and 5% CO_2 gas as well as humidity need to be provided throughout the video session. Homemade and commercial microscope environmental chambers as well as heat and CO_2 flow rate controllers need to be used. As regards the heat, because the immersion objectives act as heat sink thereby creating a decrease of temperature at the interface between the objective and the sample, it is important to use an objective heater in the environmental top stage chamber while a stage heater is also good. We had also positive experience using the compact Chamlide incubator top stage system from Live Cell Instrument, which accommodates a range of magnetic or nonmagnetic holder settings (i.e., glass bottom dishes, chambers holding glass coverslips or well plates of various dimensions) compatible or not with liquid perfusion at controlled flow rates.

2.5 Software

MetaMorph 7.7.0.0 Molecular devices.
   Icy 1.9.5.1 http://icy.bioimageanalysis.org/
   ImageJ 1.51j8 https://imagej.nih.gov/ij/.
   UCSF ChimeraX 0.1 https://www.rbvi.ucsf.edu/chimerax/

3 Methods

3.1 Plating Cells on Coated Glass-Coverslips

Twenty-four to forty-eight hours prior to recording invasion events, adherent cells are plated by default on poly-L-Lysine (100 μg/ml dH$_2$O) -coated glass coverslips or MatTek glass bottom dishes or any other systems fitting the cell chamber holders (overnight 4 °C). For specific needs, collagen (rat tail collagen 1, 50–100 μg/ml 0.02 M acetic acid), fibronectin (50 μg/ml PBS), gelatin (0.2% dH$_2$O) or specific extracellular matrix components can be used with adapted coating protocols. At the time of the invasion assay, cells must have reached ~80% confluence. Cells are washed with HBSS^{++} supplemented with 0.2–1% FCS (i.e., low amounts of FCS can help to limit autofluorescence) and calcium to 1.6 mM final concentration immediately prior transfer into the cell holder setting within the microscope chamber. The so-called Motility Buffer (MB), which allows maintaining proper osmolarity, is our reference buffer used for all comparative preinvasive and invasive behaviors. However if we extend the period of live recording post-invasion—to monitor tachyzoite replication for instances—we then replace the MB by complete medium but lacking phenol red to avoid nonspecific fluorescence in particular in the blue-yellow spectrum.

3.2 Collecting *T. gondii* Tachyzoites for Invasion Recording

The quality of the parasite preparation is essential to sample enough events in a short amount of time, thereby limiting the photosensitivity problems (*see* **Note 1**). To this end, we synchronize the parasite culture and recover the progeny within 2–4 h post–spontaneous egress in the culture medium. In the case of tachyzoite mutants impaired in their egress potential (i.e., actin knockout, [23]), we scrap the cells from the flask and mechanically disrupt them by a few passages through a 26 gauge syringe needle. The amount of parasites needed for each session is washed in the MB by gentle centrifugation, resuspended in a small volume of MB and rapidly added to the target cells under the microscope. Because we limit the volume in the cell chamber, parasite sedimentation is fast allowing to rapidly proceed for image acquisition. For the 20 min regular video sessions, we do not need to add more volume but for longer imaging periods care is taken to prevent evaporation that would change the osmolarity by filling the cell chamber with medium and keeping saturated humidity in the vicinity of the cell culture setting (i.e., in the compact or wide top-stage chambers). Importantly our priority is to maintain parasites "healthy" by limiting CO_2 and temperature fluctuations to obtain reliable phenotype analysis.

3.3 Image Acquisition and Analysis

Images are usually acquired in DIC and two fluorescent channels at optimal speeds to achieve the efficient spatiotemporal resolution. Using MetaMorph, we systematically go below 1 s per frame and to this end, for reasons mentioned earlier, we select low laser power and low time exposure while in case the camera has a "denoise" setting, we switch off the option. Once sequences have been captured over routine 20 min video-recording sessions, the sequences of interest are cropped using MetaMorph and ImageJ software. Then using the open software Icy, the researcher can access a variety of parameters of static or moving defined "fluorescent" object(s) using tools such as (*see* **Notes 2** and **3**):

- Tracking of object(s):
    - Simultaneous tracking of multiple moving and static objects.
    - Combination of different fluorescent markers' tracking.
    - Extraction of values depending on the tracking object(s) such as:
    Speed.
    Displacement.
    Surface area.
    Size measurement (perimeter, etc.).
    Circularity.
    Distance tracking between two different objects.
    Fluorescence intensity, etc.
    - Wide variety of visualization options for the tracks.
- Deformability of static object(s) overtime:
    - Size measurement (perimeter, etc.).
    - Fluorescence intensity.
    - Circularity.
    - Surface area, etc.
- 3D/4D reconstruction:
    - Volume area.
    - Fluorescence Intensity, etc.

All the data are exported in either the .xls or the .csv file which allows easy import and processing by all common software for data

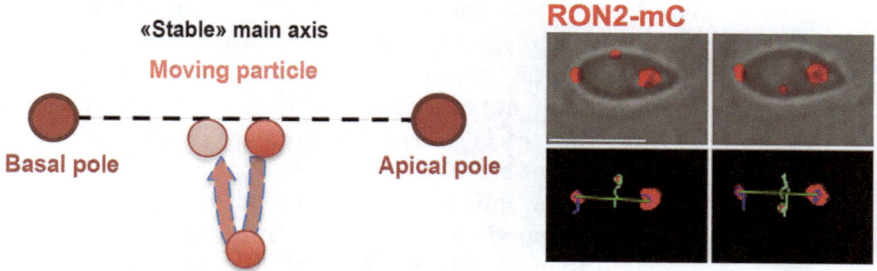

Fig. 3 Schematic representation of the object tracking that allows quantifying the twisting motion accounting for TJ closure. Right top panel shows the overlay image (DIC-RON2-mC, red) and right bottom panel shows the three objects (rhoptry, TJ, and internal vesicle) tracked using Icy software, scale bar: 5 μm

analysis. Moreover, Icy can create graphical plots of your data of interest (*see* **Note 2**).

To finalize the 3D and 4D reconstruction, we use the open source software ChimeraX.

Example: A tachyzoite that expresses RON2 fused to the mCherry tag (red) invades a host cell which expresses the hPM reporter fused to GFP (green). This **dual fluorescence** allows detecting and monitoring the (1) release of the RON complex precisely defining the t0 point of entry, (2) stretching and shrinking of the circular TJ that accommodates parasite progression into an inward hPM-derived bud that forms concomitantly, (3) the closure of the TJ ring, and (4) the birth of the PV when the bud has separated from the hPM therefore precisely defining the final time (ft). Image processing reveals that the parasite executes a rotation around its long axis which imposes a twisting motion on its basal pole, hence ensuring TJ closure and bud sealing while promoting membrane fission upstream the TJ. Interestingly, we observe after twisting the formation of micropatterns in the PV membrane (PVM), while after fission we measure a relaxation phase of the parasite body coupled with the stretching of the tightly adjusted PVM. We focus here on how image processing of the invading RON2-mC tachyzoite has allowed analyzing the final twisting motion (Fig. 3, for details, *see* [15]).

Rotation can be defined by the movement of one object around the axis that connects two objects.

In our case, we assess the rotation using the following protocol:

1. Detection of the objects in the red fluorescent channel using the *Spot detector* plugin overtime. The RON2-mC pools correspond to the rhoptry and the closing/close TJ at each pole of the parasite respectively and define the main axis of the *T. gondii* tachyzoite.

2. Tracking of these objects overtime using the *Spot tracking* plugin.

3. After **step 2**, the *Track manager* plugin window opens automatically providing the possibility to activate different subplugins (*track processors*) that can export values for speed, displacement, etc. of all the tracked objects. In our case we use the *track processor Instant speed* which shows that the reference objects at each pole of the tachyzoite have almost zero speed and the intermediate object moves with a significant speed around the main axis. *Track processor Intensity speed* is used to assess whether the object rotates around the axis (i.e., continuous 360° rotation) (left panel Fig. 3) rather than a flip-flop like movement (i.e., 180 °C back and forward rotations). In more details, the intensity of the tracked object over time decreases when the object gets out of focus and reincreases when back in focus, thereby demonstrating the continuous rotation process.

By applying filters and threshold on the images in the fluorescent channel of interest, we clearly observe the dynamics of the hPM-derived bud that tightly surrounds the invading parasite. Icy has by default the widely used filters such as *Median filter* and the interface of the intensity brightness control panel is quite useful. By using the *Intensity profile* plugin we can access the intensity distribution of the forming and newly formed PV and therefore detect any abnormal process of PV biogenesis.

We describe the relaxation of the parasite body as follows:

1. Using the same "stable" spots that have been tracked in the rotation protocol.

2. Using the *track processor Distance profiler*, the distance between the two stable spots could be recorded over time. Results showed that there was an increase in the length of the axis that connects these two spots.

4 Notes

1. *T. gondii* tachyzoites have been found sensitive to phototoxic damages when they express high amounts of soluble protein in fusion with GFP or YFP. Mammalian cells also show differential sensitivity to illumination-induced ROS. Overall, we advise to reduce the peak intensity of the laser beam even if that means extending the exposure time provided it is compatible with the temporal resolution needed to capture the multistep sequence of cell invasion. Ideally fluorescent markers should be carefully tested and compared with available alternatives. On the same line, caution is necessary to ensure that cells are maintained in good condition and are functional while on the microscope

stage with illumination in the presence of synthetic fluorophores or fluorescent proteins.

2. Icy is an open source software that gives the ability to the user to search for similar tasks or solutions to possible problems through an online interactive forum. For example, the user can create a new thread with his/her problem and then other users or the Icy software engineers can provide advice/help.

3. Not only the best phenotypic description of a parasite preinvasive and invasive skills clearly gains from a careful comparative analysis of the dynamic behavior with the current reference scheme (i.e., as described earlier), but it can also improve the model itself by highlighting specific steps within "normal" or "abnormal" sequences. It is important to be aware of continual advances in live imaging techniques/platforms, in the design of fluorescent probes and computationally efficient algorithms to increase the accuracy of the image information content we can capture and process.

References

1. Tardieux I, Baum J (2016) Reassessing the mechanics of parasite motility and host-cell invasion. J Cell Biol 214:507–515. https://doi.org/10.1083/jcb.201605100

2. Sidik SM, Huet D, Ganesan SM, Huynh M-H, Wang T, Nasamu AS, Thiru P, Saeij JPJ, Carruthers VB, Niles JC, Lourido S (2016) A genome-wide CRISPR screen in *Toxoplasma* identifies essential apicomplexan genes. Cell 166:1423–1435.e12. https://doi.org/10.1016/j.cell.2016.08.019

3. Sidik SM, Huet D, Lourido S (2018) CRISPR-Cas9-based genome-wide screening of *Toxoplasma gondii*. Nat Protoc 13:307–323. https://doi.org/10.1038/nprot.2017.131

4. Bichet M, Joly C, Henni AH, Guilbert T, Xémard M, Tafani V, Lagal V, Charras G, Tardieux I (2014) The *Toxoplasma*-host cell junction is anchored to the cell cortex to sustain parasite invasive force. BMC Biol 12:773. https://doi.org/10.1186/s12915-014-0108-y

5. Hu K, Johnson J, Florens L, Fraunholz M, Suravajjala S, DiLullo C, Yates J, Roos DS, Murray JM (2006) Cytoskeletal components of an invasion machine--the apical complex of *Toxoplasma gondii*. PLoS Pathog 2:e13. https://doi.org/10.1371/journal.ppat.0020013

6. Mondragon R, Frixione E (1996) Ca(2+)-dependence of conoid extrusion in *Toxoplasma gondii* tachyzoites. J Eukaryot Microbiol 43:120–127

7. Lourido S, Tang K, Sibley LD (2012) Distinct signalling pathways control *Toxoplasma* egress and host-cell invasion. EMBO J 31:4524–4534. https://doi.org/10.1038/emboj.2012.299

8. Lourido S, Moreno SNJ (2015) The calcium signaling toolkit of the apicomplexan parasites *Toxoplasma gondii* and Plasmodium spp. Cell Calcium 57:186–193. https://doi.org/10.1016/j.ceca.2014.12.010

9. Carey KL, Westwood NJ, Mitchison TJ, Ward GE (2004) A small-molecule approach to studying invasive mechanisms of *Toxoplasma gondii*. Proc Natl Acad Sci U S A 101:7433–7438. https://doi.org/10.1073/pnas.0307769101

10. Hakimi M-A, Olias P, Sibley LD (2017) *Toxoplasma* effectors targeting host signaling and transcription. Clin Microbiol Rev 30:615–645. https://doi.org/10.1128/CMR.00005-17

11. Graindorge A, Frénal K, Jacot D, Salamun J, Marq JB, Soldati-Favre D (2016) The conoid associated motor MyoH is indispensable for *Toxoplasma gondii* entry and exit from host cells. PLoS Pathog 12:e1005388. https://doi.org/10.1371/journal.ppat.1005388

12. Mordue DG, Desai N, Dustin M, Sibley LD (1999) Invasion by *Toxoplasma gondii* establishes a moving junction that selectively excludes host cell plasma membrane proteins on the basis of their membrane anchoring. J Exp Med 190:1783–1792

13. Charron AJ, Sibley LD (2004) Molecular partitioning during host cell penetration by *Toxoplasma gondii*. Traffic 5:855–867. https://doi.org/10.1111/j.1600-0854.2004.00228.x

14. Suss-Toby E, Zimmerberg J, Ward GE (1996) *Toxoplasma* invasion: the parasitophorous vacuole is formed from host cell plasma membrane and pinches off via a fission pore. Proc Natl Acad Sci U S A 93:8413–8418

15. Pavlou G, Biesaga M, Touquet B, Lagal V, Balland M, Dufour A, Hakimi M-A, Tardieux I (2018) *Toxoplasma* parasite twisting motion mechanically induces host cell membrane fission to complete invasion within a protective vacuole. Cell Host Microbe 24:81–96.e5. https://doi.org/10.1016/j.chom.2018.06.003

16. Fox BA, Ristuccia JG, Gigley JP, Bzik DJ (2009) Efficient gene replacements in *Toxoplasma gondii* strains deficient for nonhomologous end joining. Eukaryot Cell 8:520–529. https://doi.org/10.1128/EC.00357-08

17. Huynh M-H, Carruthers VB (2009) Tagging of endogenous genes in a *Toxoplasma gondii* strain lacking Ku80. Eukaryot Cell 8:530–539. https://doi.org/10.1128/EC.00358-08

18. Sidik SM, Hackett CG, Tran F, Westwood NJ, Lourido S (2014) Efficient genome engineering of *Toxoplasma gondii* using CRISPR/Cas9. PLoS One 9:e100450. https://doi.org/10.1371/journal.pone.0100450

19. Shen B, Brown KM, Lee TD, Sibley LD (2014) Efficient gene disruption in diverse strains of *Toxoplasma gondii* using CRISPR/CAS9. MBio 5:e01114–e01114. https://doi.org/10.1128/mBio.01114-14

20. Andenmatten N, Egarter S, Jackson AJ, Jullien N, Herman J-P, Meissner M (2013) Conditional genome engineering in *Toxoplasma gondii* uncovers alternative invasion mechanisms. Nat Methods 10:125–127. https://doi.org/10.1038/nmeth.2301

21. Bichet M, Touquet B, Gonzalez V, Florent I, Meissner M, Tardieux I (2016) Genetic impairment of parasite myosin motors uncovers the contribution of host cell membrane dynamics to *Toxoplasma* invasion forces. BMC Biol 14:97. https://doi.org/10.1186/s12915-016-0316-8

22. Rhee JM, Pirity MK, Lackan CS, Long JZ, Kondoh G, Takeda J, Hadjantonakis A-K (2006) In vivo imaging and differential localization of lipid-modified GFP-variant fusions in embryonic stem cells and mice. Genesis 44:202–218. https://doi.org/10.1002/dvg.20203

23. Egarter S, Andenmatten N, Jackson AJ, Whitelaw JA, Pall G, Black JA, Ferguson DJP, Tardieux I, Mogilner A, Meissner M (2014) The *Toxoplasma* Acto-MyoA motor complex is important but not essential for gliding motility and host cell invasion. PLoS One 9:e91819. https://doi.org/10.1371/journal.pone.0091819

Chapter 13

Experimental Approaches for Examining Apicoplast Biology

Marco Biddau, Jana Ovciarikova, and Lilach Sheiner

Abstract

Genetic manipulation is a powerful tool to study gene function but identifying the direct and primary functional outcomes of any gene depletion is crucial for this strategy to be productive. This is a major challenge for the study of apicoplast biology, because, in the absence of an efficient isolation method, apicoplast functions must be assayed in the parasite. These assays should be performed dynamically from the time of gene depletion, and include standards and controls that separate direct from indirect phenotypes. Here, we describe a pipeline for apicoplast functional analysis and highlight relevant mutant *T. gondii* cell lines and apicoplast markers that are available in the field and that enhance the specificity of phenotype description.

Key words Apicoplast, Plastid, Import, Organelle, Redox, Fluorescence, roGFP, qPCR, qRT-PCR, Live imaging

1 Introduction

T. gondii, and most other parasites from the phylum Apicomplexa, possess an organelle named the apicoplast. This parasite plastid evolved through secondary endosymbiosis of an ancestral eukaryote with a red-algal cell. Resulting from this path of acquisition the apicoplast has four compartments (Fig. 1), and understanding their distinct cellular roles and their biogenesis has important implication on our understanding of eukaryotic evolution and of cell biology outside the common model organisms. The apicoplast shares its origin with plastids found in a diverse group of organisms collectively named chromalveolates. *T. gondii* is one of the most experimentally amenable chromalveolates, and this motivated extensive research into apicoplast biology as model for the secondary plastid of this clade.

In addition, the apicoplast is essential for *T. gondii* tachyzoites in culture, as well as for any life stage of any other apicoplast containing apicomplexan studied to date. Due to this essential role and due to being unique to parasites and absent from

Christopher J. Tonkin (ed.), *Toxoplasma gondii: Methods and Protocols*, Methods in Molecular Biology, vol. 2071, https://doi.org/10.1007/978-1-4939-9857-9_13, © Springer Science+Business Media, LLC, part of Springer Nature 2020

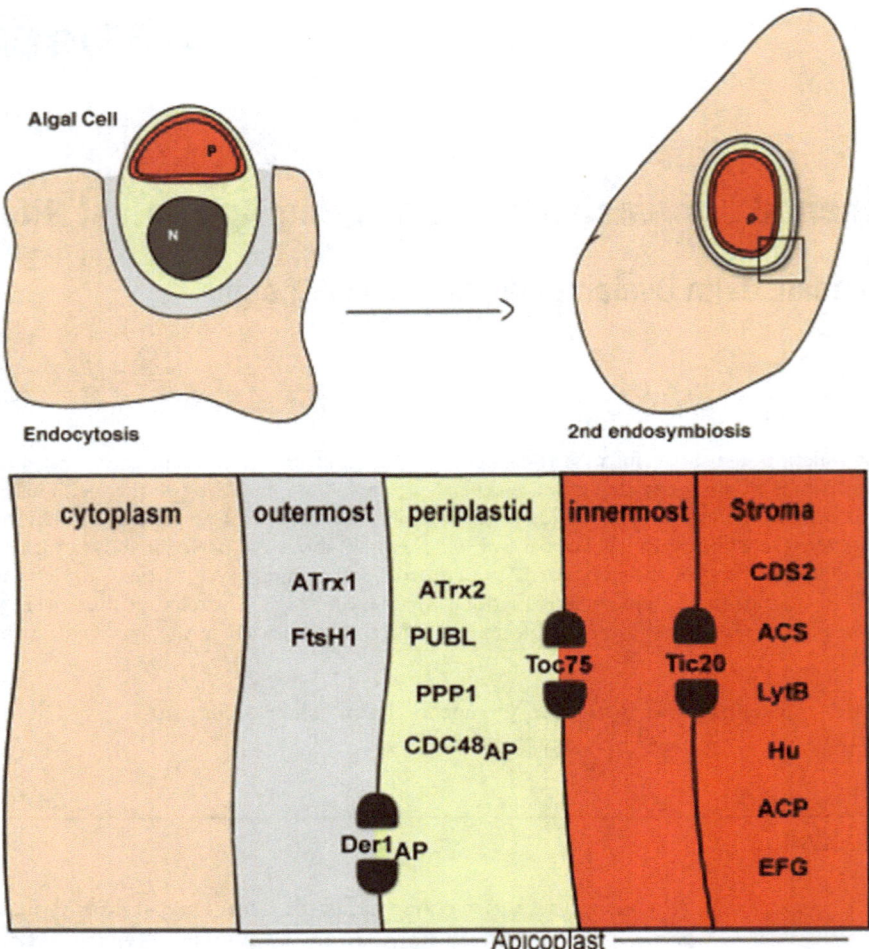

Fig. 1 An illustration of how the secondary endosymbiosis lead to the formation of each of the four apicoplast compartments. The outermost compartment (grey) originates from the endomembrane of the host; the periplastid compartment (yellow) originate from the algal symbiont's cytoplasm; the two inner compartments (red) originate from the algal symbiont's primary plastid. Each compartment in the "inset" scheme contain names of resident proteins for which a genetic depletion study was performed. Table 1 provides the detail of these studies

mammalians the apicoplast is one of the strongest candidates for anti-apicomplexan drug targets. This motivation further enhances research of apicoplast biology.

The diverse nature of chromalveolates provides power to identify apicoplast proteins encoding genes via comparative genomics and via linkage analysis between phylogenetic distribution and phylum phenotype. The strong genetics of *T. gondii* provides efficient tools to delete and deplete those genes for functional analysis. However, in the absence of an efficient apicoplast isolation method, it is not possible currently to perform direct functional studies in vitro as is standard in chloroplast research. Instead, apicoplast functions must be assayed in the context of the complete parasite. Because the apicoplast provides essential metabolites to the parasite, impairment of one apicoplast function may lead to secondary, indirect phenotypes in the parasite that complicate functional analyses. Therefore, it is critical to performed the functional analysis over a careful time scale from the moment of gene depletion, and to include standards and relevant controls that help separate direct from indirect phenotypes.

Several groups in the field, including us, analyzed an array of apicoplast functional mutants and identified and characterized a series of apicoplast proteins that function in its different pathways (Fig. 1, Table 1). Using these mutants and insights we assembled a pipeline for apicoplast functional analysis that should assist in the future analysis of new apicoplast mutants (Fig. 2). The goal of our pipeline is to start with the easier and least resource demanding methods to define the likely function in question and to work the way from there toward the more engaged and in-depth analysis of the relevant phenotype. The method relies on collective evidence showing that there is distinct order of events following the disruption of each of the apicoplast pathways. For example, when a protein import component is depleted, a protein import defect is seen first followed by reduction of organelle numbers, then leading to parasite death [1]. The method also relies upon distinct morphological outcomes of defects in different apicoplast pathways. For example, defects in apicoplast fission leads to rapid accumulation of elongated organelles [2]. The pipeline consists of several functional assays: apicoplast morphology and numbers are measured via immunofluorescence imaging and analysis; protein import into the apicoplast is assessed via examination of transit peptide processing of newly synthesized proteins; apicoplast genome integrity and transcription is analyzed through apicoplast gene specific qPCR and qRT-PCR; the course of development of a morphological defect is examined via live microscopy; the redox state in the organelle's stroma is assayed via a redox fluorescent sensor named roGFP that we recently adapted to *Toxoplasma* (Subheadings 2.4, 3.5, and 4.5). Identification of the earliest detectable defect among protein import, genome integrity, transcription and redox state is critical to defining the function of the depleted gene. A temporal analysis of phenotypes, covering time point when GOI expression levels are down but before full depletion, is critical for separating primary from secondary effects.

Table 1
A collection of published mutants whereby various apicoplast proteins with different localizations and functions were depleted

Full name	Name in Fig. 1	ToxoDB ID	Subcompartment	Type of mutant	PMID for gene mutant characterization	Function in apicoplast biology (if know)
Acetyl-CoA synthetase	ACS	TGME49_294820	Stroma	Inducible	29678960	Metabolic function—FAS
Apicoplast thioredoxin 1	ATrx1	TGME49_312110	Outermost	Inducible	29470517	Protein import
Apicoplast thioredoxin 2	ATrx2	TGME49_310770	Periplastid	Inducible	29470517	Organelle gene expression
	FTsH1	TGGT1_259260	Outermost	Small molecule inhibitor	28826494	
Plastid ubiquitin-like protein	PUBL	TGME49_223125	Periplastid	Inducible	28655825	Protein import
	CDC48AP	TGME49_321640	Periplastid	Inducible	28655825	Protein import
Patatin-like phospholipases 2	PL2	TGME49_231370		Inducible	28419631	
Cytidine diphosphate-diacylglycerol synthase 2	CDS2	TGGT1_263785		Inducible	28314772	
Glycerol 3-phosphate acyltransferase	ATS1	TGME49_270910		Inducible	27490259	Metabolic function—FAS
Translocon of the outer membrane 75	Toc75	TGME49_272390	Second inner membrane	Inducible	26381927	Protein import
Phosphatidylinositol 3 kinase	PI3K	TGME49_215700	Outermost and elsewhere	Inducible	25329540	
Ubiquitin activating, conjugating and ligating enzymes	TgE1ap TgE2ap	TGME49_226740 TGME49_304460	Periplastid	Inducible	23785288	Protein import
Myosin F	MyoF	TGME49_278870	Apicoplast vicinity	Inducible	23695356	Segregation

Full name	Abbreviation	Gene ID	Localization	Method	PMID	Function
translocon of the inner membrane	Tic22	TGME49_08605	One or more of the intermembrane spaces	Inducible	23027875	Protein import
	HU protein	TgME49_027970	Stroma	Knockout	22611021	DNA maintenance
Translation elongation factor G	EFG	TGME49_023970	Stroma	3'UTR disruption	22059956	
Periplastid protein	PPP1	TGME49_287270	Periplastid	Inducible	22144892	Protein import
Isoprenoid precursors synthesis pathway	LytB DOXPRI	TGME49_001270 TGGT1_125270	Stroma		21690250	Metabolic function—Isoprenoid precursors synthesis pathway
Apicoplast membrane-localized phosphate translocator	APT	TGME49_261070	Different apicoplast membranes	Inducible	20036630	Metabolic function—import for metabolites
Derlin 1	Der1(Ap)		Periplastid membrane	Inducible	19808683	Protein import
Dynamin-related protein	DrpA	TGME49_267800	Apicoplast surface	Inducible, protein level	19217294	Apicoplast fission
Translocon of the inner membrane	Tic20	TGME49_255370	Innermost membrane	Inducible	18757752	Protein import
Acyl carrier protein	ACP	TGME49_264080	Stroma	Inducible	16920791	Metabolic function—FAS

The corresponding lines may be used as controls during the functional analysis of new mutants

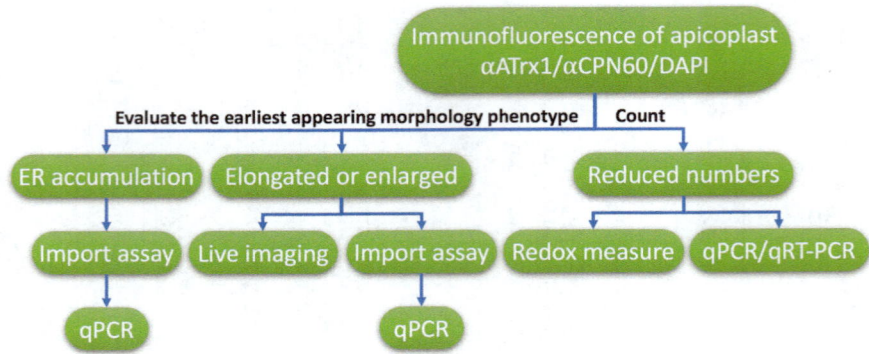

Fig. 2 A pipeline of apicoplast functional analysis using the discussed array of assays. In *T. gondii* the apicoplast has a typical morphology, thus simple immunofluorescence analysis often provides insight into the potential defect. The main morphological defects are mentioned. Suggested follow-up functional assays that would address the potential defect proposed by the morphology is mentioned below each. In the case of import defect, the assay is indirect as it analyses transit peptide processing defect as an indication for failure of the protein to reach the apicoplast. For this reason, it is suggested to examine for organelle loss via qPCR of an apicoplast genome–encoded gene. When import is the primary defect organelle loss is observed at least 24 h (4 replication cycles) after the processing defect is observed

2   Materials

2.1 Immuno-fluorescence Assay (IFA)

1. Parasites inside human foreskin fibroblasts (HFF) cultured on glass coverslips.

2. 4% (V/V, diluted from 20% commercial stock) paraformaldehyde.

3. Phosphate buffered saline (PBS).

4. Blocking buffer: PBS, 0.2%Triton X-100, 2% bovine serum albumin.

5. Washing buffer: PBS, 0.2%Triton X-100.

6. Glass slides.

7. Mounting medium of choice.

2.2 Import Assay

1. Complete cytomix.
   120 mM KCl.

   0.15 mM $CaCl_2$.

   10 mM K_2HPO_4/KH_2PO_4, pH 7.6.

   25 mM HEPES pH 7.6.

   2 mM EGTA, pH 7.6.

   5 mM $MgCl_2$.

   Adjusted with KOH to pH 7.6.

   3 mM ATP (add fresh just before transfection).

3 mM GSH (add fresh just before transfection).

2. Plasmid pBT-LytB-Ty.
   The plasmid is from [3], and contains the following elements:
   Bleomycin selectable marker.
   TUB8 promoter.
   LytB (TGME49_001270) cDNA fused to Ty tag.

3. Plasmid pTUB8-PPP1-Ty.
   The plasmid is from [1, 4], and contains the following elements:
   Bleomycin selectable marker.
   TUB8 promoter.
   PPP1 (TGME49_287270) cDNA fused to Ty tag.

2.3 qPCR and qRT-PCR of an Apicoplast Genome–Encoded Gene

2.3.1 Parasite Culturing

1. Culture medium: DMEM supplemented with 4 mM glutamine, 10% FBS, 100 U/mL penicillin, and 100 μg/mL streptomycin.

2. 6 cm culture dishes and 6-well culture plates.

3. For Tet-inducible mutants: Anhydro tetracycline stock solution at 2 mg/mL in ethanol.

4. 15 mL falcon tubes, 1.5 and 2 mL Eppendorf tubes, pipettes, micropipettes, and tips.

5. 10 mL syringes, 23G or 26G needles, 3 μm pore syringe filters.

2.3.2 gDNA Purification

1. Nuclease-free H_2O.

2. TN9 Buffer: 500 mM Tris–HCl pH 9, 2 M NaCl in dH_2O, filter-sterilized.

3. 0.5 m EDTA in H_2O, autoclaved.

4. 50 mg/mL Proteinase K, 40 μL aliquots.

5. 10% SDS.

6. Phenol–chloroform–isoamyl alcohol 25:24:1.

7. Tube shaker or spinning wheel.

8. 3 M sodium acetate (NaOAc) in dH_2O.

9. 100% isopropanol alcohol.

10. 70% ethanol (EtOH) in dH_2O.

11. Tabletop centrifuge for Eppendorf and falcon tubes.

2.3.3 RNA Purification

1. TRI-reagent.

2. QIAGEN RNeasy kit.

3. QIAGEN RNase-free DNase kit or equivalent.

2.3.4 Retrotranscription	1. RETROscript Kit or equivalent (random decamer protocol required).
	2. Thermocycler.
	3. PCR tubes.

2.3.5 qPCR	1. Power SYBR Green PCR Master Mix or equivalent.
	2. Optical 96-well reaction plates.
	3. Optical adhesive films or 96-well plates.
	4. Applied Biosystems 7500 Real-Time PCR System or equivalent.

2.4 Live Microscopy

1. Culture medium—same as that in Subheading 2.3.1.
2. Human foreskin fibroblasts grown in culture medium in Glass bottom optical dishes.
3. Microscope with heat control and CO_2 supply.

2.5 Measurement of Redox Changes Using roGFP

2.5.1 Parasite Culturing

1. Culture medium—same as point Subheading 2.3.1.
2. 6 cm culture dishes and 6-well culture plates.
3. 30 mm ⌀ circle coverslips #1.
4. For Tet-inducible mutants: Anhydro tetracycline stock solution at 2 mg/mL.
5. 15 mL falcon tubes, 1.5 and 2 mL Eppendorf tubes, pipettes, micropipettes, and tips.

2.5.2 Microscope Imaging

1. HEPES buffer: 20 mM HEPES, 130 mM NaCl, 5 mM KCl, 1 mM $CaCl_2$, 1 mM $MgCl_2$, 10 mM D-glucose. Correct pH to 7.4.
2. 1 M diamide solution.
3. 1 M DTT solution.
4. Microscope live imaging chamber.
5. Zeiss Axio Observer A1 microscope or equivalent.
6. Colibri illumination system or equivalent.
7. Axio Vision software or equivalent.

3 Methods

3.1 Immuno-fluorescence Assay (IFA) (See Note 1)

1. Parasites are cultured in HFFs on a glass coverslip inside 24-well plate.
2. Remove all media and add 300–500 µL of 4% paraformaldehyde to completely cover the coverslip.
3. Incubate for 20 min at RT.

4. Remove PFA into designated waste and wash slides 3× with PBS.

5. At this point the coverslips can be stored at 4 °C (in PBS) if necessary.

6. Add blocking and permeabilization buffer and make sure slide is fully covered.

7. Incubate for 20 min at RT.

8. Remove blocking buffer.

9. Add primary antibody in blocking buffer. You can put as little as 20 μL directly on the slide but make sure you remove majority of the buffer from blocking step.

10. Place moist (not wet!) tissue over the wells and incubate for 1 h at RT.

11. Remove antibody and wash 3 × 5 min with washing buffer. Plates may be placed on low-speed shaker to increase the efficiency of the washes.

12. Add secondary antibody in blocking buffer. You can put as little as 20 μL directly on the slide but make sure you remove majority of the buffer from washing step.

13. Incubate in dark for 45 min, RT (once again, place moist tissue over the wells).

14. Remove antibody and wash 3 × 5 min with washing buffer. Plates may be placed on low-speed shaker to increase the efficiency of the washes.

15. Wash once with PBS.

16. Mount the coverslips onto glass slides using mounting medium of your choice.
    Store slides in dark at 4 °C.

3.2 Apicoplast Protein Import Assay (See Note 2)

1. Parasites are grown in 6 cm dishes in HFFs with or without any relevant gene-depletion inducer added to the growth medium for a given period (this will depend on the dynamics of gene disruption).

2. 10×10^6 parasites (estimated fully lysed 6 cm dish) are harvested 24 h before the expected end of the desired time point. Namely, if when testing a 72-h time point, parasites are harvested 48 h after ATc treatment for this step, then incubated for additional 24 h after the transfection bellow. For -ATc we collect parasites after 24 h of growth with no ATc for this step.

3. Parasites are transiently transfected with pBT_LytB_Ty [3] or with pTUB8-PPP1-Ty [4] (see Note 3). Briefly, parasites are centrifuged ($1500 \times g$ 15 min 4 °C); growth media is aspirated gently but thoroughly (time allowed for medium to reaccumulate at the bottom of the tube after the first aspiration, then

aspirate again); 10×10^6 parasites resuspended in 700 μL complete Cytomix + 100 μL of DNA (80 μg) in Cytomix. Electroporate with the following conditions (Bio-Rad Gene-Pluser Xcell electroporator):

4 mm cuvette gap.

Voltage: 1700 V.

Pulse Length: 0.2 ms.

# of pulses: 2.

Interval: 5 s.

4. Transfected parasites are grown with or without the relevant gene-depletion inducer for an additional 24 h.

5. After 24 h parasites are harvested. The 10×10^6 transfected parasites will not have lysed a new 6 cm dish, thus harvesting requires scraping of the HFF, syringing out the parasites (26G needle) and filtering broken HFF debris (3 μm pore size filter).

6. Parasites are span down ($1500 \times g$ 15 min 4 °C). Washed once with $1\times$ PBS. Pellet is resuspended in 100 μL sample buffer (NuPAGE® Invitrogen) and boiled at 95 °C for 10 min.

7. 25 μL are used to separate by SDS-PAGE and Western blot is preformed using anti-Ty antibody (anti-Ty1 antibody, monoclonal BB2).

8. Both LytB-Ty and PPP1-Ty will show two bands: slow migrating "premature" band and faster migrating "mature" band corresponding to proteins that reached the apicoplast and lost their transit peptide. The intensities of mature and premature bands are measured (suggestion: use Western blot Odyssey CLx + Odyssey Image Studio Software) and mature–premature ratio is calculated. Noimport defect will show constant ratio between parental and gene-depleted lines as well as over time since depletion. An import defect will result in a decreasing ratio with time. A primary import defect will show a decreased ratio prior to loss of the plastid (*see* **Note 4**).

3.3 qPCR and qRT-PCR of an Apicoplast Genome–Encoded Gene

3.3.1 Parasite Culturing and Harvesting

1. Culture parasites following standard procedures using a 6 cm dish with confluent HFF monolayers for each parasite line.

2. When parasites have completely lysed the dishes, transfer 50 μL of medium containing the egressed parasites to each well of one or more wells of 6-well dish containing confluent monolayers of HFFs and 3 mL of fresh medium (*see* **Note 5**). Two wells from these plates will be used for each condition (for example: untreated control, 72 h ATc, 48 h ATc, and 24 h ATc = 8 wells in total (*see* **Note 6**)).

3. Parasites should take 3 days to completely lyse the HFF in the. Thus, if ATc induction is needed ATc is added (final

concentration 0.5 µg/mL) at a timing suitable for the desired condition. For example, for 72 h ATc is added on day 0, for 48 h on day 1, and for 24 h on day 2. On day 2 all the supernatants are replaced to remove all extracellular parasites.

4. At day 3, supernatant with egressed parasites from all the conditions are collected after resuspending the remaining infected HFF loosely attached to the well bottoms by repeated pipetting with a P1000 micropipette (*see* **Note 7**). Parasites from each two wells of the same conditions are combined, syringed through a 23G needle and filtered through a 3 µm syringe filter into a 15 mL falcon tube.

5. Parasites are spun down at $450 \times g$ for 5 min at RT.

6. The supernatant is discarded and parasite pellets are stored in the same 15 mL falcons at -20 °C until nucleic acids are extracted.

3.3.2 gDNA Purification
*(See **Note 8**)*

1. In a 2 mL Eppendorf mix:
   1160 µL dH$_2$O.

   200 µL TN9 buffer.

   400 µL 0.5 M EDTA solution.

   40 µL proteinase K (50 mg/mL).

   Add this solution to the falcon tube containing the thawed parasite pellet from above and resuspend.

2. Add 200 µL 10% SDS to the solution (*see* **Note 9**).

3. Incubate the solutions at 50 °C O/N while shaking/rotating.

4. After incubation, add 1 mL of phenol–chloroform–isoamyl alcohol and set in a shaker/spinning wheel for 1 h at RT (*see* **Note 10**).

5. Spin the mix for 10 min at $3000 \times g$ and carefully collect the upper phase in 2 mL Eppendorf tubes (max 800 µL per tube) making sure you do not disturb the bottom phases (*see* **Note 11**).

6. Add 1:30 volume of NaOAc and 0.6 volumes of isopropanol and mix by inverting 5–10 times (*see* **Note 12**).

7. Centrifuge the tubes at $16,000 \times g$ for 10 min at 4 °C.

8. Discard supernatant and wash pellets with 500 µL 70% EtOH in dH$_2$O.

9. Spin at $16,000 \times g$ for 5 min at 4 °C and remove the supernatant.

10. Gently tap the tube on a piece of paper towel to remove the remaining EtOH and leave in a chemical hood to dry (*see* **Note 13**).

11. Resuspend the pelleted DNA in 50 μL of nuclease-free H_2O and check quantity and quality using a NanoDrop and running the DNA on a gel (*see* **Note 14**).

3.3.3 RNA Purification
*(See **Note 15**)*

1. Resuspend the thawed pellet in 300 μL buffer RLT from QIA-GEN RNeasy kit and mix by pipetting.

2. Add 300 μL of TRI-Reagent and vortex for a few seconds.

3. Incubate at room temperature for 5 min.

4. Add 200 μL Chloroform and mix by inverting 5–10 times (*see* **Note 16**).

5. Incubate at room temperature for 10 min.

6. Centrifuge tubes at $16,000 \times g$ for 15 min.

7. Transfer the upper aqueous phase to a clean 2 mL tube being extremely careful not to disturb and transfer the bottom phases and the white particles between phases (*see* **Note 17**).

8. The recovered upper phase is diluted 1:1 with 70% EtOH and mixed by inversion 5–10 times.

9. Load the solution on RNeasy columns (700 μL maximum, use one column per condition) and spin at $8000 \times g$ for 15 s at RT.

10. Discard the flow through and repeat the previous step until all the solution for each condition has passed through its column.

11. Load 350 μL of buffer RW1 and spin at $8000 \times g$ for 15 s at RT.

12. On each column load a mixture of 70 μL RDD buffer and 10 μL of DNase I and incubate at RT for 15 min (*see* **Note 18**).

13. Load again 350 μL of buffer RW1 and spin at $8000 \times g$ for 15 s at RT to wash the DNase I.

14. Load 500 μL of buffer RPE and spin at $8000 \times g$ for 15 s.

15. Transfer the column to a new collection tube (provided with the kit).

16. Load again 500 μL of buffer RPE, however this time spin at $16,000 \times g$ for 2 min.

17. Transfer the column to a RNase-free tube (provided with the kit), load 30 mL of RNase-free water (also provided with the Kit) and incubate for 1–5 min at RT.

18. After incubation, spin the column in the tube at $8000 \times g$ for 1 min to elute RNA (*see* **Note 19**).

19. Estimate quantity and quality by NanoDrop and electrophoresis.

    NanoDrop reads for A_{260}/A_{280} ratio should be >1.9, while A_{260}/A_{230} ratio should be >2.0.

Electrophoresis should show two bands corresponding to the large and small subunit of the rRNA (*see* **Note 20**).

20. RNA must be stored at −80 °C!

*3.3.4 Generation of cDNA from RNA with the RETROscript Kit (See **Note 21**)*

1. From above purified RNA, transfer 1–2 μg to PCR tubes, and make sure to use the same quantity of RNA for each condition (*see* **Note 22**).

2. Bring the volume to 10 μL with nuclease-free H_2O and add 2 μL of Oligo(dT) (to retrotranscribe mRNA only) or Random Decamers (to retrotranscribe all RNAs). These reagents are provided with the RETROscript kit. Mix and spin briefly.

3. Place tube in a thermocycler for 3 min at a temperature between 70 and 85 °C (the higher the RNA GC content the higher the temperature).

4. When incubation is complete, place tubes on ice and spin briefly.

5. Add the following reagents to the tube on ice:
    (a)   2 μL 10× RT Buffer.
    (b)   4 μL dNTP mix.
    (c)   1 μL RNase inhibitor.
    (d)   1 μL MMLV-RT.
    Mix and spin briefly.

6. Incubate for 1 h in a thermocycler at 42 °C followed by a 10 min 92 °C inactivating incubation.

7. Proceed with the RT-qPCR or store at −20 °C for a few weeks or −80 °C for a few months.

8. As a rule of thumb, your reaction has virtually converted all your RNA to cDNA (*see* **Note 23**), thus a rough cDNA concentration would be RNA starting concentration.

*3.3.5 Testing the qPCR Primers (See **Note 24**)*

Example for primers used in qPCR to follow apicoplast DNA content and transcription [4]:

Housekeeping nuclear gene (actin):

Forward: GGGACGACATGGAGAAAATC.

Reverse: AGAAAGAACGGCCTGGATAG.

Apicoplast-encoded tested target (TogoCr29):

Forward: GCCCGTACTAAAACTGACACAAG.

Reverse: AGGCATCCTTTATCCCGAAG.

1. Primers for your nuclear housekeeping gene (e.g., Actin1) and for your apicoplast gene of interest (e.g., TogoCr29) must be tested to apply the $2^{-\Delta\Delta CT}$ relative quantification method [5].

2. Dilute your gDNA (qPCR) or your cDNA (RT-qPCR obtained from retrotranscription) from your untreated condition to a starting concentration of 50 ng/μL (*see* **Note 25**).

3. Make 1:5 dilutions of this templates to have 6 dilutions (e.g., 50, 10, 2, 0.4, 0.08, and 0.016 ng/μL).

4. Prepare a master mix containing the primers diluted in nuclease-free H_2O at a concentration of 0.75 μM. You should prepare enough master to make triplicates of each template dilution and to run controls using your housekeeping gene primer couple (e.g., 6 dilutions × 3 replicates × 4 μL used for each reaction = 72 μL; therefore, you should prepare about 100 μL for each primer couple tested).

5. Load your master mix in a qPCR optical 96-well plate and to each well add (*see* **Note 26**):

   (a) 1 μL template dilution (DNA or cDNA).

   (b) 5 μL Power SYBR Green PCR Master Mix.

6. Leave one to three wells for the H_2O control, using the housekeeping gene primers master mix and replacing the template dilution with water (remember to add the SYBR green Master Mix as on point 5).

7. Only if you are testing primers for RT-qPCR, leave one to three more wells for your RNA control. In this case, your template will be replaced by a dilution (e.g., 50 ng/μL) of the RNA (and not the cDNA) from the untreated condition (*see* **Note 27**).

8. Seal the plate close with an adhesive plate seal. Use a plastic spatula being careful to completely stick the foil while avoiding piercing it.

9. Briefly spin the plate in a centrifuge to collect the reagent at the bottom of the wells and release any air bubbles.

10. Place in the qPCR machine and run with a standard protocol, if a primer dissociation step test is available, make sure to include it to your run.

11. Once the run is completed, check the dissociation steps for each primer couple and make sure only one peak is displayed for each reaction. The presence of multiple peaks or abnormally shaped peaks is an indication of aspecific binding or self-binding of the primers and, therefore, this primer couple should be replaced.

12. For each suitable primer couple, export the C_t values and make averages for each triplicate condition at each dilution (50, 10, 2, 0.4, 0.08 and 0.016 ng) and plot them in a scatter plot with C_t averages on the y-axis and $\log_{10}$ of the concentrations in the y-axis (you can do this on, e.g., Microsoft Excel or similar software).

13. Calculate the trendline passing by the C_t average points and obtain the slope value from the line equation (e.g., if $y = mx + b$ the slope value is m).

14. Apply the following formula to calculate the percentage of primer efficiency:

$$\left[\left(10^{\frac{1}{m}}\right) - 1\right]100$$

   where m is the slope obtained from the trendline equation.

15. Primers couples with efficiency between 90% and 110% can be used for qPCR. The difference between the compared housekeeping and target gene primer couple efficiency should not be higher than 5%.

3.3.6 Setting up the qPCR/RT-qPCR Reactions

1. Similar to the previous section, prepare a master mix for each primer couple you want to use diluting them in nuclease-free H_2O to a concentration of 0.75 μM. In this case, you will need only 3 replicates for each condition (e.g., if three times point with ATc are tested, you will have 3 repetitions each containing three time points and an untreated control = 12 reaction. In this case, you will need about 60 μL of the master mix (*see* **Note 28**).

2. Load 4 μL of your master mixes in each well of a qPCR optical 96 well plate and to each well add (*see* **Note 29**):

   (a) 1 μL of your DNA (qPCR) or cDNA (RT-qPCR) at 10 ng/μL.

   (b) 5 μL Power SYBR Green PCR Master Mix.

3. Two quality controls should be added to your run using the housekeeping gene primers. In the first one, you should replace DNA or cDNA with water. The second one is only required in RT-qPCR and consists of replacing the cDNA with a similar dilution of the RNA used as template (*see* **Note 30**).

4. Seal the plate with an adhesive plate seal as above.

5. Spin the plate briefly and run it in the qPCR machine, again, add the primer dissociation step if available.

6. When the run is complete, check the dissociation tests to evaluate if the primer couples worked fine.

7. Export your C_t values for further calculations.

8. To evaluate the fold change in relative expression using the $2^{-\Delta\Delta CT}$ method, calculate the average C_t for all the triplicate values. These values should represent the housekeeping gene in the untreated condition (HU), the housekeeping gene in the treated conditions (in our example—H24, H48, H72), the gene of interest in the control line (IU) and the gene of interest in all the conditions (in our example—I24, I48, I72).

9. Calculate the differences between the treatments for the gene of interest and the housekeeping gene (I24-H24; I48-H48 and I72-H72 to respectively obtain ΔCT24, ΔCT48, and ΔCT72).

10. Calculate the difference between the gene of interest and housekeeping in the untreated condition (IU-HU) to obtain the ΔCTU.

11. Calculate the difference between each condition and the control, so ΔCT24-ΔCTU; ΔCT48-ΔCTU and ΔCT72-ΔCTU to respectively obtain the ΔΔCT24, ΔΔCT48 and ΔΔCT72.

    Calculate the value of $2^{-\Delta\Delta CT}$ for each of the $\Delta\Delta C_T$, this value represents the fold change in relative expression for the gene of interest at each condition when normalized for the housekeeping gene expression (*see* **Note 31**).

3.4 Live Microscopy

1. Seed parasites onto confluent HFF monolayer in optical dishes. One approach is to put the parasites into the optical dishes, spin at $300 \times g$ for 5 min at RT, incubate at 37C, 5% CO_2 for 30–60 min and gently wash with culture medium. This approach results in large number of single intracellular parasites allowing for imaging of endodyogeny in small vacuoles. Alternatively, parasites can be incubated in the live dish overnight to have larger vacuoles for imaging. In general, smaller vacuoles are easier to image as the organelles and the parasites are more likely to be all in focus.

2. Regardless of seeding method, wash the dish gently several times with culture medium to remove majority of extracellular parasites. Keep the parasites in the culture medium for the imaging.

3. Preheat microscope imaging chamber to 37 °C. The time will vary based on the size of the imaging chamber.

4. Once preheated, place dish with the parasites onto microscope and switch on CO_2 supply setting it at 5%.

5. Find focus and then allow the dish to sit for at least 30 min prior to imaging.

6. If your parasites are fluorescent, focus on a vacuole and find the minimum exposure time and minimum light (LED light) amount that allows you to visualize your protein (*see* **Note 32**).

7. Find a new vacuole and snap a few images to make sure all is in focus. It may take several attempts to find a vacuole where all the parasites are well aligned and organelles can be seen.

8. Start imaging. The longer the total imaging time the longer the interval between time points. In general, 15 min time points for 4–6 h imaging do not seem to cause any harm to the parasites (*see* **Note 33**).

9. Parasites will likely move during the imaging. Before each time point put them back in focus as much as possible using as little light as possible.

10. Process the file using program of your choice.

3.5 Measurement of Redox Changes Using roGFP

3.5.1 Parasite Culturing

1. In a 6-well plate with 30 mm ⌀ coverslips in each well seed HFF and allow growth to a confluent monolayer on the coverslip.

2. Grow parasites following standard procedures, then infect the monolayer on the coverslip. Plan to have freshly lysed parasites from a 6 cm dish 24 h before the experimental endpoint (consider this if needed to grow in, e.g., ATc).

3. Use parasites obtained from each fully lysed plate to transfect a suitable expression plasmid containing apicoplast-targeted roGFP (e.g., pTUB8-FNR-roGFP(6)), and use it to inoculate three wells of a 6-well with coverslips, each with different parasite dilutions (*see* **Note 34**).

4. Culture parasites for an additional 24 h.

5. Use standard light microscope to select wells with a high number of vacuoles but no monolayer lysis yet (*see* **Note 35**).

3.5.2 Microscope Chamber Setup (See **Note 36**)

1. Remove medium from the well you want to test.

2. Gently wash the well with 1 mL HEPES buffer twice.

3. Add 2 mL of HEPES buffer to the well.

4. Lift the coverslip (*see* **Note 37**) and transfer it in a petri dish containing HEPES buffer, gently swirl the plate.

5. Transfer the coverslip to a second petri dish containing HEPES and swirl gently again.

6. Put the coverslip on a piece of paper to dry the bottom, the cell monolayer must face up without touching the paper.

7. Mount the coverslip onto the live imaging chamber and assemble according to the manufacturer's instructions.

8. Pipet 1 mL of HEPES buffer in the chamber and test leakage by placing the chamber on a fresh piece of tissue paper (*see* **Note 38**).

9. Gently wash the bottom of the coverslip with Milli-Q H_2O in the chamber to remove salts.

10. Empty the chamber and add 800 μL of HEPES buffer.

3.5.3 Imaging of the Parasites

1. A Zeiss Axio Observer A1 inverted microscope is used to image the cells.

2. Set the microscope revolver to the 60× or 100× objective, place a drop of immersion oil on it and place the chamber onto the microscope stage touching the oil (*see* **Note 39**).

3. Focus on the parasites in the monolayer using white light.

4. Once in focus, place a dark cover on top of the chamber and check the fluorescent signal at 385 and 470 nm excitation wavelengths.

5. Focus on the fluorescent parasites and start imaging.

6. Fluorescence excitation light is generated and monitored by the Colibri illumination system coupled to the computer-controlled AxioVision software, which alternated the excitation wavelength between 385 and 470 nm.

7. Following the software manufacturer's instructions zoom on several apicoplast areas and draw containing circles for several regions of interest and for an area of background (*see* **Note 40**).

8. Fluorescence emission at 510 nm is recorded for regions of interest which were defined above.

9. For the acquisition define an interval of 1 min and start imaging in both wavelengths.

10. At 3 min, add 0.8 μL of 1 M diamide, and continue imaging.

11. At 6 add 8 μL of 1 M DTT, continue imaging for 2–4 more minutes.

12. Throughout the imaging the software records the intensities from each wavelength and the ratio between them, and generates a graph of the ratio changes over time. The difference between the ratios found after diamide addition and after DTT addition is the dynamic rage of the roGFP-fusion tested in the corresponding compartment. The ratio detected at the start of the experiment reflects the probe's steady state (*see* **Note 41**).

4   Notes

The apicoplast functional analysis pipeline presented here has several experimental components. Notes are provided for each of these components:

1. Apicoplast compartments can behave differently from one another in a given cell-line. For example, enlargement only of the outer membrane, while the stroma remains wild type size [6]. Thus, when using immunofluorescence to score apicoplast loss or to evaluate morphology changes it is imperative to label different components: DAPI for the genome, ATrx1 [7] for the outer membrane, CPN60 [8] for the stroma.

2. This assay is designed to monitor the transit peptide processing of apicoplast proteins that are synthesized after the depletion of the gene of interest. Processing is an indication of delivery to the suitable apicoplast compartment. The transient expression

of tagged apicoplast proteins allows detection of newly synthesized proteins expressed after the given period of depletion. The abundance of the tagged apicoplast targeted protein will depend on the efficiency of the transient transfection, and therefore cannot be compared between samples. Rather, the ratio of the preprocessed and processed bands indicates the extent of import. If equal signals between lanes is desired nevertheless, it is possible to run a second SDS-PAGE and blot where loading is adjusted to equalize the protein based on its expression level in each sample.

3. This assay can be adapted to apicoplast markers other than LytB and PPP1. In order to validate each new marker, one would be encouraged to examine its import (via this same method) in *Toxoplasma* mutants with apicoplast import defect (e.g., Toc/Tic mutants, e.g., [9, 10]) and with apicoplast mutants that are not impaired in import (e.g., [3]). The inducible knockdown of the translocon components: Tic20 [10], Toc75 [9] and Der1AP [8] could be used as positive control; while negative control would use a with apicoplast biogenesis defect but no apicoplast protein import defect like the PI3K inducible knockdown [6].

4. An alternative way to look at processing or modification of apicoplast proteins that are synthesized after the depletion of a gene of interest is via pulse chase labeling followed by immunoprecipitation of apicoplast proteins [1, 10]. Note that one of the modifications tested is lipoylation, however this protocol used an anti-lipoic antibody that was discontinued. In the hands of these authors, the pulldown has not worked with any new anti-lipoic acid antibody.

5. The inoculum of freshly lysed parasites use to pass to each well of the 6-well plate depends on the rate of growth of the given line and may need adjustment. Generally, using 50 µL taken from a fully lysed 6 cm dish with 5 mL culture, to inoculate a well of a 6-well dish would result in parasites lysis after 72 h.

6. Parasites from 1 fully lysed well are generally sufficient to obtain enough RNA for one experiment. However, using 2 wells provides a better amount of nucleic acids with the possibility to repeat some of the steps in case a technical replicate is required.

7. If intracellular parasites are required, lower numbers of parasites should be inoculated (this may require adjustment) on day 0. At collection, the culture medium should be replaced with $1\times$ PBS before harvesting the parasites by scrape, syringe and filter of the infected HFF monolayers. Since parasites with growth defect are typically slower in growth, higher inoculum may be required at day 0.

8. Purification of gDNA is performed using phenol–chloroform–isoamyl alcohol procedure to maximize the gDNA yield. Alternatively, a DNA extraction commercial kit can be used following the manufacturer's instructions.

9. Adding SDS last avoids parasite precipitation.

10. Phenol–chloroform–isoamyl alcohol is a toxic reagent that can cause burns if it gets in contact with skin. Always use gloves and work in a fume hood. Read the manufacturer safety information before use. Discard chlorinated waste per your institute's health and safety regulations. Never use polystyrene pipettes to aliquot chloroform containing solution; only use 1000 μL filter tips or glass Pasteur pipettes.

11. Phase lock gel can be used to facilitate the upper phase recovery. About 100 μL of the gel should be placed at the bottom of a 15 mL falcon tube by brief centrifugation. Lysis solution and chloroform should then be added on top. The gel will migrate at the interface between upper and lower phase avoiding carry on of the lower phase. A cheaper alternative is high vacuum grease, which has similar properties but should be autoclaved before use.

12. A lump of gDNA could be visible at this stage floating in the tube. If not, a tiny vitreous pellet will appear after centrifugation.

13. A small white pellet should be visible at this stage. The drying step should not be prolonged excessively but just until evaporation of the remaining liquid. Properly dried pellet maintains vitreous edges while over drying produces completely white pellets that are difficult to redissolve in nuclease-free H_2O.

14. NanoDrop reads of a good quality DNA have a 260/280 ratio > 1.8 and a 260/230 ratio > 2.0. Quality of gDNA should also be evaluated by electrophoresis, where no smears should be noticed but just a band >10.0 kb.

15. In this protocol, a combination of TRI-reagent and silica columns is used to maximize yield and purity. Alternatively, silica columns only can be used to purify total RNA. TRI-reagent is toxic; therefore, the provider's safety information should be read, and disposal of any waste containing this reagent should be done according to your institute's health and safety regulations.

16. Care should be taken while handling chloroform and waste should be disposed according to your institute's regulations. Always work in a fume hood and use 1000 μL filter tips or glass Pasteur pipettes to aliquot chloroform.

17. As explained in (see **Note 11**), phase lock gel or high vacuum grease can simplify this step.

18. Follow the manufacturer's instructions to generate aliquots and for details on how to store them. Any other brand equivalent DNase I and buffer kit can be used as an alternative (use at least 50 μL of working solution containing 5–10 U of DNase I).

19. Respin the flow-through in the column may increase the final yield.

20. If purity of RNA is poor, RNA can be precipitated by addition of 1:30 volumes of NaOAc and 2.5 volumes of EtOH, this can be incubated at −80 °C between 30 min and overnight and then centrifuged at 16,000 × g for 20 min at 4 °C. Pellets are then washed once or twice with 70% EtOH and dried to be then resuspended in nuclease-free H_2O. This procedure may slightly reduce yield but significantly increases RNA quality. An alternative may be to respin the RNA solution in the same RNeasy column but this may not help if the column is saturated by contaminants.

21. Any equivalent kit can be used for this so long as the random primer (decamers) protocol and reagents are provided.

22. If your RNA is not concentrated enough, you can precipitate and resuspend it in a smaller amount of nuclease-free H_2O as explained in **Note 16**.

23. Unfortunately, there is not a straightforward way to check your cDNA quality. The best test is to evaluate the qPCR amplification of your cDNA template. For this reason, it is crucial to use very high-quality RNA for your retrotranscription reaction.

24. When using the $2^{-\Delta\Delta CT}$ method it is crucial to test the primer pairs' efficiency in advance to infer if it is reasonable to make comparison between different primer couples. Therefore, this step is essential for both cDNA and gDNA templates.

25. Obviously, if you use gDNA you will be performing a qPCR, while if you are using cDNA you will be performing a RT-qPCR. Having a good quantification of your samples is crucial here; using a NanoDrop can be helpful.

26. A suggestion on order of loading the plate: have three columns for each primer couple (A1 to F1; A2 to F2; A3 to F3; etc.) and a line for each untreated template dilution (gDNA or cDNA). This allows testing 5 primer couples in a single run by loading an additional primer couple in lines G and H and leaving 6 wells for the RNA and H_2O controls.

27. The no template control identifies any contamination in the reagent used, while, the RNA control identifies DNA contamination in your RNA due to inefficient DNase treatment. These controls are crucial and should be performed for every qPCR.

A good negative control should show a $C_t > 30$ or undetectable.

28. It is always better to prepare a slightly bigger amount of the master mix (4–5 reactions more) to avoid running out. Using the same master mix for all reactions helps to better standardize the results. A master mix with all the components could also be used. However, this will increase the number of different master mixes and be a source of confusion while loading the plate.

29. A proposed order of loading is having the different primer pairs in each column triplicates and the different templates in each line, placing the untreated template on line A and all the conditions in the lines underneath.

30. This is like what is done in the primer test, *see* **Note 27** for details.

31. To simplify these steps, an automated Excel sheet can be used. Some templates are available online.

32. A major technical challenge with live imaging is balancing parasite survival with signal intensity and time-lapse resolution. Long and repeating exposure to light (LED light) is toxic to the parasites. It is advised to dedicate the set-up before imaging to define the minimal exposure sufficient for generating interpretable signal (while considering potential bleaching over time). It is beneficial to identify the minimal number of stacks needed.

33. When imaging for a long period (hours), observation of parasite division is a good indication for viability at the end of the imaging.

34. To dilute you can transfer a third of the transfection to the first well and mix with the 3 mL fresh medium in the well. Take 1 mL of this medium and pass it to the next well and repeat for the third dilution.

35. Vacuoles containing 2–4 parasites are the best to read so wells having the highest number of these should be imaged.

36. Obviously, these steps vary per microscope/chamber in use. Alternatively, optical petri dishes can be used.

37. Lifting the coverslip can be challenging due to adherence to the bottom of the well. Use a 1000 μL tip to gently release the coverslip and slip a tweezer underneath to lift it out of the well.

38. Pipet the buffer gently, while touching the wall of the chamber and avoiding directing the flow onto the monolayer.

39. To enable accurate measure of apicoplast redox via roGFP it is imperative to image with high magnitude (using ×60 or ×100 objective) and to ensure that each of the regions being measured is fully contained within the organelle. This may be

challenging: due to the high magnitude, small organelle size and movement of the host cells, of the parasites and of the organelle, the region of interest is often rapidly shifted from its original target during imaging. The solution is simple: image analysis is performed post imaging and while repositioning the region in every frame.

40. As apicoplasts are small, zooming in on the image as when selecting regions of interest increases accuracy.

41. Different roGFP variants have varying dynamic ranges of reactivity to redox levels, and the fusions to a targeting signal may affect this range. A sensor that is fully oxidized or fully reduced in its compartment cannot respond to further changes and thus cannot report on those changes. It is advised to generate a series of targeting signal/roGFP variant fusion combinations to enhance the chances of identifying a sensor with suitable range for its target compartment.

References

1. Sheiner L, Demerly JL, Poulsen N, Beatty WL, Lucas O, Behnke MS, White MW, Striepen B (2011) A systematic screen to discover and analyze apicoplast proteins identifies a conserved and essential protein import factor. PLoS Pathog 7(12):e1002392

2. van Dooren GG, Reiff SB, Tomova C, Meissner M, Humbel BM, Striepen B (2009) A novel dynamin-related protein has been recruited for apicoplast fission in *Toxoplasma gondii*. Curr Biol 19(4):267–276

3. Nair SC, Brooks CF, Goodman CD, Sturm A, McFadden GI, Sundriyal S, Anglin JL, Song Y, Moreno SN, Striepen B (2011) Apicoplast isoprenoid precursor synthesis and the molecular basis of fosmidomycin resistance in *Toxoplasma gondii*. J Exp Med 208(7):1547–1559

4. Biddau M, Bouchut A, Major J, Saveria T, Tottey J, Oka O, van-Lith M, Jennings KE, Ovciarikova J, DeRocher A, Striepen B, Waller RF, Parsons M, Sheiner L (2018) Two essential Thioredoxins mediate apicoplast biogenesis, protein import, and gene expression in *Toxoplasma gondii*. PLoS Pathog 14(2):e1006836

5. Livak KJ, Schmittgen TD (2001) Analysis of relative gene expression data using real-time quantitative PCR and the 2(−Delta C(T)) method. Methods 25(4):402–408

6. Daher W, Morlon-Guyot J, Sheiner L, Lentini G, Berry L, Tawk L, Dubremetz JF, Wengelnik K, Striepen B, Lebrun M (2015) Lipid kinases are essential for apicoplast homeostasis in *Toxoplasma gondii*. Cell Microbiol 17(4):559–578

7. DeRocher AE, Coppens I, Karnataki A, Gilbert LA, Rome ME, Feagin JE, Bradley PJ, Parsons M (2008) A thioredoxin family protein of the apicoplast periphery identifies abundant candidate transport vesicles in *Toxoplasma gondii*. Eukaryot Cell 7(9):1518–1529

8. Agrawal S, van Dooren GG, Beatty WL, Striepen B (2009) Genetic evidence that an endosymbiont-derived endoplasmic reticulum-associated protein degradation (ERAD) system functions in import of apicoplast proteins. J Biol Chem 284(48):33683–33691

9. Sheiner L, Fellows JD, Ovciarikova J, Brooks CF, Agrawal S, Holmes ZC, Bietz I, Flinner N, Heiny S, Mirus O, Przyborski JM, Striepen B (2015) *Toxoplasma gondii* Toc75 functions in import of stromal but not peripheral apicoplast proteins. Traffic 16(12):1254–1269

10. van Dooren GG, Tomova C, Agrawal S, Humbel BM, Striepen B (2008) *Toxoplasma gondii* Tic20 is essential for apicoplast protein import. Proc Natl Acad Sci U S A 105(36):13574–13579

Chapter 14

Measuring Solute Transport in *Toxoplasma gondii* Parasites

Esther Rajendran, Kiaran Kirk, and Giel G. van Dooren

Abstract

The uptake of host-derived nutrients is key to the growth and survival of *Toxoplasma gondii* parasites. Nutrients are acquired via solute transporters that localize to the plasma membrane of the parasites. In this chapter, we describe methodology by which the uptake of solutes via plasma membrane transporters may be monitored and characterized. These assays, used here to investigate the uptake of amino acids into parasites, have broad applicability in measuring the uptake of a diverse range of solutes.

Key words *Toxoplasma gondii*, Transporters, Amino acids, Plasma membrane

1 Introduction

1.1 Nutrient Acquisition in Toxoplasma gondii

Toxoplasma gondii belongs to a phylum of protozoan parasites called the Apicomplexa. These parasites establish an intracellular niche in their hosts in which they replicate. In the case of *T. gondii*, replication occurs by a process of endodyogeny, during which the parasite undergoes an internal budding process that leads to the formation of two daughter parasites within one parent cell [1]. Cell replication occurs every 6–8 h, and requires that the parasites double their DNA content and synthesize new organelles. *T. gondii* parasites undergo multiple cell division events within a single host cell. Ultimately, they egress from the host cell, going on to invade nearby host cells and reestablishing an intracellular infection. This cycle of invasion, intracellular replication and egress is known as the lytic cycle, and leads to the numerous disease symptoms caused by *T. gondii* [2].

Apicomplexan parasites are descended from free-living, phototrophic algal ancestors. With a bit of sunlight, some carbon dioxide and a dash of minerals, these algae synthesized all of the organic molecules required for their propagation [3]. As they evolved to become obligate intracellular parasites, ancestral apicomplexans lost the capacity to synthesize many essential organic molecules, and became reliant on their host organisms as a source for these

Christopher J. Tonkin (ed.), *Toxoplasma gondii: Methods and Protocols*, Methods in Molecular Biology, vol. 2071,
https://doi.org/10.1007/978-1-4939-9857-9_14, © Springer Science+Business Media, LLC, part of Springer Nature 2020

compounds [3–6]. The lytic cycle of *T. gondii* is a nutrient-hungry process. Energy for all stages of the lytic cycle is acquired through the catabolism of glucose and glutamine [7, 8]. Intracellular replication requires the synthesis of new proteins, nucleic acids (DNA and RNA), and numerous lipids. This requires the parasite to have access to a range of nutrients including nucleosides, amino acids, fatty acids and other lipids, and a range of vitamins and minerals [5, 9]. Although *T. gondii* has the capacity to synthesize some of these compounds, most are scavenged by the parasite from its host [10–15].

1.2 The Role of Solute Transporter Proteins in Nutrient Acquisition

T. gondii parasites endocytose material from their host, and this contributes to intracellular pools of metabolites such as amino acids [16]. However, the primary route of entry of most nutrients into the parasite is across the plasma membrane. Most nutrients are hydrophilic and, as a result, do not simply diffuse across the plasma membrane. Instead, they enter the parasite via plasma membrane-localized solute transporter proteins. Each of these transporters has one or more substrate binding sites, specific for the solute(s) that they transport. The binding of a substrate to the transporter on one side of the membrane (e.g., outside the parasite) is followed by a conformational shift in the transporter structure, resulting in the substrate being translocated to the other side of the membrane (e.g., inside the parasite).

Transporter proteins take several forms. Uniporters bind and transport one substrate molecule at a time, mediating the net transport of substrates down their concentration gradient (i.e., from an aqueous environment of higher substrate concentration to one of lower substrate concentration). Symporters and antiporters mediate the cotransport of two or more substrate molecules: symporters transport substrates in the same direction across a membrane, whereas antiporters transport the two substrates in opposite directions. Symporters and antiporters act as secondary active transporters, coupling the transport of one substrate (typically an ion such as Na^+ or H^+) down its electrochemical gradient to the transport of a second substrate (e.g., a nutrient) against its electrochemical gradient (e.g., from an aqueous environment of lower substrate concentration to an environment of higher substrate concentration). Such transporters provide a mechanism by which a cell can accumulate nutrients against a concentration gradient.

Despite the importance of transporters for parasite growth, the function of only a handful of transporter proteins have been demonstrated and characterized. These include transporters that mediate the uptake of glucose [17], nucleosides [18], and amino acids [12, 19]. Several of these known transporters have been shown to be important for progression of the *T. gondii* parasite through its lytic cycle; these include the major arginine and tyrosine transporters of the parasite [12, 19]. However, the major glucose transporter in the parasite is dispensable for in vitro growth, and even the arginine and tyrosine transporters are not essential when parasites are cultured at high concentrations of these amino acids [7, 12, 19]. This indicates that the parasite has metabolic flexibility in its energy sources, and alternative uptake pathways for the uptake of at least some amino acids [7, 12, 19, 20].

1.3 Approaches for Characterizing Solute Transporters in *T. gondii*

Establishing experimental approaches to characterize transporters in *T. gondii* has been key to elucidating their roles in parasite growth and physiology. Recent high- and medium-throughput genetic approaches allow researchers to identify transporters that fulfil important functions in the parasite [12, 21]. The powerful genetic tools available in *T. gondii* makes the generation of transporter knockouts and/or regulatable mutants feasible, and makes determining the sub-cellular localization of these proteins straightforward [7, 12, 18, 19]. Such genetically modified strains are invaluable for understanding the importance of particular transporters for parasite growth, and for their functional characterization. Many *T. gondii* transporters have orthologues in other apicomplexan parasites, including the causative agents of malaria [12, 17, 19, 22]. Insights into the function of *T. gondii* transporters may, therefore, offer valuable perspectives into the function of orthologous transporters from other parasites.

Transporter proteins are emerging as particularly efficacious drug targets [23, 24]. They appear to be overrepresented as targets in screens of diverse compound libraries of antimalarial drugs [25, 26], and it is likely that drugs targeting the uptake of essential nutrients in *T. gondii* will be effective inhibitors of parasite growth.

Recently, our group has established the function of a family of plasma membrane-localized amino acid transporters that are found in *T. gondii* and other apicomplexan parasites [12, 19]. These studies provide a template for characterizing solute transporters in *T. gondii*, setting out a three-step experimental approach to determine the function of solute transporters, and their importance for parasite growth and virulence.

Step 1. Where does the transporter localize? This involves integrating epitope tags into the native locus of candidate transporters, then determining the localization of the tagged protein by immunofluorescence assay.

Step 2. Is the transporter important for parasite growth, in vitro *and* in vivo? This involves generating mutant parasites strains that are deficient in the transporter(s) of interest, then measuring parasite growth. Mutants can be generated in a variety of ways. We have generated gene knockouts using traditional crossover recombination approaches [19], and gene disruptions by more modern CRISPR-based approaches [12]. If genes are not amenable to such disruption approaches, they can be targeted using regulatable approaches. We have generated regulatable transporter mutants by introducing an anhydrotetracycline-regulated promoter upstream of the target gene [19], or by fusing auxin-inducible degron domains onto target transporters (Hapuarachchi, Kirk, Lehane, and van Dooren, unpublished). Once a mutant is generated, parasite growth can be measured in vitro using either plaque assays or fluorescence growth assays. The importance of a transporter for parasite virulence, in vivo, can be measured through mouse infection experiments [12, 19].

Step 3. What does the transporter transport? This is perhaps the most difficult question to answer, and addressing it ideally involves a multipronged approach.

Metabolomics. Initial insights into transporter function may be gained using targeted or untargeted metabolomic approaches [12]. A depletion of a particular metabolite in parasites defective in the candidate transporter may, for example, suggest a role for the transporter in the uptake of that particular metabolite.

Heterologous expression. Heterologous expressions studies represent the gold standard for gaining a detailed understanding of the functional characteristics of a transporter protein. Parasite plasma membrane transporters can be expressed in a range of heterologous systems. *Xenopus laevis* oocytes have proven particularly useful in this regard, providing valuable insights into substrate specificities and transporter kinetics for a range of *T. gondii* transporter proteins [12, 17–19]. Expression of transporters in the oocyte system is achieved through the injection of RNA encoding the target transporter into the oocyte. After confirming that the transporter is targeted to the plasma membrane of the oocyte, the uptake of candidate substrates is measured. This is typically achieved by incubating oocytes in a solution containing a radiolabeled (e.g., ^{3}H- or ^{14}C-labeled) form of the substrate of interest, and measuring the time-dependent accumulation of radioactivity in the oocytes. In some cases (if the transport process is "electrogenic"; i.e., generates an electrical current) transport may be measured electrophysiologically, by impaling the oocyte with electrodes [19]. If the transporter functions as an exchanger (e.g., an antiporter), oocytes may be preloaded with candidate exchange substrates [12].

Parasite transport assays. A third approach for characterizing plasma membrane transporters entails measuring the uptake of candidate substrates into the parasites themselves. This typically involves incubating parasites in a solution containing a radiolabeled form of the candidate substrate and measuring the time-dependent uptake of radiolabel. Comparing the uptake of radiolabeled substrate between wild type and mutant parasites not expressing the transporter of interest provides a powerful test for whether that transporter plays a role in the uptake of the substrate into parasites under the particular conditions in which the measurements are carried out [12, 19]. Such assays can also be used to characterize the kinetics and substrate selectivity of particular transporters, even if the molecular identities of those transporter are unknown [27].

In this chapter, we describe step-by-step approaches for undertaking such radiolabel uptake assays in *T. gondii* parasites, providing detailed protocols for:

(a) Measuring the time-dependent uptake of candidate substrates across the parasite plasma membrane.

(b) Characterizing transporter kinetics.

(c) Investigating transporter substrate selectivity.

The methodologies described below are those used in studies that we and others have undertaken to characterize the uptake of numerous substrates into the related *P. falciparum* parasites including sugars, nucleosides, amino acids, vitamins, polyamines, and inorganic ions (reviewed in [28]). We have used the same approaches to measure the uptake of amino acids across the plasma membrane of *T. gondii* [12, 19], with the techniques involved being generally applicable to the characterization of the transport of a broad range of aqueous substrates.

2   Materials

2.1   Preparation of Solutions

1. Calculate the volume of **parasite suspension** and volume of **2× radiolabeled substrate solution** (i.e., a solution containing radiolabeled substrate at 2× the desired final concentration) required for the experiment. Typically, a volume of 200 µl (a mixture of 100 µl parasite suspension and 100 µl of 2× radiolabeled substrate solution) is used per data point, and we typically acquire two "technical replicates" for each data point. If performing a timecourse experiment with ten time points, each to be done in duplicate, then 2 ml each of parasite suspension and radiolabel solution is required (*see* **Note 1**).

2. Prepare the radiolabeled substrate solution containing 2× the final concentration of the test substrate in sterile Phosphate-Buffered Saline-Glucose (PBS-Glucose). PBS-Glucose consists of PBS (e.g., Dulbecco's PBS, Sigma, D8537) supplemented with 10 mM D-glucose. For [^{3}H]-labeled (*see* **Note 2**) and [^{14}C]-labeled substrates, we typically use final radiolabel concentrations of 1 µCi ml^{-1} and 0.1 µCi ml^{-1}, respectively (*see* **Note 3**). We typically supplement the radiolabeled substrate in the substrate solution with unlabeled substrate (*see* **Note 4**).

3. Store the 2× radiolabeled substrate solution and PBS-glucose required to resuspend parasites in a 37 °C water bath until required.

4. Aliquot 250 μl of an oil mix consisting of 84% v/v PM125 high temperature silicone bath fluid (Clearco, PM-125) and 16% v/v light mineral oil (Sigma, M5904; *see* **Note 5**) into labeled 1.5 ml tubes (*see* **Note 6**). The oil is chosen to have a density intermediate between that of the parasites and the aqueous medium in which the parasites are suspended (*see* **Note 5**). Add the oil mix to as many 1.5 ml tubes as there are experimental timepoints or conditions.

2.2 Parasite Preparation

For uptake assays with extracellular tachyzoites, a fully egressed parasite culture is preferred in order to obtain the maximum number of cells possible. The volume of the cell culture should be scaled according to the number of data points required for the assay. In a typical experiment, we aim for $1-2 \times 10^7$ cells per technical replicate, with each data point to be averaged from two technical replicates.

1. Filter a fully egressed parasite culture through a 3 μm polycarbonate membrane filter to remove host cell debris.

2. Count the parasite number using a hemocytometer.

3. Centrifuge the parasite suspension at $1500 \times g$ for 10 min to pellet the parasites.

4. Wash the parasites by resuspension of the pellet in 1 ml PBS-Glucose, transfer the suspension to a 1.5 or 2 ml centrifuge tube, then centrifuge at $12,000 \times g$ for 1 min to repellet the cells.

5. Resuspend the parasites in PBS-Glucose at a concentration of $1-2 \times 10^8$ cells ml^{-1} and keep at 37 °C until required. 100 μl of this solution is used for each technical replicate.

3 Methods

3.1 Radiolabeled Substrate Uptake Time Course Experiment

In this section we describe the design of an experiment to measure the time-dependent uptake of a radiolabeled substrate into *T. gondii* parasites. This is typically the starting point for characterizing the transport of a substrate across the parasite plasma membrane. Such an experiment provides information about whether, and, if so, at what rate, a substrate is taken up by the parasites under the conditions tested.

The assay is typically performed in tubes incubated in a water bath set to 37 °C (*see* **Note 7**).

1. To commence the assay, combine equal volumes of **2× radiolabeled substrate solution** and **parasite suspension** (we will refer to this mixture as the **reaction mixture**). Start timer immediately.

2. 10–15 s before each predetermined timepoint, transfer 200 μl of the **reaction mixture** to a 1.5 ml microcentrifuge tube that contains the oil mix and that is sitting in the rotor of a micro-centrifuge (*see* Subheading 2.1; *see* **Note 8**). The reaction mix-ture should be layered on top of the oil. When the timepoint is reached, close the lid of the 1.5 ml tube lid and commence centrifugation. Centrifuge at $12,000 \times g$ for 30 s. To account for variation in sample handling, we perform uptake assays in duplicate (i.e., aliquot two samples at each timepoint), and treat these as technical replicates during data processing (*see* Subheading 3.2). The centrifugation separates the parasites from the uptake solution (*see* **Note 5**), and uptake is considered to have "stopped" at the time at which the microcentrifuge is started.

3. Remove the tubes from the centrifuge, place them in a separate rack, and proceed to the other timepoints (*see* **Note 9**).

4. Repeat the sampling step for all timepoints. To avoid parasites settling over time, mix the uptake solution gently before removing samples (either by inverting the tube or using a pipette). If the timepoints are greater than 5 min apart, gently invert (or "flick") the tube 3–4 times to mix every 5 min then return the tube to the water bath.

5. Once the final timepoint sample has been taken, the samples are processed. First, the aqueous radiolabeled solution above the oil layer is removed from each tube, leaving at least some of the oil layer intact. We do this using a vacuum-based aspiration device (*see* **Note 10**). Each tube is then washed three times with water, with the remnant oil layer protecting the parasite pellet from exposure to the water (*see* **Note 10**). The purpose of the wash step is to remove any residual radiolabel that is left on the walls of the tube, above the oil layer. Following the washes, the remaining oil mixture is removed without disturbing the para-site pellet.

6. Add 500 μl of 0.1% (v/v) Triton X-100 in water to each tube. This solubilizes the parasites and any radiolabel that was taken up by the parasite during the timecourse. Leave the tubes at room temperature for >1 h to ensure that the parasites are fully solubilized (we often leave this overnight).

7. Transfer the tube contents to a scintillation vial (*see* **Note 11**). Add 1.5 ml of scintillation fluid, secure with a lid, label then vortex the tube to ensure that the Triton X-100 extract and the scintillation fluid are well mixed.

8. In addition to the timepoints, there are two other samples that must be collected during these experiments: a **"trap"** and a **"standard"**.

9. The **"trap"** sample provides a measure of the amount of unincorporated radiolabeled substrate that is centrifuged through the oil layer (i.e., the "background" radiolabel in the experiments). This is the radiolabel that is present in the extracellular medium "trapped" between cells within the cell pellet following centrifugation of the parasites through the oil mixture. The radioactivity in the trap sample is subtracted from the total radioactivity in the cell pellet to provide a measure of the amount of radioactivity that has actually been taken up by the parasite (*see* Subheading 3.2).

   The simplest way to measure the trap is to acquire a timepoint at the very outset of the experiment (i.e., at "time-zero"). However, there may be significant uptake of radiolabeled substrates in the short time that it takes to acquire a sample (i.e. in the time that it takes to add the radiolabel to the parasites, aliquot the parasite mixture onto the oil layer, and to centrifuge the parasites through the oil), resulting in an overestimate of the trap. Our preferred method of obtaining a trap value is to take a sample as rapidly as possible, using an uptake solution to which a large excess of unlabeled substrate has been added (i.e., at a concentration manyfold higher than that of the radiolabeled substrate). The unlabeled substrate present in the solution competes with the radiolabeled substrate for the transporter, thereby minimizing the uptake of radiolabel during the short time required to take and process the sample. If an inhibitor of the transport process being characterized is available, this provides an alternate means of minimizing the uptake of substrate during the short sampling and processing period.

   To obtain the trap sample, mix the parasites and the radiolabel solution containing excess unlabeled substrate or inhibitor, and immediately transfer an aliquot onto an oil layer in a 1.5 ml tube, then centrifuge. This sample is then processed as for all others. Given its importance in the subsequent data analysis, we always obtain a minimum of three trap values for each experiment. The average of these trap values is then subtracted from the radioactive counts obtained at each timepoint (*see* Subheading 3.2).

10. The **"standard"** is a measurement of the amount of radiolabel in a defined volume of the uptake solution. The measurement enables the calculation of the **amount** of substrate taken up from the **measured radioactivity** associated with each sample (*see* Subheading 3.2). To obtain the standard, pipette three 10 μl aliquots of the $2\times$ radiolabeled substrate solution used for uptake into three separate scintillation vials (i.e., the measurement is done in triplicate). Add 500 μl of 0.1% (v/v) Triton X-100 so that the contents of the scintillation tube are as close

as possible to those of all the samples, then add 1.5 ml of scintillation fluid, secure the lid, label and vortex to mix.

11. Measure the radioactivity present in each of the samples (typically for 1 min) with a scintillation counter, using a suitable protocol, according to manufacturer's instructions.

3.2 Data Analysis for Radiolabel Uptake Experiments

1. To illustrate how the data acquired in such an experiment are analyzed, we present here an example of an experiment we conducted, in which we measured the time-dependent uptake of the amino acid L-lysine into *T. gondii* parasites.

2. The first step in estimating the amount of substrate taken up into the parasites at each timepoint is to subtract the "trap" (i.e., background) value from the total radioactivity associated with each sample (*see* Subheading 3.1, **step 9**). The radioactivity measurements from the scintillation counting are recorded as "counts per minute" (cpm). The average cpm for the three trap samples is subtracted from the cpm obtained for each individual timepoint sample, to yield an estimate of the cpm taken up into the parasites. If the radiolabel has been diluted in generating the $2\times$ radiolabeled substrate solution for the trap, it will be necessary to take this (typically negligible) dilution into account.

3. Substrate uptake rates are typically expressed in terms of "amount of substrate taken up, by a given number of cells, in a given length of time" (e.g., mol per cell number per min). This enables direct comparisons between different studies. To estimate the amount of substrate taken up during an experiment, we first need to calculate the relationship between the measured radioactivity (in units of cpm) and the amount of substrate. In other words, in our experiment, we need to know how much L-lysine (labeled and unlabeled) each cpm equates to.

   In calculating this, we first calculate the total concentration of L-lysine in the $2\times$ radiolabeled substrate solution. In the example we are considering, the $2\times$ radiolabeled substrate solution contained $100\,\mu M$ unlabeled L-lysine, and $0.2\,\mu Ci\,ml^{-1}$ of $[^{14}C]Lys$. The $[^{14}C]Lys$ was obtained from a stock solution containing $0.1\,\mu Ci\,\mu l^{-1}$ $[^{14}C]Lys$, with a specific activity of $318{,}800\,\mu Ci\,mmol^{-1}$. The stock solution therefore has a $[^{14}C]$ Lys concentration of $1/318800 \times 0.1 = 3.14 \times 10^{-7}\,mmol\,\mu l^{-1} = 314\,\mu M$. To prepare the $2\times$ radiolabeled substrate solution, this $314\,\mu M$ stock solution was diluted 1:500. The radiolabeled L-lysine therefore contributed a concentration of $314/500 = 0.627\,\mu M$ to the total L-lysine concentration. The total concentration of L-lysine in the $2\times$ radiolabeled

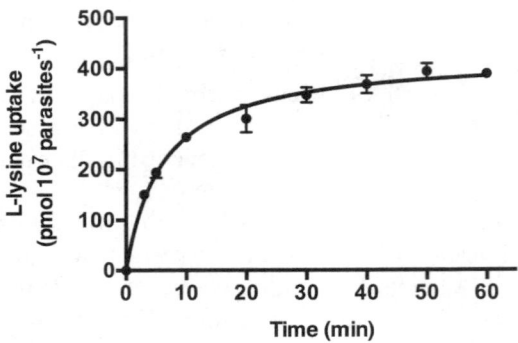

Fig. 1 Timecourse of L-lysine (Lys) uptake by wild type *T. gondii* parasites. Transport assays were performed in PBS-Glucose containing 0.1 μCi ml^{-1} [^{14}C] Lysine and 50 μM unlabeled L-lysine. Accumulation of L-lysine was monitored over 60 min. Data were derived from two independent experiments, each consisting of two technical replicates. Error bars represent the range/2 of the two biological data points. The line is derived from a single exponential function fitted to the data by nonlinear least-squares regression

substrate solution is the sum of the labeled and unlabeled solution: $100\ \mu M + 0.6\ \mu M = 100.6\ \mu M$.

4. To calculate the relationship between cpm and the amount of substrate, we use the results obtained for the **standard** samples. The standard samples were prepared using 10 μl of the 2× radiolabeled substrate solution. Given that the total L-lysine concentration in the 2× radiolabeled substrate solution was 100.6 μM, the total *amount* of L-lysine in 10 μl of this solution is calculated to be 1.006×10^{-9} mol, or 1.006 nmol. If, in our example, the scintillation counter gives an average measurement of 6000 cpm in the standard sample, then we know that in our experiment 6000 cpm equates to 1.006×10^{-9} mol of L-lysine. From this we calculate the amount of L-lysine per cpm to be 1.006×10^{-9} mol/6000 cpm $= 167.7 \times 10^{-15}$ mol/cpm, or 167.7 fmol of L-lysine/cpm.

5. We can now calculate the amount of L-lysine uptake in each of the timecourse samples taken throughout the experiment. In our example, at the 5 min timepoint the radioactivity taken up into the parasites (calculated by subtracting the trap cpm from the total measured cpm in this sample) was 1193 cpm. This corresponds to 1193 cpm $\times$ 167.7 fmol cpm$^{-1} = 200$ pmol of L-lysine.

6. Next we relate the uptake of L-lysine to parasite number. The uptake assay was performed using 10^7 parasites in each sample tube. Thus, from the 5 min sample, it may be calculated that under the conditions of the experiment, after 5 min of uptake in a 50 μM L-lysine solution, the amount of L-lysine taken up was 200 pmol/10^7 parasites (Fig. 1).

7. Similar calculations for each sample provide estimates of the amount of L-lysine taken up at each timepoint. For each timepoint, we typically obtain two technical replicates, and these are averaged to generate the timecourse for that particular experiment. Experiments are repeated on multiple days, with solutions prepared independently (*see* **Note 12**).

8. The uptake of L-lysine (in pmol per 10^7 parasites) is plotted as a function of time, to generate a timecourse of the sort seen in Fig. 1. Error bars (range/2 of values from the two biological replicates in this case) provide a measure of the variation. For simple uptake experiments such as these, the data are typically fitted with a single exponential function to provide a line of best fit (Fig. 1).

9. The initial slope of the line-of-best-fit enables the calculation of **the initial rate of uptake** of the substrate. Differences in initial uptake rates between cells exposed to different conditions (e.g., the presence and absence of potentially competing substrates) can reveal important functional characteristics (e.g., substrate selectivity; *see* Subheading 3.3.2) of the transporter(s) involved. Differences in initial uptake rates between different parasites (e.g., wild type versus mutant parasites) can provide important insights into the function of the transporter proteins being characterized (e.g., [12, 19]).

3.3 Variations of the Uptake Assay

The experiments described above examine the uptake of a candidate substrate over time. In the remainder of this chapter, we consider variations on this assay, such as those used to investigate the **kinetics** and **substrate specificity** of transporters involved in the uptake of the substrates of interest.

3.3.1 Investigating Transporter Kinetics

Transporters differ in their **affinity** for a particular substrate, and in the **maximum velocity** with which they can transport that substrate across a membrane. Understanding both the substrate affinity and the maximum velocity of a transporter is important for understanding the physiological role that the transporter serves.

During the transporter-mediated translocation of solutes across a membrane, a substrate molecule first binds to a site on the transporter protein. This binding is followed by a conformational shift in the protein, which results in the translocation of the substrate across the membrane [29]. The **affinity** of the transporter binding site for a particular substrate governs the physiological concentrations at which a transporter is effective in mediating the transport of that substrate.

Transporters with **high affinity** for a particular substrate are effective at transporting that substrate across a membrane when the concentrations of the substrate are low. By contrast, transporters with a **low affinity** for a particular substrate are typically less effective at low substrate concentrations, but effective at high substrate concentrations, provided that substrates of higher affinity are not present.

Transporters that operate at a **high velocity** can mediate the uptake of large amount of substrate in a given time. This is particularly important for substrates that are consumed in large quantities in a cell (e.g., energy sources such as glucose or glutamine). Transporters that function with a **low velocity** are likely to be better suited to the uptake of substrates required in lower amounts.

The affinity and velocity of transporters mirrors similar properties of enzymes that mediate biochemical reactions. The Michaelis–Menten model was developed to describe the enzymatic conversion of substrate to product. The model describes substrate binding to (or disassociating from) an enzyme and the subsequent irreversible product formation. The Michaelis-Menten equation describes the velocity of the reaction (V, the rate of reaction progression per unit time) as a function of the maximum reaction velocity (V_{max}), the substrate concentration ($[S]$) and the Michaelis constant (K_M). The K_M is a dissociation constant that describes the affinity of the enzyme for the substrate. It equates to the concentration of substrate at which the reaction velocity reaches half the V_{max}:

$$V = V_{max}[S]/(K_M + [S]) \tag{1}$$

The Michaelis-Menten equation can often be fitted to the substrate concentration dependence of transporter-mediated substrate uptake. Although the model may be oversimplified for complex transport systems (e.g., transporters with multiple substrate binding sites), it is adequate for providing the basic parameters required to understand the kinetics of many transporters.

To determine the kinetic properties of a transporter, the rate of uptake of the substrate of interest is measured over a range of substrate concentrations. If the plot of the transport rate as a function of the substrate concentration can be fitted by the Michaelis-Menten equation, it is then straightforward to determine the V_{max} and K_M of the transporter. The substrate affinity, as exemplified by the K_M, is an inherent property of the transporter protein. Because the K_M is a dissociation constant it is *inversely* correlated with the affinity of the transporter for its substrate. Low K_M values correspond to a high affinity of a transporter for its substrate, and vice versa. Unlike the V_{max} value, K_M does not change with the abundance of a particular transporter.

Knowing the K_M value of a substrate for a particular transporter enables important comparisons to be made. Comparing the K_M values for a range of substrates provides insights into the substrate selectivity of the transporter. Comparing the K_M values for a particular substrate between two or more transporters can provide important information about the respective roles of those transporters in different physiological situations.

In this section, we use the example of L-lysine uptake in *T. gondii* to illustrate the approach to characterizing transporter kinetics. In doing so, we make the assumption that *T. gondii* has a single L-lysine transporter. We have evidence that this is the case (Rajendran, Kirk and van Dooren, unpublished); for other substrates this must be determined experimentally. In instances in which more than one transporter mediates the uptake of a substrate into a cell, kinetic properties of individual transporters should be determined when the alternative transporters for a particular substrate are inactivated, either via genetic disruption or chemical inhibition. Kinetic properties of transporters can also be determined using heterologous expression systems (e.g., *Xenopus* oocytes) that allow transporters to be studied in isolation (*see* Subheading 1.3).

Analysis of Transporter Kinetics

The following describes a determination of the kinetic properties of the *T. gondii* L-lysine transporter. Any such analysis entails measuring the rate of uptake over a range of substrate concentrations.

1. The first step involves making $2\times$ **radiolabeled substrate solutions** that contain a range of unlabeled L-lysine concentrations. To do this, we start by make two stock solutions, each containing 0.2 µCi ml^{-1} [^{14}C]Lys in PBS-Glucose (**Solutions A** and **B**).

2. **Solution A**: make 500 µl of a solution containing 0.2 µCi ml^{-1} [^{14}C]Lys *and* 5 mM unlabeled L-lysine in PBS-Glucose (this is $2\times$ the highest concentration of L-lysine to be tested in the experiment; *see* **Note 13**). Add 212.5 µl of this solution to "Tube 1" (Fig. 2).

3. **Solution B**: make 2 ml of a solution containing 0.2 µCi ml^{-1} [^{14}C]Lys (and no unlabeled L-lysine). For the [^{14}C]Lys stock that we purchased for these experiments, 0.2 µCi ml^{-1} of [^{14}C]Lys corresponded to a L-lysine concentration of 0.627 µM (*see* Subheading 3.2). Aliquot 212.5 µl of this solution into "Tubes 2–9" (Fig. 2).

4. Add 212.5 µl of solution A to Tube 2 (to produce a solution that contains 2.5 mM L-lysine; Fig. 2). Mix thoroughly, then remove 212.5 µl of this solution, add it to Tube 3 (1.25 mM L-lysine), then continue to perform two-fold serial dilutions across Tubes 4–8 (Fig. 2). This will give L-lysine concentrations of 626 µM, 313 µM, 157 µM, 79 µM and 40 µM; note that these values take into account the 0.627 µM [^{14}C]Lys in each tube. Leave Tube 9 with just solution B (i.e., without any unlabeled L-lysine; this tube will contain 0.627 µM L-lysine, the concentration of the radiolabeled L-lysine). Note that on

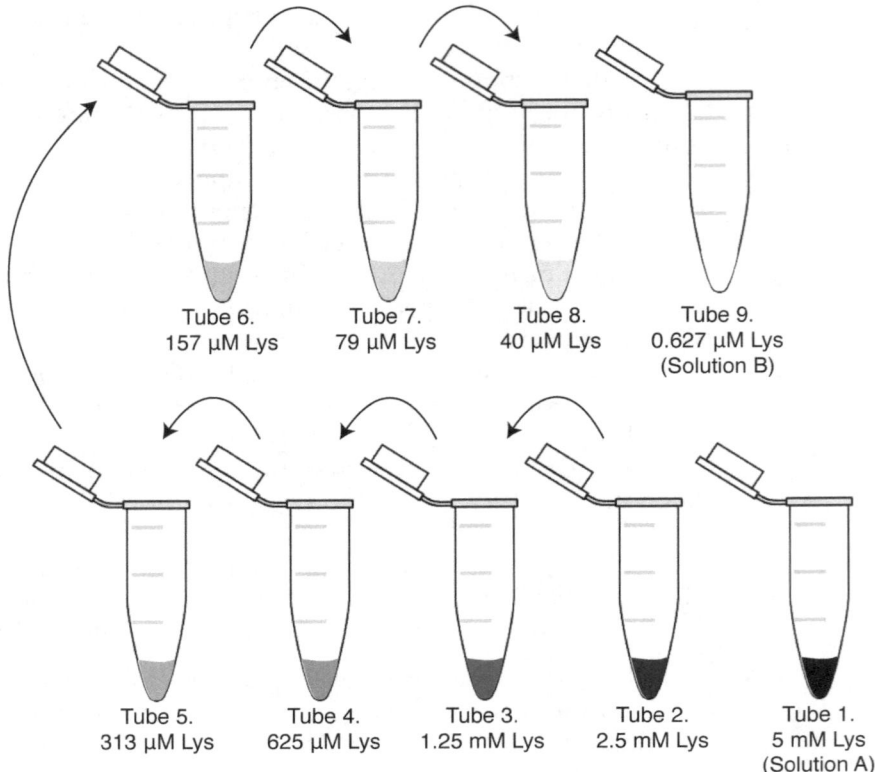

Fig. 2 A schematic showing the preparation of 2× radiolabeled substrate solutions used for the kinetic experiments described in Subheading "Analysis of Transporter Kinetics". 212.5 μl of Solution B (0.2 μCi ml⁻¹ [¹⁴C]Lys in PBS-glucose) is added to Tubes 2–9. 212.5 μl of Solution A (0.2 μCi ml⁻¹ [¹⁴C]Lys together with 5 mM unlabeled L-lysine) is added to Tube 1. 212.5 μl of solution A is added to Tube 2, and this solution is then serially diluted in Tubes 3–8. The final concentrations of L-lysine in each tube are indicated. Note that all tubes contain 0.2 μCi ml⁻¹ [¹⁴C]Lys. These tubes serve as 2× radiolabeled substrate solutions for the subsequent uptake assays

completing these dilutions, each tube will contain the same concentration of [^{14}C]Lys radiolabel (0.2 μCi ml^{-1}), but will differ in the *total* L-lysine concentration.

5. Prepare parasites as described in Subheading 2.2 (*see* **Note 7**).

6. Commence uptake by adding 212.5 μl of the **parasite suspension** to each tube containing the **2× radiolabeled substrate solution**s (*see* **Note 14**).

7. Incubate the **reaction mixture** at 37 °C for 3 min, a time chosen because it falls within the initial, approximately linear, phase of L-lysine uptake as determined in the uptake timecourse experiment (*see* Subheadings 3.1 and 3.2; Fig. 1).

8. At 3 min, transfer 2× 200 μl aliquots of each **reaction mixture** to separate tubes containing oil mixture, then centrifuge the two samples, thereby sedimenting the parasites through the oil

mix and terminating uptake. The two samples serve as technical replicates.

9. Acquire three "**trap**" samples from sample tubes containing the highest concentration of L-lysine (2.5 mM), and centrifuging the parasites through the oil layer *immediately* after adding the parasite suspension (i.e., time-zero). The 2.5 mM L-lysine concentration is chosen to maximize the extent to which the unlabeled substrate competes with the labeled substrate and thereby minimize the uptake of radiolabel.

10. Process all samples, and determine the amount of radiolabel in each by scintillation counting, as described in Subheading 3.1.

11. For the **standard** sample, transfer three 10 μl aliquots of the 2× radiolabeled substrate solutions used for uptake to separate scintillation vials. Add 500 μl of 0.1% (v/v) Triton X-100 then process and count as described in Subheading 3.1.

Data Analysis for Transporter Kinetic Experiments

The data analysis for experiments investigating the kinetics of a substrate transporter follow the same general approach describe in Subheading 3.2. Here, we go through this step-by-step, using the L-lysine transporter kinetics experiment described above as an example.

1. First, the average of the three trap cpm values is subtracted from the cpm value for each sample, to give a measure of the amount of radioactivity (in cpm) actually taken up by the parasites at each substrate concentration tested.

2. Using the cpm values obtained for the standard samples, convert the trap-corrected cpm for each sample to the amount of L-lysine taken up by the parasite during the 3 min incubation period, as described in Subheading 3.2. Average the values from the two technical replicates for each experimental condition. Note that these calculations take into account the different L-lysine concentrations in the uptake solutions from each sample. Although the cpm values will likely be highest for the uptake performed at the lowest total L-lysine concentration (because there is less unlabeled L-lysine competing with [^{14}C] Lys for the transporter), the total amount of L-lysine taken up into parasites will increase with increasing L-lysine concentration.

3. Divide the total amount of L-lysine taken up by the number of cells in each sample and by the length of the incubation period (3 min in this example) to yield an uptake rate, expressed in terms of amount of L-lysine taken up, per parasite, per min.

4. Plot the rate of L-lysine uptake as a function of the concentration of L-lysine in the extracellular solution (Fig. 3).

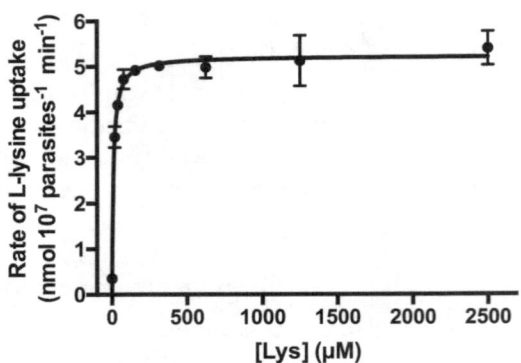

Fig. 3 Concentration-dependence of L-lysine transport in wild-type *T. gondii* parasite. [^{14}C]lysine uptake was measured over 3 min in the presence of varying concentrations of lysine (0.6 μM to 2.5 mM). The data were averaged from two independent experiments and are shown ± range/2. The Michaelis-Menten equation was fitted to the data by nonlinear regression using GraphPad Prism ($K_M = 9.9 ± 1.6$ μM; $V_{max} = 5.2 ± 0.1$ nmol 10^7 parasites^{-1} min^{-1})

5. If these data can be fitted by the Michaelis-Menten equation (Eq. 1), it is then a straightforward process to determine substrate affinity (K_M) and maximum rate or velocity of uptake (V_{max}). Curve-fitting programs such as Prism (GraphPad), SigmaPlot (Systat Software) and Origin (OriginLab) are routinely used for such data analysis. In this particular example, the estimated K_M of the L-lysine transporter in *T. gondii* is $9.9 ± 1.6$ μM and the V_{max} is $5.2 ± 0.1$ nmol 10^7 parasites^{-1} min^{-1} (*see* **Note 15**).

3.3.2 Investigating the Substrate Selectivity of a Transporter

Some transporters transport a single substrate, while others have broader substrate specificity. In *T. gondii*, for example, the *Tg*ApiAT1 transporter (also known as *Tg*NPT1) has a high selectivity for L-arginine [19]. However there is a second transporter, with broader selectivity for cationic amino acids, that transports both L-arginine and L-lysine ([19]; Rajendran, Kirk and van Dooren, unpublished). Similarly, the *Tg*ApiAT5-3 transporter has a broad selectivity for aromatic and large neutral amino acids [12].

As noted in Subheading 3.3.1, the binding of a substrate to its transporter is followed by a conformational shift in the structure of the transporter, leading to the translocation of the substrate across the membrane [29]. If the transporter binding site is capable of binding different substrates, then in the presence of these substrates there will be competition between the different substrates for binding to, and transport by, the transporter. This phenomenon provides the basis for investigating the substrate selectivity of a transporter using **competition assays**. These entail measuring the uptake of a radiolabeled form of a known substrate of the transporter of interest in the presence of an excess concentration of an alternative (unlabeled) substrate to "compete out" the uptake of the radiolabeled substrate. If the unlabeled compound inhibits the uptake of the radiolabeled substrate, then this may indicate that the compound is also a substrate of the transporter. If an excess concentration of a particular unlabeled compound does not inhibit uptake of the radiolabeled substrate, it is unlikely that the compound is a substrate of the transporter.

As with the kinetic analyses (Subheading 3.3.1), an important factor to take into account when performing these "competition" experiments is that some substrates are taken up by more than one transporter. Under these circumstances, the results of such competition assays are likely to reflect the net effects on multiple transporters, complicating the analysis. For example, in *T. gondii*, L-arginine is taken up by both the *Tg*ApiAT1 transporter and an alternative, broad-specificity cationic amino acid transporter [19]. The addition of unlabeled L-lysine inhibits the uptake of radiolabeled L-arginine through the cationic amino acid transporter but not through *Tg*ApiAT1, a transporter that is selective for L-arginine [19]. In such situations, it can be advantageous to compare the results of competition assays performed in wild type and mutant parasites lacking one of the transporters for a particular substrate. In the case of L-arginine transport in *T. gondii*, uptake is only partially inhibited by the addition of L-lysine in wild type parasites (in which the two transporters, *Tg*ApiAT1 and the broad-specificity cationic amino acid transporter, are operating), but almost completely inhibited in *Tg*ApiAT1 knockout parasites, in which arginine is taken up almost entirely via the broad-specificity cationic amino acid transporter. L-Lysine is a substrate for this transporter and unlabeled L-lysine therefore effectively competes with radiolabeled L-arginine for the transporter [19].

In this final section of this chapter we describe a competition assay designed to investigate the substrate specificity of the transporter that mediates L-lysine uptake into *T. gondii* parasites. In undertaking this assay, it is helpful to have an understanding of the kinetic parameters of the transporter of interest.

As above, initial timecourse experiments are used to determine a timepoint which falls in the initial linear phase of the uptake timecourse and which may therefore be used to estimate the initial rate of substrate uptake (*see* Subheadings 3.1 and 3.2; Fig. 1). From the kinetic analysis (*see* Subheadings "Analysis of Transporter Kinetics" and "Data Analysis for Transporter Kinetic Experiments"; Fig. 3), we know the K_M of the transport system for the substrate we are measuring. Experiments such as these are typically conducted using a substrate concentration at, or around, the K_M of the transporter.

1. Prepare stock solutions in PBS-glucose (or other suitable solvent) for each of the candidate "competitive" substrates to be

tested. In the experiment shown here, we have tested for competition by the following candidate substrates: L-glutamate, L-alanine, L-ornithine and L-arginine. Each candidate substrate was added to a final concentration of 5 mM from a 100 mM stock solution. The experiment also includes a **control** sample to which no candidate competitive substrate was added, and a **trap** sample containing 5 mM L-lysine (*see* Subheading 3.3.2, **step 8**).

2. Prepare 1.5 ml of 0.22 μCi ml^{-1} [^{14}C]Lys solution containing 111 μM unlabeled L-lysine in PBS-Glucose and aliquot 202.5 μl of this radioactive solution into 1.5 ml tubes.

3. Add 22.5 μl of the 100 mM amino acid stock solution into the corresponding tubes, giving a concentration of 10 mM (2$\times$ final concentration). Adjust the pH as necessary (*see* **Note 13**). For the control sample, add 22.5 μl of PBS-glucose. Keep all tubes at 37 °C.

4. Prepare parasites as described in Subheading 2.2.

5. Start the uptake assay by adding 225 μl of the **parasite suspension** to each tube of the **2$\times$ radiolabeled substrate solutions** (*see* **Note 14**).

6. Incubate the **reaction mixture** at 37 °C for 3 min, a time chosen as it falls within the initial linear phase of the uptake timecourse (*see* Subheadings 3.1 and 3.2; Fig. 1).

7. Transfer duplicate 200 μl aliquots from each **reaction mixture** to tubes containing oil mixture (the duplicate samples serve as technical replicates), then centrifuge the tubes to sediment the parasites beneath the oil, thereby separating the parasites from the extracellular solution and terminating uptake.

8. Acquire a **trap** sample by combining parasites and radiolabel in the presence of 5 mM (i.e., excess) L-lysine and sampling as quickly as possible (as described above).

9. For the **standard** samples, transfer three 10 μl aliquots of the 2$\times$ radiolabeled substrate solutions used for uptake to three separate scintillation vials. Add 500 μl of 0.1% (v/v) Triton X-100 then process and count as described in Subheading 3.1.

10. Process all samples as described previously. Determine the amount of [^{14}C]Lys taken up by the parasites as described in Subheading 3.1, and from this calculate the total amount of L-lysine taken up, as described in Subheading 3.2.

11. Compare the uptake of L-lysine in the control sample with that measured in the presence of each of the different candidate substrates. In the example given here, we found that the addition of excess cationic amino acids (L-arginine and L-ornithine) inhibited the uptake of L-lysine, whereas the addition of the anionic amino acid L-glutamate or the neutral amino acid L-

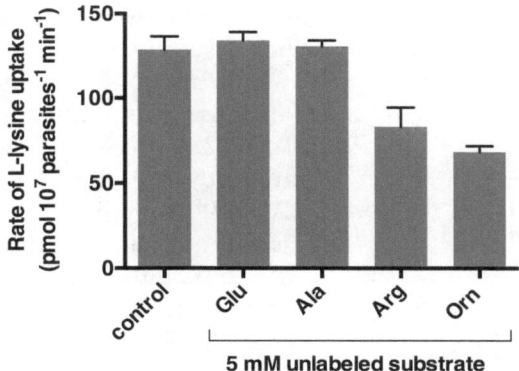

Fig. 4 Competition assays testing for the ability of various (unlabeled) amino acids to inhibit the uptake of L-lysine into wild type *T. gondii* parasites. Uptake assays were performed in PBS-Glucose containing 0.1 μCi ml^{-1} [^{14}C]lysine and 50 μM unlabeled lysine with each of the unlabeled amino acids present at 5 mM. Uptake of [^{14}C]lysine was monitored over 3 min. Data were derived from two independent experiments, each consisting of two technical replicates, and error bars represent the half range

alanine did not (Fig. 4). This is consistent with the L-lysine transporter of *T. gondii* having broad specificity for cationic amino acids, but not having a significant affinity for either neutral or anionic amino acids. This hypothesis is readily tested by carrying out direct measurements of the uptake of the candidate substrates, using radiolabeled forms of these compounds in conjunction with the methodologies described in this chapter.

4   Notes

1. It is a good idea to have an excess of the solutions and suspensions used in each experiment, to allow for the loss of small volumes of each in the course of pipetting. Typically, for a 2 ml volume, make 100-200 μl (5–10%) of extra solution.

2. If the radiolabeled substrate is in aqueous solution, the [^{3}H]-radionuclide will slowly (typically on a timescale of months) reach equilibrium with [^{1}H] from the water molecules in the solution (i.e., the ^{3}H radionuclide on the labeled substrate will be replaced with the stable ^{1}H atom of water, forming unlabeled substrate and tritiated water (^{3}H$_2$O)). The older the [^{3}H]-substrate stock, the more of this replacement will have taken place.

3. Radiolabeled substrate is used as a tracer in uptake assays. The goal is to have a small but measurable amount of the substrate (in order to minimize both the cost of the experiment and the

amount of radioactive waste produced). The volume of radiolabeled substrate used varies between substrates and even between vials purchased from the same company. Radioactivity is expressed in either Curie (Ci) or Bequerel (Bq; $1 \text{ Bq} = 2.7 \times 10^{-11}$ Ci or 60 disintegrations per minute, dpm). We have used Ci in this chapter. One μCi equals 2.22×10^6 dpm. The half-life of the radioisotope and age of the stock of radiolabeled substrate, the specific activity of the substrate (i.e., the radioactivity per amount of substrate; e.g., Ci mmol^{-1}), and the concentration of radioactivity (e.g., mCi ml^{-1}) all need to be taken into account when designing an experiment.

4. The rate at which the radiolabeled substrate is taken up is dependent on a range of factors, including the concentration of substrate in the medium (*see* Subheading 3.3.1). Increasing the extracellular concentration of substrate will generally increase the total uptake of substrate (the higher the extracellular concentration, the higher the rate of uptake, except under conditions in which the transporter is "saturated"). In experiments in which the substrate concentration is varied, this may be achieved by varying the concentration of radiolabeled substrate in the medium. However, radiolabeled substrate is expensive. An alternative, and usually preferred, approach involves keeping the concentration of radiolabeled substrate constant (and low), and varying the concentration of unlabeled substrate. A complicating factor is that unlabeled substrate will compete with the labeled substrate for the transporter(s), thereby decreasing the amount of radiolabel taken up (*see* Subheading 3.3.2). In any such experiment, the relative amounts of radiolabeled and unlabeled substrate must therefore be optimized to obtain a measurable amount of radiolabeled uptake while keeping the amount of radiolabeled substrate used as low as possible.

5. The oil mixture used in these experiments is designed to be intermediate in density between the (more dense) parasite and the (less dense) aqueous solution in which the parasites are suspended, such that when a parasite suspension is layered on top of the oil and centrifuged the parasites are pelleted beneath the oil and the aqueous extracellular solution remains on top of the oil, thereby effectively stopping substrate uptake. The ratio of PM125 to light mineral oil used in these *T. gondii* "oil-stop" experiments was described in a paper by [30]. The PM125 oil and light mineral oil do not mix readily. To ensure uniform mixing, incubate the mixture in a 15 or 50 ml tube on a rotating wheel for ~30 min. The mixture can be stored at room temperature for long-term use.

6. The high viscosity of the oil results in the oil taking longer to load and dispense than is the case for aqueous solutions. To assist in dispensing the viscous oil mixture, cut the end of a 1 ml pipette tip (~2–3 mm) to widen the opening, and allow sufficient time for each pipetting step, ensuring that the pipette tip remains in the oil mixture until the flow into the pipette tip stops, thereby ensuring that air bubbles are not formed in the oil mixture.

7. A circulating water bath is ideal for this assay as it allows for effective heat exchange and uniform temperature control throughout the water bath. If a water bath is not available, heat blocks are an alternative. Ensure that the temperature of both parasite suspension and the radiolabeled solution is 37 °C before the start of the experiment. Transporter function is temperature-dependent and it is important that this parameter is kept constant.

8. Care should be taken when pipetting live parasites to avoid the risk of infection. Ideally, parasite pipetting should occur in a Class 2 biosafety cabinet, or, if one is not available, the researcher should wear a face-shield or safety glasses.

9. If the timepoints are less than 2 min apart, it is useful to have more than one centrifuge for this assay.

10. A pump or vacuum driven aspirator is used for aspirating the radioactive extracellular solution from above the oil layer, and for aspirating the oil layer after the washes are complete. For the addition of water during wash steps, we use two different methods. One entails using a pipette to add ~1 ml of water on top of the oil mixture. The other entails simply immersing the tube in a container/beaker of continuously running water placed in the sink (the oil layer prevents water from mixing with the parasite sample beneath the oil). The advantage of the second method is that it saves time. However, this can only be used if the rules on radioactive waste management in the investigator's country/state allows for low level radioactive wastes to be diluted and discarded down designated sinks. All washes are repeated three times to remove any residual radioactive solution remaining above the oil layer. Ensure that some oil is left before the last wash to prevent the wash water from coming into contact with the parasite pellet (which, if it happens, can cause cell lysis and inaccuracy in uptake measurements).

11. Make sure the parasite pellet is fully dissolved before transferring the solution to a scintillation vial. Avoid vortexing the sample at this stage; vortexing will cause the mixture to froth, making the transfer of the sample to the scintillation vial difficult.

12. Radiolabeled substrate transport assays should be performed a minimum of three times, with the results reported as averaged data together with the calculated error. In the event that the variation between experiments is large, the experiment should be repeated until the experimenter has confidence in the observed pattern or in the value of the parameter under investigation.

13. Keep in mind that the pH of the uptake solution may change with different concentrations of a substrate, or in the presence of potentially competing substrates. Variations in pH may have a profound effect on uptake rates, particularly (but not only) when measuring uptake via H^+-coupled transporters. Measure the pH of the solution from which you make the substrate stock, and adjust as necessary.

14. Stagger the addition of the parasite suspension to each of the $2\times$ radiolabeled substrate solution tubes to enable enough time for the subsequent processing of each sample.

15. The substrate concentrations used for such a kinetic analysis should include multiple concentrations below the K_M of the transporter, and multiple concentrations at which the transporter is operating at close to V_{max}. Achieving this may involve some optimisation. In the particular example shown in Fig. 3, V_{max} is reached at concentrations above ~300 μM L-lysine, and we have several data points above this value. However, we have only one data point below the K_M of the transporter. This is not ideal. The accuracy of the K_M estimation would be improved by including some substrate concentrations between 0.6 and 20 μM.

Acknowledgments

Work in this area in our laboratories was supported by a grant from the Australian Research Council (DP150102883) to K.K. and G.v. D.

References

1. Striepen B, Jordan CN, Reiff S, van Dooren GG (2007) Building the perfect parasite: cell division in apicomplexa. PLoS Pathog 3(6):e78

2. Montoya JG, Liesenfeld O (2004) Toxoplasmosis. Lancet 363(9425):1965–1976

3. Woo YH, Ansari H, Otto TD, Klinger CM, Kolisko M, Michalek J et al (2015) Chromerid genomes reveal the evolutionary path from photosynthetic algae to obligate intracellular parasites. Elife 4:e06974

4. Janouskovec J, Keeling PJ (2016) Evolution: causality and the origin of parasitism. Curr Biol 26(4):R174–R177

5. Tymoshenko S, Oppenheim RD, Agren R, Nielsen J, Soldati-Favre D, Hatzimanikatis V (2015) Metabolic needs and capabilities of *Toxoplasma gondii* through combined computational and experimental analysis. PLoS Comput Biol 11(5):e1004261

6. van Dooren GG, Striepen B (2013) The algal past and parasite present of the apicoplast. Annu Rev Microbiol 67:271–289

7. Blume M, Rodriguez-Contreras D, Landfear S, Fleige T, Soldati-Favre D, Lucius R et al (2009) Host-derived glucose and its transporter in the obligate intracellular pathogen *Toxoplasma gondii* are dispensable by glutaminolysis. Proc Natl Acad Sci U S A 106 (31):12998–13003

8. MacRae JI, Sheiner L, Nahid A, Tonkin C, Striepen B, McConville MJ (2012) Mitochondrial metabolism of glucose and glutamine is required for intracellular growth of *Toxoplasma gondii*. Cell Host Microbe 12(5):682–692

9. Coppens I (2014) Exploitation of auxotrophies and metabolic defects in *Toxoplasma* as therapeutic approaches. Int J Parasitol 44 (2):109–120

10. Charron AJ, Sibley LD (2002) Host cells: mobilizable lipid resources for the intracellular parasite *Toxoplasma gondii*. J Cell Sci 115 (Pt 15):3049–3059

11. Fox BA, Gigley JP, Bzik DJ (2004) *Toxoplasma gondii* lacks the enzymes required for de novo arginine biosynthesis and arginine starvation triggers cyst formation. Int J Parasitol 34 (3):323–331

12. Parker KER, Fairweather SJ, Rajendran E, Blume M, McConville MJ, Bröer S et al (2019) The tyrosine transporter of *Toxoplasma gondii* is a member of the newly defined apicomplexan amino acid transporter (ApiAT) family. PLoS Pathog 15(2):e1007577

13. Pernas L, Bean C, Boothroyd JC, Scorrano L (2018) Mitochondria restrict growth of the intracellular parasite *Toxoplasma gondii* by limiting its uptake of fatty acids. Cell Metab 27 (4):886–97 e4

14. Pfefferkorn ER (1984) Interferon gamma blocks the growth of *Toxoplasma gondii* in human fibroblasts by inducing the host cells to degrade tryptophan. Proc Natl Acad Sci U S A 81(3):908–912

15. Schwartzman JD, Pfefferkorn ER (1982) *Toxoplasma gondii*: purine synthesis and salvage in mutant host cells and parasites. Exp Parasitol 53(1):77–86

16. Di Cristina M, Dou Z, Lunghi M, Kannan G, Huynh MH, McGovern OL et al (2017) *Toxoplasma* depends on lysosomal consumption of autophagosomes for persistent infection. Nat Microbiol 2:17096

17. Joet T, Holterman L, Stedman TT, Kocken CH, Van Der Wel A, Thomas AW et al (2002) Comparative characterization of hexose transporters of *Plasmodium knowlesi*, *Plasmodium yoelii* and *Toxoplasma gondii* highlights functional differences within the apicomplexan family. Biochem J 368(Pt 3):923–929

18. Chiang CW, Carter N, Sullivan WJ Jr, Donald RG, Roos DS, Naguib FN et al (1999) The adenosine transporter of *Toxoplasma gondii*. Identification by insertional mutagenesis, cloning, and recombinant expression. J Biol Chem 274(49):35255–35261

19. Rajendran E, Hapuarachchi SV, Miller CM, Fairweather SJ, Cai Y, Smith NC et al (2017) Cationic amino acid transporters play key roles in the survival and transmission of apicomplexan parasites. Nat Commun 8:14455

20. Nitzsche R, Zagoriy V, Lucius R, Gupta N (2016) Metabolic cooperation of glucose and glutamine is essential for the lytic cycle of obligate intracellular parasite *Toxoplasma gondii*. J Biol Chem 291(1):126–141

21. Sidik SM, Huet D, Ganesan SM, Huynh MH, Wang T, Nasamu AS et al (2016) A genome-wide CRISPR screen in *Toxoplasma* identifies essential apicomplexan genes. Cell 166 (6):1423–1435

22. Carter NS, Ben Mamoun C, Liu W, Silva EO, Landfear SM, Goldberg DE et al (2000) Isolation and functional characterization of the *Pf*NT1 nucleoside transporter gene from *Plasmodium falciparum*. J Biol Chem 275 (14):10683–10691

23. Cesar-Razquin A, Snijder B, Frappier-Brinton-T, Isserlin R, Gyimesi G, Bai X et al (2015) A call for systematic research on solute carriers. Cell 162(3):478–487

24. Lin L, Yee SW, Kim RB, Giacomini KM (2015) SLC transporters as therapeutic targets: emerging opportunities. Nat Rev Drug Discov 14(8):543–560

25. Hapuarachchi SV, Cobbold SA, Shafik SH, Dennis AS, McConville MJ, Martin RE et al (2017) The malaria parasite's lactate transporter PfFNT is the target of antiplasmodial compounds identified in whole cell phenotypic screens. PLoS Pathog 13(2):e1006180

26. Lehane AM, Ridgway MC, Baker E, Kirk K (2014) Diverse chemotypes disrupt ion homeostasis in the malaria parasite. Mol Microbiol 94(2):327–339

27. De Koning HP, Al-Salabi MI, Cohen AM, Coombs GH, Wastling JM (2003) Identification and characterisation of high affinity nucleoside and nucleobase transporters in *Toxoplasma gondii*. Int J Parasitol 33 (8):821–831

28. Kirk K, Lehane AM (2014) Membrane transport in the malaria parasite and its host erythrocyte. Biochem J 457(1):1–18

29. Colas C, Ung PM, Schlessinger A (2016) SLC transporters: structure, function, and drug discovery. Medchemcomm 7(6):1069–1081

30. Schwab JC, Afifi Afifi M, Pizzorno G, Handschumacher RE, Joiner KA (1995) *Toxoplasma gondii* tachyzoites possess an unusual plasma membrane adenosine transporter. Mol Biochem Parasitol 70(1-2):59–69

Chapter 15

Toxoplasma gondii: Bradyzoite Differentiation In Vitro and In Vivo

Joshua Mayoral, Manlio Di Cristina, Vern B. Carruthers, and Louis M. Weiss

Abstract

Toxoplasma gondii, a member of the Apicomplexa, is known for its ability to infect an impressive range of host species. It is a common human infection that causes significant morbidity in congenitally infected children and immunocompromised patients. This parasite can be transmitted by bradyzoites, a slowly replicating life stage found within intracellular tissue cysts, and oocysts, the sexual life cycle stage that develops in domestic cats and other Felidae. *T. gondii* bradyzoites retain the capacity to revert back to the quickly replicating tachyzoite life stage, and when the host is immune compromised unrestricted replication can lead to significant tissue destruction. Bradyzoites are refractory to currently available *Toxoplasma* treatments. Improving our understanding of bradyzoite biology is critical for the development of therapeutic strategies to eliminate latent infection. This chapter describes a commonly used protocol for the differentiation of *T. gondii* tachyzoites into bradyzoites using human foreskin fibroblast cultures and a CO_2-limited alkaline cell media, which results in a high proportion of differentiated bradyzoites for further study. Also described are methods for purifying tissue cysts from chronically infected mouse brain using isopycnic centrifugation and a recently developed approach for measuring bradyzoite viability.

Key words *Toxoplasma*, Bradyzoite, Tissue cyst, Differentiation, Stress, In vitro, In vivo

1 Introduction

The term *bradyzoite* is classically used to describe a slow-growing life stage of certain organisms belonging to a subclass of apicomplexans known as the Coccidia [1]. In the case of *Toxoplasma gondii*, bradyzoites are 7×1.5 μm crescent-shaped organisms found within intracellular tissue cysts most commonly in neural and muscular tissue [2]. Tissue cysts vary in size and can contain from two to several thousand individual bradyzoites [2]. Within an intermediate host, when infected tissue containing tissue cysts is ingested, the released bradyzoites differentiate into tachyzoites, a quickly replicating life stage that disseminates to various organs, causing an acute infection [3]. Acute infection may also occur from

Christopher J. Tonkin (ed.), *Toxoplasma gondii: Methods and Protocols*, Methods in Molecular Biology, vol. 2071,
https://doi.org/10.1007/978-1-4939-9857-9_15, © Springer Science+Business Media, LLC, part of Springer Nature 2020

the ingestion of oocysts containing sporozoites, which differentiate into tachyzoites shortly after invasion of the host [3]. During the course of acute infection in mice, tachyzoites differentiate into bradyzoites in various tissues, with most bradyzoites appearing in the brain [4]. Chronic infection results when a competent immune response controls and clears the tachyzoite population within the host, leaving predominately the bradyzoite population intact [3]. It is thought that bradyzoites persist within their host during chronic infection by repeated cycles of tissue cyst rupture, infection of new host cells, and the formation of new tissue cysts [5]. The likelihood of an individual parasite behaving as a tachyzoite or bradyzoite can be thought of as a continuum, where a bradyzoite or a tachyzoite can be identified on the basis of specific markers, but an intermediate state cannot be easily identified. The decision to form a bradyzoite vacuole (also known as a tissue cyst) or a tachyzoite vacuole is likely an early event during the course of host cell invasion [2]. Support for this notion is provided by the finding that tissue cyst markers can be identified within vacuoles containing an individual parasite shortly after invasion [2, 6]. Although it is classically thought that bradyzoites are a quiescent life stage that replicate asynchronously, recent work has demonstrated that bradyzoites replicate in dynamic fashion during the course of chronic infection in mice [7].

In their host cells, both tachyzoites and bradyzoites reside within a specialized compartment referred to as the parasitophorous vacuole, within which the parasite scavenges nutrients and replicates [8, 9]. When imaged with transmission electron microscopy (TEM), the parasitophorous vacuoles and the morphology of bradyzoites and tachyzoites differ dramatically. Bradyzoites typically contain a posteriorly located nucleus, electron dense rhoptry organelles, and an abundance of amylopectin storage granules that stain positive with Periodic Acid-Schiff Base (PAS) [2, 10]. Within tissue cysts, bradyzoites typically reside in an electron dense matrix or ground substance [10]. Bradyzoite tissue cysts also contain an amorphous collection of proteinaceous material just beneath the limiting membrane of the parasitophorous vacuole, known as the cyst wall [11]. Cyst wall thickness varies between 50 and 500 nm depending on the age of the cyst, which is generally inferred by the size of the tissue cyst and the development of the cyst wall [12]. In contrast to bradyzoite vacuoles, tachyzoite vacuoles lack the ground substance and cyst wall that typify tissue cysts, instead residing in relatively clear vacuoles containing an intertubular (or intravacuolar) network (IVN) between individual tachyzoites [13].

Decades of research has led to the identification of several stage-specific cytoplasmic and secreted proteins in bradyzoites that can be identified during the course of differentiation in vitro (illustrated in Fig. 1) (*see* ref. [14]). The small heat shock protein

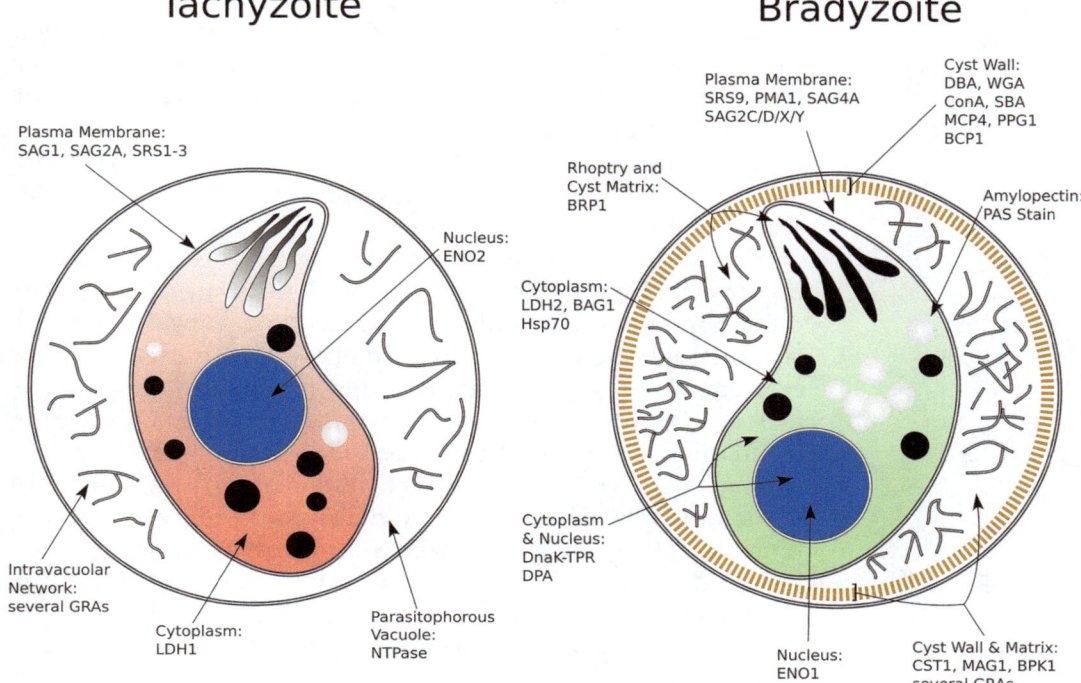

Fig. 1 Markers used to distinguish tachyzoites and bradyzoites. Note that certain markers appear earlier than others during the course of tachyzoite-to-bradyzoite differentiation. Modified from ref. [14] with permission from Elsevier

BAG1 (formerly known as BAG5) was one of the earliest identified bradyzoite markers, shown to localize to the cytoplasm of brady-zoites as early as 1 day postdifferentiation by alkaline media induction [15, 16]. A few cyst wall proteins that play an important role in cyst wall rigidity and bradyzoite persistence have been described, such as BPK1 and CST1 [17, 18]. It is well known that the bradyzoite-derived cyst wall is glycosylated, as various lectins have been shown to react with the cyst wall and are commonly used as markers for bradyzoite differentiation [19–21]. The use of trans-genic reporter strains also allows bradyzoites to be identified in vitro and in vivo through the use of fluorescent proteins and enzymes expressed under the control of stage-specific gene promoters [22, 23]. It is important to note that not every bradyzoite protein marker is expressed at the same time during the course of tachyzoite to bradyzoite conversion. The bradyzoite proteins BAG1 and CST1 appear to be expressed early following in vitro induction, whereas the proteins SRS9 and LDH2 tend to be expressed at later time points following in vitro induction [16, 18, 22, 24].

In vitro derived cysts and in vivo derived cysts have shown some differences in protein localization. One particular cyst wall protein,

BCP1, was shown to exhibit punctate localization within in vitro derived tissue cysts [25]. In contrast, this same protein was shown to localize to the cyst wall and was translated into a protein of larger size within in vivo derived cysts [25]. While this suggests that not every observation made using the in vitro model of bradyzoite differentiation is true of bradyzoites that differentiate in vivo, the in vitro model has proven to be a useful tool in the field, identifying several bradyzoite antigens whose size and localization has been confirmed using tissue cysts isolated from in vivo sources. Hence, in vitro models are powerful, but need to be interpreted with caution and should be confirmed with additional in vivo assays.

Although the markers described above have proven useful in characterizing bradyzoite differentiation, it is worth noting that the most sensitive marker in identifying *mature* bradyzoite tissue cysts is determination of the prepatent period in felines; that is, the time to oocyst release by a cat following ingestion of parasites (3–10 days in the case of bradyzoite tissue cyst ingestion) [26]. Most laboratories do not have access to felines for bioassays or are not well equipped to work with oocysts; therefore, such assays are not commonly used.

The factors governing tachyzoite to bradyzoite differentiation (and vice-versa) have been the subject of intense research, and several reviews exist addressing this topic [27–29].

It is clear from collective observations that bradyzoite differentiation is in response to stress, either perceived through the infected host cell or directly on the parasite itself. Examples of stressful stimuli, which have all been demonstrated as feasible in vitro induction methods, include gamma-interferon treatment, induction of host cell nitric oxide, heat-shock, nutrient deprivation, and alterations in pH [29]. Several chemical compounds have also been shown to induce bradyzoite differentiation through various mechanisms, reviewed in [30]. The cell type that is infected can also influence bradyzoite differentiation, as postmitotic cells such as neurons or skeletal muscle cells have been shown to facilitate bradyzoite differentiation more so than tachyzoite replication [31, 32]. Indeed, neurons have been shown to be the most common cell type to harbor tissue cysts within the brain [11, 33, 34].

Work on the cellular mechanisms within the parasite responsible for stage conversion between tachyzoites and bradyzoites is still ongoing. Apicomplexan AP2 proteins (ApiAP2), as well as the phosphorylation status of the parasite eukaryotic initiation factor-2 (eIF2), have been shown to play important roles in facilitating or repressing tachyzoite to bradyzoite differentiation [35, 36].

Excellent protocols on the isolation of in vivo bradyzoites from mouse brain and the differentiation of bradyzoites in vitro are available elsewhere [37, 38]. The focus of this chapter is to describe three separate methods. The first is a simple approach toward obtaining differentiated bradyzoites in vitro through the use of human foreskin fibroblasts cultures and an alkaline, CO_2-depleted media in the absence of gaseous CO_2, which appears to be the most common approach for in vitro bradyzoite induction in modern *Toxoplasma* research. This method is reproducible and results in a large proportion of differentiated bradyzoites, which can be confirmed through the use of reporter strains or via immunofluorescence of bradyzoite specific markers. The second method describes isopycnic separation of *T. gondii* tissue cysts from chronically infected mouse brains using a Percoll buffer, originally described by Cornelissen et al. [39]. This approach ultimately results in a pellet containing tissue cysts that can be used for further experimentation and analysis. Finally, we describe an approach for assessing viability of bradyzoites based on quantitative PCR (qPCR) combined with a plaque assay.

2 Materials

2.1 Cell Culture

1. Human Foreskin Fibroblasts, HFF-1 (ATCC®SCRC-1041™).

2. Dulbecco's Modified Eagle Medium (DMEM) supplemented with 10% fetal bovine serum (FBS) and 2 mM L-glutamine. A 1:200 dilution of a 10,000 U/mL penicillin and streptomycin stock can be added if desired (these help prevent bacterial contamination of the media).

3. *T. gondii* strain/transgenic line of choice (*see* **Note 1**).

4. Tissue culture vessels of choice.

5. Tissue culture CO_2 incubators.

6. 5 μm filters and Luer-Lock syringes.

2.2 Bradyzoite Differentiation

1. Differentiation Media: Gibco™ High glucose DMEM powder, 50 mM HEPES, 1% FBS. Media adjusted to pH 8.2. A 1:200 dilution of 10,000 U/mL penicillin and streptomycin stock can be added if desired (these help prevent bacterial contamination of the media). Prepare 1 L of differentiation media by dissolving 1 packet of DMEM powder with 11.91 g HEPES powder in 800 mL ultrapure water. Adjust the pH to 8.2 by measuring with a pH probe and adding freshly made 1 M NaOH. Adjust final volume accordingly with ultrapure water. Filter solution through a 0.45 μm or 0.22 μm bottle-top filter. Add FBS after filtration, as well as penicillin/streptomycin if desired. Store differentiation media at 4 °C until needed (*see* **Note 2**). Warm the media to 37 °C before use.

2. 1 M NaOH.

3. Ultrapure water (e.g., Milli-Q® filtered water).

4. pH probe.

5. Bottle-top filters (0.45 μm or 0.22 μm).

2.3 In Vivo Tissue Cyst Purification

1. Mouse strain of choice chronically infected with *T. gondii* strain/transgenic line of choice.

2. Sterile dissection instruments (e.g., scissors, forceps, and spatula).

3. Equipment for euthanasia (e.g., CO_2 chamber).

4. Luer-Lock syringe (10 mL or larger).

5. Petri dishes (large enough to hold more than 10 mL).

6. Thomas® Pestle Tissue Grinder Assembly, using either a Teflon® pestle or a size B glass pestle. Items should be autoclaved before use.

7. Percoll® (P1644 Sigma).

8. $1\times$ Phosphate Buffered Saline (PBS).

9. 70% ethanol.

10. Centrifuge capable of speeds up to $26{,}600 \times g$.

11. Centrifuge tubes (resistant to breaking at $26{,}600 \times g$).

12. 50 mL conical tubes.

2.4 Bradyzoite Viability Assay

1. Tissue culture 6-well plates.

2. Hank's Balanced Salt Solution (HBSS) (without Ca^{2+} and Mg^{2+}).

3. Cell scrapers.

4. 10 mL Luer-Lock syringe.

5. 25 or 27 gauge needles.

6. Pepsin solution $2\times$: 340 mM NaCl, 120 mM HCl, 0.52 mg/mL pepsin (porcine gastric mucosa $\geq$250 units/mg solid). To prepare 50 mL of pepsin solution $2\times$, dissolve 26 mg pepsin and 0.993 g of NaCl in 45 mL ultrapure water, adjust pH to 2.0, and bring the solution to 50 mL with ddH_2O. Filter the solution using a 0.2 μm filter and store at 4 °C. Prepare fresh solution for each use.

7. Neutralization buffer $2\times$: 188 mM Na_2CO_3. To prepare 50 mL of neutralization buffer $2\times$, dissolve 1 g Na_2CO_3 in 50 mL ultrapure water. Filter the solution using a 0.2 μm filter and store at 4 °C.

8. Genomic extraction kit.

9. qPCR machine.

10. qPCR reagents.

11. Primers for qPCR. TUB-for 5′-GCG TCT TGG ATT TGG AG-3′ and TUB-rev 5′-TGG AGA CCA GTG CAG TTG TC-3′.

12. 15 mL conical polystyrene tubes.

3   Methods

3.1   Cell Culture

1. *T. gondii* tachyzoites can be maintained in confluent HFF monolayers grown in supplemented DMEM media within 37 °C incubators at 5% CO_2. When the majority of host cells have lysed and freshly egressed parasites are seen, the tachyzoites can be passaged by inoculating a fresh confluent HFF monolayer.

3.2   Bradyzoite Differentiation

1. Collect freshly egressed tachyzoites via filtration through a 5 μm filter. If the culture has not fully lysed, the culture can be scraped with a cell scraper and passed through needles of increasingly smaller diameter (up to 27.5 gauge) with a syringe before filtration. Freshly egressed tachyzoites and lysed intracellular parasites have similar rates of differentiation.

2. Count the filtrate in a hemocytometer. Calculate the amount of parasites needed to achieve the desired multiplicity of infection (MOI) (*see* **Note 3**).

3. Infect an HFF monolayer plated in a tissue culture vessel of choice with the appropriate amount of filtered parasites. Place the infected culture in a 37 °C incubator at 5% CO_2.

4. Two hours postinfection (*see* **Note 4**), replace the media in the culture with differentiation media (*see* Subheading 2.2) and transfer the culture to a 37 °C incubator set at 0% CO_2 (ambient air, *see* **Note 5**).

5. Replace media every 1–2 days with fresh differentiation media. This reduces the likelihood of bradyzoites reverting to tachyzoites.

6. Visualize or collect bradyzoites for desired assay as needed at a given time point postdifferentiation (*see* **Notes 3** and **6**). After 3 days in culture, the ME49 or Prugniaud *T. gondii* strains have over 90% of vacuoles expressing bradyzoite markers. The proportion of differentiated bradyzoites can be confirmed with reporter strains and/or immunofluorescence assays using antibodies to bradyzoite specific markers (*see* Fig. 1).

3.3   In Vivo Tissue Cyst Purification

1. Collect mice chronically infected with *T. gondii* (*see* **Notes 7** and **8**), and sacrifice following an approved animal euthanasia protocol.

2. After mice have been sacrificed, transfer mice to a biosafety cabinet and spray down the skin of the head with 70% ethanol.

3. Remove the skin of the head by cutting from the base of the neck down to the nose, further removing skin with forceps if necessary.

4. Make a single incision at the base of the skull, cut along the base of the skull on both the right and left side, starting at the initial incision. The skull can usually be peeled away with forceps after these cuts are made. Collect the brain with a spatula, severing the connection to the olfactory bulbs in the process. If desired, the sacrificed mouse can be decapitated prior to skull dissection. Repeat for other mice.

5. Transfer the brains into a 50 mL conical tube, and rinse the brains several times with prechilled PBS to remove erythrocytes.

6. Transfer brains onto a petri dish, and homogenize the brains using a Luer-Lock syringe without an attached needle in 10 mL of PBS (no more than five brains should be homogenized in 10 mL). After homogenization and if desired, check the Petri dish for intact tissue cysts under a microscope.

7. Collect the homogenate with a syringe and transfer into the Thomas® Pestle Tissue Grinder Assembly (see **Note 9**). Homogenize further by grinding with at least ten full passes. Keep the homogenate on ice.

8. Make 50 mL of a 45% Percoll solution (22.5 mL Percoll in 27.5 mL PBS).

9. Divide 25 mL of the 45% Percoll solution into two centrifuge tubes. Add 5 mL of the homogenized cyst solution into each tube.

10. Centrifuge the two solutions at $26,600 \times g$ for 20 min at $4\,°C$.

11. Carefully remove 3 mL from the bottom of each tube and discard (see **Note 10**).

12. Carefully remove the next 20 mL from the bottom of each tube, and place into new 50 mL conical tubes. Fill up each tube to 50 mL with PBS.

13. Centrifuge the solutions at $130 \times g$ for 10 min at $4\,°C$.

14. The tissue cysts should form a pellet at the bottom of the tubes by this step. Aspirate the supernatant and resuspend the pellet in 500 µL PBS. Take a small aliquot (e.g., 10 µL) of these solutions and make a wet mount with a coverslip and microscope slide, counting the number of cysts present in the aliquot and determining the total number of cysts in the pellet. If cysts are to be used for murine infection the appropriate amount of cysts can be used directly from this suspension.

15. Concentrate the cysts again by centrifuging the samples at $1400 \times g$ for 4 min at room temperature.

16. Remove the supernatant. At this stage, the pellet can be stored in $-80\,°C$ for future analysis or fixed for electron microscopy.

3.4 Bradyzoite Viability Assay

1. Differentiate bradyzoites as described in Subheading 3.2.

2. After 7 days, parasites are largely converted into bradyzoites. If any treatment is to be tested on fully converted bradyzoites, it should start on day 7 postinfection. Change media every day or two with fresh differentiation media (supplemented with fresh drug if applying a treatment) until the selected time point (s) (*see* **Note 11**).

3. At the time point(s) selected to perform the viability assay (*see* **Note 12**) remove media from the infected monolayers and then wash infected monolayers three times with HBSS (without Ca^{2+} and Mg^{2+}).

4. Add 2 mL of HBSS, scrape the monolayer with a cell scraper and then syringe up and down four times with a 25 or 27 gauge needle.

5. Recover the media containing scraped cells from each well, transfer to a 15 mL conical tube, wash the well with 1.5 mL of HBSS, and add to the same 15 mL tube.

6. Add 3.5 mL of pepsin solution 2×, mix and incubate samples in a water bath for 30 min at 37 °C.

7. Stop the reaction by adding 7 mL of neutralization buffer 2× (final concentration 94 mM Na_2CO_3).

8. Centrifuge 1800 × *g* for 10 min at RT.

9. Very carefully pour off the supernatant and then resuspend in 1 mL of supplemented DMEM.

10. Count parasites (add trypan blue, to avoid counting dead parasites killed by pepsin treatment) in the control (untreated) sample using a hemocytometer.

11. Take 100, 1000 and 5000 parasites (based on the number from the control) and infect HFF monolayers grown in 6-well plates in triplicate for plaque assay (in 3 mL of fresh supplemented DMEM).

12. Incubate the 6-well plates undisturbed for 10–14 days (depending from the parasite strain) in a humidified 37 °C incubator with 5% CO_2.

13. After the incubation period, check the 6-well plates on an inverted microscope with a low power objective for plaques. If present, stain with crystal violet, and count plaques (*see* **Note 13**).

14. To perform qPCR to normalize the total number of bradyzoites added to 6-well plates for plaque assay (*see* **Note 14**), spin 800 μL bradyzoites from **step 9** and centrifuge the samples at 1800 × *g* for 10 min at RT.

15. Carefully remove with a pipette all the supernatant without disturbing the pellet.

16. Purify nucleic acids gDNA using NucleoSpin Tissue kit (Macherey-Nagel, cat. no. 740952) or any other commercial genomic extraction kit (the pellets can be frozen at $-80\ ^\circ C$ for future purification).

17. In parallel, prepare a reference gDNA from a known number of parasites (e.g., 10^7 or 10^8 tachyzoites). Dilute the reference gDNA to have a concentration of DNA corresponding to 10^5, 10^4, 10^3, 10^2, and 10^1 tachyzoites/µL to generate a standard curve.

18. Perform qPCR using the TUB-for and TUB-rev primers for the *tubulin* gene (or primers to amplify any other genomic fragment). Use the highest volume suggested by the manufacturer of the qPCR machine being utilized. In addition, generate a standard curve with six reference points using gDNA and using sterile ultrapure water as a negative control.

19. Utilize a dual step cycle of $98\ ^\circ C/5$ s and $68\ ^\circ C/30$ s for 40 cycles. Set a melting curve from 58 to $95\ ^\circ C$, 5 s/step, $0.5\ ^\circ C$ increments to assess that your primers produce only one amplicon.

20. Use the reference curve generated to calculate how many parasite genomes went into the 6-well plates for the plaque assay to obtain the number of plaques formed from X number of parasite genomes.

4   Notes

1. Type II and III strains differentiate into bradyzoites more readily compared to Type I. All strains display varying degrees of spontaneous differentiation in the absence of added stress (albeit at low rates). Type II strains are very amendable to in vitro differentiation protocols, as previously described [27].

2. Differentiation media remains effective for several months if stored at $4\ ^\circ C$.

3. Depending on the MOI used, bradyzoites can be maintained in culture for several days, even weeks. We have observed greater amounts of parasite egress and reinvasion with MOIs of 3:1 and greater. Therefore, depending on the nature of the experiment, the MOI should be chosen carefully to prevent premature HFF monolayer lysis. We have also observed less egress in the ME49 Type II strain compared to the Prugniaud Type II strain when equal MOIs are used.

4. Bradyzoite differentiation may be induced earlier than 2 h postinfection if desired (e.g., at the time of invasion). The media of the HFF monolayer to be infected can be replaced with differentiation media, after which filtered tachyzoites can

be pelleted and resuspended in differentiation media, followed by inoculation of the HFF monolayer with the resuspended parasites.

5. The absence of CO_2 in differentiating cultures plays an important role in parasites lacking the UPRT gene, as it is thought these parasites exhibit increased sensitivity to CO_2 starvation due to the need for CO_2 in the de novo synthesis of pyrimidine, as described in [40]. Additionally, removing CO_2 prevents its dissolution in the differentiation media, which could acidify the media and relieve alkaline stress.

6. If passaging of in vitro differentiated bradyzoites is desired, the culture should be scraped with a cell scraper and passed through needles of increasingly larger gauge (up to 27.5 gauge) with a syringe, followed by filtration through a 5 μm filter. We have found that the liberation of individual bradyzoites from in vitro tissue cysts can be challenging depending on the age of the cysts. Several passes through syringe needles may be needed for effective cyst disruption.

7. The strain of mouse/parasite, life stage of parasite inoculum, route and amount of inoculum, as well as antiparasite treatment during infection are all important considerations when generating in vivo tissue cysts, reviewed in [41]. Generally, Type II tissue cysts passaged between mice orally or intraperitoneally (or Type II tachyzoites taken from tissue culture in vitro and inoculated intraperitoneally) result in higher cyst yields in most strains of mice compared to other parasite types [37]. However, as noted by Watts et al., tissue cyst yield can be quite variable even between identical mouse strains infected with the same dose of parasites for the same length of time [37].

8. In mice, chronic infection with *T. gondii* begins after the immune response removes most replicating tachyzoites in the body, leaving predominately the bradyzoite population intact 3 weeks post-infection [10]. Therefore, bradyzoite tissue cysts from the mouse brain are usually harvested no earlier than 3 weeks postinfection.

9. Thomas® Pestle Tissue Grinder Assemblies are available in various sizes. We find those with a 30 mL capacity work well for homogenizing 10 mL volumes. Pestle clearance is important to minimize cyst breakage during tissue homogenization. We have found that the "B″" size of glass pestles or Teflon pestles are useful for cyst purification.

10. For pipetting we use a 4 in. (or longer) 14 gauge blunt dispensing needle and a syringe, which facilitates selective aspiration from the bottom of the tube.

11. Converted parasites can be kept in culture as long as 5 weeks postinfection, depending on the strain used. PruΔku80 shows

good viability 4 weeks postconversion, whereas Prugniaud and ME49 lose most of their viability beyond 2 weeks postconversion.

12. In principle, this viability assay can also be applied to cysts purified from the brains of chronically infected mice as described in Subheading 3.3.

13. Some *T. gondii* strains do not form plaques that are visible with crystal violet. In this case count the number of infective areas using an optical microscope.

14. qPCR measures the total number of bradyzoites regardless of whether they are dead or alive. This is an important advantage of qPCR over counting parasites in a hemocytometer, since in our experience dead bradyzoites can be deformed and are not easily identified by microscopic methods.

Acknowledgments

This work was supported by 1F31AI136401 (J.M.), R01AI134753 (L.M.W.), and R21AI123495 (L.M.W.).

References

1. Frenkel JK, Smith DD (2003) Determination of the genera of cyst-forming coccidia. Parasitol Res 91:384–389

2. Dubey JP, Lindsay DS, Speer CA (1998) Structures of *Toxoplasma gondii* tachyzoites, bradyzoites, and sporozoites and biology and development of tissue cysts. Clin Microbiol Rev 11:267–299

3. Montoya JG, Liesenfeld O (2004) Toxoplasmosis. Lancet 363:1965–1976

4. Di Cristina M, Marocco D, Galizi R, Proietti C, Spaccapelo R, Crisanti A (2008) Temporal and spatial distribution of *Toxoplasma gondii* differentiation into bradyzoites and tissue cyst formation in vivo. Infect Immun 76:3491–3501

5. Rougier S, Montoya JG, Peyron F (2017) Lifelong persistence of *Toxoplasma* cysts: a questionable dogma? Trends Parasitol 33:93–101

6. Sahm M, Fischer HG, Gross U, Reiter-Owona-I, Seitz HM (1997) Cyst formation by *Toxoplasma gondii* in vivo and in brain-cell culture: a comparative morphology and immunocytochemistry study. Parasitol Res 83:659–665

7. Watts E, Zhao Y, Dhara A, Eller B, Patwardhan A, Sinai AP (2015) Novel approaches reveal that *Toxoplasma gondii* bradyzoites within tissue cysts are dynamic and replicating entities in vivo. MBio 6: e01155–e01115

8. Dou Z, McGovern OL, Di Cristina M, Carruthers VB (2014) *Toxoplasma gondii* ingests and digests host cytosolic proteins. MBio 5: e01188–e01114

9. Caffaro CE, Boothroyd JC (2011) Evidence for host cells as the major contributor of lipids in the intravacuolar network of *Toxoplasma*-infected cells. Eukaryot Cell 10:1095–1099

10. Ferguson DJ, Hutchison WM (1987) An ultrastructural study of the early development and tissue cyst formation of *Toxoplasma gondii* in the brains of mice. Parasitol Res 73:483–491

11. Ferguson DJ, Hutchison WM (1987) The host-parasite relationship of *Toxoplasma gondii* in the brains of chronically infected mice. Virchows Arch A Pathol Anat Histopathol 411:39–43

12. Fortier B, Coignard-Chatain C, Soete M, Dubremetz JF (1996) Structure and biology of *Toxoplasma gondii* bradyzoites. Comptes rendus des seances de la Societe de biologie et de ses filiales 190:385–394

13. Sibley LD, Niesman IR, Parmley SF, Cesbron-Delauw MF (1995) Regulated secretion of multi-lamellar vesicles leads to formation of a tubulo-vesicular network in host-cell vacuoles

occupied by *Toxoplasma gondii*. J Cell Sci 108:1669–1677

14. Tu V, Yakubu R, Weiss LM (2017) Observations on bradyzoite biology. Microbes Infect 20:466–476

15. Bohne W, Gross U, Ferguson DJ, Heesemann J (1995) Cloning and characterization of a bradyzoite-specifically expressed gene (hsp30/bag1) of *Toxoplasma gondii*, related to genes encoding small heat-shock proteins of plants. Mol Microbiol 16:1221–1230

16. Parmley SF, Weiss LM, Yang S (1995) Cloning of a bradyzoite-specific gene of *Toxoplasma gondii* encoding a cytoplasmic antigen. Mol Biochem Parasitol 73:253–257

17. Buchholz KR, Bowyer PW, Boothroyd JC (2013) Bradyzoite pseudokinase 1 is crucial for efficient oral infectivity of the *Toxoplasma gondii* tissue cyst. Eukaryot Cell 12:399–410

18. Tomita T, Bzik DJ, Ma YF, Fox BA, Markillie LM, Taylor RC, Kim K, Weiss LM (2013) The *Toxoplasma gondii* cyst wall protein CST1 is critical for cyst wall integrity and promotes bradyzoite persistence, e1003823. PLoS Pathog 9

19. Sethi KK, Rahman A, Pelster B, Brandis H (1977) Search for the presence of lectin-binding sites on *Toxoplasma gondii*. J Parasitol 63:1076–1080

20. Caffaro CE, Koshy AA, Liu L, Zeiner GM, Hirschberg CB, Boothroyd JC (2013) A nucleotide sugar transporter involved in glycosylation of the *Toxoplasma* tissue cyst wall is required for efficient persistence of bradyzoites. PLoS Pathog 9:e1003331

21. Tomita T, Sugi T, Yakubu R, Tu V, Ma Y, Weiss LM (2017) Making home sweet and sturdy: *Toxoplasma gondii* ppGalNAc-Ts glycosylate in hierarchical order and confer Cyst Wall rigidity. MBio 8:e02048–e02016

22. Yang S, Parmley SF (1997) *Toxoplasma gondii* expresses two distinct lactate dehydrogenase homologous genes during its life cycle in intermediate hosts. Gene 184:1–12. 23

23. Unno A, Suzuki K, Batanova T, Cha SY, Jang HK, Kitoh K, Takashima Y (2009) Visualization of *Toxoplasma gondii* stage conversion by expression of stage-specific dual fluorescent proteins. Parasitology 136:579–588

24. Kim SK, Boothroyd JC (2005) Stage-specific expression of surface antigens by *Toxoplasma gondii* as a mechanism to facilitate parasite persistence. J Immunol 174:8038–8048

25. Milligan-Myhre K, Wilson SK, Knoll LJ (2016) Developmental change in translation initiation alters the localization of a common microbial protein necessary for *Toxoplasma* chronic infection. Mol Microbiol 102:1086–1098

26. Dubey JP, Speer CA, Shen SK, Kwok OC, Blixt JA (1997) Oocyst-induced murine toxoplasmosis: life cycle, pathogenicity, and stage conversion in mice fed *Toxoplasma gondii* oocysts. J Parasitol 83:870–882

27. Weiss LM, Kim K (2000) The development and biology of bradyzoites of *Toxoplasma gondii*. Front Biosci 5:D391–D405

28. Lyons RE, McLeod R, Roberts CW (2002) *Toxoplasma gondii* tachyzoite-bradyzoite interconversion. Trends Parasitol 18:198–201

29. Luder CGK, Rahman T (2017) Impact of the host on *Toxoplasma stage* differentiation. Microb Cell 4:203–211

30. Sullivan WJ Jr, Jeffers V (2012) Mechanisms of *Toxoplasma gondii* persistence and latency. FEMS Microbiol Rev 36:717–733

31. Luder CG, Giraldo-Velasquez M, Sendtner M, Gross U (1999) *Toxoplasma gondii* in primary rat CNS cells: differential contribution of neurons, astrocytes, and microglial cells for the intracerebral development and stage differentiation. Exp Parasitol 93:23–32

32. Swierzy IJ, Luder CG (2015) Withdrawal of skeletal muscle cells from cell cycle progression triggers differentiation of *Toxoplasma gondii towards* the bradyzoite stage. Cell Microbiol 17:2–17

33. Cabral CM, Tuladhar S, Dietrich HK, Nguyen E, MacDonald WR, Trivedi T, Devineni A, Koshy AA (2016) Neurons are the primary target cell for the brain-tropic intracellular parasite *Toxoplasma gondii*. PLoS Pathog 12:e1005447

34. Melzer TC, Cranston HJ, Weiss LM, Halonen SK (2010) Host cell preference of *Toxoplasma gondii* cysts in murine brain: a confocal study. J Neuroparasitology 1:pii: N100505

35. Hong DP, Radke JB, White MW (2017) Opposing transcriptional mechanisms regulate *Toxoplasma* development. mSphere 2:e00347-16

36. Holmes MJ, Augusto LDS, Zhang M, Wek RC, Sullivan WJ Jr (2017) Translational control in the latency of apicomplexan parasites. Trends Parasitol 33:947–960

37. Watts EA, Dhara A, Sinai AP (2017) Purification *Toxoplasma gondii* tissue cysts using percoll gradients. Curr Protoc Microbiol 45:20c.2.1–20c.2.19

38. Tobin C, Pollard A, Knoll L (2010) *Toxoplasma gondii* cyst wall formation in activated bone marrow-derived macrophages and bradyzoite conditions. J Vis Exp 12(42):2091

39. Cornelissen AW, Overdulve JP, Hoenderboom JM (1981) Separation of *Isospora (Toxoplasma) gondii* cysts and cystozoites from mouse brain tissue by continuous density-gradient centrifugation. Parasitology 83:103–108

40. Bohne W, Roos DS (1997) Stage-specific expression of a selectable marker in *Toxoplasma gondii* permits selective inhibition of either tachyzoites or bradyzoites. Mol Biochem Parasitol 88:115–126

41. Szabo EK, Finney CA (2017) *Toxoplasma gondii*: one organism multiple models. Trends Parasitol 33:113–127

Chapter 16

Three-Dimensional Reconstruction of *Toxoplasma*–Neuron Interactions In Situ

Carla M. Cabral, Emily F. Merritt, and Anita A. Koshy

Abstract

How tissue and cellular architecture affects host cell–microbe interactions in vivo remains poorly defined because imaging these interactions in complex tissue is difficult and standard in vitro cultures do not mimic whole organ architecture. Here we describe a method that combines new tissue clearing techniques, high-resolution imaging, and three-dimensional reconstruction to overcome these barriers and allow in situ imaging of host cell–microbe interactions in complex tissue. We use the interactions between neurons and *Toxoplasma gondii*, a ubiquitous, protozoan parasite that establish a lifelong central nervous system (CNS) infection in mice and humans, as a model for this technique. This method aims to provide an easy, reproducible way to visualize the complex relationship between host cells and intracellular pathogens within a whole organ.

Key words *Toxoplasma*, Confocal microscopy, 3-D reconstruction, Tissue clearing, Host-microbe interactions

1 Introduction

For over 100 years, scientists have been developing methods to render tissue transparent to better understand how cells and systems function and interact. Without clearing, light refracts off components within the tissue, making it difficult to obtain clear, high-resolution images of the entire tissue. To circumvent this issue, thin sections are generally imaged, but these images do not offer a full understanding of the dynamics within the intact tissue. Serial reconstructions from the thinner sections is possible but time consuming and loses information at the interface of sections. Using techniques such as electron microscopy or serial block face sectioning for whole brain reconstructions renders the tissue unusable for any other evaluation. Early clearing protocols overcame a number of these issues, but imaging technology lagged in its ability to

Carla M. Cabral and Emily F. Merritt contributed equally.

Christopher J. Tonkin (ed.), *Toxoplasma gondii: Methods and Protocols*, Methods in Molecular Biology, vol. 2071, https://doi.org/10.1007/978-1-4939-9857-9_16, © Springer Science+Business Media, LLC, part of Springer Nature 2020

capture images deep within the tissue in a time-efficient manner. Today, however, this field is growing at a rapid pace with a number of new protocols for clearing and staining thick tissue sections (reviewed in [1–4]). Advances have also been made in imaging technology including confocal, multiphoton, and light sheet microscopy as well as longer working distance objectives to obtain the high-resolution images necessary for accurate reconstructions. In addition, the endogenous expression of fluorescent proteins has overcome the need for antibody penetration through thick tissue, another key step in imaging deep tissues. The final advancement is the continued development of image analysis software ranging from open-source programs such as ImageJ [5] to more specialized software such as IMARIS (Bitplane). Combining these advancements allows for unprecedented insight into intact biological systems.

This protocol focuses on imaging the interactions between the obligate intracellular parasite *Toxoplasma gondii* and the brain. *Toxoplasma* is a protozoan parasite that naturally establish a lifelong infection in the central nervous system (CNS) of a number of intermediates hosts, including humans and rodents. This tropism for and long-term persistence in the CNS underlies the symptomatic disease *Toxoplasma* can cause in the immunodeficient as well as enabling *Toxoplasma*'s ability to pass between intermediate hosts. Yet CNS persistence remains relatively poorly understood, especially in vivo. Our ability to visualize the CNS–parasite interactions is made possible by using parasites that both express a fluorescent protein at all life cycle stages and that trigger host cell expression of a second fluorescent protein ([6]). The protocol described here combines high-resolution confocal imaging with 3-D reconstruction of *Toxoplasma* infected, cleared mouse brain tissue sections, allowing for visualization of individual parasites inside whole neurons in situ. Optimized tissue clearing techniques and better optics now allow for routine capture and analysis of areas up to 1 mm × 1 mm × 200 µm, with high resolution at the level of the single infected neuron. In addition, we provide protocols for immunofluorescent staining of the thick tissue using standard techniques with increased incubation times making the completed protocol a 7-day process and as an optional microwave technique that reduces the completed protocol to 2 days (Fig. 1). The ability to stain cleared tissue enables one to potentially use tissue and parasites with no endogenous fluorescent protein expression as well as allowing one to develop reconstructions that include multiple cell types. While this protocol has been optimized for *Toxoplasma* and brain tissue, it should be modifiable for any complex tissue and microbe.

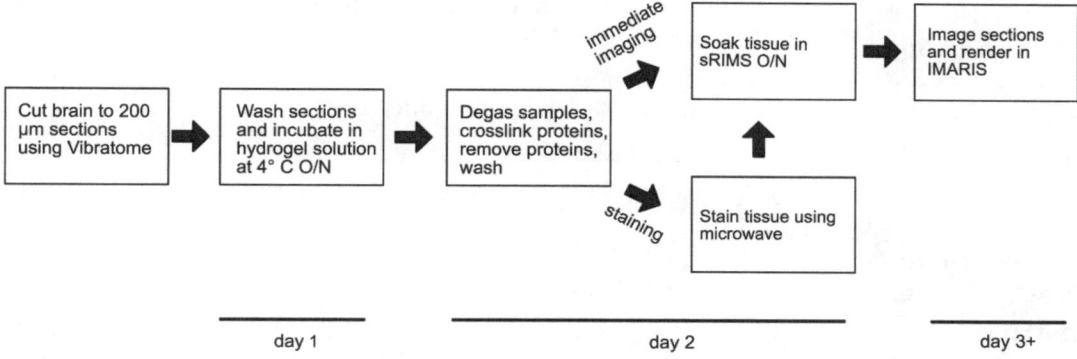

Fig. 1 Schematic of the thick brain section clearing and imaging process. The amount of time required to image sections and make 3-D renderings using IMARIS software will be user and application dependent

2   Materials

2.1   General Materials

1. Glass vials, 1 ¾ in. × ½ in. Other containers can be used (e.g., conical tubes); however, this protocol is for the specified glass vials. Users will need to adjust the protocol for containers of different dimensions.

2. Nitrogen gas.

3. 23 gauge 1 ½" needle.

4. Parafilm.

5. 100 mm petri dish.

6. Paint brush.

7. Microscope slides.

8. #1.5 cover glass.

2.2   Materials for Immunofluorescence Staining

1. Transfer pipettes.

2. 24-well plates.

2.3   Reagents Required

1. 2,2′-Azobis[2-(2imidazolin-2-yl)propane] dihydrochloride (Wako Chemicals USA, Inc., Cat. # VA-044) referred to as "Azo-initiator."

2. 40% Acrylamide (RPI, Corp., Cat. # A11265).

3. Dimethyl Sulfoxide [DMSO] (Fisher Scientific, Cat. # BP231).

4. Phosphate buffered saline [PBS], 10× Solution (Fisher Scientific, Cat. # BP399).

5. Sodium azide [NaN_3] (Acros Organics, Cat. # 19038).

6. Sodium dodecyl sulfate [SDS] (Sigma, Cat. # L3771).

7. Sodium phosphate dibasic heptahydrate [Na_2HPO_4] (Sigma-Aldrich, Cat. # S7907).

8. Sodium phosphate monobasic monohydrate [NaH_2PO_4] (Sigma-Aldrich, Cat. # S9638).

9. Sorbitol (Fisher Scientific, Cat. # BP439).

10. Triton X-100 (Fisher Scientific, Cat. # BP151).

2.4 Solutions to Be Prepared for Tissue Clearing

1. 1× PBS (1 L). Combine 900 ml Milli-Q H_2O (MQ H_2O) with 100 ml 10× PBS.

2. 0.1 M Phosphate Buffer (500 ml) [PB]. Dissolve 1.55 g NaH_2PO_4 and 5.45 g Na_2HPO_4 in 400 ml MQ H_2O then pH to 7.5. Bring to 500 ml with MQ H_2O, filter sterilize and store at 4 °C.

3. 0.02 M PB (1 L). Combine 800 ml MQ H_2O and 200 ml 0.1 M PB. Store at 4 °C.

4. Wash solution (1 L). Dissolve 5 ml Triton X-100 (0.5%) and 0.4 g NaN_3 (0.04%) in 900 ml 1× PBS. pH to 7.5 then bring to 1000 ml with 1× PBS. Store at 4 °C covered from light.

5. 4% Acrylamide (500 ml) [A4P0]. Combine 50 ml of 40% Acrylamide and 50 ml of 10× PBS in 350 ml MQ H_2O then pH to 7.5. Bring to 500 ml with MQ H_2O and store at 4 °C covered from light.

6. Hydrogel monomer solution. For every 1 ml of A4P0 solution, add in 2.5 mg Azo-initiator. Stir until dissolved and use immediately (*see* **Note 1**).

7. 8% SDS (500 ml). Add 40 g SDS to 350 ml 0.1 M PB (*see* **Notes 2** and **3**). Heat and stir slowly to dissolve then pH to 7.5. Bring to 500 ml with 0.1 M PB and store at room temperature covered from light.

8. Sorbitol Refractive Index Matching Solution (500 ml) [sRIMS]. Add 70% Sorbitol (w/v) (350 g) and 0.01% NaN_3 (0.05 g) to 400 ml 0.02 M PB. Stir to dissolve, pH to 7.5 then bring to 500 ml with 0.02 M PB. Store at room temperature.

2.5 Antibodies and Reagents for Tissue Staining

1. Normal goat serum (Jackson ImmunoResearch, Cat. # 005-000-121).

2. Mouse anti-NeuN, biotin conjugated (Millipore, Cat# MAB377B).

3. Streptavidin Cy5 (Invitrogen, Cat. # 434316).

4. NeuroTrace 435/455 blue-fluorescent Nissl stain (Thermo Fisher Scientific, Cat. # N21479).

2.6 Solutions to Be Prepared for Tissue Staining

1. Permeabilization solution. Add 10 ml Triton X-100 (2%), 100 ml DMSO (20%) and 0.2 g NaN_3 (0.04%) to 390 ml 1× PBS. Stir to dissolve. Store at 4 °C covered from light.

2. Blocking solution. Add 10 ml normal goat serum (10%), 0.5 ml Triton X-100 (0.5%) and 0.04 g NaN_3 (0.04%) to 89.5 ml 1× PBS. Stir to dissolve. Store at 4 °C covered from light.

3. Primary antibody solution. NeuN (1:200) antibody in wash solution or NeuroTrace 435/455 blue-fluorescent Nissl (1:200) in wash solution.

4. Secondary antibody solution. For NeuN staining only, dilute Streptavidin 647 (1:200) in wash solution.

3 Methods

Detailed protocols for infection of Cre-reporter mice with *Toxoplasma*-Cre parasites, harvesting of brains, sectioning of brain tissue and creation of spacer slides can all be found on Jove.com [7]. As fluorescence is quenched by light, the tissue should be kept covered/protected from light during the entire protocol.

3.1 Tissue Clearing

1. Transfer tissue sections to vials containing 1× PBS (*see* **Note 4**).

2. If tissue sections have been stored in media other than PBS, wash tissue sections in fresh 1× PBS for 3 × 5–10 min at room temperature on rotator. On last wash, make hydrogel monomer solution.

3. Aspirate PBS from vials and fill with hydrogel monomer solution.

4. Incubate sections in hydrogel monomer solution overnight at 4 °C on rotator.

5. Degas solution. Take cap off vial and cover vial opening with parafilm. Parafilm needs to be tight, but not pulled so thin that it tears easily. Gently place 23 g needle through the parafilm, into the hydrogel monomer solution, and bubble Nitrogen gas through the solution for 3 min (*see* **Note 5**).

6. Incubate sections in hydrogel monomer solution for 1–2 h at 42 °C on rotator. Solution should appear very viscous if polymerization occurs.

7. Transfer sections to new vials with wash solution. Wash tissue in wash solution for 1 × 5–10 min, then 3 × 20 min at room temperature on rotator (*see* **Notes 6** and **7**).

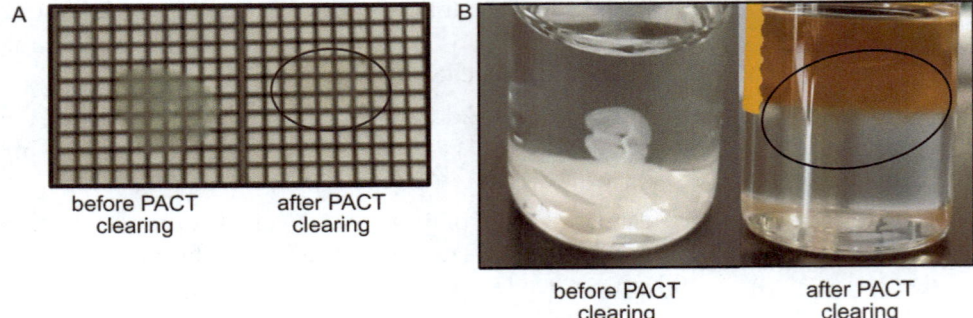

Fig. 2 PACT clearing thick sections (**a, b**). Representative images of 200 μm thick brain sections before and after PACT clearing (**step 10**). Left images are brain section(s) prior to clearing, and right images are after PACT clearing and saturation in sRIMS. For right images, circle outlines sections, which are difficult to visualize because of the clearing. For (**b**) sections are in PBS in left image and are in sRIMS in right image

8. Aspirate wash solution and then add 8% SDS solution. Incubate at 45 °C on rotator until tissue appears clear (*see* **Note 8**).

9. Aspirate SDS solution. Then wash sections in wash solution for 1 × 10 min, then 3 × 20 min at room temperature on rotator. If planning to stain sections immediately, please skip to Subheading 3.2 or Subheading 3.3 as appropriate. If not staining immediately, store tissue in 1× PBS rather than wash solution.

10. If not continuing to stain tissue, aspirate wash solution and then fill vial with sRIMS. Incubate sections in sRIMS at room temperature for 30 min to 1 h on rotator. Then take vials off rotator and allow sections to incubate in sRIMS at room temperature overnight. After sections have been saturated in sRIMS, they will have achieved maximum clarity (Fig. 2). Mount tissue sections in fresh sRIMS, not from the vial, on spacer slide with cover glass (*see* **Notes 6, 9, 10**).

11. After imaging, wash tissue sections in 1× PBS to remove sRIMS. Tissue may be stored long term in 1× PBS at 4 °C (*see* **Notes 11** and **12**).

3.2 Tissue Staining Without Microwave

1. Fill wells of 24-well plate with 500 μl permeabilization solution (*see* **Notes 13** and **14**).

2. Move tissue sections into 24-well plate (no more than three sections per well) containing permeabilization solution.

3. Incubate tissue for 2 h at room temperature on an orbital shaker.

4. Aspirate permeabilization solution. Then, to each well, add appropriate volume of primary antibody solution to cover sections. Parafilm around plate. Incubate tissue for 3 days at 37 °C on an orbital shaker (*see* **Note 15**).

5. Aspirate primary antibody solution and then add 500 μl wash solution. Wash sections for 3 × 20 min on an orbital shaker.

6. Aspirate wash solution and then add appropriate volume of secondary antibody solution to each well. Parafilm around plate. Incubate tissue overnight at 37 °C on an orbital shaker.

7. Aspirate secondary antibody solution and then add 500 μl wash solution. Wash sections for 3 × 20 min on an orbital shaker.

8. Aspirate wash solution and then move tissue sections to vials with sRIMS.

9. Incubate sections in sRIMS at room temperature for 30 min to 1 h on rotator. Then take vials off rotator and allow sections to incubate in sRIMS at room temperature overnight.

10. Mount tissue sections in fresh sRIMS, not from the vial, on spacer slide with cover glass.

11. After imaging, wash tissue sections in 1× PBS to remove sRIMS. Tissue may be stored long term in 1× PBS at 4 °C (*see* **Notes 16** and **17**).

3.3 Tissue Staining with Microwave

1. For this protocol, we used a PELCO BioWave® Pro+ microwave from Ted Pella Inc. The number of steps and time per step needs to be tested and optimized by each investigator. Here we discuss microwave staining of 200 μm thick sections using the primary antibody, NeuN, or the intracellular stain, Nissl. Additional primary and secondary antibodies can be used simultaneously to stain for other antigens as long as care is taken to use antibodies raised in different species from the primary. Fill wells of 24-well plate with 500 μl permeabilization solution.

2. Move tissue sections into 24-well plate (no more than three sections per well).

3. Place 24-well plate into vacuum chamber in microwave.

4. Continue with the following microwave settings aspirating prior solution and adding next solution (300–500 μl) at each "User Prompt On" step.

   (a) Antibody staining using NeuN: Add biotinylated NeuN (1:200) to primary antibody solution. Add Streptavidin Cy5 (1:200) to secondary antibody solution.

   (b) Intracellular staining using Nissl: Add Neurotrace 435/455 blue fluorescent Nissl (1200) to secondary antibody solution when staining for multiple markers. If only staining using Nissl, microwave protocol **steps 4–20** can be omitted (*see* **Notes 17** and **18**).

Step#	Description	User prompt	Time (min)	Power (watts)
1	Permeabilization on	On	2	150
2	Permeabilization off	Off	1	150
3	Permeabilization on	Off	2	150
4	Block on	On	2	150
5	Block off	Off	1	150
6	Block on	Off	2	150
7	Primary Ab on	On	6	150
8	Primary Ab off	Off	4	150
9	Primary Ab on	Off	6	150
10	Primary Ab off	Off	4	150
11	Primary Ab on	Off	6	150
12	Primary Ab off	Off	4	150
13	Primary Ab on	Off	6	150
14	Primary Ab off	Off	4	150
15	Primary Ab on	Off	6	150
16	Primary Ab off	Off	4	150
17	Primary Ab on	Off	6	150
18	Wash	On	2	150
19	Wash off	Off	1	150
20	Wash	On	2	150
21	Secondary Ab on	On	6	150
22	Secondary Ab off	Off	3	150
23	Secondary Ab on	Off	6	150
24	Secondary Ab off	Off	3	150
25	Secondary Ab on	Off	6	150
26	Secondary Ab off	Off	3	150
27	Secondary Ab on	Off	6	150
28	Secondary Ab off	Off	3	150
29	Secondary Ab on	Off	6	150
30	Secondary Ab off	Off	3	150
31	Secondary Ab on	Off	6	150
32	Wash	On	2	150
33	Wash off	Off	1	150
34	Wash	On	2	150

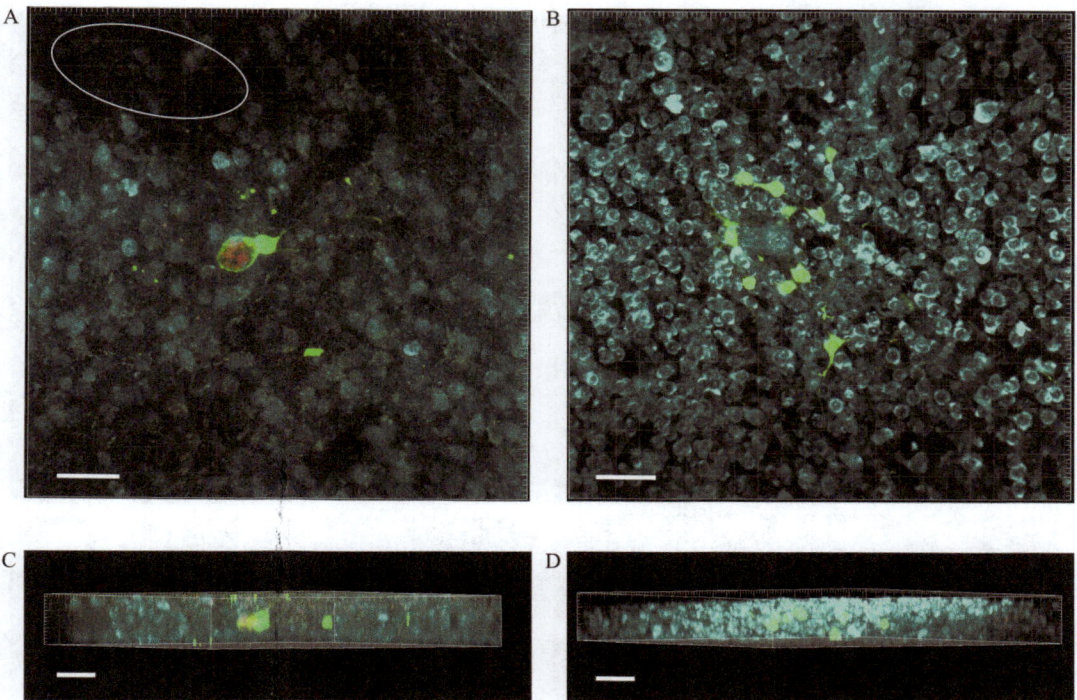

Fig. 3 Antibody versus dye staining of 200 μm thick brain section. *Toxoplasma* infected brain sections cleared using PACT, then stained with the anti-NeuN antibody using the microwave protocol (**a, c**) or Nissl staining (**b, d**), a common stain used to identify neurons. Nissl staining stains RNA, including rough ER. Antibody staining provides neuron-specific staining compared to Nissl; however, in *Toxoplasma* infected tissue we see some areas that have lost NeuN antigenicity. This loss of antigenicity prevents antibody from binding in these "dead zones," preventing antibody cell labeling (white circle in panel **a**). This problem can be avoided by using an intracellular stain, such as Nissl, which will stain many cell types. (**a**) Maximum projection image of center 60 μm from 200 μm thick section stained with anti-NeuN antibodies. Blue color represents NeuN staining of neuron nuclei. Green fluorescence is from *Toxoplasma* injected neurons (TINs); red fluorescence is from mCherry expressing parasites that have formed a cyst within the infected neuron. (**b**) Colors as in (**a**) but now orthogonal view of NeuN stained tissue. (**c**) Maximum projection image of 68 μm stack from 200 μm thick section stained with Nissl. Colors as in (**a**) except that blue color represents Nissl staining. (**d**) Orthogonal view of Nissl stained tissue. Orthogonal views (**b, d**) show that both NeuN antibody and Nissl stain are able to penetrate and stain throughout the tissue section. Maximal projection images representing the entire 200 μm thick section lack clarity due to the abundance of cells/staining being projected onto a 2-D image. Scale bar = 50 μm

5. Aspirate wash solution and then move tissue sections to vials with sRIMS.

6. Incubate sections in sRIMS at room temperature for 30 min to 1 h on rotator. Then take vials off rotator and allow sections to incubate in sRIMS at room temperature overnight.

7. Mount tissue sections in fresh sRIMS, not from the vial, on spacer slide with cover glass.

8. After imaging, wash tissue sections in 1× PBS to remove sRIMS. Tissue may be stored long term in 1× PBS at 4 °C (Fig. 3).

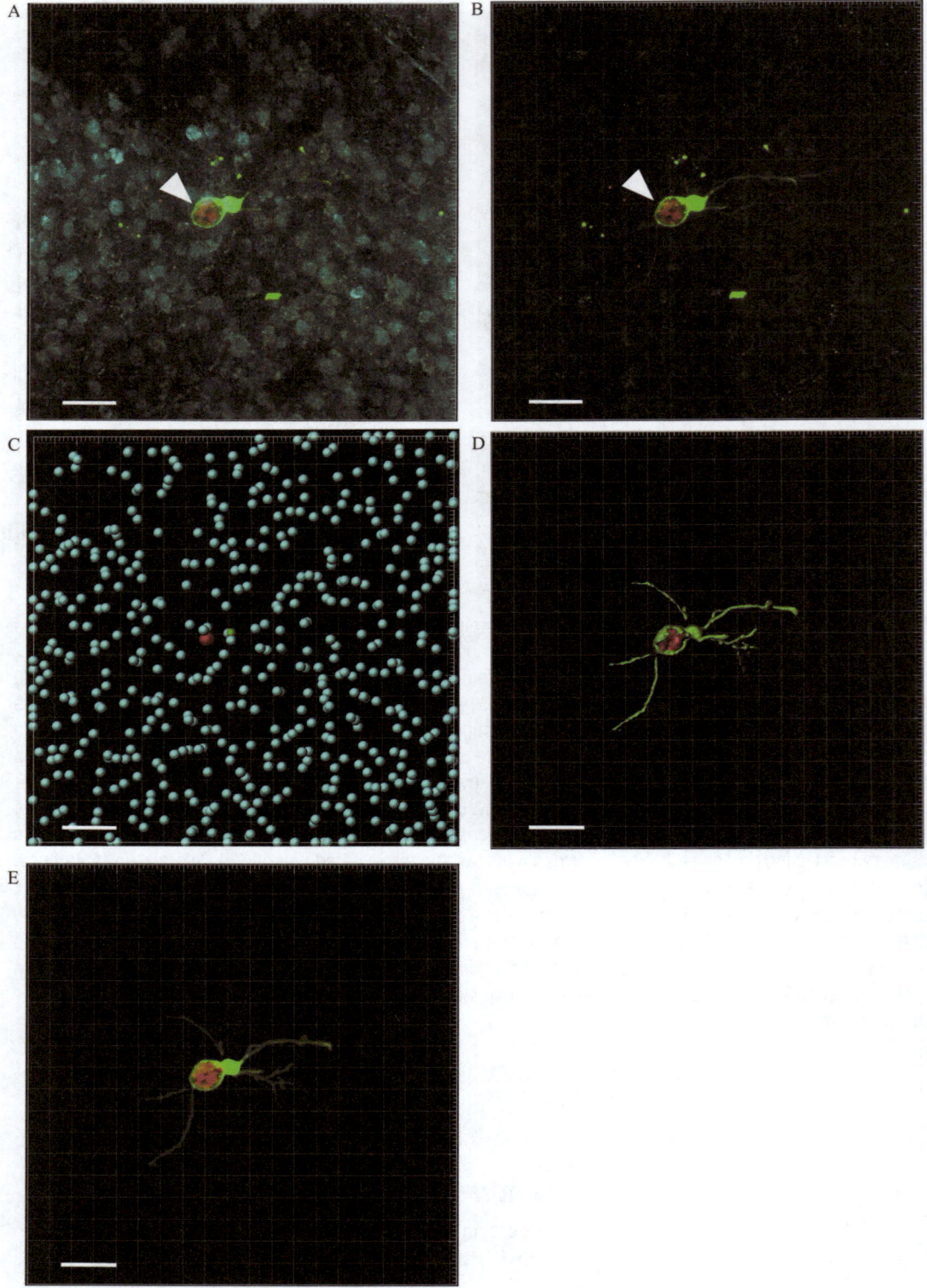

Fig. 4 3-D reconstruction of 200 μm thick brain section. *Toxoplasma* infected brain sections cleared using PACT and stained for bystander neurons using NeuN (blue) with the microwave method. Green cell is

3.4 Imaging Tissue Sections

Images of tissue processed by the above protocol were obtained on a Zeiss LSM 880 inverted confocal microscope using a Plan-Apochromat $20\times/0.8$ (WD = 0.55 mm) objective and Zen Black software interface. Z-stack images through the entire thickness of the tissue were obtained (*see* **Note 15**).

3.5 3-D Reconstruction of Confocal Images

Confocal images were loaded into IMARIS image analysis software (Bitplane) for 3-D reconstruction. Depending on the project, we rendered images with either filaments or surfaces or spots to obtain different data (Fig. 4).

4 4. Notes

1. Hydrogel monomer solution must be made fresh just prior to use. Polymerization and crosslinking of the solutions components occurs when it is heat activated and can also begin if left at room temperature for more than a few hours.

2. SDS powder should be opened, weighed, and dissolved in fume hood.

3. SDS must be kept at room temperature or it will precipitate out.

4. May use conical tubes or other containers for clearing and staining of tissue.

5. During degassing step (flooding vial with nitrogen gas), it is important to avoid creating a large hole in the parafilm, as the goal is to prevent oxygen from reentering the vial. Oxygen will impede the polymerization and crosslinking. Quickly place cap back on vial to prevent reintroduction of oxygen into the sample. Be careful to not tear parafilm during the recapping. If the nitrogen pressure is too high or the volume of solution in the vial is too great, solution will bubble out of the parafilmed vial. If done correctly, solution should become very viscous after incubation.

Fig. 4 (continued) a *Toxoplasma* injected neuron (TIN); red fluorescence is from mCherry expressing parasites that have formed a cyst within the infected neuron. (**a**) Original image obtained on a Zeiss 880 Confocal microscope and then imported as a CZI file. (**b**) Original image with noninjected, bystander neurons removed. Due to the thickness of the tissue and density of neurons within the section, the blue can be overwhelming for visualizing TINs in their entirety. White arrow indicates *Toxoplasma* cyst within TIN. (**c**) 3-D rendering of original image using IMARIS spots tool, which converts each cell into a single "spot" based on size inclusion criteria. Blue spots are bystander neurons, the green spot is the GFP$^+$ neuron's cell body, and the red spot is the *Toxoplasma* cyst within the GFP$^+$ neuron. The spots tool can be used to generate *X, Y, Z* coordinates for each individual cell. (**d**) 3-D rendering generated using surfaces tool in IMARIS and with bystander neurons removed. Surfaces allows only the cells of interest to be rendered while removing pixels that are not to be rendered. (**e**) Final 3-D rendering of infected, GFP$^+$ neuron generated from surfaces tool. Scale bar = 50 μm

6. The easiest way to transfer sections from the thick hydrogel monomer solution to new vials for mounting or washing is to dump out the solution into a petri dish and pick up the tissue with a paint brush. Any size vials or petri dishes may be used depending on the scale of your project.

7. During the clearing process, tissue will increase in size and become more gelatinous in nature making it difficult to pick up and transfer. It is best to use a flat headed paint brush when manipulating the tissue from this point forward.

8. The amount of time it takes for tissue to clear is dependent on the type of tissue and how well the hydrogel monomer solution saturated and solidified in the tissue. For our 200 μm thick mouse brain tissue sections, we achieve full clearance in 20 min. When starting this protocol, it is advised to look at your tissue every 10 min to gauge the level of tissue transparency.

9. May use other materials to make spacer slides.

10. You may soak tissue sections in sRIMS for less time if you need to image right away but allowing the solution to fully saturate the tissue provides better refractive index matching throughout the tissue, which results in clearer images.

11. We have noted that mounted tissue should be imaged within a few days or a precipitate may form around edges of the slide or sRIMS may begin to evaporate.

12. The amount of time tissue may be stored in $1\times$ PBS at 4 °C varies but we have sections that have been stored for over 1 year.

13. Optional—use different size plate or container for staining depending on volume of tissue to be stained.

14. When adding solution to the 24-well plate, use the amount of solution needed to appropriately cover the tissue sections. Depending on how many sections are in each well, you may need more or less solution.

15. Primary and secondary antibody concentrations as well as incubation time will need to be tested and optimized for each antibody and tissue type and thickness used.

16. Images may be obtained on any confocal microscope system using any objective that is capable of capturing high-resolution images through your tissue type and thickness. Settings such as laser power, pinhole size, dimensions, gain, and offset were optimized for each experiment. For single parasites inside neurons, we found that image frames obtained at a resolution of 1024×1024 pixels with a pixel dwell time of 2.06 μs gave an optimum result for 3-D reconstruction, but we found that a 512×512 pixel resolution with a pixel dwell time of 4.12 μs was enough for 3-D detection of single cells. For all

experiments, we used the optimal z-step size as calculated by the Zen software unless otherwise noted. All settings will need to be optimized for each investigator.

17. Quality of PACT clearing greatly affects tissue staining. If images do not stain as expected it is likely due to tissue not being fully cleared and antibodies unable to penetrate thick sections.

18. If additional staining is desired, Nissl can be diluted in PBS (1:200), added to tissue, and placed on orbital shaker at 37 °C, overnight. After incubation, wash tissue in PBS 3 × 10 min on orbital shaker at room temperature prior to placing in sRIMS.

References

1. Silvestri L, Costantini I, Sacconi L et al (2016) Clearing of fixed tissue: a review from a microscopist's perspective. J Biomed Op 21:81205–81208

2. Seo J, Choe M, Kim S-Y (2016) Clearing and labeling techniques for large-scale biological tissues. Mol Cells 39:439–446

3. Azaripour A, Lagerweij T, Scharfbillig C et al (2016) A survey of clearing techniques for 3D imaging of tissues with special reference to connective tissue. Prog Histochem Cytochem 51:9–23

4. Vigouroux RJ, Belle M, Chédotal A (2017) Neuroscience in the third dimension: shedding new light on the brain with tissue clearing. Mol Brain 10:33

5. Schindelin J, Arganda-Carreras I, Frise E et al (2012) Fiji: an open-source platform for biological-image analysis. Nat Methods 9:676–682

6. Koshy AA, Dietrich HK, Christian DA et al (2012) *Toxoplasma* co-opts host cells it does not invade. PLoS Pathog 8:e1002825

7. Cabral CM, Koshy AA (2014) 3-D imaging and analysis of neurons infected *in vivo* with *Toxoplasma gondii*. JoVE 94:e52237

Chapter 17

Model Systems for Studying Mechanisms of Ocular Toxoplasmosis

Justine R. Smith, Liam M. Ashander, Yuefang Ma, Elise Rochet, and João M. Furtado

Abstract

The most common human disease caused by infection with *Toxoplasma gondii* is ocular toxoplasmosis, which typically is manifest as recurrent attacks of necrotizing retinal inflammation with subsequent scarring. The multilayered retina contains specialized cell populations, including endothelial cells, epithelial cells, neurons and supporting cells, all of which may be involved in this condition. In vitro investigations of basic mechanisms operating in human ocular toxoplasmosis use cellular and molecular methods that are common to the study of many pathological processes, and the novel aspect of this research is the use of human retinal cell subsets. Most in vivo research on ocular toxoplasmosis is conducted in the laboratory mouse. Experimental models involve local or systemic inoculation of parasites to induce acute disease, or sequential systemic and local parasite inoculations to trigger recurrent disease. We present methods for in vitro and in vivo studies of ocular toxoplasmosis, including dissection of the human eye, and culture and infection of differentiated cell populations from the retina, as well as induction of mouse ocular toxoplasmosis by intraocular, or sequential systemic and intraocular, inoculations, and imaging of toxoplasmic retinal lesions.

Key words Ocular toxoplasmosis, *Toxoplasma*, Eye, Retina, Human, Mouse

1 Introduction

In humans, ocular toxoplasmosis is the most common medical presentation of an infection with *Toxoplasma gondii* [1]. In over 90% of presentations, this condition is characterized by recurrent attacks of necrotizing inflammation based in the retina (i.e., retinitis) that may be associated with inflammation of other intraocular tissues, including the adjacent choroid and the vitreous (Fig. 1) [2, 3]. Clinical manifestation of ocular toxoplasmosis reflects in part the infection with the parasite, and in part the host immune response, which frequently involves exuberant inflammation. While an intraocular infection is usually aggressive in those persons who are immunocompromised (e.g., patients treated with immunosuppressive drugs or patients with immunodeficiency conditions, such

Christopher J. Tonkin (ed.), *Toxoplasma gondii: Methods and Protocols*, Methods in Molecular Biology, vol. 2071,
https://doi.org/10.1007/978-1-4939-9857-9_17, © Springer Science+Business Media, LLC, part of Springer Nature 2020

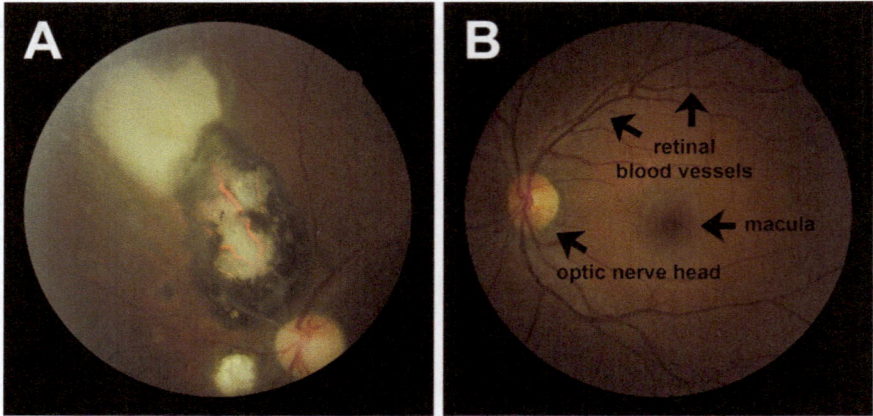

Fig. 1 (**a**) Clinical photograph taken through the dilated pupil of the left eye in a patient with active toxoplasmic retinitis. There is fluffy white focus of retinal inflammation, adjacent to a pigmented retinochoroidal scar, both located superior to the optic nerve head. An additional retinochoroidal scar is present, situated temporal to the optic nerve head. (**b**) Clinical photograph of a healthy posterior left eye

as acquired immunodeficiency syndrome) or individuals who contract the infection in utero, the majority of people who present with ocular toxoplasmosis are otherwise healthy adults [4]. Past teaching was that most infections were contracted in utero and presented later in life at the time of a reactivation; on the contrary, thorough reevaluation of multiple clinical studies indicates most infections are contracted after birth [5]. Genotyping of parasites isolated from patients with ocular toxoplasmosis indicates that both virulent and avirulent strains may be responsible for the disease in immunocompetent persons [6–9].

After entering the human body, the primary route by which *T. gondii* accesses organs is the bloodstream and lymphatic system [10]. The eye is protected by blood-ocular barriers that exist at a cellular level. The blood-retinal barrier is constituted by [1] a vascular endothelium with endothelial cells lacking fenestrations and connected by tight junctions and adherens junctions, which is reinforced by pericytes, glial cells and neurons (i.e., "the neurovascular unit of the retina"); and [2] an epithelium with pigment epithelial cells, also tightly connected by junctional complexes, and located on the substantial Bruch's membrane [11, 12]. The vast majority of published descriptions of human pathology in ocular toxoplasmosis detail cases of aggressive, end-stage disease, but rare reports of recent-onset ocular toxoplasmosis indicate that the condition has its origin in the inner retina [13, 14]. Given that the retinal vascular endothelium is based on the surface of the inner retina, while the pigment epithelium marks the limit of the outer retina, these observations are most consistent with *T. gondii* accessing the retina across the vascular endothelial barrier. A direct comparison between different endothelial cell subpopulations

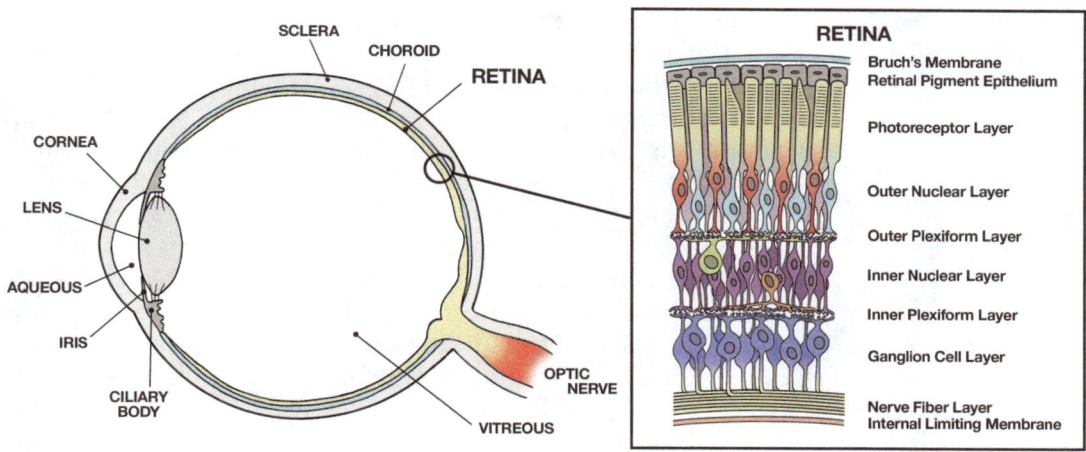

Fig. 2 Cartoon of the human eye, including cellular level detail of the retina, drawn in cross section. An external limiting membrane is situated between the photoreceptor and outer nuclear layers. Drawings were generated by Mr. David Heinrich (Flinders Medical Centre Medical Illustration & Media Unit, Adelaide, Australia)

suggests retinal endothelial cells are relatively susceptible to infection with *T. gondii* tachyzoites [15], and studies utilizing Boyden chamber transwell assays indicate both free tachyzoites and dendritic cells infected with tachyzoites are capable of migration across human retinal endothelial monolayers [16, 17].

With responsibility for visual processing, the retina is constituted of ten layers: three layers of neuronal cell bodies; four layers of neuronal processes, including the photoreceptor segments; two "membranes" that are formed by cellular structures; and the pigment epithelium (Fig. 2). Multiple retinal cell populations are highly differentiated for specialized functions. Photoreceptors detect light photons, and subsequently the visual signal is processed by other neuronal subsets (i.e., bipolar cells, ganglion cells, horizontal cells, and amacrine cells) prior to exiting the retina via ganglion cell axons, which constitute the optic nerve [18]. Mueller glial cells are specialized supporting cells that extend from outer to inner retina; other supporting cells include pericytes associated with the retinal vessels, astrocytes and microglia [11, 19]. The retinal pigment epithelium has diverse functions: an essential role in the visual cycle of retinal; provision of nutrition to and recycling of segments from photoreceptors; source of growth factor proteins; maintenance of ocular immune privilege; and protection of the eye by absorption of light [20]. In vitro studies conducted with human retinal explants suggest that following arrival in the retina, tachyzoites may navigate through the multilayered retina, and thus gain access to any cell population [21]. However, while *T. gondii* has the ability to infect all nucleated cells, a comparison of tachyzoite growth in neurons and Mueller cells indicates there are differences in susceptibility of retinal cell types to infection with the parasite [21]. Clearly the function(s) of any given retinal cell type will determine the impact of *T. gondii* infection, with potential to influence retinal structure and/or function more broadly. Thus, while investigations of basic mechanisms operating in human ocular toxoplasmosis use cellular and molecular methods that are common to the study of many pathological processes, the novel aspect of the work is the use of the specialized human retinal cell populations.

Experimental models of ocular toxoplasmosis were first reported in sulfadiazine-treated golden hamsters infected with tachyzoites delivered by subcutaneous or intraperitoneal injection [22], and in albino or pigmented rabbits infected by intracarotid or suprachoroidal injection of tachyzoites [23, 24]. Subsequently, ocular disease has been produced by systemic or local inoculation of different forms of *T. gondii* in a range of mammals [25]. However, the human retina demonstrates highly specialized cell topography, with a fovea in the area of retina corresponding to the central visual field; amongst mammals, the fovea exists only in Haplorrhine primates [26]. In order to faithfully replicate the human phenotype of ocular toxoplasmosis, a nonhuman primate model is required. Experimental toxoplasmosis following injection of tachyzoites into the central retina under direct visualization has been achieved previously in several monkey species [27], but today such work raises ethical debate and poses considerable expense and logistical challenges. Currently, as in other fields of ophthalmic research, the vast majority of in vivo research on ocular toxoplasmosis is conducted in the laboratory mouse, reflecting practical reasons, but also present capability for genetic manipulation, plus the wide range of reagents and equipment developed for this species. Fortunately there is opportunity to reconcile results obtained in mouse models with investigations conducted using human retinal tissue. Although a wide variety of mouse models of ocular toxoplasmosis have been described, the majority involve a local inoculation (i.e., intraocular injection of tachyzoites) or a systemic inoculation (i.e., intraperitoneal injection or peroral delivery of bradyzoites, or intraperitoneal injection of tachyzoites) to produce acute disease [25]. Ocular immune privilege may be breached prematurely by intraocular injection, but this route most reliably induces vigorous retinitis. Sequential systemic and local parasite inoculations have also been used, and provide the opportunity to study reactivation of ocular toxoplasmosis [28]. Different strains of inbred mouse demonstrate different susceptibilities to experimental ocular toxoplasmosis [29]. However, selection of strain is also impacted by outcome measures of the investigation, since pigmentation of tissues, including the choroid and retinal pigment epithelium, may complicate interpretation of some ocular histopathological changes but conversely may facilitate clinical visualization of retinal lesions.

In vivo studies of disease models typically include clinical outcome measures, in parallel with histopathological and molecular results. Technologies for mouse ocular imaging are well progressed, facilitating clinical assessment of experimental ophthalmic diseases. The rodent microscope that is manufactured by Phoenix Research Labs has been applied to the study of diverse mouse retinal pathologies [30–32]. This system provides anterior and posterior eye color photography, plus more sophisticated options for evaluating the retina, including angiography, optical coherence tomography and electroretinography. A draw back of the rodent microscope is its cost: in 2018, the Phoenix Micron IV Retinal Imaging Microscope base model retailed at approximately USD80,000. For clinical evaluation of experimental ocular toxoplasmosis in particular, posterior eye color photography is sufficient. Thus, the investigator may look to simple imaging systems that are readily assembled in-house and relatively low in cost. One mouse-specific setup—topical endoscopic fundus imaging (TEFI) [33, 34]—has been widely applied in the evaluation of a range of retinal disease models, including ocular toxoplasmosis (Fig. 3) [28, 35–37]. This system, which costs less than USD8,000 to build, is composed of an endoscope connected in parallel to a light source and a photographic camera.

In this chapter, we present methods that have specific application for in vitro and in vivo studies of ocular toxoplasmosis. We describe dissection of the human eye, to obtain retina for explants or for further processing to isolate retinal cells. We also describe the isolation and culture of differentiated cell populations from human retina, including endothelial cells, pigment epithelial cells, and Mueller cells, and the preparation of dissociated retinal cultures, in which Mueller cells support the growth of neurons. These are methods that we have either developed in-house (i.e., endothelial cells [38]) or adapted from methods published by independent research groups (i.e., pigment epithelial cells [39–41], Mueller cells [42] and dissociated retinal cultures [43, 44]). Since some researchers may not have access to human eyes, we have included a list of primate retinal cell lines that are widely available (Table 1). We provide methods for mouse experimental ocular toxoplasmosis induced by intraocular inoculation using a technique adapted from that used by retinal stem cell biology researchers [45], as well as sequential systemic and intraocular inoculation. There are many minor technical variations for these models. In addition, we describe the application of TEFI for visualization of toxoplasmic retinal lesions, including an explanation of how the retinal images may be processed.

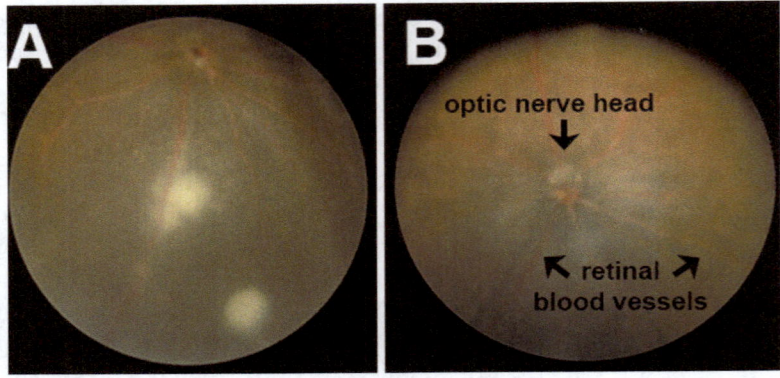

Fig. 3 (**a**) Topical endoscopic fundus image taken through the dilated pupil of the right eye of a C57BL/6 mouse with experimental ocular toxoplasmosis. There are two fluffy white foci of retinal inflammation, both located inferior to the optic nerve head, with retinal vasculitis. The view is hazy due to secondary inflammation of the vitreous. (**b**) Topical endoscopic fundus image of the saline-infected right eye of a C57BL/6 mouse

Table 1
Description of widely studied human and nonhuman primate retinal cell lines

Retinal cell	Designation (source)	Notes
Endothelial	RF/6A (ATCC)	Rhesus macaque choroid-retina origin: Immortalized spontaneously [49]; Grown in EMEM with 10% FBS
Pigment epithelial	ARPE-19 (ATCC, Manassas, VA)	Immortalized spontaneously [50]; Grown in 1:1 DMEM: Ham's F-12 Nutrient Mixture with 10% FBS; cellular and molecular phenotypes vary with culture conditions [51, 52]
Neuron	Y79 (ATCC)	Retinoblastoma origin [53]; Grown in RPMI-1640 medium with 10–20% FBS (in suspension)
	WERI-Rb-1 (ATCC)	Retinoblastoma origin [54]; Grown in RPMI-1640 medium with 10–20% FBS (in suspension)
Mueller	MIO-M1 (University College London, Institute of Ophthalmology, London, UK; subject to material transfer agreement)	Immortalized spontaneously [42]; Grown in DMEM with 10% FBS

ATCC American Type Culture Collection, *EMEM* Eagle's Minimum Essential Medium, *FBS* Fetal Bovine Serum, *DMEM* Dulbecco's Modified Eagle's Medium, *RPMI* Roswell Park Memorial Institute Medium

2 Materials

2.1 Dissection of Human Posterior Eyecups

1. A pair of human posterior eyecups (provided by eye bank following removal of cornea for use in corneal transplantation).

2. Dulbecco's phosphate buffered saline (without calcium or magnesium, pH 7.2) [PBS].

3. PBS with 100 U/mL penicillin–100 μg/mL streptomycin (Thermo Fisher Scientific-GIBCO, Grand Island, NY: catalog number 10131).

4. Holding buffer: PBS with 2% fetal bovine serum [FBS]. Store at 4 °C for up to 2 months. Use chilled.

5. Dissecting instruments (i.e., scalpels, microscissors, microforceps).

6. Tissue culture dishes (6 cm diameter).

7. Plastic tubes (50 mL).

2.2 Dissociated Human Retina Culture

1. Papain (Sigma-Aldrich, St. Louis, MO: catalog number P5306): 2 mg/mL solution in Dulbecco's Modified Eagle's Medium (with glucose and L-glutamine) [DMEM] (Thermo Fisher Scientific-GIBCO: catalog number 11965). Store at −20 °C for up to 6 months.

2. Deoxyribonuclease [DNase] I (Sigma-Aldrich: catalog number DN25): 0.7 mg/mL solution in DMEM. Store at −20 °C for up to 6 months.

3. Retina medium: 50% DMEM and 50% Ham's F-12 Nutrient Mix [F-12] (Thermo Fisher Scientific-GIBCO: catalog number 11765) with 2% FBS and 100 U/mL penicillin–100 μg/mL streptomycin.

4. Poly-L-lysine hydrobromide (Sigma-Aldrich: catalog number P4707): 16 μg/mL solution in sterile water.

5. Laminin (Sigma-Aldrich: catalog number L4544): 16 μg/mL solution in Hank's balanced salt solution [HBSS].

6. Straight-blade scissors.

7. Serological pipettes (5 mL).

8. Plastic tubes (15 mL).

9. "FluoroDish" tissue culture dishes (35 mm diameter, glass-bottomed) (World Precision Instruments, Sarasota, FL: catalog number FD35). Coat culture surfaces sequentially with poly-L-lysine hydrobromide and laminin for 15 min each at 1 μg/cm² (250 μL). Dry for 2 h at 37 °C. Store at 2–8 °C for up to 1 month.

2.3 Human Retinal Endothelial Cell Culture

1. Collagenase II (Thermo Fisher Scientific-GIBCO: catalog number 17101): 1 and 0.5 mg/mL solutions in holding buffer (*see* Subheading 2.1, **item 4**). Store 10 mg/mL solutions in PBS at −20 °C for up to 6 months.

2. Endothelial cell medium: MCDB-131 medium (Sigma-Aldrich: catalog number M8537) with "EGM-2 SingleQuots" (Clonetics-Lonza, Walkersville, MD: catalog number CC-4176) supplements (omitting FBS, hydrocortisone and gentamicin) and 2% or 10% FBS.

3. PBS.

4. 0.05% w/v trypsin–EDTA (Thermo Fisher Scientific-GIBCO: catalog number 25300).

5. FBS (undiluted).

6. Holding buffer: *see* Subheading 2.1, **item 4**.

7. Endothelial cell isolation beads: Dynabeads M-450 Epoxy (Thermo Fisher Scientific-Invitrogen DYNAL, Oslo, Norway: catalog number 14011) coated with mouse anti-human CD31 antibody (BD Biosciences-Pharmingen, San Diego, CA: catalog number 555444), according to manufacturer's instructions. Store in 3×10^7 beads/mL suspension in PBS at 4 °C for up to 6 months.

8. "MACS SmartStrainers" disposable cell strainer (30 μm pores) (Miltenyi Biotec, Auburn, CA: catalog number 130-098-458).

9. "Dynabeads MPC-S" magnet (Thermo Fisher Scientific-Invitrogen DYNAL: catalog number A13346).

10. Micropipettes (1000 μL).

11. Plastic tubes (15 mL).

12. Collagen I (Santa Cruz Biotechnology, Santa Cruz, CA: catalog number: sc-29009): 50 μg/mL solution in 0.01 M hydrochloric acid.

13. Tissue culture dishes (6 cm and 10 cm diameter). Coat culture surfaces with collagen I for 2 h. Air-dry at room temperature. Store at 4 °C for up to 1 month.

2.4 Human Retinal Pigment Epithelial Cell Culture

1. Collagenase IA/Collagenase IV: Single solution of collagenase 1A and collagenase IV (Sigma-Aldrich: catalog numbers C9891 and C5138, respectively), both at 0.5 mg/mL, in HBSS. Store at −20 °C for up to 6 months.

2. Holding buffer: *see* Subheading 2.1, **item 4**.

3. Sucrose medium: 15% w/v solution in 50% DMEM and 50% F-12 with 10% FBS. Store at −20 °C for up to 6 months.

4. Epithelial cell medium: 50% Minimum Essential Medium Eagle alpha modification (with sodium bicarbonate) [MEM] (Sigma-

Aldrich: catalog number M4526), 25% DMEM and 25% F-12 with N1 Medium Supplement ($1\times$) (Sigma-Aldrich: catalog number N6530), nonessential amino acid solution ($1\times$) (Thermo Fisher Scientific-GIBCO: catalog number 11140), GlutaMAX Supplement ($1\times$) (Thermo Fisher Scientific-GIBCO: catalog number 35050), 0.25 mg/mL taurine (Sigma-Aldrich, catalog number T0625), 0.02 μg/mL hydrocortisone (Sigma-Aldrich, catalog number H0396), 0.013 ng/mL 3,3′,5-triiodo-L-thyronine sodium (Sigma-Aldrich, catalog number T5516), 2% or 10% FBS, and 100 U/mL penicillin-100 μg/mL streptomycin.

5. 0.25% w/v trypsin–EDTA (Thermo Fisher Scientific-GIBCO: catalog number 25200).

6. Dissecting instruments (i.e., razor blade, spatula).

7. Plastic tubes (15 mL).

8. Micropipettes (200 μL).

9. Tissue culture dishes (6 cm diameter).

2.5 Human Retinal Mueller Cell Culture

1. Dispase II (Thermo Fisher Scientific-GIBCO: catalog number 17105): 0.5 mg/mL solution in PBS. Store 10 mg/mL solutions in PBS at −20 °C for up to 6 months.

2. Holding buffer: *see* Subheading 2.1, **item 4**.

3. Mueller cell medium: DMEM with nonessential amino acid solution ($1\times$), GlutaMAX Supplement ($1\times$), 1 mM sodium pyruvate (Thermo Fisher Scientific-GIBCO: catalog number 11360), 10% FBS and 100 U/mL penicillin–100 μg/mL streptomycin.

4. Straight-blade scissors.

5. Micropipettes (1000 μL).

6. "EasyStrainer" disposable cell strainer (100 μm pores) (Greiner Bio-One, Frickenhausen, Germany: catalog number 542000).

7. Tissue culture dishes (10 cm diameter).

2.6 Infection of Human Retinal Cells with T. gondii

1. *T. gondii* tachyzoites (in 48-h passage in human foreskin fibroblast cultures at 37 °C and 5% CO_2 in air).

2. Human foreskin fibroblasts (available from multiple retailers, including ATCC, Manassas, VA: catalog number PCS-201-010): confluent cell monolayers in tissue culture flasks, selected to produce required number of tachyzoites.

3. Tachyzoite medium: DMEM with 1% FBS.

4. Infection medium (*see* **Note 24** plus: retina: Subheading 2.2, **item 3**; endothelial cells: Subheading 2.3, **item 2**; epithelial cells: Subheading 2.4, **item 4**; Mueller cells: Subheading 2.5, **item 3**).

5. Filter assembly: "Nuclepore" 47 mm diameter polycarbonate membrane with 3.0 μm pores and "Swin-Lok" membrane holder (GE Healthcare-Whatman, Buckinghamshire, UK: catalog numbers 111112 and 420400), plus 10 mL slip-tip syringe and 15 mL tube.

6. Plastic tubes (15 mL).

2.7 Mouse Ocular Toxoplasmosis: Acute Disease Model

1. *T. gondii* tachyzoites (in 48-h passage in human foreskin fibroblast cultures at 37 °C and 5% CO_2 in air).

2. Human foreskin fibroblasts: confluent cell monolayers in tissue culture flasks, selected to produce required number of tachyzoites.

3. Tachyzoite medium.

4. Adult C57BL/6 mice (female).

5. PBS.

6. Tropicamide 1% w/v eye drops (Alcon, Fort Worth, TX).

7. Phenylephrine hydrochloride 2.5% w/v eye drops (Bausch & Lomb, Bridgewater, NJ).

8. Goniovisc 2.5% eye gel (HUB Pharmaceuticals, Plymouth, MI).

9. Needles (30 G).

10. Hamilton syringes (25 μL) or equivalent plastic syringe (with 1 μL graduations).

11. Glass needles: 1.5 mm glass capillaries (World Precision Instruments: catalog number 1B150), pulled manually in flame or on automated puller.

12. Flexible plastic tubing (1.5 mm internal diameter).

2.8 Mouse Ocular Toxoplasmosis: Recurrent Model

1. Type II strain *T. gondii* bradyzoite cysts (maintained by gavage inoculation of adult Swiss-Webster mice (female) and harvested from brain 8 weeks after infection): One mouse brain should yield at least 200 cysts, which is sufficient to infect 40 mice. Store at 4 °C. Use within 24 h of harvest.

2. *T. gondii* tachyzoites (in 48-h passage in human foreskin fibroblast cultures at 37 °C and 5% CO_2 in air).

3. Human foreskin fibroblasts: confluent cell monolayers in tissue culture flasks, selected to produce required number of tachyzoites.

4. Tachyzoite medium.

5. Adult C57BL/6 mice (female).

6. PBS.

7. Needles (21 G and 30 G).

8. Plastic syringes (1 mL).

9. Tropicamide 1% w/v eye drops.

10. Phenylephrine hydrochloride 2.5% w/v eye drops.

11. Goniovisc 2.5% eye gel.

12. Hamilton syringes (25 μL) or equivalent plastic syringe (with 1 μL graduations).

13. Glass needles: 1.5 mm glass capillaries (World Precision Instruments) pulled manually in flame or on automated puller.

14. Flexible plastic tubing (1.5 mm internal diameter).

2.9 Mouse Retinal Photography

1. D90 or D7000 series cameras (Nikon Corporation, Tokyo, Japan).

2. Minitripod modeled for camera.

3. 60 mm f/2.8 D lens (Nikon Corporation).

4. 62-52 step-down ring (available from most camera retailers).

5. Storz 590-44 coupling adaptor (Karl Storz, Tuttlingen, Germany).

6. Storz 481C halogen light with optical fiber cable (Karl Storz).

7. Storz 1218 tele-otoscope (Karl Storz).

8. Tropicamide 1% w/v eye drops.

9. Phenylephrine hydrochloride 2.5% w/v eye drops.

10. GenTeal Tears eye gel (Alcon).

2.10 Processing Mouse Retinal Images

1. ViewNX 2 software (Nikon Corporation). Available at no charge from Download Center: http://downloadcenter. nikonimglib.com/en/products/166/ViewNX_2.html.

3 Methods

3.1 Dissection of the Human Posterior Eyecups

1. Disinfect each posterior eyecup by immersing for 20 min in a 50 mL tube of PBS with 100 U/mL penicillin–100 μg/mL streptomycin. Rinse the eyecup twice in additional tubes of PBS alone to remove antibiotics.

2. Transfer the eyecup to a tissue culture dish. Use a scalpel to make a small incision through the sclera and into the cup, just behind the ora serrata. Extend this incision around the entire cup with scissors, to remove the remains of the anterior segment, including the iris and the lens (*see* **Note 3**).

3. Tip the eyecup on its side so the vitreous partially pours out. Grasping the upper rim of the cup with one microforceps, gently tease the vitreous out of the cup with a second microforceps (*see* **Note 4**).

4. Continuing to hold the rim of the eyecup with one microforceps, gently pick up the neural retina at the rim and gently pull the tissue inwards to detach it from the underlying retinal pigment epithelium (*see* **Note 5**).

5. Cut the neural retina free from the eyecup close the optic nerve head with microscissors and rinse this in chilled holding buffer in a clean tissue culture dish, in advance of cell isolation procedures (*see* **Note 6**).

6. Again holding the rim of the eyecup with one microforceps, gently peel the retinal pigment epithelium with adherent choroid from the underlying sclera with a second microforceps.

7. Cut the retinal pigment epithelium-choroid free from the eyecup close the optic nerve head with microscissors and rinse these in chilled holding buffer in a clean tissue culture dish, ahead of isolation of pigment epithelial cells.

3.2 Dissociated Human Retina Culture

1. Following dissection of the neural retina, this tissue is placed in holding buffer (*see* Subheading 3.1, **step 7**). Move the tissue to a clean tissue culture dish containing 2 mL of papain and cut into 2 mm squares with scissors.

2. Incubate the retina for 30 min at 37 °C and 5% CO_2 in air, shaking the dish gently every 5 min.

3. End the digestion by adding 1 mL of FBS, followed by 4 mL of DNase I.

4. Triturate the tissue by passing through the serological pipette six times. Place the retina suspension in a 15 mL tube and allow the tissue to settle for 1 min.

5. Collect the supernatant and centrifuge this at $150 \times g$ for 5 min at room temperature. Discard the supernatant and resuspend the cell pellet in 5 mL of retina medium.

6. Count the cells by hematocytometer and dilute the cell suspension in additional retina medium to bring this to 2×10^6 cells/mL.

7. Seed tissue culture dishes with 1 mL of cell suspension (10^6 cells), and culture the cells undisturbed for 5 days at 37 °C and 5% CO_2 in air (*see* **Note 7**).

8. After 5 days in culture, replenish the retina medium. Change the medium on the culture twice a week until cultures become confluent (*see* **Note 8**).

9. When dissociated retina cultures reach confluence, they should appear as a mat of spindle shaped glial cells with scattered small neuronal cell bodies atop. (Photomicrograph is presented in ref. 21.) Cell types may be distinguished on expression of neuron-specific enolase [NSE] (neurons) and glial fibrillary acidic protein [GFAP] (glial cells) (Table 2).

Table 2
Human retinal cell markers and information on antibodies used for phenotyping cells by immunocytochemistry

| Cell marker | Antibody | | | | |
	Supplier	Catalog number	Description	Working concentration	Label
CD31	Dako	M0823	Monoclonal mouse IgG1κ	10 μg/mL	Surface
CRALBP	Thermo Fisher Scientific-Invitrogen	PA5-29759	Polyclonal rabbit IgG	2 μg/mL	Cytoplasmic
CK8	Abcam	ab53280	Monoclonal rabbit IgG	0.15 μg/mL	Cytoplasmic
GFAP	R&D Systems	AF2594	Polyclonal sheep IgG	10 μg/mL	Cytoplasmic
GS	Sigma-Aldrich	G2781	Polyclonal rabbit IgG	15 μg/mL	Cytoplasmic
NSE	Thermo Fisher Scientific	PA5-29759	Rabbit antiserum	NA (1:500 dilution)	Cytoplasmic
RPE65	Novus Biologicals	NB100-355	Monoclonal mouse IgG1κ	4 μg/mL	Cytoplasmic
α-SMA	Abcam	ab5694	Polyclonal rabbit IgG	2 μg/mL	Cytoplasmic
VIM	Merck Millipore-Chemicon	MAB3400	Monoclonal mouse IgG1	1 μg/mL	Cytoplasmic
VWF	DAKO	A0082	Polyclonal rabbit IgG	15 μg/mL	Cytoplasmic
ZO-1	Thermo Fisher Scientific-Invitrogen	40-2200	Polyclonal rabbit IgG	2.5 μg/mL	Junctional

CRALBP Cellular retinaldehyde-binding protein, *CK* Cytokeratin, *GFAP* Glial fibrillary acidic protein, *GS* Glutamine synthetase, *NSE* Neuron-specific enolase, *RPE* Retinal pigment epithelium-specific protein, *SMA* Smooth muscle actin, *VIM* Vimentin, *VWF* von Willebrand factor, *ZO* Zonula occludens, *NA* Not applicable
Working concentrations are a guide and should be verified by the researcher for the laboratory

3.3 Human Retinal Endothelial Cell Culture

1. Following dissection of the neural retina, this tissue is placed in holding buffer (*see* Subheading 3.1, **step** 7). Rinse twice with holding buffer to remove any adherent retinal pigment epithelium. Transfer to a clean tissue culture dish with 3 mL of collagenase II (1 mg/mL) and incubate on an orbital shaker for 15 min at 37 °C and 5% CO_2 in air (*see* **Note 9**).

2. Dissociate the digested retina by gentle pipetting with the micropipette, and transfer the tissue suspension to a 15 mL tube (*see* **Note 10**).

3. Centrifuge the retina suspension at $150 \times g$ for 1 min. Collect the supernatant to a new tube.

4. Centrifuge the supernatant at $280 \times g$ for 5 min. Discard the resulting supernatant, and resuspend the cell pellet in endothelial cell medium (with 2% FCS). Transfer the suspension to a 6 cm diameter tissue culture dish and incubate this at 37 °C and 5% CO_2 in air.

5. Resuspend the original cell pellet in 4 mL of collagenase II (0.5 mg/mL) in a fresh tissue culture dish. Again dissociate the digested retina by gentle pipetting and incubate on an orbital shaker for 15 min at 37 °C and 5% CO_2 in air.

6. View the suspension at the microscope. If the retina is well digested (i.e. there are no cell clumps), centrifuge at $280 \times g$ for 5 min. Discard the resulting supernatant, and resuspend the resulting cell pellet in endothelial cell medium (with 2% FBS). Transfer the suspension to a 10 cm diameter tissue culture dish and incubate this at 37 °C and 5% CO_2 in air. If the tissues are not well digested, repeat **steps 5** and **6**, and collect additional dishes (*see* **Note 11**).

7. After 1–2 days in culture, replenish the endothelial cell medium (with 2% FBS). Change the medium on the culture every 2–3 days. Monitor the cultures daily for any nonendothelial, contaminating cells, and if detected, remove by these cells by scrapping, followed by aspiration.

8. Proceed with endothelial cell purification after 7–10 days of culture, after nonendothelial, contaminating cells are visible, but before they dominate the culture. Aspirate endothelial cell medium from the cultures and rinse them with PBS. Add trypsin to the cultures (2 mL for 10 cm diameter dish), and incubate them for 3 min at 37 °C and 5% CO_2 in air (*see* **Note 12**).

9. Stop the activity of the trypsin with undiluted FBS (one-third of trypsin volume). Break cell clumps by gentle pipetting with the micropipette, and pass the cell suspension through the cell strainer into a 50 mL tube.

10. Centrifuge the cell suspension at $280 \times g$ for 5 min. Discard the supernatant, and resuspend the cell pellet in holding buffer (300 µL per 10^6 cells).

11. Add endothelial cell isolation beads to cell suspension in bead–cell volume ratio of 3:1 (i.e. add 100 µL of beads to 10^6 cells). Mix well and incubate on ice for 15 min, swirling the tube every 5 min (*see* **Note 13**).

12. Transfer the tube to the magnet. Allow 2 min for separation, and transfer the holding buffer to a new 50 mL tube. Wash the

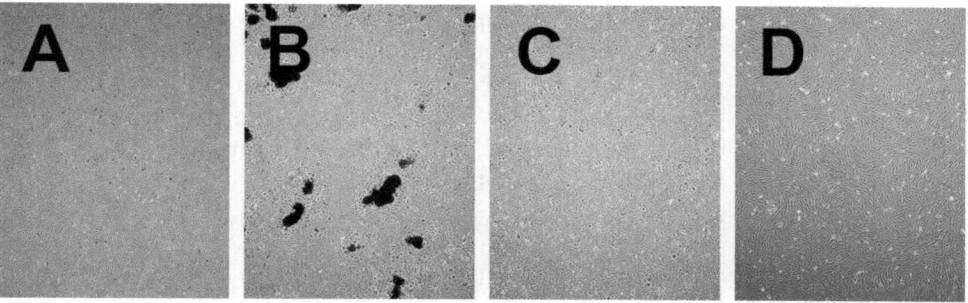

Fig. 4 Photomicrographs of confluent cultured cells that have been isolated from human retina, including (**a**) endothelial cells, (**b**) pigment epithelial cells, (**c**) subcultured pigment epithelial cells, and (**d**) Mueller cells. Original magnification: 40×

beats vigorously with holding buffer to remove nonendothelial cells approximately five times until there are no cells without beads.

13. Resuspend the cells in 8 mL of endothelial cell medium (with 10% FBS), transfer them to a clean 6 cm or 10 cm diameter tissue culture dish, depending on cell number, and incubate this at 37 °C and 5% CO_2 in air (*see* **Note 14**). Repeat the purification procedure with any additional cultures collected in **step 6**.

14. Change the medium on the cultures every 2–3 days until they become confluent (*see* **Note 15**).

15. When retinal endothelial cells reach confluence, they should form a cobblestone monolayer (Fig. 4). Cell phenotype and purity may be confirmed on expression of CD31 and von Willebrand factor [VWF] (Table 2).

3.4 Human Retinal Pigment Epithelial Cell Culture

1. Following dissection of the retinal pigment epithelium-choroid, this tissue is placed in holding buffer (*see* Subheading 3.1, **step 7**). Replace the holding buffer with 3 mL of collagenase IA/collagenase IV. Cut the tissue into 2 quadrants with a razor blade and flatten it.

2. Incubate the retinal pigment epithelium-choroid for 30 min at 37 °C and 5% CO_2 in air. Subsequently, remove the collagenase IA/collagenase IV, and rinse the tissue with holding buffer (*see* **Note 16**).

3. Working under a dissecting microscope, gently scrape sheets of retinal pigment epithelium off Bruch's membrane with a spatula (*see* **Note 17**). Collect the sheets into a 15 mL tube containing holding buffer (*see* **Note 18**).

4. Centrifuge the sheet suspension at $150 \times g$ for 1 min. Discard the supernatant and gently resuspend the sheet pellet in 3 mL of holding buffer (*see* **Note 19**).

5. Layer the holding buffer with sheets onto 3 mL of sucrose medium, and incubate this for 15 min at room temperature to allow any single cells to separate from the sheets. Discard the upper half of the volume, and centrifuge the lower half of the volume at $10 \times g$ for 1 min. Discard the supernatant and resuspend the pellet in holding buffer.

6. Centrifuge the sheet suspension again at $10 \times g$ for 5 min and resuspend the pellet in epithelial cell medium with 10% FBS. Distribute the sheets in tissue culture dishes to cover approximately half of the surface. Break apart large sheets by gently pipetting using a 200 μL micropipette (see **Note 20**).

7. Culture the cells at 37 °C and 5% CO_2 in air for 24 h and then change FBS supplement in epithelial medium to 2% (see **Note 21**).

8. Change the epithelial medium on the culture twice a week. Monitor the cultures daily for any nonepithelial, contaminating cells, and if detected, remove by these cells by scrapping, followed by washing with PBS.

9. When retinal pigment epithelial cells reach confluence, they should have a hexagonal shape and be pigmented (Fig. 4). Cell phenotype and purity may be confirmed on expression of cytokeratin-8, retinal pigment epithelium-specific protein [RPE]65, cellular retinaldehyde-binding protein [CRALBP]; and zonula occludens [ZO]-1, but not α-smooth muscle actin [SMA], which indicates mesenchymal differentiation (Table 2). Measurement of transepithelial resistance may be performed to indicate polarization [39].

3.5 Human Retinal Mueller Cell Culture

1. Following dissection of the neural retina, this tissue is placed in holding buffer (see Subheading 3.1, **step 7**). Wash three times with holding buffer to remove any adherent retinal pigment epithelium. Move the tissue to a clean tissue culture dish containing 2 mL of dispase II and cut into 2 mm squares with scissors.

2. Incubate the retina on an orbital shaker for 10 min at 37 °C and 5% CO_2 in air.

3. Triturate the tissue by passing through the micropipette. Subsequently strain the tissue suspension through the cell strainer.

4. Centrifuge the cell suspension at $280 \times g$ for 5 min at room temperature. Discard the supernatant and resuspend the cell pellet in 8 mL of Mueller cell medium.

5. Transfer the cell suspension to a tissue culture dish, and culture the cells undisturbed for 5 days at 37 °C and 5% CO_2 in air.

6. Change the medium on the culture after 5 days, and subsequently twice a week until the culture becomes confluent (*see* **Note 22**).

7. When retinal Mueller cells reach confluence, they should have a spindle shape (Fig. 4). Cell phenotype and purity may be confirmed on expression of glutamine synthase [GS], CRALBP and vimentin [VIM]; cultured Mueller cells also express GFAP (Table 2).

3.6 Infection of Human Retinal Cells with T. gondii

1. Pass tachyzoites to fresh fibroblast monolayers 48 h before the infection.

2. After 24 h, assess the infection by light microscopy. Over 90% of fibroblasts should be visibly infected with replicating tachyzoites. Replace the tachyzoite medium to remove nonviable, extracellular tachyzoites.

3. Examine the fibroblasts for lysis after a further 24 h, and harvest a tachyzoite suspension when approximately 70–90% of fibroblasts have lysed (*see* **Note 25**).

4. Remove cell debris from the tachyzoite suspension by filtering. Insert the filter membrane into the membrane holder, shiny side down, and build the filter assembly. Draw up the entire volume of tachyzoite suspension into a 10 mL syringe. Place the filter assembly onto the 15 mL centrifuge tube with the outlet port inside the tube; insert the slip tip into the filter assembly inlet port; and gently depress the syringe plunger until the entire volume is expelled.

5. Centrifuge the tachyzoite suspension at $400 \times g$ for 10 min at 18 °C. Discard the supernatant and resuspend the tachyzoite pellet in 1 mL of infection medium.

6. Count the tachyzoites by hematocytometer, and dilute the tachyzoite suspension in additional infection medium to achieve the required multiplicity of infection (*see* **Note 26**).

7. Add infection medium with tachyzoites to the human retinal cell cultures (or human retinal explants) and return the cultures to incubation.

8. After sufficient time for cell invasion (typically 4 h for cells, and longer for explants), wash cultures with and replace the infection medium to remove any extracellular tachyzoites.

3.7 Mouse Ocular Toxoplasmosis: Acute Disease Model

1. Prepare tachyzoites following the method described in Subheading 3.6, **steps 1–5**, with the exception that the tachyzoite pellet is resuspended in PBS.

2. Count the tachyzoites by hematocytometer, and dilute the tachyzoite suspension in additional PBS to achieve the required

number/mL, calculated for an intraocular injection volume of 2 μL, but allowing for wastage (*see* **Notes 29** and **30**).

3. Anesthetize the C57BL/6 mouse (*see* **Notes 31** and **32**).

4. Instill tropicamide and phenylephrine eye drops to dilate the pupil. Apply Goniovisc eye gel over the cornea.

5. Connect the rubber tubing to the syringe and glass pipette. Draw up over 2 μL of tachyzoite suspension into the syringe (*see* **Notes 33** and **34**).

6. Viewing the eye under a surgical microscope or with the aid of surgical loupes, and grasping the head above and below the eyelids with thumb and index finger, make a tiny incision through the sclera, 1 mm behind the limbus in the outer-upper quadrant with a 30 G needle. Angle the needle backwards, in a line that passes between the lens and the retina.

7. Insert the tip of the glass pipette along the path created by the needle and into the vitreous, watching through the dilated pupil to ensure the tip does not touch the lens or the retina.

8. When the tip is positioned within the vitreous, slowly depress the syringe plunger, injecting 2 μL of tachyzoite suspension (*see* **Note 36**).

3.8 Mouse Ocular Toxoplasmosis: Recurrent Disease Model

1. Harvest tissue cysts from brain of infected Swiss-Webster mice and homogenize this tissue in 1 mL of PBS.

2. Count the cysts in a 20 μL volume, using a microscope slide and coverslip. Dilute the cyst suspension in additional PBS to achieve the required number/mL, calculated for an intraperitoneal injection volume of 100 μL, but allowing for wastage (*see* **Note 38**).

3. Inoculate the C57BL/6 mouse by intraperitoneal injection of 100 μL of cyst suspension using a 21 G needle mounted on a 1 mL syringe.

4. Challenge is performed 28 days after the primary infection. Prepare and inject tachyzoites, as described in Subheading 3.7 (*see* **Note 40**).

3.9 Mouse Retinal Photography with TEFI

1. Set the camera to manual and select the following settings:

   (a) Shutter speed: 1/25–1/30 s. Longer speeds result in brighter images, but increase the possibility of motion artifact.

   (b) Aperture: ƒ/2.8.

   (c) ISO: up to 800.

   (d) Image quality: RAW. This selection records images as NEF files.

2. Mount the camera on the minitripod. Use the step-down ring and coupling adaptor to connect the camera lens with the tele-otoscope. Attach the otoscope to the light via the cable. When the light is on, images from the otoscope appear on the camera screen.

3. Anesthetize the mouse (*see* **Note 41**).

4. Instill tropicamide and phenylephrine eye drops to dilate the pupil. Apply GenTeal Tears gel on the cornea.

5. Bring the viewing tip of the tele-otoscope in contact with the gel on the cornea. Direct the lower half of the tip (providing the illumination) toward the region of the retina to be imaged (e.g., the lower half of the tip is placed at 3 o'clock to image the nasal retina of the right eye). Adjust position of the mouse as required. Take at least one image of the central retina and one image each of the superior, nasal, inferior and temporal retinal quadrants.

6. After retinal photography is completed, reapply GenTeal tears gel to the cornea while the mouse remains anesthetized.

3.10 Processing Mouse Retinal Images

1. Open ViewNX2. Select the folder that contains the images to be edited from the folder list on the left side of the screen. Click on an image, which will be displayed in the middle of the screen.

2. On the right side of the screen, select "Adjustments."

3. Change "White Balance" box from "Recorded Value" to "High Color Rendering Fluorescent."

4. Adjust the lightness of the image by moving the "Exposure Comp." cursor.

5. Adjust the contrast of the image by moving the "Contrast" cursor.

6. Save the edited image and select the "Convert File" icon at the top of the screen. Select the required file format (e.g., JPEG, TIF), plus the folder in which the image should be stored, and click "Convert."

4   Notes

Dissection of Human Eye

1. Human eyes should be held in 4 °C until use, but dissected as soon as possible to minimize autolysis of the tissue. Similarly, cell isolation procedures should begin immediately after the dissection to maximize yields.

2. All steps should be performed in a biological safety cabinet, following standard precautions and aseptic technique.

3. Successful retinal pigment epithelial culture is dependent on obtaining intact sheets that preserve cell connections. Therefore, when incising, the blade must be sufficiently sharp that no pressure is required and the eye is not deformed.

4. Ensure that vitreous is removed completely from the posterior eye cup, as residual vitreous may interfere with dissociation of the retina for cell isolation.

5. Neural retina is a delicate tissue and may tear during removal, but this will not impact the success of subsequent cell isolation procedures.

6. When collecting neural retina, cut the tissue as close as possible to the optic nerve head to collect the large vessels at this location, in order to maximize yield of endothelial cells, and take care not to disturb the retinal pigment epithelium.

Dissociated Human Retina Culture

7. Cells may be seeded in standard tissue culture dishes. However, superior imaging of immunolabeled cells is achieved when the cells were plated in glass-bottomed FluoroDish dishes.

8. If large amounts of cell debris become attached to the tissue culture dish, wash the dish gently several times in PBS. However, cell debris is also removed when the medium is changed.

Human Retinal Endothelial Cell Isolation

9. If tissue suspension contains obvious cell clumps, indicating an accumulation of extracellular DNA, DNase I may be added to the collagenase solution.

10. There is a fine line between pipetting sufficiently to dissociate the retina and pipetting excessively and impacting cell viability and overall yield.

11. It is important to not over-digest the retina. Both duration of digestion and concentration of collagenase are critical: do not digest for more than 60 min.

12. Trypsin is toxic to endothelial cells, and attempting to dislodge every cell from the tissue culture dish may jeopardize viability of cells that are already in suspension. Several quick knocks may free additional cells from the dish.

13. Purification is a balance between not losing endothelial cells and having too few beads per cell. If too many beads bind, cells will not attach to tissue culture dish, but if too few beads bind, cells will not be collected. Check bead-cell binding at the microscope during each separation and stop when the bead–cell ratio exceeds 3:1.

14. Endothelial cells should not be seeded too sparsely during the isolation or after passaging the cells. Maintain the cells at a minimum of 40% confluent at all times.

15. At confluence, the endothelial cell cultures should be 99% pure. If they are not, the purification procedure may be repeated.

Human Retinal Pigment Epithelial Cell Isolation

16. Removing the collagenase IA/collagenase IV is essential to prevent excessive digestion of the retinal pigment epithelium-choroid, which frees cells from the choroid that may subsequently contaminate the epithelial cell culture.

17. Take care not to perforate Bruch's membrane to reduce the risk of contaminating the epithelial cell culture with choroidal cells.

18. Do not collect any pieces of choroid to avoid contamination of the epithelial cell culture with choroidal cells.

19. The freshly isolated retinal pigment epithelial sheets are very fragile and any pipetting must be gentle.

20. The density at which the retinal pigment epithelial sheets are plated is critical for a successful culture. Sparse plating promotes de-differentiation of the cells, and dense plating results in a multilayered culture. Large sheets may roll in culture, which prevents attachment.

21. If cells attach slowly, the reduction in FBS supplementation may be performed at 48 or 72 h.

Human Retinal Mueller Cell Culture

22. Replace half the medium only at each change to maintain retinal Mueller cell-derived trophic factors in the culture.

Infection of Human Retinal Cells with *T. gondii*

23. Decontaminate all equipment, consumables and liquid waste in 70% ethanol. Filter assemblies may be autoclaved for reuse after ethanol decontamination.

24. If not standard procedure, heat-inactivate the FBS that is used for the infection medium, by heating at 55 °C for 30 min, and reduce the concentration to no more than 5% for the 4-h invasion step.

25. Fibroblasts also may be lysed mechanically at 24 h after infection, by passage through a 25 G needle.

26. The multiplicity of infection is typically 5 for natural *T. gondii* isolates, which exhibit relatively low viability in the laboratory [46].

27. A plaque assay should be performed in parallel with any infection study, in order to assess tachyzoite viability.

Mouse Ocular Toxoplasmosis: Acute Disease Model

28. Female mice are preferred in studies of mouse toxoplasmosis as they are more susceptible to the infection than male mice [47].

29. The number of tachyzoites and parasite strain may be adjusted to alter the course of the intraocular inflammation. Robust inflammation occurs within 1 week after intravitreal injection of 10^4 RH strain tachyzoites.

30. Intravitreal injection of normal saline causes retinal lesions, which may be confused with toxoplasmic retinitis.

31. The pigmented eyes of C57BL/6 mice are ideal for imaging of toxoplasmic retinal lesions. The C57BL/6N substrain mice carry a mutation of the *Crb1* gene known as the *rd8* mutation, which results in a retinal degeneration, and should not be used for experimental models of ocular toxoplasmosis [48]. This mutation is not present in the C57BL/6J substrain, which therefore is suitable for this research.

32. Inhalational anesthesia with isoflurane is relatively safe and permits rapid recovery.

33. A 30 G needle is an alternative to the glass needle and plastic tubing. However, this set-up requires greater operator dexterity during the injection procedure.

34. Working with an assistant, who plunges the syringe, permits the operator to remain focused on the position of the glass pipette in the eye.

35. The mouse lens is proportionately larger than the human, and a common complication of intravitreal injection is cataract caused by pipette-lens touch, which prevents subsequent imaging by TEFI. Before undertaking the procedure, researchers may benefit from reviewing anatomical images of the mouse eye.

36. To avoid backflow of the tachyzoite suspension after intravitreal injection, which is related to a temporary increase in intraocular pressure, the cornea may be punctured with a 30 G needle immediately ahead of injection to release aqueous and reduce the pressure.

37. A plaque assay should be performed in parallel with any infection study, in order to assess tachyzoite viability.

Mouse Ocular Toxoplasmosis: Recurrent Disease Model

38. The number of cysts and parasite strain may be varied. Systemic infection is achieved reliably by approximately 2 weeks after injection of 5 PRU strain cysts.

39. Anticipate transient signs of systemic infection in C57BL/6 mice during the second week following infection, such as hunching and hair bristling.

40. The number of tachyzoites and parasite strain may be adjusted to alter the course of the intraocular inflammation. Robust inflammation occurs within 1 week after intravitreal injection of 2000 PRU strain tachyzoites.

Mouse Retinal Photography with TEFI

41. Inhalational anesthesia with isoflurane is relatively safe and permits rapid recovery.

42. The retina of an anesthetized adult mouse with normal pupil dilation and no corneal, lens or vitreous opacity may be photographed in under 3 min.

43. A clear view of the retina is essential to obtaining quality photographs of the mouse retina. View may be reduced by posterior synechiae (adhesions between iris and lens which limit pupil dilation) or vitritis associated with the retinitis and/or corneal or lens opacities induced during the imaging procedure.

44. Timing of photography can be planned around the anticipated course of the inflammation. Within the week following intravitreal injection of tachyzoites, intraocular inflammation is largely confined to the retina.

45. Corneal opacity may be caused by drying and/or by abrasion or burn from the tele-otoscope viewing tip. The use of GenTeal Tear eye gel reduces the risk of these complications. Lens opacity may be caused by light exposure, and minimizing the duration and number of examinations limits this complication.

Processing Mouse Retinal Images

46. White balance and exposure may be adjusted only for images that are in NEF file format, not images that are in JPEG or TIF file format.

Acknowledgments

This work was supported in part by the Australian Research Council (FT130101648 to JRS) and the National Health and Medical Research Council (GNT1066235 to JRS).

References

1. Dubey JP (2010) Toxoplasmosis of animals and humans, 2nd edn. CRC Press, Taylor & Francis Group, Boca Raton, FL

2. London NJ, Hovakimyan A, Cubillan LD et al (2011) Prevalence, clinical characteristics, and causes of vision loss in patients with ocular toxoplasmosis. Eur J Ophthalmol 21:811–819

3. Holland GN (2004) Ocular toxoplasmosis: a global reassessment. Part II: disease manifestations and management. Am J Ophthalmol 137:1–17

4. Lum F, Jones JL, Holland GN, Liesegang TJ (2005) Survey of ophthalmologists about

ocular toxoplasmosis. Am J Ophthalmol 140:724–726

5. Holland GN (2003) Ocular toxoplasmosis: a global reassessment. Part I: epidemiology and course of disease. Am J Ophthalmol 136:973–988

6. Vallochi AL, Muccioli C, Martins MC et al (2005) The genotype of *Toxoplasma gondii* strains causing ocular toxoplasmosis in humans in Brazil. Am J Ophthalmol 139:350–351

7. Switaj K, Master A, Borkowski PK et al (2006) Association of ocular toxoplasmosis with type I *Toxoplasma gondii* strains: direct genotyping from peripheral blood samples. J Clin Microbiol 44:4262–4264

8. Fekkar A, Ajzenberg D, Bodaghi B et al (2011) Direct genotyping of *Toxoplasma gondii* in ocular fluid samples from 20 patients with ocular toxoplasmosis: predominance of type II in France. J Clin Microbiol 49:1513–1517

9. Herrmann DC, Maksimov P, Hotop A et al (2014) Genotyping of samples from German patients with ocular, cerebral and systemic toxoplasmosis reveals a predominance of *Toxoplasma gondii* type II. Int J Med Microbiol 304:911–916

10. Barragan A, Sibley LD (2003) Migration of *Toxoplasma gondii* across biological barriers. Trends Microbiol 11:426–430

11. Runkle EA, Antonetti DA (2011) The blood-retinal barrier: structure and functional significance. Methods Mol Biol 686:133–148

12. Antonetti DA, Klein R, Gardner TW (2012) Diabetic retinopathy. N Engl J Med 366:1227–1239

13. Nicholson DH, Wolchok EB (1976) Ocular toxoplasmosis in an adult receiving long-term corticosteroid therapy. Arch Ophthalmol 94:248–254

14. Yeo JH, Jakobiec FA, Iwamoto T et al (1983) Opportunistic toxoplasmic retinochoroiditis following chemotherapy for systemic lymphoma. A light and electron microscopic study. Ophthalmology 90:885–898

15. Smith JR, Franc DT, Carter NS et al (2004) Susceptibility of retinal vascular endothelium to infection with *Toxoplasma gondii* tachyzoites. Invest Ophthalmol Vis Sci 45:1157–1161

16. Furtado JM, Bharadwaj AS, Ashander LM et al (2012) Migration of *Toxoplasma gondii*-infected dendritic cells across human retinal vascular endothelium. Invest Ophthalmol Vis Sci 53:6856–6862

17. Furtado JM, Bharadwaj AS, Chipps TJ (2012) *Toxoplasma gondii* tachyzoites cross retinal endothelium assisted by intercellular adhesion molecule-1 in vitro. Immunol Cell Biol 90:912–915

18. Masland RH (2012) The neuronal organization of the retina. Neuron 76:266–280

19. Vecino E, Rodriguez FD, Ruzafa N et al (2016) Glia-neuron interactions in the mammalian retina. Prog Retin Eye Res 51:1–40

20. Strauss O (2005) The retinal pigment epithelium in visual function. Physiol Rev 85:845–881

21. Furtado JM, Ashander LM, Mohs K et al (2013) *Toxoplasma gondii* migration within and infection of human retina. PLoS One 8:e54358

22. Frenkel JK (1955) Ocular lesions in hamsters; with chronic *Toxoplasma* and Besnoitia infection. Am J Ophthalmol 39:203–225

23. Hogan MJ (1951) Ocular toxoplasmosis. Columbia University Press, New York, NY

24. Nozik RA, O'Connor GR (1968) Experimental toxoplasmic retinochoroiditis. Arch Ophthalmol 79:485–489

25. Dukaczewska A, Tedesco R, Liesenfeld O (2015) Experimental models of ocular infection with *Toxoplasma gondii*. Eur J Microbiol Immunol (Bp) 5:293–305

26. Provis JM, Dubis AM, Maddess T, Carroll J (2013) Adaptation of the central retina for high acuity vision: cones, the fovea and the avascular zone. Prog Retin Eye Res 35:63–81

27. Culbertson WW, Tabbara KF, O'Connor R (1982) Experimental ocular toxoplasmosis in primates. Arch Ophthalmol 100:321–323

28. Rochet E, Brunet J, Sabou M et al (2015) Interleukin-6-driven inflammatory response induces retinal pathology in a model of ocular toxoplasmosis reactivation. Infect Immun 83:2109–2117

29. Lu F, Huang S, Hu MS, Kasper LH (2005) Experimental ocular toxoplasmosis in genetically susceptible and resistant mice. Infect Immun 73:5160–5165

30. Chen J, Qian H, Horai R et al (2013) Use of optical coherence tomography and electroretinography to evaluate retinal pathology in a mouse model of autoimmune uveitis. PLoS One 8:e63904

31. Wigg JP, Zhang H, Yang D (2015) A quantitative and standardized method for the evaluation of choroidal neovascularization using MICRON III fluorescein angiograms in rats. PLoS One 10:e0128418

32. Fuma S, Nishinaka A, Inoue Y et al (2017) A pharmacological approach in newly established retinal vein occlusion model. Sci Rep 7:43509

33. Paques M, Guyomard JL, Simonutti M et al (2007) Panretinal, high-resolution color photography of the mouse fundus. Invest Ophthalmol Vis Sci 48:2769–2774

34. Xu H, Koch P, Chen M et al (2008) A clinical grading system for retinal inflammation in the chronic model of experimental autoimmune uveoretinitis using digital fundus images. Exp Eye Res 87:319–326

35. Copland DA, Wertheim MS, Armitage WJ et al (2008) The clinical time-course of experimental autoimmune uveoretinitis using topical endoscopic fundal imaging with histologic and cellular infiltrate correlation. Invest Ophthalmol Vis Sci 49:5458–5465

36. Chen M, Forrester JV, Xu H (2011) Dysregulation in retinal para-inflammation and age-related retinal degeneration in CCL2 or CCR2 deficient mice. PLoS One 6:e22818

37. Furtado JM, Davies MH, Choi D et al (2012) Imaging retinal vascular changes in the mouse model of oxygen-induced retinopathy. Transl Vis Sci Technol 1:5

38. Bharadwaj AS, Appukuttan B, Wilmarth PA et al (2013) Role of the retinal vascular endothelial cell in ocular disease. Prog Retin Eye Res 32:102–180

39. Blenkinsop TA, Salero E, Stern JH, Temple S (2013) The culture and maintenance of functional retinal pigment epithelial monolayers from adult human eye. Methods Mol Biol 945:45–65

40. Fernandez-Godino R, Garland DL, Pierce EA (2016) Isolation, culture and characterization of primary mouse RPE cells. Nat Protoc 11:1206–1218

41. Sonoda S, Spee C, Barron E et al (2009) A protocol for the culture and differentiation of highly polarized human retinal pigment epithelial cells. Nat Protoc 4:662–673

42. Limb GA, Salt TE, Munro PM et al (2002) In vitro characterization of a spontaneously immortalized human Muller cell line (MIO-M1). Invest Ophthalmol Vis Sci 43:864–869

43. Gaudin C, Forster V, Sahel J et al (1996) Survival and regeneration of adult human and other mammalian photoreceptors in culture. Invest Ophthalmol Vis Sci 37:2258–2268

44. Romano C, Hicks D (2007) Adult retinal neuronal cell culture. Prog Retin Eye Res 26:379–397

45. Lu B, Malcuit C, Wang S et al (2009) Long-term safety and function of RPE from human embryonic stem cells in preclinical models of macular degeneration. Stem Cells 27:2126–2135

46. Khan A, Behnke MS, Dunay IR et al (2009) Phenotypic and gene expression changes among clonal type I strains of *Toxoplasma gondii*. Eukaryot Cell 8:1828–1836

47. Roberts CW, Cruickshank SM, Alexander J (1995) Sex-determined resistance to *Toxoplasma gondii* is associated with temporal differences in cytokine production. Infect Immun 63:2549–2555

48. Mattapallil MJ, Wawrousek EF, Chan CC et al (2012) The Rd8 mutation of the Crb1 gene is present in vendor lines of C57BL/6N mice and embryonic stem cells, and confounds ocular induced mutant phenotypes. Invest Ophthalmol Vis Sci 53:2921–2927

49. Lou DA, Hu FN (1987) Specific antigen and organelle expression of a long-term rhesus endothelial cell line. In Vitro Cell Dev Biol 23:75–85

50. Dunn KC, Aotaki-Keen AE, Putkey FR, Hjelmeland LM (1996) ARPE-19, a human retinal pigment epithelial cell line with differentiated properties. Exp Eye Res 62:155–169

51. Ahmado A, Carr AJ, Vugler AA et al (2011) Induction of differentiation by pyruvate and DMEM in the human retinal pigment epithelium cell line ARPE-19. Invest Ophthalmol Vis Sci 52:7148–7159

52. Samuel W, Jaworski C, Postnikova OA et al (2017) Appropriately differentiated ARPE-19 cells regain phenotype and gene expression profiles similar to those of native RPE cells. Mol Vis 23:60–89

53. Reid TW, Albert DM, Rabson AS et al (1974) Characteristics of an established cell line of retinoblastoma. J Natl Cancer Inst 53:347–360

54. McFall RC, Sery TW, Makadon M (1977) Characterization of a new continuous cell line derived from a human retinoblastoma. Cancer Res 37:1003–1010

Chapter 18

Using BioID for the Identification of Interacting and Proximal Proteins in Subcellular Compartments in *Toxoplasma gondii*

Peter J. Bradley, Shima Rayatpisheh, James A. Wohlschlegel, and Santhosh M. Nadipuram

Abstract

BioID is an in vivo biotinylation system developed to examine the proximal and interacting proteins of a bait protein within a subcellular compartment. This approach has been exploited in *Toxoplasma* for protein–protein interaction studies and proteomic characterizations of intracellular compartments. The BioID method requires constructing a translational fusion between a protein of interest and the promiscuous biotin ligase BirA* (a mutant of the *E. coli* protein BirA) which enables trafficking of the protein to the correct intracellular compartment and association with its partners. Proximity labelling occurs upon addition of biotin to the media and the biotinylated target proteins are then be purified using stringent conditions via streptavidin chromatography. In this chapter, we describe the methodology to fuse BirA* (or the newer variant BioID2) to a bait protein using endogenous gene tagging in *Toxoplasma* and then identify the proximal and interacting proteins using in vivo biotinylation, streptavidin purification and mass spectrometric analysis.

Key words BioID, Protein–protein interaction, Proteome, Mass spectrometry

1 Background and Introduction

Toxoplasma gondii is a remarkable parasite that contains a number of unique subcellular compartments that play critical roles in its intracellular lifestyle [1, 2]. These include the regulated secretory organelles such as the micronemes, rhoptries, and dense granules that play roles in host cell invasion and manipulation of host functions as well as the plastid-like apicoplast, the inner membrane complex (IMC) and the plant-like vacuole. Determining the complete protein composition and protein–protein interactions within these compartments is crucial to understanding their functions. Standard techniques to identify organellar protein constituents such as organelle isolation, monoclonal antibody screens, and

Christopher J. Tonkin (ed.), *Toxoplasma gondii: Methods and Protocols*, Methods in Molecular Biology, vol. 2071,
https://doi.org/10.1007/978-1-4939-9857-9_18, © Springer Science+Business Media, LLC, part of Springer Nature 2020

bioinformatic approaches have been utilized in *Toxoplasma* [3–6]. Similarly, protein–protein interaction methods such as coimmunoprecipitation, in vitro assays with recombinant proteins, and yeast two-hybrid approaches have also been employed [7–9]. However, each of these can be particularly challenging for subcellular compartments that are refractory to isolation or for the study of protein–protein interaction studies of membrane proteins, or those attached to the unique cytoskeletal meshwork of the parasite [1].

The development of proximity-dependent biotin identification (BioID) provided a simple and powerful tool that is able to circumvent problems with traditional protein-protein interaction approaches [10, 11]. The BioID method utilizes a mutant form of the biotin ligase BirA (named BirA∗) whose mutagenesis converts the enzyme from one that biotinylates a lysine residue on a specific 15 amino acid "biotin acceptor peptide" to a promiscuous enzyme that is able to biotinylate proximal and interacting proteins. Biotinylation occurs on targets within an approximate 10 nM radius of the bait protein and only requires the fusion protein targeted to the correct compartment and the addition of biotin to the media. Because BioID labels both proximal and interacting proteins, the method can be used to identify proteomes or subproteomes in the subcellular compartment of interest as well as bona fide interactors with the bait protein (Fig. 1). Examples of exploiting the BioID system for discovery of organellar protein composition in *Toxoplasma* include its use in the IMC and in the secreted contents of the parasitophorous vacuole. While these studies yielded large numbers of new proteins in their compartments (as well as likely interactors with the bait proteins), they are certainly not complete proteomes which could be further investigated with additional BioID experiments using different bait proteins or BirA∗ fused to minimal organellar targeting signals [12, 13]. The utility of BioID for identifying bona fide interactors was shown with discovery of a number of targets of the kinase TgCDPK3, which would likely have been challenging using conventional approaches [14]. Distinguishing interactors from proximal proteins was improved in a recent study of the conoid using SFINX software analysis which mathematically predicts protein–protein interactions from mass-spectrometry data [15]. Together, these studies highlight the utility of the system to understand protein composition and interaction in the unique compartments of *Toxoplasma* and related apicomplexan parasites.

A number of recent improvements to the BioID approach suggest that the system will become even more important in the future. The first advance was the development of BioID2, which exploited a smaller biotin ligase from *Aquifex aeolicus* which lacks the DNA binding domain present in *E. coli* BirA [16]. BioID2 showed more selective biotinylation of target proteins and required less biotin supplementation for efficient labelling. In the same report, the biotinylation range of BioID2 was enhanced by the

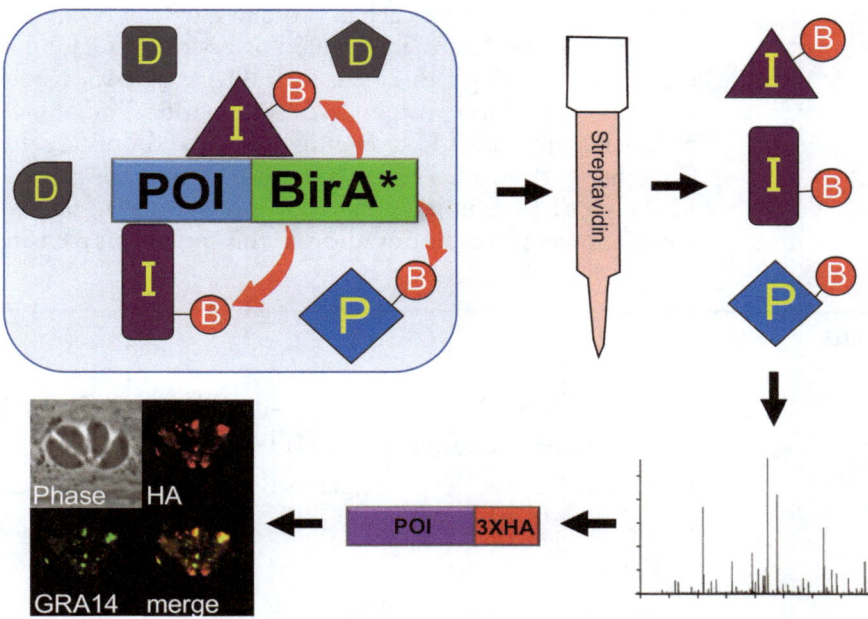

Fig. 1 Standard workflow of BioID experiments in *Toxoplasma gondii*. A protein of interest (POI) is fused with the promiscuous biotin ligase BirA∗. In the presence of biotin added to the media, BirA∗ biotinylates interacting proteins and proximal proteins (labeled "I" and "P") in its subcellular compartment while more distal proteins (labeled D) are not biotinylated. After 24 h of incubation, the parasites (and host cells) are lysed under stringent conditions and proteins are purified by streptavidin chromatography. The purified fraction is analyzed directly on the beads by tryptic digestion and mass spectrometry. Candidate proteins are curated from the analysis and verified by C-terminal endogenous epitope tagging and immunofluorescence (example: GRA33 [HA/red] with GRA14 comarker [green])

addition of a 25-nm flexible linker consisting of 13 repeats of the sequence GGGGS. An intriguing twist on the BioID approach was provided by the development of Split-BioID in which two inactive portions of the enzyme are fused to two bait proteins in a protein complex [17, 18]. Biotinylation occurs once the portions are brought in close enough proximity to assemble into an active enzyme. This approach can thus be used to probe different sub-complexes of enzymes and expose the protein–protein interactions of each subcomplex. The most recent development is TurboID, which used directed evolution to produce a BirA that can label target proteins in as little as 10 min [19]. This resolves one of the main criticisms of the standard BioID approaches which require 18–24 h on labelling time and thus cannot be used for dynamic processes that occur in short time periods. There is yet another method of in vivo protein biotinylation using an ascorbate peroxidase named APEX2 which uses an alternative reagent (biotin-phenol) for biotinylation of interacting and proximal proteins. This system has the advantage of a short labeling time which may provide results most similar to TurboID, although direct comparisons with identical bait proteins have not been reported. In this chapter, we describe a detailed protocol for tagging a gene of interest at its endogenous locus with BirA∗, assessing biotinylation activity of the fusion protein, large scale purification of biotinylated products, and mass spectrometric identification of target proteins. Together with another recently published methods paper of BioID in *T. gondii*, we hope to provide users with a simple detailed approach to in vivo biotinylation in this important parasite [20].

2   Materials

- *T. gondii*: RHΔ*ku80*Δ*hxgprt* strain, PRUΔ*ku80*Δ*hxgprt* strain.
- Human foreskin fibroblasts (HFFs).
- T4 DNA Ligase (New England Biolabs™ Cat#M0202S).
- T4 DNA polymerase (New England Biolabs™ Cat#M0203S).
- Pfu DNA polymerase.
- Restriction endonucleases: BsaI-HF, PvuI-HF, and PacI (New England Biolabs™).
- LB broth.
- Ampicillin.
- Plasmid Miniprep kit.
- Plasmid Gel isolation kit.
- Plasmid Midiprep kit.
- Trypsin 0.05% EDTA for tissue culture.
- Pyrimethamine (powder).
- Formaldehyde 37%.
- Bovine serum albumin, Fraction V.
- Mouse monoclonal anti-HA.11 antibody (suggested dilution 1:2000).
- Mouse anti-FLAG antibody (suggested dilution 1:2000).
- Goat anti-mouse IgG (H + L) Secondary Antibody Conjugated with Alexa Fluor™ 594 (ThermoFisher™ Cat#A32723, suggested dilution 1:2000).
- Streptavidin Alexa Fluor™ 488 conjugate (ThermoFisher™ Cat#S11227, (suggested dilution 1:2000).
- Streptavidin HRP conjugate.
- 20% DMSO
- Streptavidin high-capacity agarose (Pierce™) (ThermoFisher™ Cat#20359).

- D-biotin (Sigma-Aldrich™ Cat#47868).
- Tris.
- Sodium chloride.
- Triton X-100.
- NP-40.
- Sodium deoxycholate (DOC).
- Sodium dodecyl sulfate (SDS).
- Calcium chloride ($CaCl_2$).
- Potassium phosphate dibasic (K_2HPO_4).
- Potassium phosphate monobasic (KH_2PO_4).
- Phosphate buffered saline (PBS).
- Protease inhibitor tablets (Pierce™) (ThermoFisher™ Cat#88265).
- Tris(2-carboxymethyl)-phosphine-hydrochloride (TCEP-HCl) (Pierce™, Cat# 20490).
- Iodoacetamide (Sigma™, Cat# I1149-25G).
- Lysine-C sequencing grade (Lys-C) (Princeton Separations™ Cat # EN-130).
- Trypsin Protease (Pierce™) (ThermoFisher™, Cat#90057).
- Formic Acid, LC MS grade (Pierce™,) (ThermoFisher™, Cat#85178).
- Acetonitrile, LC MS grade (Pierce TM) (ThermoFisher™, Cat#TS51101).
- *Plasmids available at* https://www.addgene.org/ *or the Peter Bradley lab, UCLA.*
- pU6-Universal (Addgene Plasmid #52694) [21].
- p.LIC.3xHA.BirA∗.DHFR.
- p.LIC.3xHA.BioID2.DHFR.
- u6 Sequencing primer for sgRNA ligation verification (GTGCGCTCTTCGAAGGGGCTTT).

2.1 Recipes

Cytomix

- KPO_4 Buffer: 43.4 mL 1 M K_2HPO_4 + 6.7 mL 1 M KH_2PO_4 + Water to 500 mL.
- 10 mM KPO_4 Buffer.
- 120 mM KCl.
- 5 mM $MgCl_2$.
- 25 mM HEPES.
- 2 mM EDTA.

7.5 mM $CaCl_2$ stock solution for use with cytomix ($50\times$)

- Dissolve $CaCl_2$ in water.

10 mM Pyrimethamine stock solution ($10,000\times$)

- Dissolve pyrimethamine in 100% ethanol.

D-Biotin Stock (50 mM)

- Dissolve in water, pH to 7.5 with 1 N NaOH.

Lysis buffer #1 (noncytoskeletal prep, RIPA)

- 150 mM NaCl.
- 50 mM Tris pH 7.5.
- 1% NP-40 (or NP-40 substitute).
- 0.5% DOC.
- 0.1% SDS.

Lysis buffer #2 (cytoskeletal prep, TX-100)

- 150 mM NaCl.
- 50 mM Tris pH 7.5.
- 1% Triton-X 100.
- 1% SDS lysis buffer
- 150 mM NaCl.
- 50 mM Tris pH 7.5.
- 1% SDS 100.

8 M urea buffer (make fresh on the day of experiment)

100 mM Tris–HCl (pH 8.0).

8 M urea.

Adjust pH to 8.0.

100 mM Tris (pH 8.5)

Dissolve in water and pH to 8.5.

100 mM $CaCl_2$

Dissolve in water.

Lys-C stock for digestion of protein off streptavidin agarose resin Dissolve to 0.1 mg/mL in water.

Trypsin stock for digestion of protein off streptavidin agarose resin Dissolve to 0.4 mg/mL in water.

Acetonitrile

Dissolve in water to 50%.

2.2 Equipment	• Syringes 3 cc, 10 cc, and 20 cc.
	• 27 G blunt needle.
	• 0.2 cm electroporation cuvettes.
	• 24- and 96-well tissue culture plates.
	• 25cm² cell culture flasks.

2.2 Equipment

- Syringes 3 cc, 10 cc, and 20 cc.
- 27 G blunt needle.
- 0.2 cm electroporation cuvettes.
- 24- and 96-well tissue culture plates.
- $25cm^2$ cell culture flasks.
- 150 mm diameter cell culture treated dishes.
- Glass coverslips: No. 1.5, 13 mm diameter.
- Hemacytometer and weighted coverslip.
- Cryogenic vials.
- 15 mL conical centrifuge tubes
- 1.5 mL microcentrifuge tubes
- Centrifuge tube filters for 1.5 mL microcentrifuge— 0.22 μm pore.
- C18 pipette tips (100 μL).
- Heat block.
- Centrifuge.
- Microcentrifuge.
- Upright microscope.
- Inverted microscope.
- Thermocycler.
- SDS-PAGE apparatus.
- Western blot transfer apparatus.
- Gel imager.
- Electroporator: Bio-Rad Gene Pulser II (Bio-Rad™ catalog# 165–2109).
- Incubator for tissue culture (5% CO_2, 37 °C).
- Rotary (orbital) shaker.
- UltiMate 3000 HPLC (ThermoFisher).
- Orbitrap Fusion Lumos Tribrid mass spectrometer (ThermoFisher).

2.3 Software

- Plasmid editor (ApE, gene strider, snapgene, etc.).
- Internet browser (Chrome, Firefox, or Edge).
- Xcalibur™ (ThermoFisher™).

3 Methods (Before Beginning—*See* Notes 1 and 2)

(A) Design and generation of LIC plasmid with C-terminal gene fragment for endogenous gene tagging using ligase independent cloning (**Option #1**)—For CRISPR/Cas9 tagging, skip to option #2 (**step B**).

(a) Plasmid preparation:

  i. Linearize the LIC.3xHA.BirA* or LIC.3xHA.BioID2 plasmid using 20 µg of plasmid and *PacI* restriction endonuclease. We recommend digesting overnight (12–18 h) at 37 °C for complete digestion.

  ii. Isolate linearized plasmid by gel purification and measure concentration by spectrometry.

  iii. T4 preparation: this step is to create single-stranded ends for ligase independent cloning. **SPECIAL NOTE: dGTP should be used for the plasmid.**

Ingredient	Volume/amount
Plasmid (DNA)	1200–1800 ng (adjust volume)
NEB buffer 2.1 (10×)	6 µL
100 mM **dGTP**	2.4 µL
T4 DNA polymerase	1.5 µL
Water	Add to 60 µL total volume

Mix reaction on ice.

Incubate reaction using thermocycler: 30 min at 22 °C then 20 min at 75 °C (to heat-inactivate T4 enzyme).

  iv. Store at −20 °C until needed.

(b) C-terminal fragment generation and preparation.

  i. In http://toxodb.org/toxo/, search for your gene of interest by gene number in the "gene ID" box (top left-hand corner). Alternatively, you can search by gene text or by using the sequence retrieval tool.

  ii. In the gene page, copy the genomic sequence into a plasmid editing software tool.

  iii. To design the primers for amplification of the C-terminal fragment (using plasmid editing software):

   1. Choose a reverse primer 18–21 bp in length which terminates just upstream of the stop codon (DO NOT include the stop codon). The reverse

complement of this sequence should be attached 3′ end of the AS LIC sequence: 5′-tcctccacttccaattttagc [*insert reverse primer*]-3′.

2. To choose a forward primer:

   (a) Choose an 18–21 bp sequence 1000–2000 bp upstream from the stop codon. Examine the fragment generated by these primers: there should be There should at least one restriction endonuclease site which is >300 bp upstream of the stop codon; this site should NOT be present in the BirA∗ (or BioID2) plasmid—this will be used to linearize the entire finished plasmid prior to transfection into parasites.

   (b) The forward primer should be attached 3′ end of the sequence:

   5′-tacttccaatccaattta[*insert fwd primer*]-3′

iv. Amplify C-terminal fragment using *Toxoplasma gondii* genomic DNA as template. Note: be sure this genomic template is the same as your choice of strain from the gene page (and the strain into which you will transfect) (*see* **Note 3**).

v. Isolate PCR fragment and purify using gel electrophoresis and gel purification and measure concentration by spectrometry.

   1. Calculate picomolar concentration using a standard conversion formula, or by using this calculator: https://www.promega.com/a/apps/biomath/

vi. T4 polymerase processing: this step is to create single-stranded ends for ligase independent cloning. **SPECIAL NOTE: dCTP should be used for the insert (fragment).**

Ingredient	Volume/amount
Fragment (DNA)	~0.2 pMol
NEB buffer 2.1 (10×)	2 μL
100 mM **dCTP**	0.8 μL
T4 DNA polymerase	0.5 μL
Water	To 20 μL

Mix reaction on ice.

Incubate reaction using thermocycler: 30 min at 22 °C then 20 min at 75 °C (to heat-inactivate T4 enzyme)

vii. Store at $-20\ ^\circ$C until needed.

(c) Ligase-independent cloning, and verification of final construct.

   i. Mix the T4 prepared plasmid and c-terminal fragment in the following proportion:

Ingredient	Volume
C-terminal fragment	3 μL
Plasmid (BirA∗ or BioID2)	1 μL
Water	6 μL

   Mix with a pipette and incubate for 10 min at room temperature (benchtop)

   ii. Transform and plate on LB/ampicillin agar plates. Incubate overnight.

   iii. Chose four colonies after growth, place in 5 mL LB/ampicillin cultures for growth overnight.

   iv. Miniprep DNA from bacteria and examine by diagnostic restriction endonuclease digest.

      1. Choose one enzyme which is present in the original LIC plasmid, the second should be the enzyme which you will use to linearize the final construct: Examine for the presence of a dropout of the correct size.

      2. Alternatively, the correct construct can be verified by sequencing.

   v. Choose a construct which contains the c-terminal fragment; amplify the bacteria colony containing this construct and midi-prep to obtain 50–100 μg of plasmid DNA.

   vi. Linearize 50–100 μg of plasmid using the previously chosen restriction nuclease. Purify by phenol/chloroform extraction and store in freezer until transfection.

(B) CRISPR/Cas9 approach: Design of sgRNA scaffold to target a gene for C-terminal endogenous gene tagging with 3×HA-BirA∗ and generation of Cas9/sgRNA plasmid (**Option #2**).

   (a) sgRNA selection,

      i. In http://toxodb.org/toxo/, search for your gene of interest using the "Sequence Retrieval" tool. Download the genomic sequence from the start codon to 1500 bp downstream of the stop codon.

ii. Copy the portion of the gene sequence that comprises the first 1500 bp following the stop codon (3′ UTR) and paste into the Eukaryotic Pathogen CRISPR guide RNA/DNA Design Tool (EuPaGDT) at http://grna.ctegd.uga.edu/. Enter a job name, select the *T. gondii* lineage database, and keep all other default settings.

iii. From the generated list of sgRNA sequences, select a 20 nucleotide sgRNA sequence that has a 3′ NGG protospacer adjacent motif (PAM) motif. The sgRNA sequence can be either on the forward or reverse DNA strand. **Criteria for selection: the higher the efficiency score, the better. We recommend using an sgRNA site which is approximately 50–200 bp downstream of the stop codon**.

(b) Generation of Cas9/U6/sgRNA plasmid for C-terminal endogenous tagging.

i. Order DNA oligos for insertion into the Cas9/U6 plasmid: The "Forward" sequence must be the same as the sgRNA generated from EuPaGDT. Copy this sequence into the ∗∗∗ of CRISPR_F oligonucleotide sequence (AAGTT∗∗∗G). Copy the reverse-complement of the sgRNA sequence into the ∗∗∗ of CRISPR_R oligonucleotide sequence (AAAAC∗∗∗A).

ii. If the U6 plasmid is not already linearized and prepared:

1. Digest u6 plasmid using BsaI-HF restriction endonuclease (*see* **Note 4**).

2. Gel purify linearized plasmid.

3. Dilute U6 plasmid to 100 ng/μL.

iii. Construct gRNA template double-stranded DNA template with BsaI overhangs.

1. After obtaining gRNA template DNA oligonucleotides, normalize each to 100 μM.

2. Dilute in a 1.5 mL tube with water to a 25 μM concentration of the single stranded oligos:

Water: 16 μL

25 μM CRISPR_F: 2 μL.

25 μM CRISPR_R: 2 μL.

Boil this mixture (100 °C) for 10 min, remove from heat and allow to cool to 23 °C.

iv. Ligate gRNA double-stranded DNA template into U6 plasmid with the following mix:

U6 plasmid (100 ng/µL)	0.5 µL
gRNA double-stranded DNA	3 µL
10× NEB ligase buffer	1 µL
NEB ligase (4,000,000 units/mL)	0.5 µL
Water	5 µL
Total	**10 µL**

v. Ligate for 1–3 h (or overnight) at room temperature (23 °C).

vi. Transform 5 µL into DH5α E. *coli* bacteria and plate onto LB/Ampicillin agar plates.

vii. Interrogate U6-universal/gRNA construct.

   1. Select four bacterial colonies to grow in 5 mL LB/Ampicillin [2–4] overnight.

   2. Next day—miniprep 5 mL cultures to obtain plasmid DNA.

   3. Examine plasmids by restriction endonuclease digest using enzymes: BsaI-HF+ PvuI-HF and examination of digest products on agarose gel (*see* **Note 5**).

      • If construct is correct, it should linearize with NO DROPOUT (7791 bp).

      • If construct is incorrect (no gRNA) the construct should be cut into two pieces (1170 bp + 6601 bp).

      • verify proper plasmid construction using sequencing. Sequencing primer is "u6 sequencing primer" in the ingredients section.

      • Choose a correct plasmid from the selected minipreps, and grow a large scale culture with the source bacterial colony (50 mL)—miniprep this large culture and concentrate to make a 50–100 µg aliquot of 25–50 µL (1–2 µg DNA per µL) (verify by spectrometry). Store at −20 °C until ready for transfection into *T. gondii*.

(c) Homology directed repair flanks for endogenous gene tagging with BirA∗.

   i. Construct the forward primer by selecting 40 bp of the gene sequence JUST UPSTREAM of the stop codon of your gene of interest (do not include the stop codon) and adding this to the 5′ end of the universal flanks tag/drug forward primer: ([fwd primer 40 bp]–GGAAGTGGAGGACGGGAATTC).

ii. Construct the reverse primer by selecting 38 bp within the 3′ UTR of your gene of interest anywhere DOWNSTREAM (3′) of the sgRNA sequence used above—add the REVERSE COMPLEMENT of this 38 bp sequence to the 5′ end of the universal flanks tag/drug reverse primer ([rev primer 38 bp]–CG ACGGCCAGTGAATTGTAATA) (we recommend normalizing primers to 100 μM concentrations).

iii. Amplify the homology directed repair flanks using as a template p.LIC.3xHA.BirA∗.DHFR or p.LIC.3xH A.BioID2.DHFR plasmid using PCR (400 μL total). Begin by mixing primers (16 μL Water+2 μL FWD + 2 μL REV).

Component	100 μL mix	400 μL mix
Template DNA (30 ng/μL)	2 μL	8 μL
Pfu 10× polymerase buffer	10 μL	40 μL
FWD/REV primer mix	4 μL	16 μL
dNTPs (10 mM)	4 μL	16 μL
Pfu polymerase	4 μL	16 μL
Water	76 μL	304 μL

iv. For two transfections (30–60 μg DNA), mix 400 μL of the above reaction, divide into 100 μL aliquots (using four [4] 200 μL PCR tubes) and place into thermocycler.

v. Amplify in thermocycler. Recommended annealing temperature: 58 °C, recommended elongation time: 5:30 per cycle, 30 cycles total. **Tip: hot start reaction**.

vi. Verify the PCR product by gel electrophoresis.

vii. Clean and concentrate the PCR product using phenol/chloroform and ethanol precipitation—resuspend the final product in 40 μL (for single transfection) or 80 μL (to divide into two transfections). Usually, this reaction provides between 30 and 60 μg total of DNA after cleaning and concentrating.

(C) Generation of BirA∗-tagged parasite lines.

(a) Prepare RHΔ*hpt*Δ*ku80* or PRUΔ*ku80*Δ*hxgprt* parasites as per transfection protocol in Cytomix transfection media.

i. Dilute 50× $CaCl_2$ to 1× in Cytomix (e.g., 0.1 mL $CaCl_2$ + 4.9 mL Cytomix).

ii. Scrape parasites which are ~80% lysed (usually 24–48 h after passage) from a T25 and lyse remaining host cells by passaging media and cells through a 3 mL syringe and 27 G needle.

iii. Transfer to a 15 mL conical and centrifuge parasites (2400 × g for 5 min). Aspirate media from pellet and wash ×1 using Cytomix. Centrifuge once again (2400 × g for 5 min), aspirate wash, and resuspend parasites in 1.6 mL of cytomix. This will suffice for four separate transfections (0.4 mL each).

(b) Transfect DNA by electroporation using:

i. 50 μg of linearized LIC plasmid (option #1) OR.

ii. 50μgrams of U6/sgRNA plasmid + All or half of HDR flanks/tag/drug linear DNA (option #2).

iii. 400 μL (0.4 mL) of parasites resuspended in cytomix.

iv. Mix in 0.2 cm electroporation cuvette and electroporate using the following parameters in Bio-Rad Gene Pulser II:

Voltage: 1.5 kV.

Capacitance: 25 μFaraday.

Pulse x1—time constant should result between 0.16 and 0.2 ms^{-1}.

(c) If desired, remove 40–80 μL of transfected parasites from electroporation cuvette to infect HFFs on a coverslip.

i. These parasites can be examined by immunofluorescence with anti-FLAG antibodies in 24–48 h after infection to examine for efficiency of uptake of U6 vector—the signal should be present in the nuclei of the parasites.

(d) Place remaining parasites from cuvette into a T25 flask with a confluent HFF monolayer.

(e) 18–24 h after transfection, replace media with cDMEM with 1 μM pyrimethamine for selection. Passage these parasites in T25 flask HFF monolayers for 7–10 days (2–3 passages).

(f) After 2–3 passages, verify gene tagging and proper localization of the POI-BirA∗ (or –BioID2) fusion by immunofluorescence assay. Probe using anti-HA.11 antibody (against the 3×HA epitope tag) for localization.

i. Pipette 20–30 μL of lysed parasites into [2] 24-well plate wells containing coverslips with HFF monolayers.

    ii. Incubate for 24 h.

    iii. Wash the coverslips x1 with PBS, and fix in 3.7% formaldehyde (diluted from 37% stock in PBS) for 15 min.

    iv. Block and permeabilize coverslips in blocking buffer (PBS/3%BSA/0.2%Tx-100) for 30 min.

    v. Primary antibody: incubate with mouse anti-HA.11 antibody.

    vi. Secondary antibody: Alexa Fluor goat-anti-mouse antibody 594 (red).

    vii. Visualize, examining for proper predicted localization of your protein of interest (looking for HA signal).

(g) After 2–3 passages, clone parasite by serial dilution using a 96-well plate and obtain a single clone. (this can be performed before or after verification of the BirA∗-POI fusion and biotinylation activity (below).

(D) Verification of in vivo biotinylation activity and localization of BirA∗-POI (protein of interest) fusion.

  (a) Immunofluorescence.

    i. After BirA∗ tagged parasites have been passaged for at least 2–3 passages, place 20–30 µL of lysed parasites into two (2) 24-well plate wells containing coverslips with HFF monolayers.

      1. For one coverslip/well, add D-Biotin to 150 µM (3 µL of 50 mM D-biotin stock per 1 mL cDMEM).

      2. For the other (control), do not add biotin.

    ii. Incubate for 24 h.

    iii. Wash the coverslips ×1 with PBS, and fix in 3.5% formaldehyde/PBS for 15 min.

    iv. Block and permeabilize coverslips in blocking buffer (PBS/3%BSA/0.2%Tx-100) for 30 min.

    v. Primary antibody: incubate with mouse anti-HA.11 antibody.

    vi. Secondary antibodies: goat-anti-mouse antibody 594 (red) and streptavidin 488 (green).

    vii. Visualize, examining for proper predicted localization of your protein of interest (looking for HA signal) and biotinylation of the predicted organellar space (streptavidin) (i.e., IMC, vacuole, etc.). Ideally these two signals should colocalize (Fig. 2a).

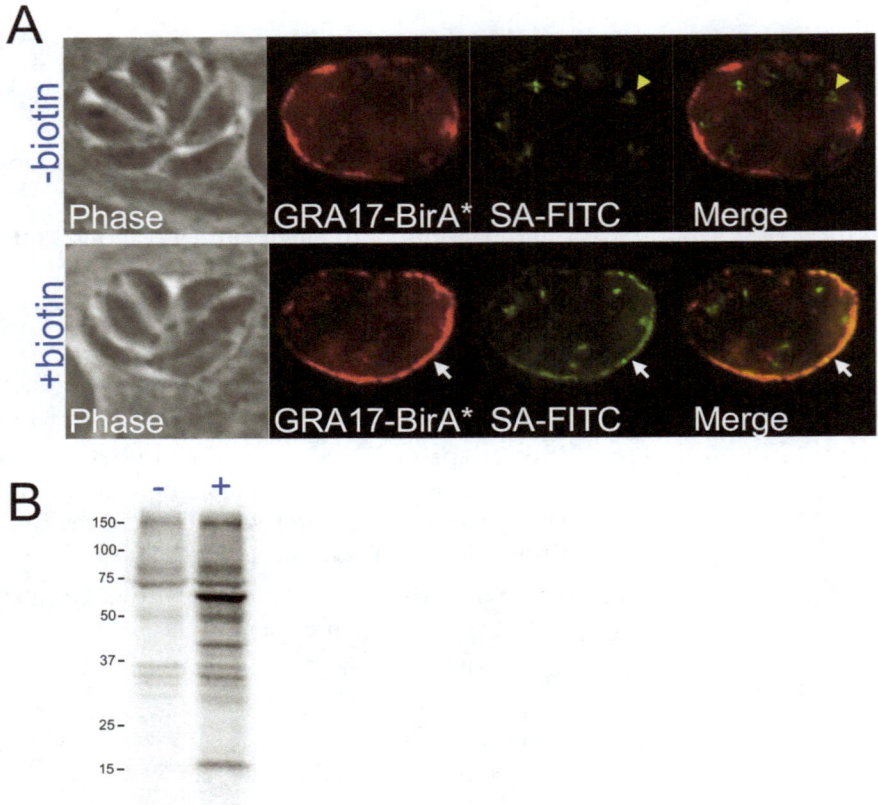

Fig. 2 Verification of the activity of BioID. GRA17-BirA∗ secreted into the vacuole is used as an example. (**a**) Immunofluorescence assay demonstrating that GRA17-BirA∗ localizes appropriately to the parasitophorous vacuole by HA staining (red). In the absence of excess biotin (top panel) streptavidin only labels the endogenously biotinylated proteins in the apicoplasts (arrowheads). However, when excess biotin is added for 24 h (bottom panel), BirA∗ is shown to be active in the parasitophorous vacuole with a bright signal along the parasitophorous vacuole membrane by streptavidin-FITC staining (arrow). (**b**) Western blot using streptavidin-HRP probe demonstrating newly biotinylated proteins in *Toxoplasma gondii* whole-cell lysates when excess biotin was incubated for 24 h

(b) Western Blot.

i. Passage BirA∗-tagged parasites into two separate T25 flasks with HFF monolayers.

- For one T25, add D-biotin to 150 μM (3 μL of 50 mM D-biotin stock per 1 mL cDMEM).
- For the other T25 (control) do not add biotin.

ii. Scrape HFF/parasites in T25 flask.

iii. For extracellular parasites—liberate parasites from HFF by serial passaging through a syringe with 27-gauge needle.

iv. Centrifuge cells/parasites at $3000 \times g$ for 10 min to pellet cells. Wash and centrifuge $\times 2$ with ice cold PBS.

v. Remove PBS and lyse in Sample Buffer for 10 min.

vi. Examine by SDS-PAGE and Western Blot by blotting with Streptavidin-HRP. **Tip: Use 5% Bovine Serum Albumin (BSA) rather than milk for blocking and blotting as milk often contains free biotin**.

1. Separately, the presence of the POI-BirA∗ fusion can be examined and verified by blotting with mouse anti-HA antibody, and goat-anti-mouse-HRP antibody (the fusion should be approximately 40 kDa larger than the POI alone).

2. The streptavidin signal for the parasite line supplemented with D-biotin should reveal multiple protein bands in addition to the endogenously biotinylated proteins present in the control lysate (Fig. 2b) (*see* **Note 6**).

(E) Large-scale BioID experiment (biotinylation of proteins and purification) (*see* **Note 7**).

(a) Definitions:

i. *Experimental line:* the BirA∗- or BioID2-fusion-transgenic parasites.

ii. *Control line:* parental parasites (RH∆*ku80*∆*hxgprt* or PRU∆*ku80*∆*hxgprt* parasites) lacking BirA∗ or BioID2.

(b) Prepare by splitting HFFs onto 150 mm tissue culture dishes and growing these to full confluence 5–7 days prior to beginning your experiment.

i. Change cDMEM on dishes 1 day prior to beginning the experiment.

(c) Using BirA∗-POI fusion line parasites, Infect HFFs in 150 mm tissue culture dishes (approximately 10^7 parasites per plate—for a multiplicity of infection of 5–10). We recommend 3–5 plates per experiment.

i. In parallel, infect the same number of plates with control parasites in the same dose. (**All steps from this point on will refer simultaneously to the control and experimental parasites lines**).

(d) Add D-biotin to each plate to 150 µM (3 µL of 50 mM D-biotin per 1 mL cDMEM).

(e) Incubate for 24–48 h.

i. For intracellular parasites, stop incubation prior to lysis (usually 24–36 h).

ii. For extracellular parasites, allow parasites to lyse completely (usually 36–48 h).

(f) Scrape plates to lift HFFs and adherent parasites using manual cell scraper. And transfer to three [3] 50 mL conical centrifuge tubes (divide volume evenly) **per experimental line**.

i. Optional for extracellular parasites: pass through 27 G needle and syringe in order to lyse host cells. (*see* **Note 8**).

(g) Centrifuge parasites/cells ($2400 \times g$ for 10 min), aspirate media, and wash/centrifuge $\times 3$ in ice-cold PBS (to reduce volume for washes, transfer parasites/cells to a 15 mL conical flask)—**After this point, keep parasites and cells on ice**.

(h) Lysis (Note: as soon as lysis buffer is added, add protease inhibitor):

i. For noncytoskeletal prep: Aspirate remaining PBS from final wash and add 15 mL lysis buffer #1. Lyse for 30 min on ice, occasionally agitating lysate with 10 mL serological pipette. Centrifuge to remove insoluble material (this will pellet). Transfer lysate to beads and proceed to binding on streptavidin beads (**step f**, iii).

ii. For cytoskeletal prep (to isolate IMC network and microtubules): Aspirate remaining PBS from final wash and add 15 mL lysis buffer #2. Lyse for 30 min, occasionally agitating lysate with 10 mL serological pipette. Centrifuge at $15,000 \times g$ for 20 min to pellet—**Retain the pellet**.

The cytoskeletal components are insoluble in TX-100—remove supernatant (store separately or discard. If it is desired, lysis supernatant can also be purified with streptavidin beads). To lyse the pellet, add 5 mL of 1% SDS buffer and lyse for 30 min—Agitate by pipetting up and down vigorously with a 5 mL serological pipette. Once the pellet is fully lysed, dilute solution in lysis buffer #2–0.1% SDS and proceed to binding.

iii. Binding. Note: prior to binding, wash and centrifuge beads $\times 3$ in the appropriate lysis buffer (#1 or #2). **100 µL bed volume per lysate is recommended**. Centrifugation should be done at $500 \times g$ for 1 min. Add 100 µL bed volume streptavidin agarose. Add the appropriate lysis buffer to fill the conical tube so that there is minimal "dry" area during binding. (use multiple tubes if volume is too great for single 15 mL conical tube). **Tip: Making sure there is minimal "dry" area stops beads from sticking to the sidewalls of the conical tube and thus being lost during binding.**

Move lysate and beads to 4 °C and rock overnight (12–18 h). (*see* **Note 9**).

iv. Centrifuge beads (500 x g for 5 min) to pellet, discard flowthrough.

v. Transfer beads in wash (buffer #1 or #2) to 1.5 mL microcentrifuge tube and wash five times in Buffer #1 for 10 min each (centrifuge between washes at 500 × g for 2 min).

vi. Wash three more times in 8 M urea buffer (see recipe).

vii. Transfer 10% of the beads from the last wash step to another 1.7 mL microfuge tube. The beads can be resuspended in sample buffer and examined by SDS-PAGE and Western Blot with Streptavidin-HRP.

viii. The remaining 90% of beads are to be submitted in 8 M Urea-100 mM Tris–HCL pH: 8.5 (Teknova) for mass-spectrometric analysis.

(F) Mass-spectrometry and analysis of biotinylated proteins (*see* **Note 10**).

(a) Digestion of proteins (On beads).

i. Add 200 mM TCEP-HCl to beads/Urea to attain a final concentration of 5 mM and shake the samples at room temperature on rotary shaker for 20 min at 1300 rpm.

ii. Add 500 mM iodoacetamide to attain to final concentration of 10 mM (always prepare fresh by suspending 0.046 g/500 μL H_2O) and shake in a dark room for 20 min at room temperature at 1300 rpm.

iii. Resuspend Lys-c in HPLC water to attain final concentration of 0.1 mg/mL.

Add Lys-C 1:100 enzyme to substrate ratio and shake in a dark room for 4 h at 37 °C at 1300 rpm.

iv. Dilute the mixture in 100 mM Tris (pH 8.5) by a factor of 4.

v. Add 100 mM $CaCl_2$ to reach to final concentration of 1 mM.

vi. Resuspend trypsin to attain final concentration of 0.4 mg/mL and add trypsin at 1:20–1:100 enzyme to substrate ratio then shake in dark room at 37 °C at 1300 rpm overnight (12–18 h).

vii. Add Formic Acid to the above solution to final concentration of 5% and shake in dark room for 5 min at room temperature at 1300 rpm.

viii. Centrifuge the samples in a microcentrifuge maximum speed (16,800 × g) at room temperature for 10 min.

ix. While the sample is centrifuging, separately wash a 0.22 μm microcentrifuge tube filter with 100 mM Tris–HCL pH:8.5 ×2 (add wash and centrifuge).

x. Transfer the supernatant from the digested sample to the filter tube. (take care not to aspirate any beads; if necessary, centrifuge again).

xi. Centrifuge for 2 min at 3000 × g.

(b) Desalting.

i. Set the pipette to 100 and secure the C18 pipette tip tightly to the end of the pipettor for optimum tip to pipettor seal and sample aspiration.

ii. Wet tip by aspirating 100 μL of 50% Acetonitrile and then discarding the solvent. Repeat ×1.

iii. Equilibrate tip by aspirating 100 μL of 5% formic acid and discard the solvent. Repeat ×1.

iv. Aspirate up to 100 μL of the sample (Adjusted to 5.0% formic acid) into the C18 tip. For maximum efficiency, dispense and aspirate sample for 20 cycles.

v. Rinse the tip by aspirating 100 μL 5% Formic Acid and discard the solvent. Repeat ×1.

vi. Elute the sample in 80 μL of 40% acetonitrile/5% formic acid. For maximum efficiency, dispense and aspirate sample for 20 cycles.

vii. Dry using speed vac.

viii. Resuspend in 10–20 μL of 5% formic acid before loading to auto sampler for Mass spectrometry analysis.

(c) Running and analysis.

i. Pack silica capillary column with C18 resin (with internal diameter of 75 micron and length of 25 cm) and run samples through the Ultimate 3000 HPLC system controlled by the Xcalibur instrument control software to be analyzed on a Orbitrap Fusion Lumos Tribrid Mass spectrometer.

ii. Elute peptides from the microcapillary column using an increasing linear gradient of acetonitrile at 300 nl/ min which are then electrosprayed directly into the mass spectrometer by applying a 2.2 kV spray voltage.

iii. The data-dependent spectral acquisition (DDA) which is composed of a repeating cycle of one full MS spectrum (m/z range = 400–1600, Resolution = 120,000) acquired using the Orbitrap mass analyzer followed by MS/MS analysis of the most abundant precursor ions from the full MS scan at 35% collision energy and 15,000 resolution.

iv. Spectra are collected using the Xcalibur data system and stored in the RAW binary file format. They are subsequently converted to the MS2 text-based format for further analysis.

v. Integrated proteomics pipeline 2 (IP2) is used to search the MS2 files against a database that contains all *Toxoplasma* protein sequences obtained from Tox-oDB. Search results are then filtered using user-defined false positive rates which are typically set to 1% at the spectral level.

vi. To isolate candidate proteins of interest for the BioID experiment, use subtractive analysis to compare the experimental parasite line proteins to the control (parental) line.

Candidate proteins can be chosen from this analysis. We recommend beginning with localization by C-terminal endogenous epitope tagging and immunofluorescence assay. In addition, one can also examine protein-protein interaction by traditional protein immunoprecipitation, "reverse" immunoprecipitation (pulling down a candidate protein, and examining for the original bait), or predicting protein-protein interactions using mathematical modeling (SFINX, or other software).

4   Notes

1. Presumably before beginning, you will have chosen a target "bait" protein to fuse with BirA* or BioID2. We found with experience that it sometimes requires a few trials of different target proteins for a particular sub-cellular organelle before finding a protein that is ideal for your purposes. Some proteins may not localize properly after fusion with BioID proteins.

Alternatively, biotinylation may not work in a given compartment. This is most likely due to misfolding and inactivation of BirA* upon fusion, disruption of biotin ligation due to the internal environment of the organelle, or poor permeability to biotin of the organellar space where the fusion traffics. We suggest having several candidate proteins of interest (POIs) selected before beginning this process. As this is a C-terminal fusion with BirA* (or BioID2) please make certain that there are no elements on the C-terminus of your POI that are essential for protein localization or trafficking before beginning this procedure.

2. We have presented two options in this protocol for using BioID. Other possibilities include: Creating a second-copy protein fused to BirA*, N-terminal fusion, or fusing BirA* variants to a protein trafficking element such as a signal peptide.

3. When designing the primers, use a calculation program such as oligocalc   (http://biotools.nubic.northwestern.edu/Oligo-Calc.html) to match the annealing/melting temperatures of the primer sequences with one another (without the extra portions for LIC processing; only the portion of the primer identical to the genomic sequence). We have found that if the GC content is approximately 30–70% and the predicted annealing temperatures of the primers (again, without the LIC portions) are approximately 62 °C, the C-terminal fragment of the gene will amplify consistently. The reverse primer is more or less "set" as the sequence should begin just upstream of the STOP codon. However, if you find that you are unable to amplify this sequence even after trying multiple different forward primers, consider excluding the final codon of the genomic sequence from your reverse primer—but make sure to keep the primer in-frame or the fusion protein will not be correct.

4. It is helpful to digest the U6 plasmid as completely as possible so that when proceeding to ligation of the sgRNA, transformation and plating, you do not have to screen as many bacterial colonies to find one that is properly ligated. To accomplish this, you may wish to digest the plasmid using the BsaI-HF enzyme twice (once overnight, and once again after gel purification of the plasmid). After completing digestion, you may wish to test the plasmid's "purity" by performing a control (false) ligation—creating a reaction with only ligase and the plasmid and transforming this reaction and plating. A clean plasmid should produce no colonies on the LB/Ampicillin plate.

5. In practice, there are many other restriction endonucleases which can be paired with BsaI-HF for this diagnostic procedure; we have chosen to use PvuI-HF due to buffer compatibility and availability of this enzyme. Other enzymes can be

used depending on which are available and compatible with the buffers used.

6. We have found in practice that it may require several different trials with bait proteins before finding a few that will function properly with BioID. At this step, you may find that your protein mislocalizes or that BirA∗ or BioID2 does not function. Before beginning with a new POI check the following: (i) be sure your POI is in-frame with the BioID enzyme (check with a plasmid editor and verify using sequencing)—if your HA tag does not appear, almost certainly there was a misstep in engineering the fusion. (ii) Be sure biotin is at a proper concentration and at a proper concentration. Biotin can be made in large stocks and stored at −20 °C for up to 6 months.

7. We suggest making up lysis buffers 1–2 days prior to the experiment and keeping these at 4 °C. 8 M Urea buffer should be made fresh the day of the experiment.

8. Syringe lysing may be difficult with large volumes using a 27-gauge needle. Serial passage through larger bore needles (21-, 23-, or 25-gauge) before passage through the 27-gauge may make this process easier.

9. We have also had success with streptavidin binding at room temperature for 4–6 h. If you wish to complete this step in 1 day, this is an option.

10. After washes are complete, optimally begin on-bead digestion and desalting within 24 h in order to prevent peptide degradation.

References

1. Blader, I.J., Coleman, B.I., Chen, C.T., and Gubbels, M.J. Lytic cycle of *Toxoplasma gondii*: 15 years later. Annu Rev Microbiol. 2015;69:463–485. doi: https://doi.org/10.1146/annurev-micro-091014-104100. PMID: 26332089; PMCID: PMC4659696

2. Sheiner L, Vaidya AB, McFadden GI (2013) The metabolic roles of the endosymbiotic organelles of *Toxoplasma* and Plasmodium spp. Curr Opin Microbiol 16(4):452–458. https://doi.org/10.1016/j.mib.2013.07.003. PMID: 23927894; PMCID: PMC3767399

3. Butler CL, Lucas O, Wuchty S, Xue B, Uversky VN, White M (2014) Identifying novel cell cycle proteins in apicomplexa parasites through co-expression decision analysis. PLoS One 9(5):e97625. https://doi.org/10.1371/journal.pone.0097625. PMID: 24841368; PMCID: 4026381

4. Gilbert LA, Ravindran S, Turetzky JM, Boothroyd JC, Bradley PJ (2007) *Toxoplasma gondii* targets a protein phosphatase 2C to the nuclei of infected host cells. Eukaryot Cell 6(1):73–83

5. Bradley PJ, Ward C, Cheng SJ, Alexander DL, Coller S, Coombs GH, Dunn JD, Ferguson DJ, Sanderson SJ, Wastling JM, Boothroyd JC (2005) Proteomic analysis of rhoptry organelles reveals many novel constituents for host-parasite interactions in *Toxoplasma gondii*. J Biol Chem 280(40):34245–34258. https://doi.org/10.1074/jbc.M504158200

6. Leriche MA, Dubremetz JF (1991) Characterization of the protein contents of rhoptries and dense granules of *Toxoplasma gondii* tachyzoites by subcellular fractionation and monoclonal antibodies. Mol Biochem Parasitol 45(2):249–259

7. Guerin A, Corrales RM, Parker ML, Lamarque MH, Jacot D, El Hajj H, Soldati-Favre D,

Boulanger MJ, Lebrun M (2017) Efficient invasion by *Toxoplasma* depends on the subversion of host protein networks. Nat Microbiol 2 (10):1358–1366. https://doi.org/10.1038/s41564-017-0018-1

8. Lamarque MH, Roques M, Kong-Hap M, Tonkin ML, Rugarabamu G, Marq JB, Penarete-Vargas DM, Boulanger MJ, Soldati-Favre D, Lebrun M (2014) Plasticity and redundancy among AMA-RON pairs ensure host cell entry of *Toxoplasma* parasites. Nat Commun 5:4098. https://doi.org/10.1038/ncomms5098

9. Alexander DL, Mital J, Ward GE, Bradley P, Boothroyd JC (2005) Identification of the moving junction complex of *Toxoplasma gondii*: a collaboration between distinct secretory organelles. PLoS Pathog 1(2):e17. https://doi.org/10.1371/journal.ppat.0010017. PMID: 16244709; PMCID: PMC1262624

10. Roux KJ, Kim DI, Burke B, May DG (2018) BioID: a screen for protein-protein interactions. Curr Protoc Protein Sci 91:19 23 1–19 23 15. https://doi.org/10.1002/cpps.51

11. Roux KJ, Kim DI, Raida M, Burke B (2012) A promiscuous biotin ligase fusion protein identifies proximal and interacting proteins in mammalian cells. J Cell Biol 196(6):801–810. https://doi.org/10.1083/jcb.201112098. PMID: 22412018; PMCID: 3308701

12. Nadipuram SM, Kim EW, Vashisht AA, Lin AH, Bell HN, Coppens I, Wohlschlegel JA, Bradley PJ (2016) In vivo biotinylation of the *Toxoplasma* parasitophorous vacuole reveals novel dense granule proteins important for parasite growth and pathogenesis. MBio 7(4). https://doi.org/10.1128/mBio.00808-16. PMID: 27486190; PMCID: PMC4981711

13. Chen AL, Kim EW, Toh JY, Vashisht AA, Rashoff AQ, Van C, Huang AS, Moon AS, Bell HN, Bentolila LA, Wohlschlegel JA, Bradley PJ (2015) Novel components of the *Toxoplasma* inner membrane complex revealed by BioID. MBio 6(1):e02357–e02314. https://doi.org/10.1128/mBio.02357-14. PMID: 25691595; PMCID: 4337574

14. Gaji RY, Johnson DE, Treeck M, Wang M, Hudmon A, Arrizabalaga G (2015) Phosphorylation of a myosin motor by TgCDPK3 facilitates rapid initiation of motility during *Toxoplasma gondii* egress. PLoS Pathog 11 (11):e1005268. https://doi.org/10.1371/journal.ppat.1005268. PMID: 26544049; PMCID: PMC4636360

15. Long S, Anthony B, Drewry LL, Sibley LD (2017) A conserved ankyrin repeat-containing protein regulates conoid stability, motility and cell invasion in *Toxoplasma gondii*. Nat Commun 8(1):2236. https://doi.org/10.1038/s41467-017-02341-2. PMID: 29269729; PMCID: PMC5740107

16. Kim DI, Jensen SC, Noble KA, Kc B, Roux KH, Motamedchaboki K, Roux KJ (2016) An improved smaller biotin ligase for BioID proximity labeling. Mol Biol Cell 27 (8):1188–1196. https://doi.org/10.1091/mbc.E15-12-0844. PMID: 26912792; PMCID: PMC4831873

17. Schopp IM, Amaya Ramirez CC, Debeljak J, Kreibich E, Skribbe M, Wild K, Bethune J (2017) Split-BioID a conditional proteomics approach to monitor the composition of spatiotemporally defined protein complexes. Nat Commun 8:15690. https://doi.org/10.1038/ncomms15690. PMID: 28585547; PMCID: PMC5467174

18. De Munter S, Gornemann J, Derua R, Lesage B, Qian J, Heroes E, Waelkens E, Van Eynde A, Beullens M, Bollen M (2017) Split-BioID: a proximity biotinylation assay for dimerization-dependent protein interactions. FEBS Lett 591(2):415–424. https://doi.org/10.1002/1873-3468.12548

19. Branon TC, Bosch JA, Sanchez AD, Udeshi ND, Svinkina T, Carr SA, Feldman JL, Perrimon N, Ting AY (2018) Efficient proximity labeling in living cells and organisms with TurboID. Nat Biotechnol 36(9):880–887. https://doi.org/10.1038/nbt.4201. PMID: 30125270; PMCID: PMC6126969

20. Long S, Brown KM, Sibley LD (2018) CRISPR-mediated tagging with BirA allows proximity labeling in *Toxoplasma gondii*. Bio Protoc 8(6). https://doi.org/10.21769/BioProtoc.2768. PMID: 29644258; PMCID: PMC5890295

21. Sidik SM, Hackett CG, Tran F, Westwood NJ, Lourido S (2014) Efficient genome engineering of *Toxoplasma gondii* using CRISPR/Cas9. PLoS One 9(6):e100450. https://doi.org/10.1371/journal.pone.0100450. PMID: 24971596; PMCID: 4074098

Chapter 19

Assays to Evaluate *Toxoplasma*–Macrophage Interactions

Debanjan Mukhopadhyay and Jeroen P. J. Saeij

Abstract

The obligate intracellular protozoan parasite *Toxoplasma gondii* can infect any nucleated cell from a warm-blooded host. However, its interaction with host macrophages plays a critical role in shaping the immune response during infection. Therefore, assessing *Toxoplasma*–macrophage interactions at a cellular level is important. In this chapter, we describe assays that can be used to characterize *Toxoplasma*–macrophage interactions. These assays can also be used to evaluate other host–pathogen interactions. We describe multiplex approaches for measuring arginase activity, indoleamine 2,3 dioxygenase activity, cell death, and parasite growth during *Toxoplasma*–macrophage interactions. These assays can be used to compare how different *Toxoplasma* strains differ in their interaction with macrophages, and we describe how to properly assess *Toxoplasma* strain differences in *Toxoplasma*–macrophage interactions.

Key words Arginase, GRA15, IDO, Inflammasome, LDH, Macrophage, Macrophage polarization, MTS, ROP16, *Toxoplasma*

1 Introduction

Cells of the macrophage–monocyte lineage are extremely plastic in nature and can be polarized into different subtypes by different exogenous stimuli [1]. The plasticity of macrophages plays a pivotal role in many diseases, including infectious, allergic, and autoimmune diseases [1]. When macrophages are stimulated by interferon gamma (IFNγ) and/or lipopolysaccharide (LPS) the NF-κB and the signal transducer and activator of transcription 1 (STAT1) signaling pathways are activated leading macrophages to become polarized toward classically activated or M1 macrophages. To get the full spectrum of macrophage microbicidal activity, it is important to stimulate macrophages with both IFNγ and LPS or IFNγ and tumor necrosis factor alpha (TNFα) [2, 3]. M1 macrophages are characterized by secretion of proinflammatory cytokines and enhanced pathogen killing ability [4]. On the contrary, macrophages that are stimulated with interleukin (IL)-4 or IL-13, which activate STAT6, become polarized toward alternatively activated or M2 macrophages. M2 macrophages have more capacity for

Christopher J. Tonkin (ed.), *Toxoplasma gondii: Methods and Protocols*, Methods in Molecular Biology, vol. 2071,
https://doi.org/10.1007/978-1-4939-9857-9_19, © Springer Science+Business Media, LLC, part of Springer Nature 2020

tissue repair and are less effective in killing intracellular pathogens [4]. Phenotypically, M1 macrophages are characterized by generation of high levels of nitric oxide (NO), reactive oxygen species (ROS), high activity of indoleamine 2,3 dioxygenase (IDO), and secretion of IL-12, which enhances type I T helper cell (Th1) responses. M2 macrophages are characterized by possessing high arginase activity, expression of mannose receptor, and secretion of cytokines such as IL-10, which enhances Th2 responses [4]. Thus, many intracellular pathogens suppress M1 macrophage polarization and activate M2 macrophages. *Toxoplasma* is an intracellular protozoan parasite that is estimated to infect ~30% of humans worldwide [5]. Many *Toxoplasma* strains exist, but in North America and Europe the majority of *Toxoplasma* strains belong to the clonal type I, II, III, and XII lineage [6]. These clonal lineages differ in many phenotypes including virulence in mice, in vitro growth rate, migration, modulation of host signaling pathways, and susceptibility to host immune responses [7]. *Toxoplasma* type II strains induce M1 macrophages in vitro with enhanced IL-12 production, whereas type I and III strains activate M2 macrophages characterized by high arginase activity, expression of the mannose receptor, and low IL-12 production [8]. This strain-specific induction of macrophage polarization is largely dependent on *Toxoplasma* proteins that are secreted into the host cell called ROPs and GRAs, which are secreted from *Toxoplasma* secretory organelles called rhoptries and dense granules. We have shown that two *Toxoplasma* proteins play a major role in the modulation of macrophage function and thereby determine the level of immune-induced inflammation. These proteins are ROP16 (a secreted kinase) and GRA15 (a secreted protein with no characterized motifs). ROP16 activates the STAT6 transcription factor resulting in M2 macrophage activation and the repression of inflammation. GRA15 activates the NF-kB transcription factor resulting in M1 macrophage activation and the activation of an inflammatory response [8]. Type I and III strain parasites have a more active version of ROP16 compared to type II strain parasites, while type II parasites have a more active GRA15 or higher expression of GRA15 compared to type I and type III strain parasites. These strain differences in ROP16 and GRA15 determine *Toxoplasma* strain differences in macrophage polarization [8–10]. It was recently shown that GRA24 also contributes to M1 macrophage polarization by activating the p38 mitogen-activated protein kinase (MAPK) pathway. Unlike the strain-specific activities of GRA15 and ROP16, GRA24 from all strains tested so far can activate p38 MAPK [11]. Thus, strain differences in GRA15 and ROP16 plays a pivotal role in determining macrophage polarization upon *Toxoplasma* infection. For many *Toxoplasma* strains the mechanism by which they modulate macrophage activation remains unknown. Furthermore, it is likely that other parasite gene products can modulate macrophage function and polarization. Thus, assessing macrophage polarization upon infection with different *Toxoplasma* strains with an easy assay is important. For this, the combined assessment of IL-12, NO, or IDO as markers for M1 activation and arginase activity as a marker for M2 activation from a single experiment can provide direct evidence for macrophage polarization by *Toxoplasma*. We will describe assays that can determine if macrophages infected with different *Toxoplasma* strains differ in their polarization profile. IL-12 can be measured from the supernatant using any commercially available ELISA kit. The arginase and IDO assay that will be described in the following section is easy to set up and perform (~2–3 h) in a 96-well plate format. Because the method described here determines the arginase activity from the cell lysate, the assay can be combined with other assays that use cell culture supernatant (e.g., assays to measure NO production or quantitate cytokines present in the supernatant).

2 Measurement of Arginase Activity from Macrophage Lysates Using a Microplate-Based Method

2.1 Materials

Prepare all solutions using deionized water and analytical or molecular biology grade reagents. Prepare and store all reagents at room temperature, unless otherwise mentioned.

2.2 Cell Culture Reagents

Macrophages are extremely sensitive to even very low levels of lipopolysaccharide (LPS) (endotoxin) from gram-negative bacteria. All solutions, buffers and media should be made with sterile, tissue culture grade, endotoxin-tested water. To avoid LPS contamination use disposable sterile plastics rather than laboratory glassware for all steps in this protocol and for storing solutions. LPS contamination can be determined with the Limulus Amebocyte Lysate assay [12]. Additionally, all the cells should be devoid of mycoplasma contamination as it can affect cell physiology, and often leads to erroneous results. Therefore, all the cells used in the study should be checked for mycoplasma contamination every 3–4 weeks either by PCR (most sensitive) or by indirect immunofluorescence assays looking for DNA-positive staining outside the host cell nucleus. For the PCR detection the following primers can be used: Fw: 5′ GGGAGCAAACAGGATTAGATACCCT 3′; Rv: 5′ TGCACCATCTGTCACTCTGTTAACCTC 3′. The following program should be used with the primers mentioned above-initial denaturation (1 min at 98 °C), denaturation (30 s at 98 °C), annealing (30 s at 55 °C), polymerization (2 min 30 s at 72 °C), repeat the cycle for 32 times and finish with a final extension (7 min at 72 °C). All mycoplasma-positive reagents should be discarded and autoclaved.

1. DMEM (Dulbecco's Modified Eagle Medium) with high glucose supplemented with 10% heat-inactivated fetal bovine serum (HI-FBS), L-Glutamine (2 mM), 100 U/mL Penicillin, 100 µg/mL Streptomycin, 20 µg/mL Gentamycin, and HEPES (1 M) (complete DMEM) is used to culture the Raw264.7 macrophage cell line. For bone marrow derived macrophages (BMDM) it is recommended to make a small batch of media containing complete DMEM complemented with 20% L929 mouse fibroblast cell culture supernatant (*see* **Note 1**), 1× nonessential amino acids (NEAA), and 1 M sodium pyruvate. To make 100 mL of medium, 20 mL of L929 medium should be added to 80 mL of complete DMEM that was supplemented with NEAA and sodium pyruvate (1 M final concentration). It is not recommended to store the BMDM medium for more than 5 days because the cytokines present in the L929 culture supernatant (*see* **Note 1**) can degrade at 4 °C. For human peripheral blood mononuclear cells (PBMCs) and monocytes, RPMI 1640 media supplemented with 10% HI-FBS, L-Glutamine (2 mM), 100 U/mL Penicillin, 100 µg/mL Streptomycin, and 20 µg/mL Gentamycin should be used. *Toxoplasma* parasites are usually maintained (*see* **Note 2**) in human foreskin fibroblasts (HFFs) in complete DMEM medium. All cells (and *Toxoplasma*) are cultured at 37 °C with 5% CO_2.

2. Sterile phosphate buffer saline (PBS).

3. Recombinant IL-4 of mouse or human origin, final concentration to be added to cells is 50 µg/mL.

4. Sterile endotoxin-free centrifuge tubes ranging from 0.5 to 50 mL volume.

5. Flat bottom 96- and 24-well plates.

6. Sterile serological pipettes 5–50 mL.

7. Cell culture incubator maintained at 37 °C with 5% CO_2.

8. Centrifuge at 4 °C with adjustable acceleration and deceleration.

2.3 Assay Reagents

1. 0.1% v/v Triton X-100 solution (this will work as a cell lysis agent; dilution should be made in deionized water). For one 96-well plate, 2.5 mL of 0.1% Triton X-100 solution is sufficient.

2. Halt protease inhibitor cocktail without EDTA (Thermo Scientific #1861284), 100× (final concentration will be 1× and dilution should be made with 0.1% Triton X-100). To make 2.5 mL of lysis buffer for one 96-well plate, 25 µL of Halt protease inhibitor cocktail and 2.5 µL of 100% Triton X-100 should be added to 472.5 µL of deionized water.

3. 10 mM Manganese chloride ($MnCl_2$) dissolved in 50 mM Tris–HCl, pH 7.5 (Can be used until the solution turns black, usually 1 week). To make 30 mL of $MnCl_2$, dissolve 0.059 g of $MnCl_2$ in 50 mM Tris–HCl, pH 7.5.

4. 1 M L-arginine, pH 9.7 (should be made fresh). To make a 3 mL solution of 1 M L-arginine, add 0.5226 g L-arginine to 3 mL of deionized water and vortex the solution to dissolve the L-arginine. Keeping the solution at 37 °C for 5–10 min will help with dissolving the L-arginine.

5. A solution of an acid mixture containing sulfuric acid/phosphoric acid/water ($H_2SO_4/H_3PO_4/H_2O$, v/v/v) in a ratio of 1:3:7 (can be stored at room temperature for at least 1 month). To make 110 mL acid mixture, add 10 mL of sulfuric acid and 30 mL phosphoric acid to 70 mL of deionized water.

6. 9% 2-isonitrosopropiophenone (ISPF) diluted in 100% ethanol (should be made fresh). For 1.5 mL solution add 0.135 g of 2-isonitrosopropiophenone to 1.5 mL of 100% ethanol and vortex the mixture to dissolve it. The solution has a semicrystalline appearance.

7. 1 M urea solution in deionized water (can be stored at 4 °C for at least 1 month). To make a 50 mL 1 M urea solution, dissolve 3 g of urea into 50 mL of deionized water and keep it at 4 °C.

2.4   Method

1. Seed 1×10^5 macrophages [13] in each well of a 96-well plate in 100 µL medium specific for the macrophage type (mentioned in cell culture reagents point 1) for at least 3 h to ensure cell adherence. For Raw264.7 macrophages, if cells are seeded the day before, seed at a density of 5×10^4 cells/well. For each condition, seed the cells in triplicate. All the outer wells should contain sterile PBS to prevent evaporation of the medium from the wells (Fig. 1a).

2. Once the parasites have grown sufficiently to create many large vacuoles that are about to lyse out of the cell, harvest parasites from infected HFFs by syringe lysis (27 and 30 G needle) should be used for maximum lysis) method (*see* **Note 2**). Remove medium from the parasite pellet after centrifugation ($570 \times g$ for 7 min) and resuspend the pellet in 1 mL of medium (same as used for culturing of macrophages). Count the parasites using a hemocytometer.

3. Infect the macrophages with *Toxoplasma* (*see* **Note 3**) using a multiplicity of infection (MOI) of 0.5–10 depending on the strain type (*see* Subheading 6) for 20–24 h. Make sure to keep the total volume per well constant by using macrophage media to adjust the total volume (Fig. 1a).

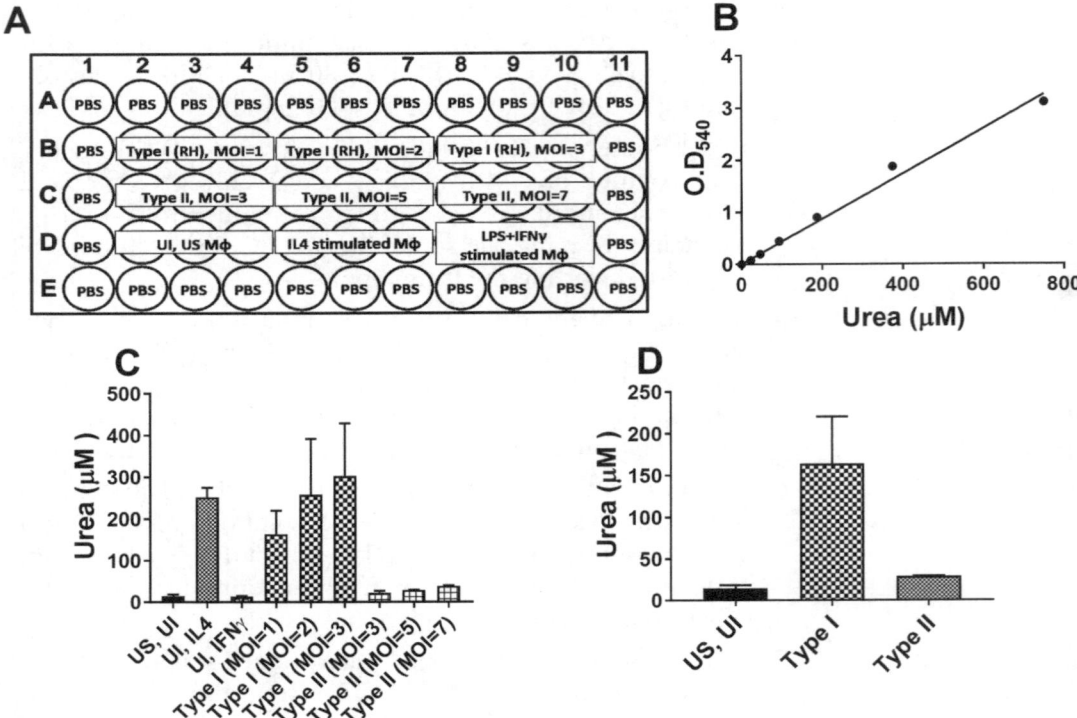

Fig. 1 Arginase assay. (**a**) A 96-well format for measuring arginase activity from macrophages. All the conditions should be performed in triplicate wells as depicted. *Mφ* macrophages, *LPS* lipopolysaccharide, *UI* uninfected, *US* unstimulated. (**b**) A standard curve of urea from which the amount of urea produced by *Toxoplasma*-infected macrophages or cytokine-treated macrophages can be derived. (**c**) Amount of urea produced from macrophages is shown where IL-4-treated cells served as positive control and IFNγ-treated cells as negative control. Different strains of *Toxoplasma* at different MOIs induced different amounts of urea. (**d**) Urea production by macrophages infected with different *Toxoplasma* strains at a similar MOI matched by plaque assay as shown in Table 1

4. Keep three wells for uninfected cells and three wells for cells stimulated with 50 μg/mL recombinant IL-4 (positive control) (*see* **Note 4**, Fig. 1a).

5. It is good practice to set up a plaque assay to determine the viability of the parasites, especially when comparing different parasite strains. The arginase activity and IL-12 production of macrophages are dependent on the infection level of the macrophages. To be able to interpret results obtained from different parasite strains or performed at different days it is therefore important to know the infectivity of your parasites. To do so, plaque assays in 24-well plates seeded with HFFs in triplicate can be used to determine the viability of the parasites (*see* **Note 5**). Without plaque assay results, potential differences between different parasites (e.g., different strains or knockout *vs.* wild type) on arginase activity or IL-12 production of

macrophages cannot be distinguished from potential influences of differences in viability.

6. After 20–24 h of infection, take the plate from the CO_2 incubator and look under the microscope to determine if there is any cell lysis caused by parasite growth. If a high degree of cell lysis occurs in some wells or with certain MOIs, it has to be noted, as this may influence the results. Following that, spin down the plates at $440 \times g$ for 5 min.

7. Transfer the supernatant to another 96-well low protein binding plate (normal 96-well tissue culture plates are OK) using a multichannel pipette and use for cytokine ELISA, lactate dehydrogenase (LDH) release assay, or NO assay.

8. Once the medium is removed, add 25 µL Triton X-100 with $1\times$ protease inhibitor cocktail to each well of the plate with the macrophages. Place the plate at −80 °C and proceed the next day with 2–3 freeze–thaw cycles, or freeze-thaw 2–3 times to ensure complete lysis of the cells and proceed same day. During freeze thaw, put two heating blocks at 60 °C.

9. Check under microscope that cells are lysed. They will appear as ghost transparent bodies.

10. Following cell lysis, add 25 µL 50 mM Tris–HCl containing 10 mM $MnCl_2$.

11. Incubate the plate containing cell and parasite lysate for 10 min at 60 °C (by sandwiching the plate between two heat blocks preheated to 60 °C).

12. After 10 min, add 25 µL 1 M L-arginine to the wells containing the 50 µL lysate.

13. After that, incubate the plate for 60 min in a 37 °C incubator (*see* **Note 6**).

14. During this 60 min incubation time, dilute 1 M urea to the following concentrations: 1500–750–375–187.5–93.8–46.9–23.4–0 µM each for triplicate wells as standards (50 µL per well). Also turn the temperature of the heating blocks up to 95 °C.

15. After 60 min, remove the plate and add 175 µL H_2SO_4–H_3PO_4–H_2O (1:3:7) to all wells. Add 200 µL to the urea dilution series in the same plate (Fig. 1a).

16. Add 12.5 µL 9% ISPF to all wells (precipitation will occur).

17. Place a high temperature resistant microplate sealing film (usually PCR plate cover) on the 96-well plate and put the 96-well plate cover on top of this.

18. Incubate for 30–60 min at 95 °C on top of a heating block with another heating block inverted on it (to prevent evaporation) and incubate till precipitation is gone and development of pink

color can be seen. The high temperature of the plates will cause damage to the plates, so keep another microplate ready (does not need to be tissue culture grade) to transfer the liquid from the heated plate to that plate.

19. After removing the plate from heating block, incubate for 10 min at room temperature in the dark. If samples are "cloudy" read later (keep plate in the dark).

20. Read the absorbance at OD at 540 and 650 nm and export the data to .txt file (*see* **Note 7**).

21. Open the txt file with excel and calculate the concentration of urea in µM from the standard curve (Fig. 1b). Subtract absorbance at OD 650 from OD 540. Determine the sample values from the urea standard curve (Fig. 1c).

3 Measurement of Host Cell Viability and *Toxoplasma* Growth in a Multiplex Assay

3.1 Introduction

Host cell death is one of several immune mechanisms for inhibiting *Toxoplasma*'s growth by destroying its replicative niche. It has been observed in human primary fibroblasts and Lewis rat macrophages [14]. IFNγ plays a pivotal role in the immune response against *Toxoplasma* in both mice and humans. Host cell death is often accompanied with restriction of parasite growth and can differ depending on the infecting *Toxoplasma* strain type [14]. Herein, we will describe a method for measuring host cell death and parasite growth from a single experiment and from the same wells using a 96-well plate assay. This assay will measure cell death by quantifying the release of the host cytoplasmic enzyme lactate dehydrogenase (LDH) into the cell culture supernatant upon cell death and measure parasite growth by measuring luciferase activity from luciferase expressing parasites. However, it should be noted that using luciferase measurements for total parasite growth has limitations as luciferase is a very stable protein and therefore signal from dead parasites could contribute to the signal. Therefore, parasite/vacuole counting should also be considered (*see* **Notes 8 and 16**). Our example will be for HFFs, but the same assay can be performed on macrophages.

3.2 Materials

Prepare all solutions using deionized water and analytical or molecular biology grade reagents. Prepare and store all reagents at room temperature, unless otherwise mentioned.

3.3 Cell Culture Reagents

1. For culturing macrophages all the reagents and equipment must be free of endotoxins as stated in the arginase assay protocol. The macrophage culture medium is the same as mentioned in the arginase assay protocol. For culturing HFFs complete DMEM should be used.

2. Any parasite strain (e.g., type I/II/III) or any transgenic strain that will be used in this assay should be genetically engineered to express luciferase [15] (*see* **Note 3**).

3. Sterile phosphate buffer saline (PBS).

4. Recombinant IFNγ of either human or mouse origin. The IFNγ should be dissolved in sterile complete DMEM media as a 100× concentrated stock solution and kept at −80 °C for storage in small aliquots to avoid repeated freeze–thaw cycles. To activate the full toxoplasmacidal activity of macrophages either LPS (10 ng/mL) or recombinant TNFα (20–100 U/ mL) should be added together with IFNγ (*see* **Note 9**).

5. Sterile endotoxin-free centrifuge tubes ranging from 0.5 to 50 mL.

6. Flat bottom 96- and 24-well plates.

7. Sterile serological pipettes 5–50 mL.

8. Cell culture incubator maintained at 37 °C and with 5% CO_2.

9. Centrifuge at 4 °C with adjustable acceleration and deceleration.

3.4 Assay Reagents

1. LDH cytotoxicity detection kit (Roche, Sigma). This system is a microplate-based method where LDH released from the dying cells can be measured from 50 to 100 μL cell culture supernatant (*see* **Note 10**).

2. Complete DMEM medium plus 2% v/v Triton X-100. This solution is used to lyse all the cells, which will be the control for maximal LDH release. To make 50 mL of this medium, 1 mL of 100% Triton X-100 should be added to 49 mL of complete DMEM medium.

3. Cell lysis buffer for the luciferase assay. To make the buffer, 1× PBS containing 2 mM Dithiothreitol (DTT) (*see* **Note 11**), 10% v/v glycerol, and 1% v/v Triton X-100 should be used. To make 50 mL of lysis buffer, 5 mL of 100% glycerol stock solution, 0.5 mL of 100% Triton X-100, and 0.1 mL of 1 M DTT solution (final concentration will be 2 mM) should mixed with 1× PBS to make the volume 50 mL. Alternatively, a 5× Luciferase Cell Culture Lysis Reagent can be purchased from Promega (Cat. Number E1500), which should be stored at −20 °C. Each time, the desired volume can be made by diluting the 5× reagent in deionized water (*see* **Note 12**).

4. Luciferase assay buffer: To make a 2× luciferase assay buffer the following reagents are required:

   (a) 500 mM (100×) magnesium chloride ($MgCl_2$) solution. To make 10 mL solution, weigh 476.05 mg of $MgCl_2$ and dissolve in deionized water. Solution can be stored at room temperature for at least 1 month.

(b) 15 mM ($100\times$) ATP solution. To prepare 10 mL solution, weigh 82.67 mg of ATP and dissolve in deionized water. Make aliquots and store at $-20\ °C$.

(c) 400 mM ($4\times$) Tris–HCl, pH 7.8 buffer. Weigh 4.85 g of Tris base and dissolve in 85 mL of deionized water. Adjust pH with 1 M HCl to pH 7.8 and make the volume up to 100 mL.

(d) To make 1 mL of fresh $2\times$ assay buffer, add the following in order: 0.5 mL Tris–HCl ($4\times$) solution, 0.02 mL of MgCl$_2$ ($100\times$), 0.02 mL of ATP ($100\times$) and adjust the volume to 1 mL with deionized water. The $2\times$ assay buffer can also be made in a large quantity and stored in small aliquots at $-20\ °C$. The day of measuring luminescence, aliquots can be thawed and diluted to $1\times$ with deionized water.

5. D-Luciferin solution: To make a $100\times$ solution (15 mg/mL) of K-Luciferin, (alternatively, Na-luciferin can also be used) dissolve 90 mg of K-luciferin in deionized water and store as small aliquots at $-80\ °C$ for up to 6 months. Aliquots can also be stored be stored at $-20\ °C$ for 2–3 weeks. Add 2 μL of D-luciferin substrate ($100\times$) to 0.198 mL of $1\times$ luciferase assay buffer on the day of measurement.

3.5   Method

1. Seed the host cells in 96-well tissue culture treated plates using 2×10^4 HFFs or 1×10^5 macrophages/well (volume = 100 μL/well) as shown in Fig. 2a. All the boundary wells should contain sterile PBS to keep the plate in moist condition for good health of the host cells and less chance of evaporation of the medium from the wells.

2. Following that, add the stimuli of interest and incubate the cells for another 16–24 h at 37 °C. IFNγ should be used at 10–100 U/mL but the activity can vary from batch to batch (*see* **Note 13**). In addition, LPS could also be added at a concentration of 10 ng/mL (the stock concentration usually is 1–10 mg/mL) or alternatively TNFα could also be added at a concentration of 10–100 U/mL (stock concentration at 10,000 U/mL).

3. After incubation with the stimuli, add luciferase expressing parasites at three different MOIs, that is, for type I (RH) strain use MOIs of 1/2/3 and for non-RH strains use MOIs of 3/5/7 (*see* Fig. 2a). Set up a plaque assay in parallel to get the real MOI (*see* **Note 13**). Let the infection proceed for 20–24 h in a 37 °C tissue culture incubator. Make sure to keep the total volume per well constant.

4. After 20–24 h of infection, remove the medium from the wells that will serve as the control for maximum cell lysis (Fig. 2a)

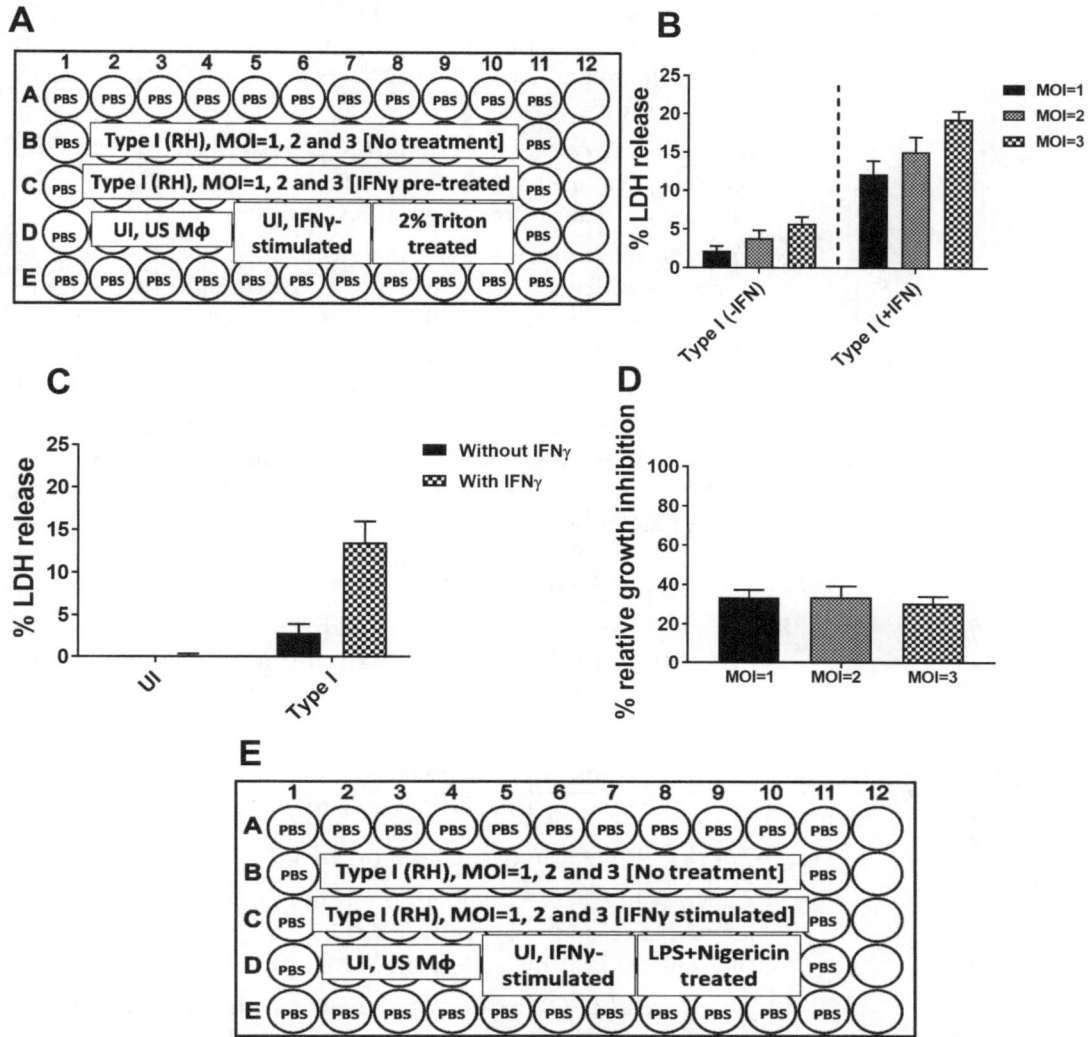

Fig. 2 Cell death assay determined by LDH release, cell viability determined by MTS-PMS assay, and parasite growth assay determined by luciferase activity measurement. (**a**) A format for 96-well plate–based multiplex assay for cell death and parasite growth measurement. *UI* uninfected, *US* unstimulated. (**b**) Bar diagram showing the normalized values of LDH release (normalized to untreated and uninfected HFFs) from the *Toxoplasma*-infected HFFs with and without IFNγ treatment (10 U/mL). (**c**) Amount of LDH release by *Toxoplasma*-infected (at a matched MOI of 1 from 3 different experiments, as determined by plaque assay) IFNγ-stimulated HFFs. (**d**) Measurement of % relative growth inhibition at MOI 1–3 of *Toxoplasma* in IFNγ-stimulated and unstimulated (US) HFFs. Here the mean luciferase reading of the triplicate wells from unstimulated cells are considered as 100% and the relative % of growth in IFNγ-stimulated cells was calculated from this value. (**e**) A format for 96-well plate–based MTS-PMS–based assay for measuring cell viability *UI* uninfected, *US* unstimulated

and replace it with complete DMEM with 2% Triton X-100 media (check under the microscope that the cells have all lysed: host cell nuclei will appear very distinct with a clear background).

5. Before taking out the medium from each well, plates should be centrifuged at $440 \times g$ for 5 min at room temperature to make sure the medium is free of parasites or cells.

6. Transfer the culture supernatant to a different 96-well plate using a multichannel pipette. To three wells add cell culture medium as a control as FBS present in medium can contain different levels of LDH (*see* **Note 14**). This plate will be used to measure cell death by measuring the amount of LDH present in the culture supernatant.

7. For the LDH assay from the culture supernatant, add the freshly prepared LDH reagent in a ratio of 1:1 to the 100 µL culture supernatant according to the manufacturer's instructions (Roche, Sigma) and incubate for 25–30 min in the dark, at room temperature.

8. The absorbance should be measured at 490 nm using a microplate reader having a filter of 490 nm or a monochromator-based plate reader. The working formula for measuring LDH release is as follows:

$$\%\text{LDH release} = \frac{[(\text{sample O.D} - \text{blank O.D}) - (\text{control O.D} - \text{blank O.D})]}{[(\text{lysis control O.D} - \text{blank O.D}) - (\text{control O.D} - \text{blank O.D})]} \times 100$$

Blank O.D.= O.D. of medium only with LDH reagent.

Control O.D. = O.D of medium from untreated and unstimulated host cells, this is supposed to have minimum absorbance if the cells are healthy.

Lysis control O.D. = Host cells treated with 2% Triton X-100 containing media which ruptures the cell membrane and releases maximum LDH. These wells will have maximum absorbance.

9. To measure the parasite growth by luciferase, add 25 µL lysis buffer mentioned in assay reagents point 3 to the cells from which the medium was removed. Seal the plate with a plate sealer and keep it at $-20\,^{\circ}\text{C}$ for 1 week or at $-80\,^{\circ}\text{C}$ for at least 1 month. Alternatively, freeze-thaw for 2–3 times and process the same day.

10. To proceed the same day for luciferase assay, after freeze thawing the lysate plate, plates should be kept at $37\,^{\circ}\text{C}$ for 30 min before reading. Two approaches can be taken for reading luminescence, either by using a luciferase plate reader or using a single channel luminometer. For plate reader-based measurement, transfer all the lysate to a white-walled plate for luminescence (e.g., Corning Costar plate, Cat. No. #3912) using a multichannel pipette followed by addition of 50 µL of

luciferase assay buffer with D-Luciferin (made fresh) as described in points 4 and 5 in assay reagents. The program for measuring luminescence should be used with 10s delay at room temperature. If a manual single channel luminometer will be used, then 50 µL of freshly made luciferase assay buffer with D-Luciferin should be first added to 1.5 mL clear centrifuge tubes (the number of tubes will be dependent on the number of wells in the plate, one tube/well). Colored centrifuge tubes should not be used. Following this, 25 µL of the lysate from one well should be added to one tube and luminescence should be recorded using 10 s delay program. This should be done sequentially for all tubes one at a time. For analysis of the result, luciferase read of non-IFNγ treated wells will be considered as 100% and relative growth inhibition of IFNγ-treated wells will be calculated accordingly. To graphically represent, either % relative growth or % relative growth inhibition (% relative growth in non-IFNγ wells − % relative growth in IFNγ-treated wells) can be plotted as shown in Fig. 2d.

4 MTS-PMS–Based Assay for Host Cell Viability: An Alternative Approach

4.1 Introduction

In addition to measuring host cell death with the LDH release assay, one can also measure the number of viable host cells. A method that is commonly used to do this is known as the MTS/PMS, [(3-(4,5-dimethylthiazol-2-yl)-5-(3-carboxymethoxyphenyl)-2-(4-sulfophenyl)-2H-tetrazolium inner salt)/phenazine methosulfate) assay [16]. This assay measures the reduction of the MTS tetrazolium compound by viable cells to generate a colored soluble formazan product. This conversion is carried out by mitochondrial dehydrogenase enzymes of metabolically active cells. The soluble formazan dye produced by viable cells can be quantified by measuring the absorbance at 490 nm [16]. This assay is rapid and can be efficiently used for measuring macrophage viability upon infection with *Toxoplasma gondii* [17].

4.2 Materials

Prepare all solutions using deionized water and analytical or molecular biology grade reagents. Prepare and store all reagents at room temperature, unless otherwise mentioned.

4.3 Cell Culture Reagents

1. For culturing macrophages all the reagents and equipment must be free of endotoxins as stated in the arginase assay protocol. The macrophage culture medium is the same as mentioned in the arginase assay protocol. For culturing HFFs complete DMEM should be used.

2. Any parasite strain (e.g., type I/II/III) or any transgenic strain that will be used in this assay should be genetically engineered to express luciferase [15].

3. Sterile phosphate buffer saline (PBS).

4. Sterile endotoxin-free centrifuge tubes ranging from 0.5 to 50 mL.

5. Recombinant IFNγ of either human or mouse origin. The IFNγ should be dissolved in sterile complete DMEM media as a 100× concentrated stock solution and kept at −80 °C for storage in small aliquots to avoid repeated freeze–thaw cycles. (*For IFNγ concentrations and stability please see* **Note 1** *of LDH assay method*).

6. Flat bottom 96- and 24-well plates.

7. Sterile serological pipettes 5–50 mL.

8. Cell culture incubator maintained at 37 °C and with 5% CO_2.

9. Centrifuge at 4 °C with adjustable acceleration and deceleration.

4.4 Assay Reagents

1. MTS stock reagent preparation: the final MTS stock concentration is 2 mg/mL to be made in sterile 1× PBS. To make 20 mL of the reagent, weigh 40 mg of the MTS powder and mix with 20 mL of sterile 1× PBS. To dissolve, vortex the solution for till the MTS is completely dissolved. When the MTS is completely dissolved, the solution will appear yellowish. Wrap the tube with aluminum foil as the solution is light sensitive. For storage, make small aliquots wrap them with aluminum foil and keep them in a cardboard box at −20 °C.

2. Preparation of PMS solution: a stock solution of PMS can be prepared in 1× sterile PBS. The concentration of the PMS stock solution is 9.2 mg/mL. To make 10 mL of solution, weigh 92 mg of PMS and mix with 10 mL of 1× sterile PBS. Small aliquots can be made, wrapped with aluminum foil, and kept in a cardboard box at −20 °C. This concentration of PMS is a 100× solution.

3. MTS-PMS reagent preparation: on the day of the experiment, take one aliquot each of MTS and PMS. First, make a 10× dilution of the PMS stock solution to get a 10× concentration (0.92 mg/mL). Mix MTS and PMS at a ratio of 10:1 in which the final concentration of PMS will be 0.092 mg/mL (1×). For instance, to make 1650 μL of final solution, mix 1500 μL of MTS with 150 μL of 0.92 mg/mL of PMS solution (10×). From this final mixture of MTS-PMS, 20 μL should be added to 100 μL of cell suspension.

4. LPS (*see* **Note 15**): Dissolve the LPS in endotoxin-free water to make a stock concentration of 1 mg/mL. Make small aliquots and keep them at −20 °C for 6 months with full functional activity. Avoid repeated freeze thawing.

5. Nigericin: Dissolve nigericin in 100% ethanol. The stock concentration of Nigericin is 1 mg/mL. Make small aliquots and keep them at −20 °C for 1 year with full functional activity. Avoid repeated freeze thawing.

4.5 Method

1. Seed the host cells in 96-well tissue culture treated plates using 1×10^5 macrophages/well (volume = 100 μL/well) as shown in Fig. 2e. All the boundary wells should contain sterile PBS to keep the plate in moist condition for good health of the host cells and less chance of evaporation of the medium from the wells.

2. Following cell seeding for 2–4 h, add the stimuli of interest and incubate the cells for another 16–24 h at 37 °C. IFNγ should be used at 10–100 U/mL but the activity can vary from batch to batch (*For IFNγ concentrations and stability please see **Note 1** of LDH assay method*).

3. After incubation with the stimuli, add parasites at three different MOIs, that is, for type I (RH) strain use MOIs of 1/2/3 and for non-RH strains use MOIs of 3/5/7 (Fig. 1a). Set up a plaque assay in parallel to get the real MOI. Let the infection proceed for 20–24 h in a 37 °C tissue culture incubator. Make sure to keep the total volume per well constant.

4. After 20 h of infection, add LPS (final concentration will be 10 ng/mL) to the designated well (Fig. 2e) for 4 h and then add nigericin (5 μM final concentration) for the final 1 h. before addition of MTS-PMS reagent (*see* **Note 16**). These wells will serve as a positive control for cell death. Add freshly prepared 20 μL of MTS-PMS solution to each well and wrap the plate with aluminum foil, and put it back in the 37 °C tissue culture incubator. Incubate for 1–2 h. Here it is important to check the color formation every 45 min to 1 h. If the red-purple formazan color is formed, measure absorbance at 490 nm. Alternatively, plate can be incubated longer for more color development. Background absorbance, which comes from spontaneous reduction of MTS-PMS by dissolved oxygen in the media, should not be more than 0.2.

5. To calculate the percentage viability of host cells the following formula can be used:

$$\% \text{viability} = \frac{[\text{sample O.D} - \text{blank O.D}]}{[\text{control O.D} - \text{blank O.D}]} \times 100$$

(a) *Blank O.D.* = O.D of medium only with MTS-PMS reagent.

(b) *Control O.D.* = O.D of medium from untreated and unstimulated host cells, this is supposed to have maximum absorbance if the cells are healthy.

5   Measurement of Indoleamine 2,3 Dioxygenase (IDO) Activity from IFNγ-Stimulated *Toxoplasma*-Infected Host Cells

5.1   Introduction

IFNγ is the major mediator of the immune response against *Toxoplasma* irrespective of host organism and cell type [18]. In humans, the mechanism of IFNγ-mediated *Toxoplasma* growth inhibition varies between cell types [14]. Among the various effector mechanisms induced by IFNγ, activation of L-tryptophan catabolism by induction of indoleamine 2,3 dioxygenase (IDO) plays an important role because *Toxoplasma* is an auxotroph for L-tryptophan [19]. Therefore, degradation of L-tryptophan is an effective mechanism for limiting parasite growth inside host cells. To assay L-tryptophan catabolism, additional L-tryptophan needs to be added to the culture media, but it should be noted that this might make it more difficult to measure parasite growth restriction due to L-tryptophan degradation. Therefore, if parasite growth restriction also needs to be assessed, culture media without additional L-tryptophan should be used in parallel. IDO is the first and rate-limiting enzyme of tryptophan catabolism through the kynurenine pathway and considered as an immunoregulatory enzyme of M1 macrophages [4]. Herein, we will describe a 96-well plate–based method for determination of IDO activity that can be combined with other assays such as cytokine measurements, cytotoxicity assays, and also parasite growth measurements. This assay will determine the L-tryptophan catabolic product Kynurenine from the culture supernatant, which correlates directly with IDO activity of the cells. Although our example is for HFFs, the same assay can be performed on macrophages.

5.2   Materials

Prepare all solutions using deionized water and analytical or molecular biology grade reagents. Prepare and store all reagents at room temperature, unless otherwise mentioned.

5.3   Cell Culture Reagents

For culturing host cells (macrophages and HFFs) all the reagents and equipment must be free of endotoxins as stated in the arginase and LDH assay protocol. The medium should contain 0.6 mM L-tryptophan. Usually DMEM contains 0.08 mM L-tryptophan; therefore, 0.52 mM L-tryptophan should be added to the medium to enhance the signal of the assay. To make 100 mL of medium, add 10.62 mg of L-tryptophan and mix and dissolve the L-Tryptophan by warming the medium in a 37 °C water bath for 10 min and then mixing again with a 25 mL serological pipette. This step must be repeated 2–3× times to completely dissolve the tryptophan in the medium. Finally, filter-sterilize the medium through a 0.22 μm filter. This medium is stable for to 2–3 weeks at 4 °C (*see* **Note 17**).

1. If parasite growth is measured by the luciferase assay, any parasite strain (e.g., type I/II/III) or any transgenic strain

that will be used in this assay should be genetically engineered to express luciferase.

2. Sterile phosphate buffer saline (PBS).

3. Recombinant IFNγ of either human or mouse origin. The IFNγ should be dissolved as stated in the LDH assay protocol.

4. Sterile endotoxin-free centrifuge tubes ranging from 0.5 to 50 mL.

5. Flat bottom and V bottom 96-well plates and 24-well plates.

6. Sterile serological pipettes 5–50 mL.

7. Cell culture incubator maintained at 37 °C and with 5% CO_2.

8. Centrifuge at 4 °C with adjustable acceleration and deceleration.

5.4 Assay Reagents

1. 30% w/v trichloroacetic acid (TCA). To make 100 mL of solution of TCA add 30 mL of 6.1 N TCA (Sigma-Aldrich, cat. number T0699) to 70 mL of deionized water. This solution is stable 4 °C for at least 1 month.

2. 5 mM L-Kynurenine solution. This solution will be diluted to prepare the standard curve for the assay. To prepare a 5 mL solution of 5 mM L-Kynurenine solution, weigh 5.2 mg and dissolve it in deionized water. Make aliquots and store them at −20 °C. Solution is stable for 1 year at −20 °C.

3. Ehrlich's reagent: Ehrlich's reagent is 1.2% p-dimethylaminobenzaldehyde in glacial acetic acid solution. This reagent should be made fresh on the day of the assay. To make 25 mL of Ehrlich's reagent, weigh 300 mg of p-dimethylaminobenzaldehyde and dissolve it in 25 mL of glacial acetic acid solution. This solution is light sensitive and has a light green color. So, after preparation, wrap the tube with aluminum foil.

5.5 Method

1. Seed the host cells in 96-well tissue culture treated plates using 2×10^4 HFFs or 1×10^5 macrophages/well (volume = 150 μL/well) as shown in Fig. 3a. All the boundary wells should contain sterile PBS to keep the plate in moist condition for good health of the host cells and less chance of evaporation of the medium from the wells.

2. Following this, add the stimuli of interest and incubate the cells for a further 16–24 h at 37 °C. IFNγ should be used at 10–100 U/mL (*see* **Note 9**).

3. After incubation with the stimuli, add luciferase expressing parasites at three different MOIs, that is, for type I (RH) strain use MOIs of 1/2/3 and for non-RH strains use MOIs of 3/5/7. Set up a plaque assay in parallel to get the real MOI (*see* **Note 5**). Infection should proceed for 18–24 h at 37 °C in a tissue culture incubator. Make sure, to keep the total

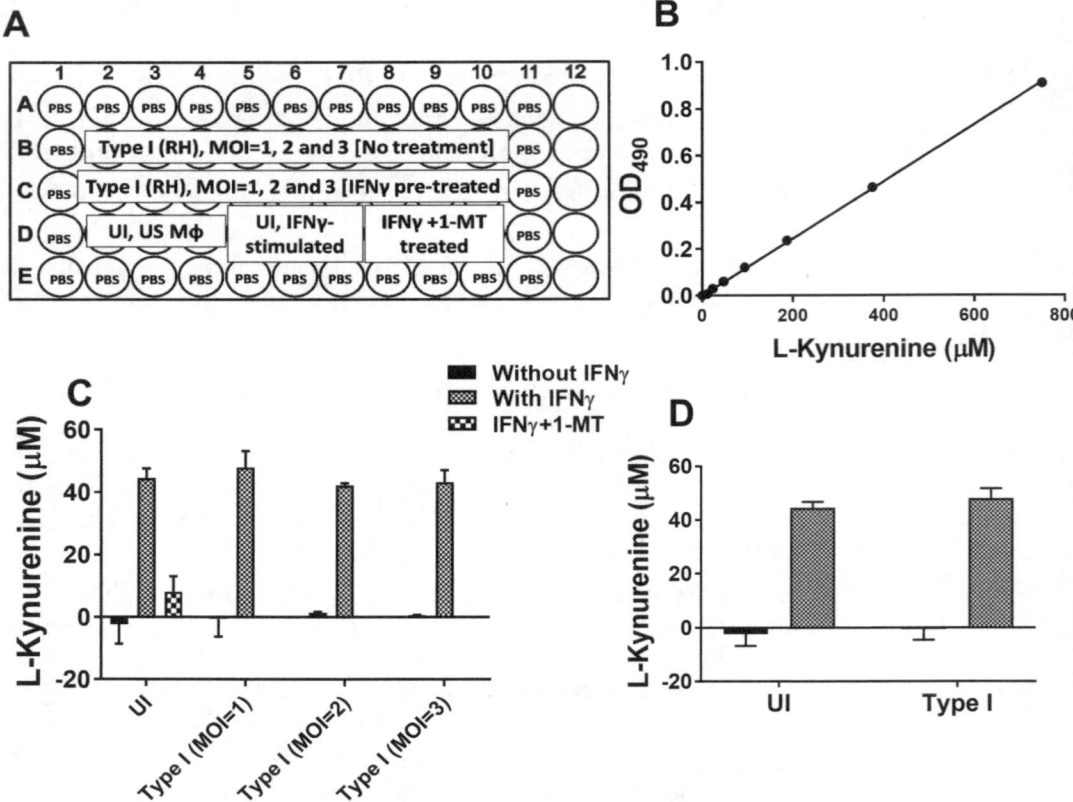

Fig. 3 Measurement of indoleamine 2,3 dioxygenase assay from the culture supernatant of IFNγ-stimulated cells. (**a**) A 96-well plate format for designing the IDO measurement experiment in IFNγ-stimulated *vs.* unstimulated *Toxoplasma*-infected cells. (**b**) Standard curve of L-kynurenine for calculation of L-kynurenine values from the supernatants collected from IFNγ-treated and untreated *Toxoplasma*-infected cells. (**c**) Bar diagram showing the amount of L-kynurenine produced from IFNγ-treated and untreated *Toxoplasma*-infected cells. (**d**) Comparison of L-kynurenine production between IFNγ-treated uninfected HFFs with IFNγ-treated and *Toxoplasma*-infected (at MOI of 1) HFFs

volume per well constant. The total volume should be 200 μL per well (Fig. 3a).

4. After 20–24 h of incubation, centrifuge the plate at 500 × *g* for 5 min at room temperature to make sure the medium is free of parasites and cells.

5. Transfer the 200 μL culture supernatant to a different 96-well plate using a multichannel pipette. In the original plate, where the cells and parasites have been incubated, add 25 μL lysis buffer mentioned in assay reagents point 3 (LDH assay protocol) to the wells to measure the parasite growth by luciferase. Seal the plate with a plate sealer and keep it in −20 °C for 1 week or at −80 °C for at least 1 month. Alternatively, freeze-thaw for 2–3 times and process the same day.

6. Now, transfer 150 μL of the culture supernatant to a 96-well V bottom plate and add 20 μL of TCA to all the wells of the V bottom plate. After sealing the plate with a plate sealer, incubate the plate at 50 °C for 30 min using a heating block. This incubation is to hydrolyze the N-formyl kynurenine produced from the catabolism of L-tryptophan to L-kynurenine. During this time, to the remaining 50 μL of the culture supernatant, add 50 μL of freshly prepared LDH reagent for measuring cell death or that plate could be stored at 4 °C for 1–2 weeks to measure the LDH activity later.

7. After 30 min of incubation, take out the plate and centrifuge the plate for 10 min at $600 \times g$. During this time dilute 5 M L-kynurenine to the following concentrations: 1500–750–375–187.5–93.8–46.9–23.4–11.72–5.86–0   μM each for triplicate wells as standards (100 μL per well). A typical standard curve of L-kynurenine is shown in Fig. 3b where the concentration of L-kynurenine is indicated on the X-axis and the net OD is indicated on the Y-axis.

8. Following centrifugation, transfer 100 μL of supernatant, taking care to not touch the bottom of the plate, to a new 96-well flat bottom plate. This is important because at the bottom of the wells, TCA precipitated proteins will be present. Therefore, to avoid protein contamination, it is recommended not to touch the bottom of the wells.

9. Add 100 μL of Ehrlich's reagent (1:1 ratio with the supernatant) to the wells and incubate for 10 min.

10. Measure the absorbance at 490 nm using a plate reader. The concentration of L-Kynurenine can be determined using the standard curve of L-KYNURENINE (Fig. 3c, d).

6   Notes

1. Differentiation of bone marrow-derived macrophages (BMDM) from bone marrow in vitro requires macrophage colony-stimulating factor (M-CSF). L929 is a murine fibroblast cell line that produces and secretes M-CSF and the filtered supernatant is described as L929 conditioned media, which needs to be added for the differentiation of BMDMs. Because the amount of M-CSF in L929 conditioned media can differ from batch to batch, it is recommended that the M-CSF is made in a large batch and its concentration is measured by ELISA. This batch should be frozen as 50 mL aliquots at −20 °C.

2. *Toxoplasma gondii* is an obligate intracellular parasite; therefore, it is usually cultured in a host cell for instance in HFFs. To

harvest a good number of viable parasites from the host cells, it is important to harvest parasites in large vacuole from intact HFFs (especially when working with non-RH parasites that are less viable outside a host cell). These infected cells can be lysed while passing the cells through a 27 and 30 G needle consecutively after scraping the cells from a T25 flask.

3. *Toxoplasma* type I (RH), type II (ME49), and type III strains (CEP) expressing GFP and luciferase can be used for the assay [15]. RH always grows faster than the other two types, so to synchronize the growth of parasite strains, always pass more parasites from previous flasks of parasites for type II and III compared to the RH strain. Also, during the infection type I RH parasites have a higher infectivity than type II and III; therefore, the MOIs used for RH should be lower than for type II and III. For instance, an MOI 3/5/7 for type II and III whereas for type I RH an MOI of 1/2/3 is used. A better choice for a type I strain might be the GT1 strain, as it is more similar to the type II and III strains in terms of infectivity.

4. IL-4 is a cytokine that when bound to its prototype receptor IL4R alpha (IL4Rα) triggers the phosphorylation and activation of STAT6. STAT6 activation induces macrophages to convert to M2 macrophages. STAT6 induces the expression of arginase in macrophages and dendritic cells [20].

5. Because *Toxoplasma* rapidly dies extracellularly (especially non-RH strains) the intended MOI determined by counting parasites with a hemocytometer often does not represent the number of parasites that are capable of infecting a cell. When comparing strains, it is therefore important to set up a plaque assay to get an indication of the infectivity of the parasites because many phenotypes are correlated with the infection load. For the plaque assay, usually 100 parasites for type I strain (RH), and 200–300 parasites for non-RH strains are added to 24-well plates with monolayers of HFFs and incubated for 4/5 days (RH) or 6/7 days (non-RH strains) after which the number of plaques is counted. Here it is important to note that if all the wells of the 24-well plates need to be used it is better to keep the plate in a sterile box with wet tissue papers because the medium from boundary wells can evaporate due to prolonged incubation time (4–6 days) of the assay. The infectivity of the parasites for each strain is determined from this plaque number (keeping in mind that each plaque is derived from a single parasite). Because macrophages were infected with different MOIs the "real MOI" for each strain can be matched and used to compare the arginase activity (Fig. 1c, d). For example, in the given example (Table 1), from the plaque assay if 100 parasites of the RH strain generate 70 plaques it means that the viability is 70%, that is, intended MOI of 1 in reality is

Table 1
Plaque assay result and viability matching

Strain type	Plaque number Well A	Well B	Well C	Average	% viability	Intended MOIs 1	2	3	5	7
						Real MOIs				
Type I (100 parasites)	62	71	77	70	70	0.7	1.4	2.1		
Type II (250 parasites)	46	40	34	40	16				0.5	**0.8**	1.1

Values marked in bold are viability-matched MOIs

0.7. On the other hand, if 250 type II parasites form 40 plaques, it means that the parasite viability is 0.16%, that is, intended MOI of 5 means real MOI of 0.8, the MOI 1 of RH strain should be compared with MOI 5 of type II strain (Table 1).

6. It is important to keep the incubation time fixed because the enzyme activity in international unit (IU) is calculated using the number of min used for incubation.

7. A monochromator-based plate reader can be used where all the wavelengths including 540 and 650 nm can be set. Otherwise a filter-based plate reader could be used, where a filter of 550 and 670 nm (for the background absorbance) is present.

8. If nonluciferase strains are used for infection, then to measure parasite growth in parallel, parasite/vacuole counting can be performed as a representative assay for parasite replication. This assay is done in a 24-well plate using coverslips as described by Iaconetti et al. [21].

9. The activity of IFNγ and TNFα usually varies between manufacturers. Thus, it is recommended that for the first time, a broad range of IFNγ and TNFα concentrations be tested to find the effective dose (EC_{50}, concentration at which parasite growth is reduced to 50%) for the experiment. Usually the working concentration of IFNγ and TNFα ranges between 10 and 100 U/mL. Commonly, recombinant IFNγ and TNFα comes at 100 μg to 1 mg per vial. To achieve the concentration in "Units/mL" the following formula can be used:

$$\text{Concentration in Units/mL} = \text{specific activity in Units/mg} \times \text{Concentration in mg/mL}$$

The IFNγ and TNFα stock concentration should be made 10^4 or 10^5 U/mL. It is recommended that each time an aliquot is taken out from −80 °C, the IFNγ and TNFα concentration that gives the same or similar result as in the first experiment be determined. This is important as the activity of IFNγ and TNFα can deteriorate over time. LPS should be dissolved in endotoxin-free sterile water at a concentration of 1–10 mg/ mL and should be aliquoted and stored in −20 °C for 6 months. Avoid repeated usage of IFNγ, TNFα, and LPS from same aliquot.

10. The usual recommendation for measurement of LDH using the kit from Roche, Sigma is to use 100 μL culture supernatant with 100 μL of LDH reagent. The important feature here is to keep the culture supernatant and LDH reagent ratio at 1:1.

11. A stock solution of 1 M DTT should be made by dissolving 1.54 g of DTT to 8 mL of deionized water and then make up to 10 mL. Following that, small aliquots of 0.1 mL could be made in small centrifuge tubes, wrapped in aluminum foil, and kept at −20 °C to avoid repeated freeze–thaw cycles.

12. If the luciferase assay will be performed later, it is recommended to add protease inhibitor cocktail 1× (Halt protease inhibitor cocktail from Thermo Fisher, without EDTA) to the lysis buffer. Add 25 μL of this lysis buffer to each well of the 96-well plates.

13. For all the assays, comparison between strain types or between wild-type vs. knockout strains should be interpreted with MOI matching by plaque assay as stated in arginase assay protocol. For the example given in Fig. 2b, c, it can be clearly seen that at different MOI the values are different. It is therefore recommended to keep a near constant MOI for repeated experiments (Fig. 2b, c). Therefore, MOI matching should be done using the plaque assay results as shown in Table 1.

14. The culture supernatant can be stored at 4 °C for 1–2 weeks for LDH measurement. However, it is better to measure it the day of collection. The plates should never be stored in −20 °C as this can decrease the LDH enzyme activity. Another important consideration is the use of media with FBS. FBS contains LDH, so using 10% FBS containing media can lead to high background compared to 1% FBS containing media. However, 10% FBS containing media is better for host cell health and metabolism. Thus, keeping media only wells at the end of incubation is important as a control.

15. It is important to use ultrapure LPS (ligand for Toll like receptor-4/TLR-4) as standard LPS can contain lipoproteins, which can also activate TLR-2 along with TLR-4 and thus can influence the result of the experiment.

16. LPS is an agonist of TLR-4 and activates the nuclear factor κB (NF-κB) transcription factors, leading to upregulation of the expression of the nucleotide-binding oligomerization domain, leucine-rich repeat, and pyrin domain containing protein (NLRP) 3 inflammasome gene (signal 1). Nigericin, a

potassium ionophore, acts as a second signal for assembly of the NLRP3 inflammasome complex and activation and cleavage of caspases 1 and 4 followed by cleavage and activation of gasdermin D, which makes pores in the cell membrane. This causes the cells to die in a process known as pyroptosis [22]. Thus, wells treated with LPS and nigericin together will act as a positive control for cell death.

17. The stock solution of L-tryptophan is dissolved in 0.1 N NaOH. This stock solution can subsequently be added directly into the media. In this case, control wells containing the appropriate amount of NaOH should also be added to the experimental setup.

18. To determine the specificity of IFNγ-mediated induction of IDO activity, an inhibitor of IDO, 1-methyl-L-tryptophan (1-MT), can also be used at a concentration of 1 or 2 mM [23].

References

1. Sica A, Mantovani A (2012) Macrophage plasticity and polarization: in vivo veritas. J Clin Invest 122(3):787–795. https://doi.org/10.1172/JCI59643

2. Hassan MA, Jensen KD, Butty V, Hu K, Boedec E, Prins P et al (2015) Transcriptional and linkage analyses identify loci that mediate the differential macrophage response to inflammatory stimuli and infection. PLoS Genet 11 (10):1–25

3. Sibley LD, Adams LB, Fukutomi Y, Krahenbuhl JL (1991) Tumor necrosis factor-alpha triggers antitoxoplasmal activity of IFN-gamma primed macrophages. J Immunol 147(7):2340–2345. http://www.jimmunol.org/content/147/7/2340.abstract

4. Murray PJ, Allen JE, Biswas SK, Fisher EA, Gilroy DW, Goerdt S et al (2014) Macrophage activation and polarization: nomenclature and experimental guidelines. Immunity 41 (1):14–20. https://doi.org/10.1016/j.immuni.2014.06.008

5. Pappas G, Roussos N, Falagas ME (2009) Toxoplasmosis snapshots: global status of *Toxoplasma gondii* seroprevalence and implications for pregnancy and congenital toxoplasmosis. Int J Parasitol 39(12):1385–1394. https://doi.org/10.1016/j.ijpara.2009.04.003

6. Lorenzi H, Khan A, Behnke MS, Namasivayam S, Swapna LS, Hadjithomas M et al (2016) Local admixture of amplified and diversified secreted pathogenesis determinants shapes mosaic *Toxoplasma gondii* genomes. Nat Commun 7:10147

7. Saeij JPJ, Boyle JP, Boothroyd JC (2005) Differences among the three major strains of *Toxoplasma gondii* and their specific interactions with the infected host. Trends Parasitol 21 (10):476–481

8. Jensen KDC, Wang Y, Wojno EDT, Shastri AJ, Hu K, Cornel L et al (2011) *Toxoplasma* polymorphic effectors determine macrophage polarization and intestinal inflammation. Cell Host Microbe 9(6):472–483. https://doi.org/10.1016/j.chom.2011.04.015

9. Rosowski EE, Lu D, Julien L, Rodda L, Gaiser RA, Jensen KDC et al (2011) Strain-specific activation of the NF-κB pathway by GRA15, a novel *Toxoplasma gondii* dense granule protein. J Exp Med 208(1):195–212. https://doi.org/10.1084/jem.20100717

10. Butcher BA, Fox BA, Rommereim LM, Kim SG, Maurer KJ, Yarovinsky F et al (2011) *Toxoplasma gondii* rhoptry kinase rop16 activates stat3 and stat6 resulting in cytokine inhibition and arginase-1-dependent growth control. PLoS Pathog 7(9):e1002236

11. Braun L, Brenier-Pinchart M-P, Yogavel M, Curt-Varesano A, Curt-Bertini R-L, Hussain T et al (2013) A *Toxoplasma* dense granule protein, GRA24, modulates the early immune response to infection by promoting a direct and sustained host p38 MAPK activation. J Exp Med 210(10):2071–2086. https://doi.org/10.1084/jem.20130103

12. Hurley JC, Tosolini FA, Louis WJ (1991) Quantitative limulus lysate assay for endotoxin and the effect of plasma. J Clin Pathol 44 (10):849–854

13. Davies JQ, Gordon S (2005) Isolation and culture of murine macrophages. Methods Mol Biol 290:91–103

14. Krishnamurthy S, Konstantinou EK, Young LH, Gold DA, Saeij JPJ (2017) The human immune response to *Toxoplasma*: autophagy versus cell death. PLoS Pathog 13(3):1–6

15. Boyle JP, Saeij JPJ, Boothroyd JC (2007) *Toxoplasma gondii*: inconsistent dissemination patterns following oral infection in mice. Exp Parasitol 116(3):302–305

16. Buttke TM, McCubrey JA, Owen TC (1993) Use of an aqueous soluble tetrazolium/formazan assay to measure viability and proliferation of lymphokine-dependent cell lines. J Immunol Methods 157(1–2):233–240

17. Cirelli KM, Gorfu G, Hassan MA, Printz M, Crown D, Leppla SH et al (2014) Inflammasome sensor NLRP1 controls rat macrophage susceptibility to *Toxoplasma gondii*. PLoS Pathog 10(3):e1003927

18. Saeij JP, Frickel EM (2017) Exposing *Toxoplasma gondii* hiding inside the vacuole: a role for GBPs, autophagy and host cell death. Curr Opin Microbiol 40:72–80

19. Pfefferkorn ER, Guyre PM (1984) Inhibition of growth of *Toxoplasma gondii* in cultured fibroblasts by human recombinant gamma interferon. Infect Immun 44(2):211–216

20. Sica A et al (2012) Mphage_M1-M2_rev_JCI2012. J Clin Invest 122 (3):787–795

21. Iaconetti E, Lynch B, Kim N, Mordue DG (2012) Determination of *Toxoplasma gondii* replication in naïve and activated macrophages. Bio Protocol 2(22):e289. https://doi.org/10. 21769/BioProtoc.289

22. Broz P, Dixit VM (2016) Inflammasomes: mechanism of assembly, regulation and signalling. Nat Rev Immunol 16(7):407–420

23. Niedelman W, Sprokholt JK, Clough B, Frickel EM, Saeij JPJ (2013) Cell death of gamma interferon-stimulated human fibroblasts upon *Toxoplasma gondii* infection induces early parasite egress and limits parasite replication. Infect Immun 81(12):4341–4349

Chapter 20

Methods for the Measurement of Early Events in *Toxoplasma gondii* Immunity in Mouse Cells

Catalina Alvarez, Ana Claudia Campos, Jonathan C. Howard, Joana Loureiro, Urs Benedikt Müller, and Ana Lina Rodrigues

Abstract

Critical steps in resistance of mice against *Toxoplasma gondii* occur in the first 2 or 3 h after the pathogen has entered a cell that has been exposed to interferon γ (IFNγ). The newly formed parasitophorous vacuole is attacked by the IFNγ-inducible IRG proteins and disrupted, resulting in death of the parasite and necrotic death of the cell. Here we describe some techniques that we have used to describe and quantify these events in different combinations of the host and the parasite.

Key words *Toxoplasma gondii*, Parasitophorous vacuole, Mouse, Innate immunity, IRG proteins, Interferon-γ, Diaphragm-derived cells, Reactive necrosis, Flow cytometry, Immunofluorescence

Abbreviations

CO_2	Carbon dioxide
DMEM	Dulbecco's modified Eagle's medium
EDTA	Ethylenediaminetetraacetic acid
FACS	Fluorescence-activated cell sorting
FBS	Fetal bovine serum
H_2O_2	Hydrogen peroxide
HEPES	4-(2-Hydroxyethyl)-1-piperazineethanesulfonic acid)
HFFs	Human foreskin fibroblasts = Hs27 cells
HI-FBS	Heat-inactivated fetal bovine serum
IFNγ	Interferon (IFN)-gamma
MMS	Multichannel microscope slide
MOI	Multiplicity of infection
NEAA	Nonessential amino acids
P/W buffer	Permeabilization/wash buffer (for intracellular staining for FACS)
PBS	Phosphate-buffered saline
PFA	Paraformaldehyde
RCF	Relative centrifugal force
RT	Room temperature

Christopher J. Tonkin (ed.), *Toxoplasma gondii: Methods and Protocols*, Methods in Molecular Biology, vol. 2071, https://doi.org/10.1007/978-1-4939-9857-9_20, © Springer Science+Business Media, LLC, part of Springer Nature 2020

SAG1   *Toxoplasma* major surface antigen 1 or P30
Sta   Staurosporine
T. gondii, Tg   *Toxoplasma gondii*
WD   Working dilution

1   Introduction

Our laboratory has concentrated on the early phases of tachyzoite invasion and residence in the parasitophorous vacuole with specific reference to the mouse IRG protein-based resistance mechanism. From this study it has become apparent that *Toxoplasma gondii* and the mouse coexist in an interesting evolutionary balance, due, presumably, to the fact that the *T. gondii* sexual stage now takes place largely in domestic cats, putting the house mouse in the firing line as an evolutionarily significant intermediate host for the parasite [1].

We present here some techniques that have facilitated this work over the last years. Protocols for isolation of mouse diaphragm cells and quantification of IRG loading on the PVM have been published in outline before but are shown here in more detailed or improved fashion. In addition, we describe a novel fluorescent necrosis reporter for use in live-cell microscopy and a flow cytometry-based method for quantifying host cell necrosis. We hope these techniques may be useful for the community and especially for newcomers to the field.

When a *Toxoplasma* tachyzoite enters a mouse cell it is enclosed in a vacuole whose membrane, the parasitophorous vacuole membrane or PVM, has just been invaginated from the host cell plasma membrane [2]. Since the entry itself takes less than 20 s, the PVM immediately after entry is probably in some respects similar to the plasma membrane, at least in lipid composition. However it differs both qualitatively and quantitatively from the plasma membrane in its protein content thanks to the action of the "moving junction" proteins at the point of entry [3]. These deplete certain classes of membrane protein from the PVM. The early PVM has also been detached from the cortical cytoskeleton of the host plasma membrane. Finally, components released from secretory organelles of the parasite into the host cell cytosol [4, 5] during entry associate rapidly with the cytosolic face of the PVM. Thus, the PVM, even a mere 20 s after its formation, is already distinctive in its properties and can no longer be considered representative of the plasma membrane. Most relevant for this study is that the recently formed PVM is now permissive for the binding of IRG proteins, unlike the plasma membrane from which it came. IRG proteins are interferon-inducible cytoplasmic GTPases that activate and assemble rapidly on the cytosolic face of the PVM of newly invaded *T. gondii*

[6]. They are essential for mouse survival following infection with all strains of *T. gondii*. By an unknown mechanism involving GTP hydrolysis, IRG proteins contribute to the deformation and ultimately the disruption of the PVM, resulting in death of the parasite and necrotic death of the infected cell [7].

Our studies have largely been conducted in mouse embryonic fibroblasts and other mesothelial cell types derived from disaggregated tissues. We have observed no distinctive behavior of tachyzoite entry or residence that appears to be related to the cell type involved. The literature indicates that macrophage lineage cells may be different from fibroblastic cells since the loading of the IRG resistance GTPases onto the PVM seems to be less efficient in inflammatory macrophages, where frequencies of vacuoles loaded with Irgb6 as low as 15% were reported [8], compared with up to 90% in our fibroblast assays [9].

During the hours following loading of IRG proteins the PVM becomes disrupted [6, 7], exposing the parasite to the cytosol and releasing whatever material may have been contained within the vacuole. Approximately 30 min after the disruption of the vacuolar membrane the permeability barrier of the parasite breaks down and cytosolic protein markers introduced into the infected cell, which until then, have been excluded from the parasite, suddenly enter the organism. We define this event as the death of the parasite. The infected cell itself is now committed to necrotic death, which follows within about 3 h after the disruption of the PVM.

These dramatic events are dependent on the genotypes of both the parasite and the host cell. Typically, genetic combinations in which IRG proteins load efficiently onto the PVM and disrupt it are "avirulent" in vivo, and favor a lifelong latent infection [7] while genetic combinations in which IRG proteins fail to load onto the PVM are "virulent" in vivo and are usually lethal for the host. Thus, hosts that successfully load IRG proteins onto the parasite can survive but their resistance is evidently not adequate to produce sterile immunity, and enough parasites survive to differentiate into bradyzoites and encyst in the brain.

The correlation between IRG protein loading, followed by vacuole disruption and host cellular necrosis is strong, and any or all of these events can be used to monitor the efficacy of a given *Toxoplasma*–host genetic combination without resorting to prolonged and ethically challenging lethality experiments in vivo. It is not yet clear whether every vacuole that is coated by IRG proteins eventually disrupts, although it seems unlikely since the intensity of IRG loading onto individual vacuoles is extremely variable, even within a single cell, from very intense to undetectable, with at least 10% of vacuoles appearing completely free from IRG proteins [9]. At least some organisms in nonloaded vacuoles escape from cells heading to necrosis and presumably survive, differentiate into bradyzoites and perhaps contribute preferentially to the formation of brain cysts. No explanation has yet been offered for the variation in the intensity of IRG loading onto individual vacuoles but it seems likely that it is adaptively regulated.

It is important to emphasize that necrosis assays, performed at 6–8 h after infection, in which necrosis is negatively correlated with virulence [7, 9], are completely distinct from plaque assays performed 5–7 days after infection, in which plaque number, representing cells disrupted by *Toxoplasma* multiplication and egress, is positively correlated with virulence [10].

2   Preparation of Diaphragm-Derived Cells (DDC) for *T. gondii* Infection (Catalina Alvarez and Urs Benedikt Mueller)

Fibroblasts such as mouse embryonic fibroblast (MEFs) or human foreskin fibroblasts (HFF) are commonly used for in vitro experiments to characterize cell-autonomous immunity to *Toxoplasma gondii*. However, MEFs are inconvenient cells to obtain for several reasons, including the requirement for timed pregnancies [11]. This can be a problem for mice recently derived from the wild, which do not breed as freely in laboratory conditions as laboratory strains, and timed pregnancies are hard to monitor. For our particular purpose we also needed a suitable cell line for in vitro experiments for characterizing individual freshly caught wild mice. We therefore modified a published methodology [12] to isolate fibroblasts from the diaphragm of single adult mice, which we term *d*iaphragm-*d*erived *c*ells or DDCs [13]. The diaphragm is a roughly triangular muscular membrane that separates the thoracic cavity from the abdominal organs in mammals (Fig. 1). We isolated pleural mesothelial cells (fibroblasts) from fresh diaphragm. We subsequently immortalize the cells by transfection with a plasmid containing the SV40 T-antigen.

It is important to appreciate that, like MEFs, DDCs are derived from a complex cell population, including macrophages. For at least two reasons the populations eventually obtained following the protocol below may show population-specific differences. First, the number of primary colonies from a single diaphragm is probably low, representing a small subset of the cells and cell populations in the original tissue. Second, the transfection procedure selects only a few cells from this complex population. In our experience the presumed heterogeneity in terms of cell subsets is not important for experiments on early *T. gondii* infection. But the ability of some DDC populations to adhere to glass cover slips does seem to be a variable, and weakly adherent cells can be hard to work with experimentally, especially for immunofluorescence. Efficient transfection with the immortalization plasmid is important to generate the most heterogeneous DDC populations. Long-term culture of immortalized DDCs undoubtedly adds another phase of selection and loss of heterogeneity. Similar considerations of course also apply to fresh and transformed MEFs.

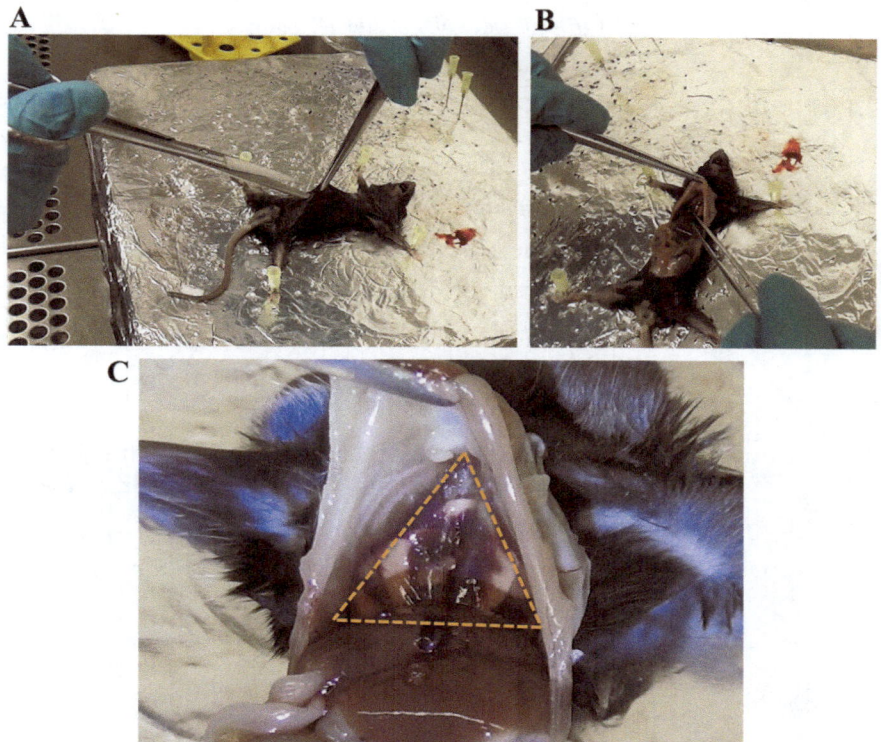

Fig. 1 Mouse diaphragm dissection. (**a**) Opening of the peritoneal cavity. (**b**) Visualization of the diaphragm membrane. (**c**) Triangular shaped-diaphragm membrane

2.1 Materials

Prepare all cell culture materials under sterile conditions and preferably work with autoclaved surgical instruments. If this is not possible, rinse instruments with ethanol and burn with a Bunsen burner before use.

Tissue isolation material

1. Isoflurane.

2. Surgical tools: forceps, scissors, and scalpel blades.

3. Ethanol 70% (EtOH).

Tissue digestion

4. Collagenase (0.1 U/ml)/Dispase (0.8 U/ml). Working solution: 100 mg/ml. Roche Diagnostics.

5. 1× trypsin–EDTA sterile filtered.

6. Syringe filter Acrodisc (25 mm), sterile, membrane pore size 0.2 μm.

7. 5 ml sterile syringe.

Cell plating and cell culture material

8. Dulbecco's modified Eagle's medium (DMEM), high glucose w/o L-glutamine w/o sodium pyruvate. N.B. *DMEM contains 3.7 g/l NaHCO₃and is buffered to pH 7.4 in an atmosphere of 10% CO₂at 37°C.*

9. Heat-inactivated fetal bovine serum (HI-FBS).

10. L-glutamine (200 mM).

11. Sodium pyruvate (100 mM).

12. 100× MEM nonessential amino acids w/o L-glutamine (NEAA).

13. 100× penicillin–streptomycin.

    Growth medium: DMEM supplemented with 10% HI-FBS, 1× NEAA, 1× penicillin–streptomycin, 1 mM sodium pyruvate, and 2 mM L-glutamine.

14. 1× phosphate-buffered saline (PBS) sterile w/o calcium and magnesium.

15. Flat bottom tissue-culture treated 6-well plates.

16. Sterile 6 cm petri dishes.

17. Pipette filter tips (20, 200, and 1000 μl).

18. Serological pipettes (5 and 10 ml).

19. 1.5 ml sterile microcentrifuge tubes.

20. Cell culture incubator maintained at 37 °C with 10% CO₂.

21. Eppendorf ThermoMixer® at 37 °C with at least two speeds: 900 and 750 rpm.

22. Centrifuge at RT for microcentrifuge tubes.

Cell immortalization

23. ScreenFect®A Transfection Reagent kit (InCella) [14].

24. Plasmid DNA: pSV3-neo plasmid [15]. ATCC reference 37,150 (https://www.addgene.org/vector-database/4267/).

2.2 Methods

2.2.1 Isolation of DDCs

1. Anesthetize the mouse using Isoflurane and kill it, normally by cervical dislocation. Spray the abdomen of the mouse with 70% EtOH.

2. Cut the abdominal skin to expose the muscle wall and peel away from the abdominal surface. Open the peritoneal cavity by holding the mouse skin with tissue forceps and cutting through the peritoneal wall with fine scissors (Fig. 1a). Pull down the abdominal organs that impede a clear view of the diaphragm (liver, stomach, intestine, etc.) to reveal the diaphragm, which is the thin membrane separating the peritoneal cavity from the thoracic cavity (Fig. 1b). Hold the sternum up

with forceps to stretch the triangular diaphragm and start cutting from bottom to top with fine scissors (Fig. 1c).

3. Wash the diaphragm with 3–5 ml of sterile $1\times$ PBS in the lid of a 6 cm dish to remove erythrocytes and transfer it to the base of the dish.

4. Using fine scissors, cut the diaphragm tissue into small pieces, as small as possible. It is advisable to use a pair of small sharp scissors for cutting with one hand and forceps in the other to hold the dish in place.

5. Add 1 ml of Collagenase/Dispase 1 mg/ml (25 µl of stock solution (100 mg/ml) in 2.5 ml of DMEM growth medium but without HI-FBS, filter with 0.2 µm syringe filter before adding to cells) to the diaphragm fragments in the dish. Cut the tip off a 1000 µl filter tip to take up all the Collagenase/Dispase along with the diaphragm fragments and transfer to a sterile 1.5 ml microcentrifuge tube.

6. Incubate the fragments of diaphragm in Collagenase/Dispase for 1 h at 37 °C using a ThermoMixer®. Shake the tube at 900 rpm and every 15 min remove the tube from the mixer and manually flip it a couple of times. Put the microcentrifuge tube back on the mixer.

7. Spin the microcentrifuge tube at low speed $(100 \times g$—800 rpm) for 10–15 s to pellet debris and transfer supernatant to a fresh sterile microfuge tube. The debris will form a smear on the side of the microfuge tube; it does not matter if some small pieces of debris come along with the supernatant.

8. Add 500 µl of sterile $1\times$ PBS to the remaining diaphragm debris, shake vigorously and spin again at low speed $(100 \times g$—800 rpm) for 10–15 s. Transfer supernatant to the tube with supernatant from **step 7**.

9. Add 1 ml of sterile $1\times$ Trypsin–EDTA solution to diaphragm debris and incubate for 1 h at 37 °C in the ThermoMixer®, shaking at 750 rpm for 1 h. Every 15 min flip the tube by hand a couple of times and put it back on the mixer.

10. In the meantime, spin down the tube containing the supernatants from the first incubation for 6 min at $(500 \times g$—1800 rpm). Take off supernatant (leave approximately 500 µl) carefully to avoid disturbing the cellular pellet.

11. Resuspend the pellet (it might look like a smear in a microfuge tube) in residual supernatant and plate out in one well of a 6-well plate. Add 2.5 ml of fresh complete DMEM growth medium with HI-FBS for a final volume of 3 ml per well.

12. To the suspension from **step 9**, add 500 µl of DMEM growth medium and plate out as a whole (diaphragm-debris + Trypsin–EDTA + DMEM growth medium) in another well. Add

1.5 ml of fresh DMEM growth medium to the well, for a final volume of 3 ml. Place the plate in a cell culture incubator at 37 °C (10% CO_2).

13. Change the medium from each well once a day for 3–4 consecutive days. After 24 h of incubation, there will be a lot of debris that will obscure growing cells that are attached to the plate surface. Therefore, from the second day resuspend the debris with a pipette and remove it with the supernatant before adding fresh medium.

14. Approximately 3–4 days after plating you will start to see small cell colonies growing. Cells might take up to 2 weeks to reach 60–80% confluence. At this point, cells are ready either to be frozen or immortalized.

2.2.2 Immortalization of DDCs by Transfection with pSV3-Neo Plasmid

1. The appropriate time to begin the transfection procedure is when the DDCs have reached 60–80% confluence. If cells have reached more than 80% confluence, it is recommended to detach them with 1× Trypsin–EDTA, split them 1:2, replate in growth medium in two new wells of a 6-well plate and allow them to reach 60–80% confluence.

2. Once cells are ready to be transfected, follow the manufacturer's instructions for the ScreenFect®A Transfection Reagent kit (*see* **Notes 1** and **2**) [14]. For this immortalization protocol we use the pSV3-neo plasmid. The transfection of fibroblasts with the pSV3-neo plasmid has been widely used for immortalization [16]. The kanamycin-resistant plasmid carries genes coding for the immortalizing SV40 large T-antigen and neomycin resistance as a dominant eukaryotic selection marker (which is not exploited in this protocol) [15].

   The plasmid DNA amount for cells growing in one well from a 6-well plate is 1000 ng. If you have a low number of cells, it is recommended to perform this transfection protocol in a 24-well plate format instead. The plasmid DNA amount in this case must be scaled down accordingly.

3. Place the plate in a cell culture incubator at 37 °C (10% CO_2) and replace the medium after 48 h.

4. Passage cells to a bigger container (e.g., cell culture flasks T25) and subculture them at least five times more to ensure all cells are indeed immortalized.

5. Cells are resuspended in 10% dimethyl sulfoxide (DMSO) in FCS and frozen at −80 °C under standard cell-freezing conditions, and a week later transferred to liquid nitrogen for long-term storage.

3   Measuring the Loading of IRG Proteins onto the Parasitophorous Vacuole Membrane (Ana Lina Rodrigues)

Much of our work in this field has been concerned with quantitative aspects of the loading of IRG proteins on to the parasitophorous vacuole membrane: its timing, its intensity, and cooperativity between different IRG proteins. Some of these experiments can be done with a simple "yes/no" read-out by direct microscopical observation of individual vacuoles and IRG proteins made visible via specific anti-IRG reagents and fluorescent second-stage detection reagents. However, while the determination of a strong "yes" is usually clear, a "no" may be harder to determine. The resolution of such an approach depends on the level of background, and this varies from antibody to antibody and from IRG protein to IRG protein. To provide a more objective criterion, it is appropriate to use a quantitative method that gives a numerical readout of the brightness of the PVM compared with the adjacent cytosol representing background. The method we describe below is designed to provide this data.

Slides are prepared carrying *Toxoplasma gondii*-infected cells, normally MEFs, DDCs (see protocol above) or other cells with a flat profile optimal for quantitative microscopy, fixed either with paraformaldehyde or occasionally with methanol. These cells are then permeabilized and stained with antibody reagents specific for one or more IRG proteins, followed by an appropriate fluorescent second stage reagent. Infected cells are photographed in a standard fluorescence photomicroscope (recently we have been using quasi-monochromatic illumination from a Zeiss Colibri system, outlined below) and subsequent analysis is conducted from stored images. Using stored images for the analysis has advantages and disadvantages. The principal advantage is that prolonged inspection and photography of individual cells in real time causes fluorescence fading. Furthermore, survey images can be collected at relatively low magnification, from which individual vacuoles can subsequently be identified for quantitation from a single image. The disadvantage in using survey images is that the focal plane may not be ideal for all vacuoles, leading to lack of resolution and loss of signal intensity, and images may be pixelated following enlargement for quantitative analysis.

These competing objectives can be reconciled with scanning at higher magnification to identify vacuoles using an antibody system to detect intracellular organisms with an excitation wavelength distant from the absorption optimum of the fluorochrome-conjugated second antibody detecting the IRG-specific antibody under test (*see* below).

A disadvantage intrinsic to this approach in general is vacuole selection. There are several criteria that need to be satisfied for a valid measurement, including: orientation of the vacuole, integrity of the PVM, and the definition of intracellularity. Choosing among these increases subjectivity that can damage the scientific outcome. Fully automatic software-mediated approaches to vacuole identification avoid subjectivity at the scanning stage but need great care in validation.

The best defense against subjective bias as well as fading fluorochromes is to use different fluorochromes to identify intracellular organisms, and to quantify IRG protein loading. We use the secreted *T. gondii* dense granule protein, GRA7, which rapidly accesses the cytosolic face of the PVM after parasite entry, is closely colocalized with IRG proteins at the PVM [6], and appears to be expressed by all intracellular *T. gondii*. We use a rat monoclonal antibody against GRA7, detected with a fluorescent secondary anti-rat Ig reagent excited at 647 nM, in the far red, and detection of IRG proteins with a secondary anti-Ig reagent excited at 488 nM. With quasi-monochromatic excitation using the Zeiss "Colibri" there is no cross-excitation and therefore no fading in the green channel. To minimize bias with this approach, the observer commits to score IRG proteins on any vacuole that is selected based on GRA7 expression.

It is difficult to stress adequately the absolute necessity of counting IRG-positive vacuoles or estimating their fluorescence intensity on coded slides. Without this security, subjective considerations play an alarmingly important role in such an analysis. However, in this context, a fully automated method for quantification of the amount and to some extent also location of fluorescent protein on the PV of *T. gondii* has been described recently [19]. The HRMAn (Host Response to Microbe Analysis) system is an open-source image analysis platform based on machine learning algorithms that quantifies the radial fluorescence intensity distribution around a vacuole. With this versatile system identification of the PV itself is also fully automatic. The identification of individual vacuoles may be subject to machine bias but this is certainly preferable to observer bias. We have not yet implemented this approach, but it could be useful in analyzing future data sets.

In our first quantitative analysis of the loading of the *T. gondii* PVM with IRG proteins we used a simple manual method allowing reading of maximum pixel intensities at the PVM itself [9]. The method had limitations, being sensitive to the focal plane and to small variations in fluorescence intensity at the PVM. More recently we have been using a semiautomated system for the measurement of fluorescence at the PVM, using the Image J Fiji toolbox [20]. The approach concentrates on proteins optically in focus at the PVM, however it also includes some out of focus and scattered light associated with the vacuole.

Fields of view were selected for photography on the basis of expression of the *T. gondii* secreted protein, GRA7, indicating intracellular organisms. Images of infected cells were then captured automatically in all relevant channels at ×40 or ×63 magnifications. To automate the measurement of fluorescence in the PV, PVM and the host cytosol in the immediate vicinity of the PVM, we created an ImageJ macro (Appendix 3). The macro assumes images were loaded into ImageJ in composite mode (all relevant colors) after achromatic pixel-shift correction to optimize overlay. The following operations are performed:

1. Defining the PV: Parasite images, identified by the observer and indicated by a mouse click, are segmented. The observer defines the PV manually by varying the "tolerance." The macro extends the definition of the PV by 0.1 μm into the cytosol to generate a Region of Interest (ROI), visible as a line corresponding to the identified PV. The ROI is then stored in ImageJ's ROI manager with the designation "PV."

2. Defining the cytosol: The macro creates a new ROI corresponding to the band of 1 μm of cytoplasm around the ROI PV (Fig. 2). The new ROI is stored in ROI manager as "Cytosol"—this will be used to obtain an estimate of the background signal in the cytosol. *See* caption to Fig. 2 for further detail.

3. Defining the PVM: The macro now creates automatically another ROI corresponding to a band of 0.8 μm of PV inside the ROI "PV" stored in ROI as "PVM."

The macro is fully documented and can easily be customized to other imaging scenarios, for example, when the order of channels is different or if the user wants a band around the PV of a different width. The table with results contains several different measurements (PV, PVM, and cytosol). These include fluorescence intensities (Mean, StDev, Min, Max, and Modal fluorescence intensities; in arbitrary units) and shape descriptors such as Feret's diameter (max and min; in microns) and circularity.

3.1   Methods

1. Open the software Fiji. Create a new Macro with the script available in Appendix 3 (copy/paste or type it).

2. Open the composite fluorescent or confocal image in the .Czi or .Tif format.

3. Run the Macro and follow the instructions given by Fiji.

4. Turn off unwanted channels and leave the reference channel.

5. Define the channel to detect PV, normally GRA7 in far red.

6. Click on the PV.

7. Double click and activate the wand tool to segment semiautomatically the PV. Adjust the tolerance if is necessary. You can also use freehand selections to draw the PV.

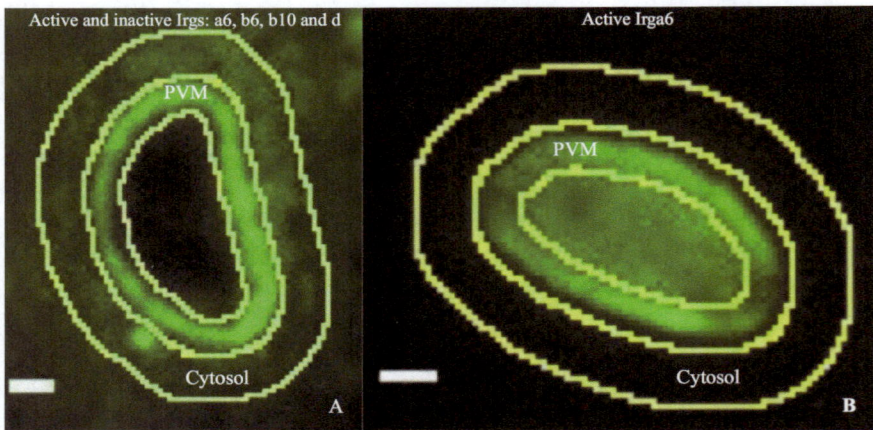

Fig. 2 Quantification of IRG proteins present on the PVM of avirulent *T. gondii* in IFNγ-stimulated mouse cells. Fluorescence intensity of IRG proteins at the PVM was quantified in intracellular (GRA7-positive) vacuoles using the 165, 141, 940, and 81 rabbit antibodies against Irga6, Irgb6, Irgb10, and Irgd, respectively, simultaneously detected with a fluorescent secondary anti-rabbit Ig reagent (**a**); and the mouse monoclonal antibody 10D7 against vacuolar Irga6 detected with a fluorescent secondary anti-mouse Ig reagent (**b**). The scale bar represents 1 μm. To measure the intensity of IRG signal on *T. gondii* PVs, we employed Fiji 2.0.0-rc69/1,52i software and a MACRO designed to allow parasite segmentation from the cytosol and rapid analysis of numerous PVs (see main text for details). The pixel intensity was defined as the total excess pixel intensity on the PVM after background subtraction. The background signal in the cytosol is an important variable. In panel (**a**) Irga6, Irgb6, Irgb10, and Irgd proteins were detected together using rabbit antisera that detect cytosolic, inactive IRG proteins as well vacuolar, activated proteins. In this example, the cytosolic background is markedly brighter than the out-of-focus center of the vacuole, which appears black, although the excess signal on the PVM is still clear. This high background is a composite of cytosolic IRG proteins and nonspecific binding of the four rabbit antisera employed. In panel (**b**) Irga6 was detected using the mouse monoclonal antibody, 10D7, which detects only activated Irga6 at the vacuolar membrane [21]. In this case, the cytosol is black, and the out-of-focus center of the vacuole is clearly visible. To deal with these important technical variations, the MACRO defines and excludes the center of the vacuole from the estimation of brightness, so only the in-focus vacuolar membrane ring is compared only with the cytosolic background

8. Transfer the results to a Microsoft Excel file. The vacuole brightness is given as the total brightness over the area of the "PVM" ROI minus the mean of the cytosolic intensity values per unit area of the "Cytosol ROI" calculated over the total area of the PVM ROI. The value is used as readout for the amount of protein recruited to each PVM (Fig. 2).

$$\text{Corrected brightness of vacuole} = x - Ay/B$$

where $x =$ total light from PVM ROI, $y =$ total light from cytosol ROI, $A =$ area of PVM ROI and $B =$ area of cytosol ROI.

4 Necrotic Death of *T. gondii*-Infected Cells: Quantification by Live-Cell Microscopy (Ana Lina Rodrigues and Joana Loureiro)

4.1 Necrosis Quantification by Live-Cell Microscopy Using Propidium Iodide (PI) (Ana Lina Rodrigues)

Because the disintegration and permeabilization of the nuclear membrane in necrotic cells allows the red-fluorescent DNA-intercalating agent PI to access the nucleus, we can calculate a necrosis rate based on the number of nuclei which become stained by PI over time by live-cell microscopy.

4.1.1 Cell Culture Reagents

1. Cells (MEFs, DDCs, HFFs, etc.) are cultured in complete DMEM (DMEM supplemented with 10% heat-inactivated fetal bovine serum or HI-FBS, 2 mM glutamine, 1 mM sodium pyruvate, nonessential amino acids, and penicillin/streptomycin).

2. *T. gondii* tachyzoites.

3. Sterile Phosphate buffer saline (PBS).

4. Stock solution of mouse (Cat. 315-05 Peprotech) or human IFNγ (Cat. SRP3058 Sigma-Aldrich) (*see* **Note 3**).

5. Multichannel microscope slides (MMS) (6-channel μ-Slide VI$^{0.4}$ slides from IBIDI Cat No. 80606). Crucially, an MMS allows growth and/or infection of host cells under different conditions in parallel assays and simultaneous live-cell imaging.

6. Sterile endotoxin-free centrifuge tubes ranging from 0.5 to 50 ml.

7. Sterile serological pipettes (5 and 10 ml).

8. Cell culture incubator maintained at 37 °C and with 10% CO_2.

9. Centrifuge at 20 °C with adjustable acceleration and deceleration.

10. 3 μm pore size filter (Nucleopore Cat No. WHA110612).

11. Plastic filter holders (Whatman Swin-Lok^{TM} WHA420200).

4.1.2 Assay Reagents

1. PBS.

2. PI solution (WD = 0.1 mg/ml). The PI stock solution should be at 1 mg/ml and kept in the dark in small aliquots at 4 °C.

3. HEPES solution (WD = 20–25 mM). The HEPES 1 M stock solution should be kept at 4 °C at 7.2–7.5 pH.

4. Hoechst 33342 (WD = 1 μg/ml). A stock solution at 1 mg/ml should be kept in the dark and at 4 °C.

4.1.3 Methods

Preparation of Cells
for Necrosis Quantification
Using PI

Day -2. Seed primary or immortalized adherent cells: 2×10^4 Immortalized MEFs, 1.5×10^4 DDCs/well or 2.5×10^4 HFFs per well of an IBIDI μ-Slide VI$^{0.4}$ multichannel microscope slide.

Day -1. Where appropriate, stimulate cells with mouse IFNγ at 40 ng/ml (200 U/ml) or human IFNγ at 50 ng/ml for 18–24 h.

Day 0. Infect cells with the appropriate strain of *T. gondii* tachyzoites at the desired multiplicity of infection (MOI) (*see* **Note 4**) and image.

1. Prior to infection of mouse/human cells, the tachyzoite suspension obtained from Hs27 cell cultures is filtered through a 3 μm pore size filter. This step ensures that only "clean" parasites, that is, parasites free of host cell debris, namely nuclei, are used, as the latter could interfere with the quantification of dead cells.

2. Add an appropriate amount of the filtered tachyzoites in complete DMEM supplemented with 0.1 mg/ml of PI, Hoechst 33342 at 1 μg/ml, and 25 mM HEPES (*see* **Note 5**) to target cells. Whereas PI accumulates only within necrotic cells, the cell-permeant nuclear counterstain Hoechst 33342 is used to assess the total number of cells, facilitating determination of the percentage of necrotic cells in real-time.

Acquisition of Images
for Necrosis Quantification
Using PI

Until such time as you wish to begin necrosis monitorization, cells can be returned to the incubator. To initiate live-cell imaging of parasite infection and host cell necrosis, place the IBIDI plate on the stage of an epifluorescence microscope equipped with a digital camera and imaging software and a heat source to maintain cells at 37 °C (*see* **Note 6**). Allow the microscope to acquire images at the appropriate time intervals. We typically perform live cell imaging of the infected cells with pictures taken at ~4–5.5 min intervals for no longer than up to ~8–10 h postinfection. Snap pictures of several positions within different channels of the plate to include proper controls and an adequate number of samples and events for necrosis quantification. This method allows quantification of necrosis in IFNγ-stimulated C57BL/6J DDCs infected with avirulent *T. gondii* (Fig. 3).

Quantification of Necrotic
Cells Using PI

Use Image J, Fiji or other software to count red nuclei.

1. Open the red channel of the Image time 0.

2. In the software use a Color Threshold option and establish the value that adapts better to your cell's nuclei size and analyze particles (red nucleus). Do the same for the last time point.

3. The total of necrotic cells is given as the total of necrotic cells observed in the images taken at the last time-point minus the total seen at time 0. Perform the same procedure for each position.

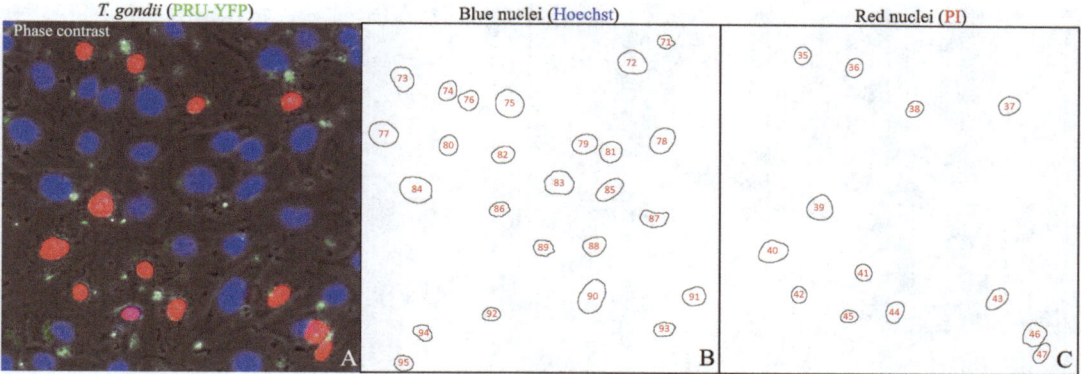

Fig. 3 Live-cell microscopy-based dual parameter tracking of IFNγ-dependent fibroblast necrosis in response to *T. gondii* infection. C57BL/6J mouse DDCs were infected with ME49 tachyzoites (MOI = 3). 100 μg/ml PI and 1 μg/ml Hoechst were added to identify necrotic and intact nuclei, respectively. Panel (**a**) shows merged images obtained from the combination of the Hoechst channel (blue), the PI channel (red), and the phase contrast channel of DDCs at 3 h after infection. Particles in the blue and red channels were defined by color threshold using Fiji 2.0.0-rc69/1,52i software and absolute numbers of blue nuclei in panel (**b**) or red nuclei in panel (**c**) were counted to obtain a necrosis proportion within the cell population (see text)

4. To obtain a necrosis rate, besides the number of necrotic cells one must determine the total number of cells: the latter can be gauged by counting the number of blue (Hoechst) labeled nuclei using the UV channel. Repeat **steps 1** and **2** for time point 0. The proportion of necrotic cells is given as the Total of Necrotic cells × 100 divided by the total of cells in time 0.

$$\%NC = \frac{TNC \times 100}{TC}.$$
TNC = Total necrotic cells.
TC = Total cells.
NC = Necrotic cells.

4.2 Discrimination of Live and Necrotic Cells by Live-Cell Microscopy Using an HMGB1-GFP Reporter (Joana Loureiro)

Release of the chromatin-binding high mobility group Box 1 protein (HMGB1) from the nucleus of cells with a damaged permeability barrier is an established marker for necrotic death [22]. Indeed HMGB1 was found in supernatants of IFN-γ-stimulated mouse fibroblasts undergoing necrosis induced by *T. gondii* infection [23]. We therefore decided to use a green fluorescent protein (GFP)-tagged HMGB1 fusion protein as a convenient live-cell microscopy reporter to monitor necrosis of *Tg*-infected cells in real time. HMGB1-GFP, released from necrotic cell nuclei, can thus become a necrosis marker complementary to propidium iodide staining, which is a positive marker for the same process.

An HMGB1-GFP fusion protein was demonstrated to be fully functional [24] and therefore we developed a reporter construct consisting of the murine HMGB1 gene with an in-frame C-terminal eGFP moiety. A detailed description of the cloning strategy for the HMGB1-GFP fusion protein is provided in Fig. 3.

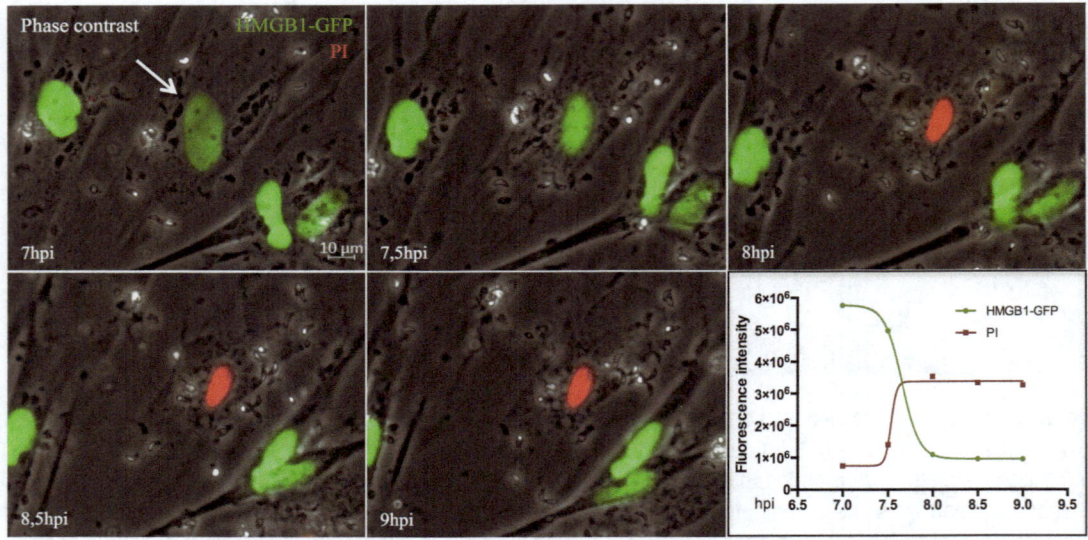

Fig. 4 Nuclear HMGB1-GFP leaks from the nuclei of IFNγ-stimulated fibroblasts undergoing necrosis upon infection with avirulent *T. gondii*. Representative images of a live-cell microscopy experiment using HFFs stably expressing the HMGB1-GFP reporter after infection with ME49 tachyzoites (MOI = 5). Time after tachyzoite addition to Hs27 cells is shown in hours postinfection (hpi). 100 μg/ml PI was added to identify necrotic nuclei. Shown are merged images obtained from the combination of the HMGB1-GFP channel (green), the PI channel (red), and the phase contrast channel. Note that several parasites seem to egress from the dying cell. The graphic inset depicts quantification of the HMGB1-GFP and PI levels in the nucleus of an individual cell undergoing necrosis (white arrow). Green or red channel fluorescence intensity was measured over time using Fiji 2.0.0-rc69/1,52i software. Shown are integrated curves of the green and red pixels found in the indicated nucleus over time

Use of the reporter necessitates generation of cell lines expressing the HMGB1-GFP fusion protein. We tested both transfection and retroviral vector-mediated transduction as methods for gene delivery for the mammalian cell lines we most frequently use (MEFs, DDCs, HFFs, HeLa). We found retroviral transduction to be the best method. We detail the protocols for packaging the HMGB1-GFP-retrovirus in competent HEK293T cells and for infecting target cells, as well as the analysis of fusion protein expression in mammalian cells in Fig. 9.

Expression of the HMGB1-GFP fluorescent reporter in murine or human fibroblasts and live-cell microscopy analysis allows the simultaneous monitoring of the cellular disintegration features that accompany necrosis [28] and HMGB1 release from necrotic cell nuclei. Additional use of (red) PI staining provides a dual fluorescence parameter-based assessment: as nuclear HMGB1-GFP (green) fluorescence is lost, necrotic cell nuclei become PI-positive (red) (Fig. 4).

The percentage of necrotic cells can be quantified, as shown in Fig. 5, by application of the procedure detailed in Fig. 4c.

We have validated this method in conditions in which necrosis or apoptosis of murine/human fibroblasts are chemically induced:

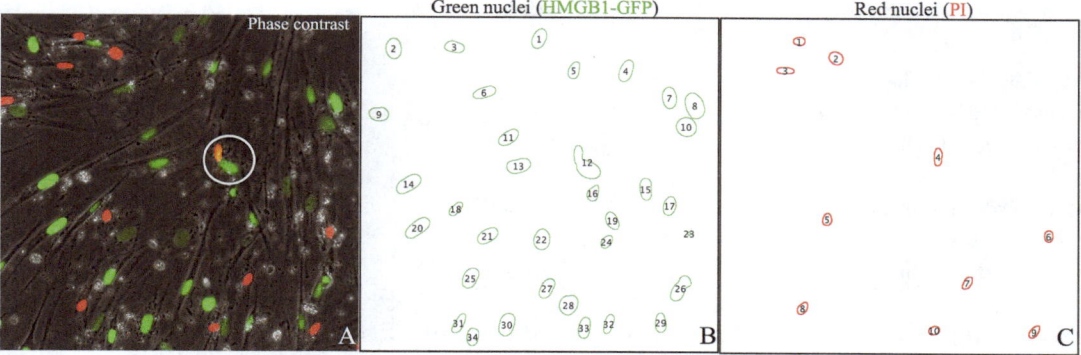

Fig. 5 Live-cell microscopy-based tracking of nuclear HMGB1-GFP leakage from fibroblasts undergoing necrosis in response to *T. gondii* infection. Panels represent the quantification method used to assess necrosis at 7–9 h after *Tg* infection of HMGB1-GFP reporter-expressing HFFs used in the experiment depicted in this figure. Panel (**a**) shows merged images obtained from the combination of the HMGB1-GFP channel (green), the PI channel (red), and the phase contrast channel. Elements in the green and red channels were defined by color threshold using Fiji 2.0.0-rc69/1,52i software and absolute numbers of green nuclei in panel (**b**) or red nuclei in panel (**c**) are counted to obtain a necrosis proportion within the cell population (see text). The adjacent pair of cells highlighted in the white circle is not resolved in the green channel, which counts only a single nucleus. Such anomalies are easy to resolve by eye since we do not use this protocol to analyze very large numbers of cells. A more complex algorithm could resolve such anomalies automatically but as it stands this is a valuable opportunity to check the results with the raw data

leakage of the HMGB1-GFP reporter occurs from the nuclei of most cells within 2–4 h of addition of high levels of hydrogen peroxide, a known necrosis trigger, but is rare in cells treated with apoptosis-inducing amounts of staurosporine (data not shown).

4.2.1 Material

1. Cell lines (derived from MEFs, DDCs, HFFs, HeLa) expressing HMGB1-GFP following retroviral transduction. These are cultured in complete DMEM growth medium (DMEM supplemented with 10% heat-inactivated fetal bovine serum or HI-FBS, 2 mM glutamine, 1 mM sodium pyruvate, nonessential amino acids, and penicillin/streptomycin) containing the antibiotic blasticidin.

2. Multichannel microscope slides (MMS) (we use 6-channel μ-Slide VI$^{0.4}$ slides, IBIDI Cat No. 80606). These slides allow growth and/or infection of host cells under different conditions in parallel assays and simultaneous live-cell imaging.

3. Mouse (Cat. 315-05 Peprotech) or human IFNγ (Cat. SRP3058 Sigma-Aldrich) (*see* **Note 3**).

4. *T. gondii* tachyzoites.

5. Epifluorescence microscope equipped with a digital camera and imaging software (*see* **Note 3** below).

6. Microscope enclosure incubation chamber (with temperature and/or CO$_2$ control) (*see* **Note 5**).

7. Propidium iodide (optional).

4.2.2 Methods

Preparation of cells for
monitoring HMGB1-GFP
leakage (see Fig. 4a)

Acquisition of images for
monitoring HMGB1-GFP
leakage (see Fig. 4b)

Quantification of necrotic
cells monitoring HMGB1-
GFP leakage and/or PI

Use Image J, Fiji or other software to count red nuclei.

1. Open the red channel of the Image time 0.

2. In the software use a Color Threshold option and establish the value that adapts best to your cell's nuclei size and analyze particles (red nucleus). Do the same for the last time point.

3. The total of necrotic cells is given as the total of necrotic cells observed in the images taken at the last time-point minus the total seen at time 0. Perform the same procedure for each position.

4. To obtain a necrosis rate, besides the number of necrotic cells one must determine the total number of cells, given by counting the number of green (HMGB1-GFP)-labeled nuclei using the green channel at time 0. Repeat **steps 1** and **2** for time point 0. The proportion of necrotic cells (%NC) is given as the Total of Necrotic cells (TNC) × 100 divided by the total of cells in time 0.

$$\%NC = \frac{TNC \times 100}{TC}.$$

TNC = Total Necrotic cells.
TC = Total cells at Time 0.
NC = Necrotic cells.

5   A Flow Cytometric Method for Quantifying Host Cell Necrosis in Response to *T. gondii* Infection (Joana Loureiro)

5.1 Discrimination of Live and Necrotic Cells by Flow Cytometry

Microscopy-based methods allow elegant observation and timing of necrosis induced by infection of IFNγ-induced cells with avirulent *T. gondii*. We sought to develop a faster and more quantitative assay of *T. gondii*-induced necrosis using flow cytometry, with scatter characteristics and membrane permeability as criteria [28, 29]. Many institutions, including ours, do not have a flow cytometer inside a BCL level 2 containment, requiring us to fix infected cell preparations before fluorescence-activated cell sorting (FACS) analysis [30] and thus preventing use of propidium iodide as a simple live/dead discriminator in FACS. To overcome this limitation, we replaced PI with the Thermo Fisher Scientific LIVE/DEAD® fixable dead cell stains for flow cytometry, which are designed to assess membrane integrity in samples after fixation.

5.1.1 A Fixation-Permissive Method for Detecting Necrosis by Flow Cytometry

LIVE/DEAD® fixable dead cell stains, recently introduced by Thermo Fisher for light microscopic and FACS-based determination of necrosis, are non cell-permeant fluorescent amine-reactive dyes, which react with cellular proteins. In live and apoptotic cells with an intact permeability barrier, only surface proteins bind to the reactive dye, resulting in dim fluorescence; the reactive dye can enter cells with a damaged permeability barrier and label proteins in the interior of the cell, producing at least a 50-fold increase in fluorescence (Fig. 10a). The staining pattern is preserved following fixation of the sample with formaldehyde. Because the technique depends on the membrane permeabilization associated with necrosis, it does not record apoptotic cell death (Fig. 10b–d). LIVE/DEAD® dye use allows efficient identification of necrosis induced by *T. gondii* in IFNγ-stimulated mouse DDCs (demonstrated below).

5.1.2 Analysis of Necrosis and Tg Infection by Flow Cytometry

Three parameters dominate the induction of necrosis in IFN-γ-induced cells infected with *T. gondii*, the infectivity of the parasites, the identity of the target cells, and in mice the genetics of the cell/parasite combination ([13] *and our unpublished observations*). Some established cell lines have lost sensitivity to *T. gondii*-induced necrosis. Using a FACS-based assay, infection rates can be assessed directly, either using parasites tagged with a fluorescent label, or in the absence of an appropriate tagged strain, by an antibody directed against the parasite.

The FACS-based assay consists essentially of three steps: (1) incubation with a LIVE/DEAD® dye indicator of plasma membrane permeability (2) paraformaldehyde fixation, and (3) staining for a *Toxoplasma* antigen or alternatively using a parasite strain expressing a fluorescent protein. The gating strategy and analysis are schematized in Fig. 6. The initial gating screen, based on side and forward scatter, serves to eliminate free parasites and small cellular debris from the analysis (Fig. 6a). Scatter characteristics do not cleanly separate whole cells from cell debris [29]; too strict a gate may exclude some small size events due to small, rounded-up necrotic cells, while too lenient a gate may allow some acellular debris or free parasites to contaminate the data. The choice of gate is therefore at the discretion of the experimenter. If desired, putative cell doublets can also be eliminated using time of flight parameters (Fig. 6b). Cells defined by these parameters are finally analyzed in two fluorescent channels, one giving the infected status, the other giving the live/dead status (Fig. 6c–f). With appropriate gating the cell population can be resolved into two

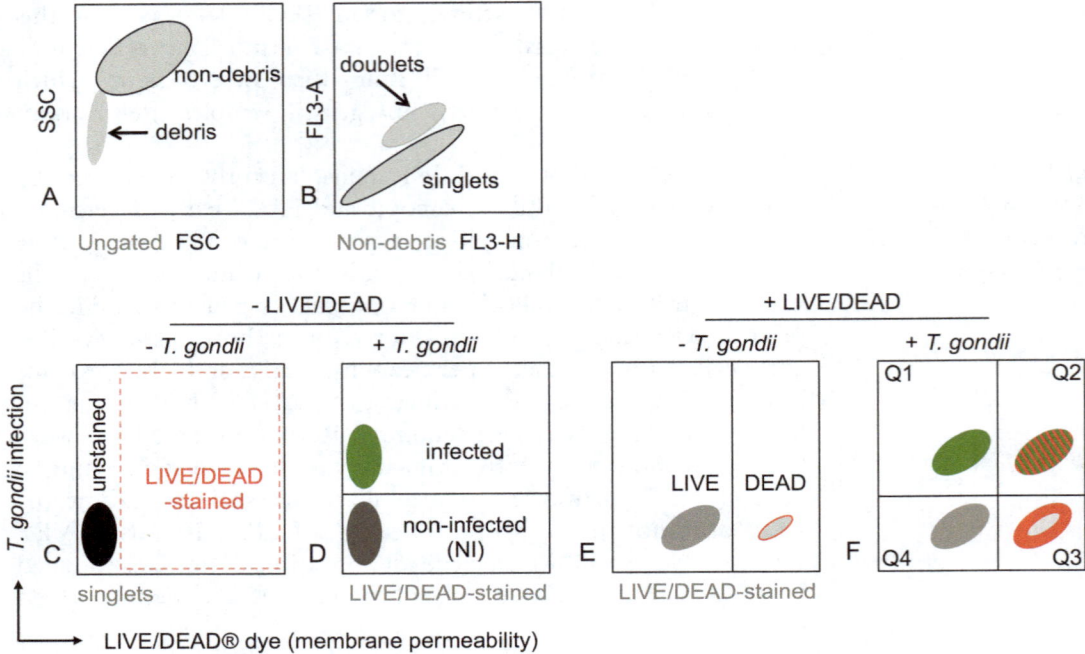

Fig. 6 Gating strategy for simultaneous detection by flow cytometry of *T. gondii*-induced necrosis and rate of infection. Using the forward scatter (FSC-H) (linear scale) and side scatter (SSC-H) (log scale) parameters, we gate out small particles (debris) (panel **a**). Cell doublets can be gated out (panel **b**) using different linear scale scatter parameters on a FORTESSA™ sorter or a fluorescent channel on a FACScalibur™. Unstained (-LIVE/DEAD), uninfected cells (*black* population) serve as a double-unstained compensation control to establish the LIVE/DEAD-stained gate (dashed red line), to which we restrict further analysis (panel **c**). We assess necrosis, that is, membrane permeability and infection levels on single cells using two-parameter (dual color fluorescence) density plots. Shown are hypothetical dot plot density profiles of cells either uninfected (− *T. gondii*) (dark grey population) or infected with Tg (+ *T. gondii*) (green population) but not incubated with LIVE/DEAD® dye (panel **d**). Panel **f** depicts hypothetical dot plots of cells incubated with the fixable LIVE/DEAD® dye (+LIVE/DEAD) prior to fixation and either uninfected (panel **e**) or infected (panel **f**). The light grey population represents the background of necrotic uninfected cells due to harvesting of adherent cells from culture dishes and manipulation during LIVE/DEAD® staining

sub-populations low or high for Tg antigen/marker (uninfected/infected, Fig. 6d) and two sub-populations low or high for live/dead (Fig. 6e). Upon gating on LIVE/DEAD-stained cells, as indicated in panel f of Fig. 6b four sub-populations arise: Quadrant Q4 contains the live, uninfected cell sub-population (dark grey), Q1 live infected cells (green), and Q2 necrotic infected cells (red and green stripes). With time after necrosis, the intracellular levels of parasite antigen or fluorescent protein from a tagged strain decrease. As a result, Quadrant Q3 contains necrotic cells that were infected and have lost the fluorescent marker (red). Quadrant Q3 also contains the background of necrotic uninfected cells found in all cell preparations harvested from plastic dishes and manipulated during LIVE/DEAD staining (Fig. 6f, light grey). The

L929 P2

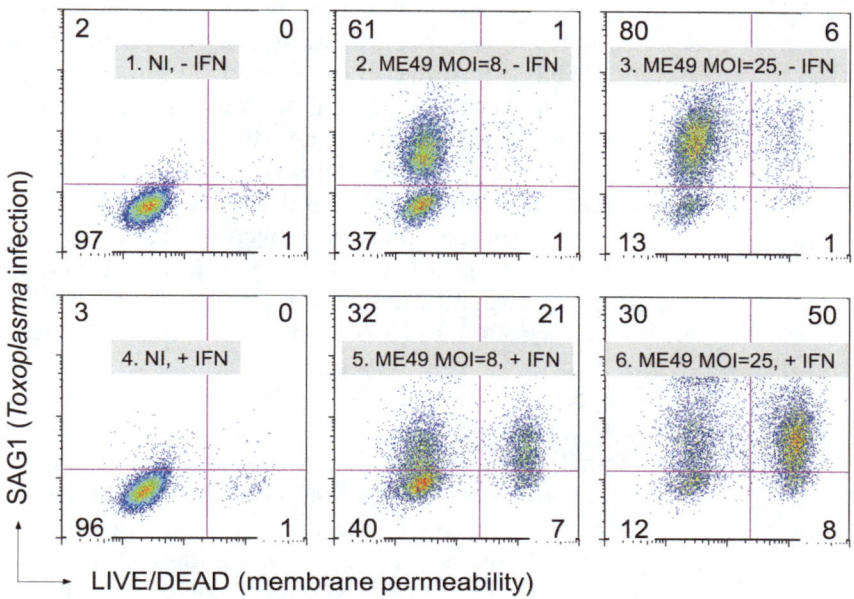

Fig. 7 The presence of IFNγ leads to host cell necrosis in response to avirulent *T. gondii* in an infection rate-dependent manner. Two-parameter pseudocolor dot plot display of L929 P2 subline fibroblasts infected with a low (MOI = 8) or high (MOI = 25) number of ME49 strain tachyzoites after 18–24 h of culture in the absence (top panels) or presence of 200 U/ml of IFNγ (bottom panels). After 8 h of infection, cells were harvested and labeled with Far Red LIVE/DEAD® stain and fixed in 4% PFA. Cells were then permeabilized and stained for *T. gondii* with the anti-p30/SAG1 TP3 MAb followed by an AF488-conjugated secondary Ab. The doubly stained population was gated as shown in Fig. 6 to eliminate free parasites and debris, as well as cell doublets. Fluorescence of 10^4 cells was measured in the FL4 (~661 nm) and FL1 (~530 nm) emission channels of a FACScalibur™ and analyzed by FlowJo 10.4 software. Control populations of uninfected cells (panels 1 and 4) and cells not induced with IFNγ (panels 1, 2, and 3) were handled similarly to determine background occupancy of the 4 analysis quadrants (Fig. 6, panel F)

proportion of infected cells is given by the ratio of Q1 + Q2 + Q3 to the total in all four quadrants, and the proportion of necrotic cells to infected live cells is given by the ratio of Q2 + Q3–Q1 + Q2 + Q3.

Figure 7 shows an example of data from analysis of necrosis in IFNγ-induced and uninduced L929 P2 fibroblasts (C3H/An strain) caused by infection with the avirulent ME49 *T. gondii* strain at two different multiplicities of infection (MOI). The infection burden within each sample is shown as intracellular levels of Tg major surface antigen 1 (SAG1 or protein P30) measured using a SAG1-specific primary antibody followed by a fluorescently conjugated secondary antibody. Unlike some L929 sublines that cannot resist *T. gondii* after induction with IFNγ, the P2 subline can control replication of the parasite [31] and, like other resistant

cells [7], dies by necrosis in the process. In this experiment uninduced L929 P2 cells showed 2% (panel 2) or 7% (Panel 3) of
necrotic cells (Quadrants 2 + 3) at the low and high MOIs of
8 and 25. The excess necrosis caused by ME49 infection in IFN-
γ-induced cells is recorded in the excess cells in Q2 and Q3 relative
to infected, live cells in Q1. Of the infected, IFNγ-induced cells
28%/60% (47%) are necrotic at an MOI of 8 (Panel 5) and 58%/
88% (66%) at an MOI of 25 (Panel 6). Increase in MOI is reflected
in a decrease in the number of uninfected cells in Q1. The small but
undoubtedly significant increase in necrotic cells in Q2 seen at high
MOI in the absence of IFNγ (Panel 3) is not explained. It may be
due to direct toxicity caused by multiple infection in these very
small cells, or to low levels of Type I IFN released by the infected
L929 P2 cells.

The proportion of cells in the background of uninfected
necrotic cells can be as low as 1–2% (as seen in this experiment in
Q3 in Panels 1 and 4) or as high as 10–15% depending on a number
of variables that are hard to control including the timing of the
experiment, the passage number and the cell type used. When the
background of uninfected necrotic cells is high it may be sensible to
correct the value in Q3 using the representation in Q3 from uninfected cells alone. With low necrotic backgrounds the correction of
Q3 is unnecessary, being well within the margin of gating error.

Figure 8 shows a similar experiment, this time with C57BL/6J
DDCs as the cells, infected alternatively with avirulent ME49 strain
(MOI = 25) or virulent RH strain (MOI = 15) parasites (the
different MOIs yielding roughly comparable infection rates were
chosen to accommodate the higher infectivity of RH strain parasites). Consistent with the fact that host cell necrosis occurs in
response to avirulent *T. gondii*, the data show a massive accumulation of IFNγ-induced cells infected with ME49 (Panel 5) in the
necrotic quadrants 2 + 3 (69%), compared with cells infected with
RH (14%) in the same two quadrants (Panel 6). The increase to
14% in necrotic cells infected with RH (Panel 6) compared with 3%
in the IFN untreated cells (Panel 3), while not large, is undoubtedly
real and presumably reflects the published observation that around
8% of RH vacuoles are fully and heavily loaded with IRG proteins,
and can be disrupted [9]. In this experiment the infection rate with
ME49 is notably higher in the IFNγ-induced cells (88% Panel 5)
than in the uninduced cells (64% Panel 2). With DDCs and MEFs
the dot clouds are more dispersed than in the case of L929 cells,
and there is a small but significant necrotic cell background of 5% in
the IFNγ-induced population (in Panel 4). In such a case it is
perhaps sensible to employ a simple correction for the uninfected
background contamination of Q3. In this example, Panel 4 showed
that a population of 88% in Q4 generates a population of 5% in Q3.
Thus in panel 6, the 33% uninfected live cells in Q4 would imply a
proportional contribution to Q3: that is, $(5/88) \times 33 = 1.9\%$. This

C57BL/6J

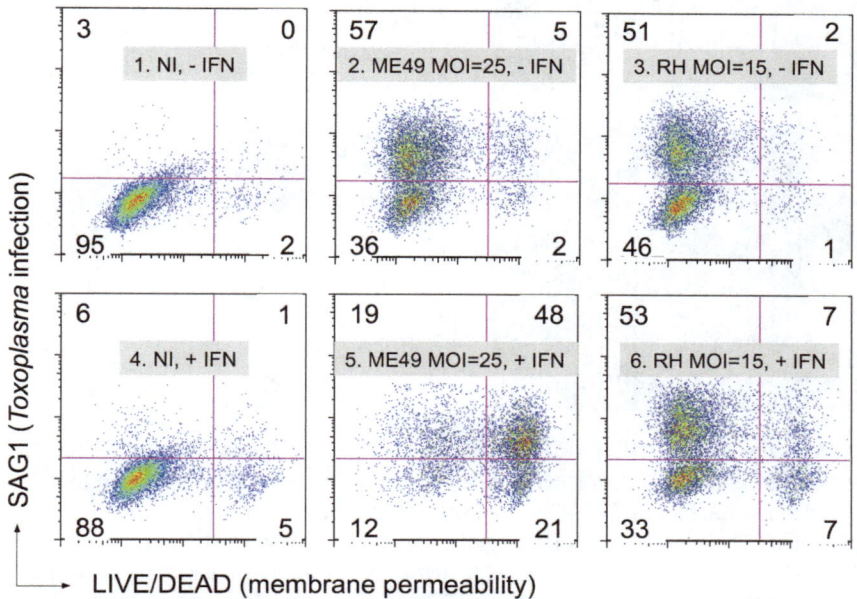

SAG1 (*Toxoplasma* infection)

LIVE/DEAD (membrane permeability)

Fig. 8 IFNγ-dependent host cell necrosis occurs in response to avirulent (ME49) but not virulent (RH) *T. gondii* tachyzoites. Two-parameter pseudocolor dot plot display of C57BL/6J DDCs infected with the indicated *T. gondii* strains after 18–24 h of culture in the absence (top panels) or presence of 200 U/ml of IFNγ (bottom panels). After 8 h of infection, cells were harvested and labeled with Far Red LIVE/DEAD® stain and fixed in 4% PFA. Cells were then handled and analyzed exactly as in Fig. 7

value can be subtracted from the raw counts of 21% and 7% in panels 5 and 6 respectively, to give corrected values of ~19% and 5% in Q3. Corrections smaller than this are hardly worth making. Furthermore there is inevitably some scatter between all panels. Our view is that it is not justified to aim for more precision.

5.2 Material

1. Complete DMEM growth medium (DMEM high glucose w/o L-glutamine w/o sodium pyruvate supplemented with 1× NEAA, 1× penicillin–streptomycin, 1 mM sodium pyruvate, and 2 mM L-glutamine) with 10% HI-FBS).

2. Mouse (Cat. 315-05 Peprotech) or human IFNγ (Cat. SRP3058 Sigma-Aldrich).

3. Adherent mouse or human cells (MEFs, DDCs, HFFs, macrophages).

4. *T. gondii* tachyzoites.

5. 1× Phosphate-buffered saline (PBS) sterile.

6. Sterile Flat bottom 12-well plates (tissue culture-treated).

7. Pipette filter tips (20, 200, and 1000 μl).

8. Serological Pipettes (5 and 10 ml).

A

B

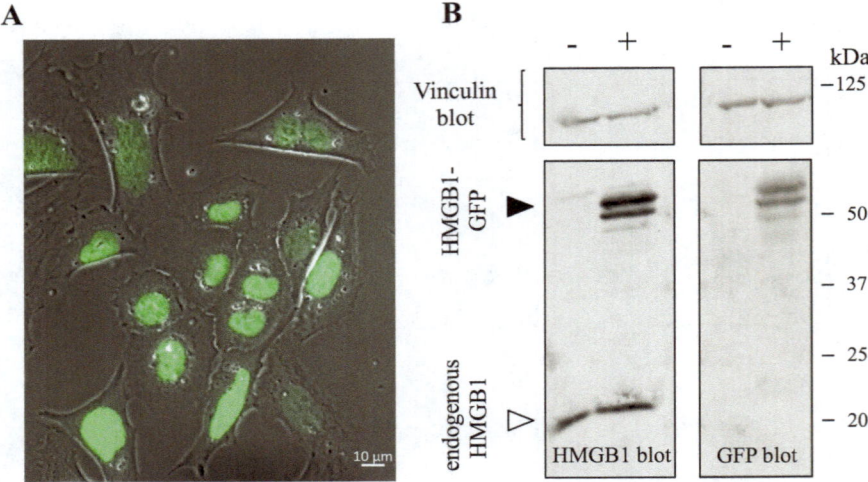

Fig. 9 Expression of the mHMGB1-GFP retroviral reporter 48 h after transduction of C57BL/6J MEFs. (**a**) Merged phase contrast and green fluorescence images of transduced MEFs. (**b**) Western blot analysis of transduced (+) and mock-transduced (−) MEFs. Replica membranes were incubated with anti-human HMGB1 or anti-GFP antibodies. The higher molecular weight portions of the two membranes (100–150 kDa) were incubated with anti-human vinculin antibody as a loading control. The molecular mass of nuclear HMGB1 is ~25 kDa, whereas cytoplasmic and extracellular HMGB1 runs at ~30 kDa, largely due to acetylation. The multiple bands in the size range for the fusion protein likely reflect posttranslational modifications (acetylation, phosphorylation, and methylation) [25–27]

9. 1.5 ml sterile microcentrifuge tubes.

10. Cell culture incubator maintained at 37 °C with 10% CO_2.

11. Accutase® cell detachment solution (BioLegend Cat No. 423201).

12. Titertube micro test tubes (Bio-Rad Cat # 223-9391).

13. Microcentrifuge suitable for RCF between 100 and 500 × *g*.

14. (Optional) V-bottom 96-well plate.

15. (Optional) Microplate centrifuge equipped with rotor and plate holders suitable for V-bottom 96 well plates.

16. BD Biosciences flow cytometry permeabilization buffer (BD Perm/Wash Buffer Cat # 554723).

17. Fixation solution (4% paraformaldehyde (PFA) in PBS).

18. Thermo Fisher Scientific LIVE/DEAD® fixable dye.

19. FACS buffer (1% BSA in PBS).

20. Anti-SAG1 antibody and fluorescent secondary antibody for detection of SAG1 antibody or fluorescent parasite strain.

21. BD FACSCalibur™ flow cytometer or FORTESSA cytometer.

22. FlowJo software.

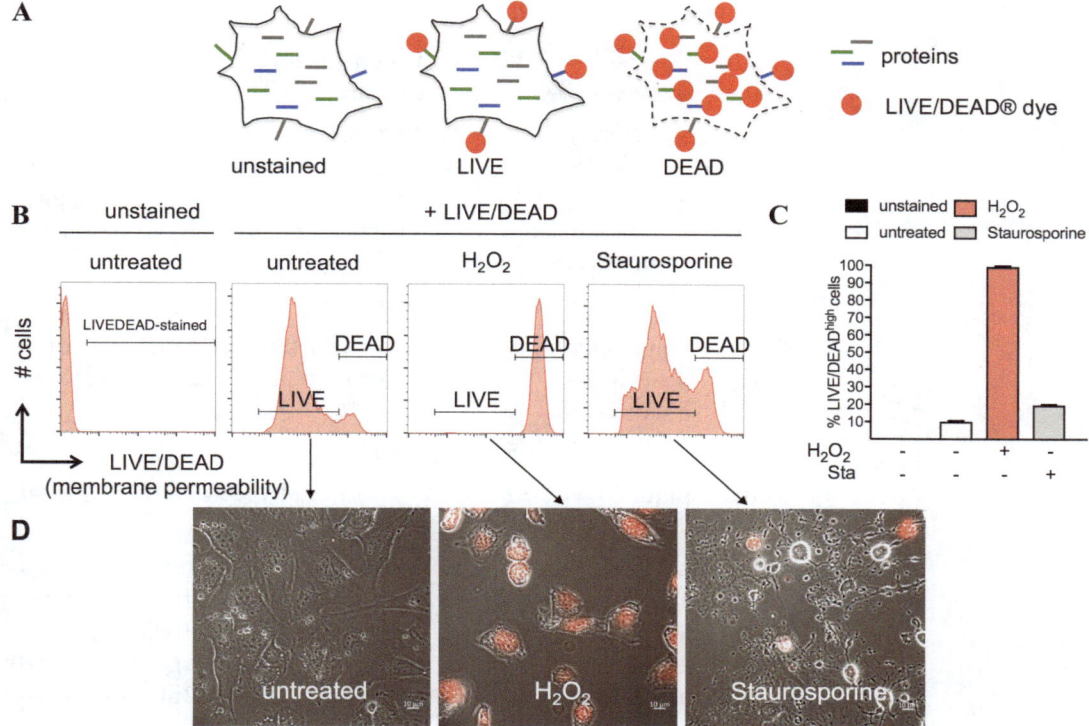

Fig. 10 A fixation-permissive method for detecting necrosis by flow cytometry. (**a**) Schematic representation of fixable LIVE/DEAD® necrosis dyes. Live cells are dimly fluorescent, whereas dead cells, with a permeable membrane (indicated by the dashed line), display higher fluorescence. (**b**) Univariate histograms depicting differential staining by LIVE/DEAD® dye of C57BL/6J DDCs left untreated or exposed to a cell death inducer. In the absence of LIVE/DEAD® stain ("unstained" panel), untreated cells show no fluorescence. LIVE/DEAD® stained, untreated cells are mostly found in the LIVE cell gate (left peak) while cells exposed to high levels (100 mM) of hydrogen peroxide (H_2O_2) which damages the permeability barrier, are found in the DEAD cell gate (right peak) of the histogram. Cells treated with 10 μM staurosporine (Sta) to induce apoptosis remain mostly within the LIVE cell gate because the permeability barrier is not broken. About 20% of cells stain heavily with the dye, presumably due to secondary necrosis after Sta-induced apoptosis. Treatment with both agents was for 3 h before preparation for FACS. Samples were analyzed by flow cytometry using 633 nm excitation and ~661 nm emission (FACScalibur cytometer, FL4 channel). (**c**) Proportion of necrotic (LIVE/DEAD^high) cells in samples shown in **b**. (**d**) The morphology and PI staining profile of C57B/L6J DDCs shown in **b** are consistent with their LIVE/DEAD staining prolife. Shown are merged images obtained from the combination of the PI (red) channel and the phase contrast channel microscopy analysis of control, 100 mM H_2O_2- or 10 μM Sta-treated cells. Changes in cell morphology range from a flat shape (untreated controls) to a round shape with enlarged nuclei and expanded cytoplasm (necrotic cells, with PI+ nuclei) to a wrinkling, stellate shape (apoptotic cells, a few PI+ nuclei)

5.3 Methods

Day 1:

Plate primary or immortalized adherent cells on 12 well plates (*see* **Note 6**).

Day 2:

Where appropriate, stimulate cells with mouse IFNγ at 40 ng/ml (200 U/ml) or human IFNγ at 50 ng/ml for 18–24 h (*see* **Note 7**).

Day 3:

1. After 20–24 h of IFNγ treatment, infect host cells with the desired *T. gondii* strain at the desired MOI.

2. For collection of host cells after infection, perform all steps at room temperature (RT). Collect host cell supernatants (containing necrotic cells that have detached from the plate). Detach adherent cells with Accutase (*see* **Note 8**) and transfer to the same Eppendorf tube.

3. Pellet cells for 5 min at 500 × *g* on a tabletop centrifuge.

4. Resuspend cells in 150 μl of PBS and transfer to microcentrifuge tubes or to a V-bottom 96 well plate if many samples are to be analyzed.

5. Pellet cells 5 min at 500 × *g* at RT.

6. Resuspend in 150 μl of PBS and pellet cells again (5 min at 500 × *g* at RT).

7. While cells are being spun down for the second time, prepare a fresh working dilution (WD) (although subject to adjustment, typically 1:200–1:300) of the desired LIVE/DEAD® dye (*see* **Note 4**, below) in PBS (always protect from light). Resuspend cells in 150 μl of LIVE/DEAD® dye (WD ~1:250) and incubate for 30 min at RT in the dark. From this step onward, the samples should be incubated in the dark.

8. Wash cells twice in 150 μl of RT PBS.

9. Resuspend in 150 μl of 4% PFA. Fix for 20 min at RT or overnight at −4 °C (*see* **Note 9**).

If you wish to analyze necrosis levels alone, go directly to FACS analysis. If you wish to analyze levels of parasite infection as well, proceed with the following steps*, unless you are using parasites expressing a fluorescent marker of an appropriate color.

*All subsequent steps must be done as far as possible in the dark, with ice-cold buffers and incubations on ice or at 4 °C.

10. Wash off PFA with two ice-cold PBS washes (5 min at 500 × *g* at 4 °C).

11. Equilibrate cells in ice-cold permeabilization/wash (P/W) buffer—BD Biosciences Perm/Wash Buffer (*see* **Note 10**)—in subsequent steps.

12. Incubate cells with an anti-SAG1 antibody dissolved in P/W buffer for 30 min at 4 °C with constant rocking. We routinely use the Santa Cruz anti-SAG1 TP3 mouse monoclonal antibody (Cat No. sc52255) (*see* **Note 10**).

13. Wash cells twice with P/W buffer.

14. Incubate cells with an appropriate fluorescent secondary antibody (*see* **Note** 7, below) dissolved in B/W buffer for 30 min at 4 °C with constant rocking.

15. Wash cells twice with P/W buffer.

16. Resuspend samples in 250 μl FACS buffer (PBS + 1% BSA) and transfer to Titertube micro test tubes for flow cytometry analysis.

6   Antisera and Monoclonal Antibodies Against Mouse and *T. gondii* Proteins for Use in These Experiments (Tables 1 and 2)

The primary antibodies might undergo property changes over time and during shipping to other labs. Therefore, working dilutions of all the primary reagents should be titrated for the cell lines being used in each lab.

Secondary immunoreagents used in immunofluorescence were diluted as suggested by the manufacturer (Life Technologies):

- Alexa 488 labeled donkey anti rabbit IgG (H + L) (A-21206).
- Alexa 488 labeled donkey anti mouse IgG (H + L) (A21202).
- Alexa 488 labeled goat anti mouse IgG (H + L) (A-11029).
- Alexa 555 labeled donkey anti rabbit IgG (H + L) (A-31572).
- Alexa 555 labeled donkey anti-mouse IgG (H + L) (A-31570).
- Alexa 647 labeled goat anti-rat IgG (H + L) (A-21247).

The reagents 4′,6-diamidino-2-phenylindole (DAPI D3571—Life Technologies) and Hoechst 33342 trihydrochloride (sc-200,908—Santa Cruz Biotechnology) were used as nuclear counterstains in fixed and live cells respectively. Propidium iodide (P4170—sigma) was used to assess cell viability in live microscopy assays.

Constructs used for retroviral expression: pM6p-HMGB1-GFP (NM_010439.4: mouse HMGB1 coding sequence with a C-terminal fusion of EGFP; Howard Lab, unpublished), pCl-Eco and pCl-10A1 [41].

7   Notes

1. There are several commercially available systems for gene delivery suitable for plasmid DNA. For this immortalization protocol we reproducibly had the highest rate of success using the ScreenFect®A Transfection Reagent kit from InCella [17]. This is a gene delivery method based on liposomal vectors (cationic thioether lipids) that show a high efficiency of transfection with

Table 1
Primary immunoreagents available from the Howard laboratory

Recognized antigen	Name	Immunogen	Type	Reference
Mouse Irga6	165/4[a]	Recombinant Mouse Irga6	Rabbit serum	[32]
Mouse Irga6	10D7[b]	Recombinant Mouse Irga6	Mouse monoclonal	[33]
Mouse Irga6	10E7[b]	Recombinant Mouse Irga6	Mouse monoclonal	[33]
Mouse Irgb6	141/3[a]	Recombinant Mouse Irgb6	Rabbit serum	[9]
Mouse Irgb6	B34	Irgb6	Mouse monoclonal	[34]
Mouse Irgb10	940/6[c]	Recombinant Mouse Irgb10	Rabbit serum	[35]
Mouse Irgd	2078	Mouse Irgd peptides CKTPYQHPKYPKVIF; CDAKHLLRKIETVNVA	Rabbit serum	[9]
Mouse Irgd	081/3[a]	Recombinant Mouse Irgd	Rabbit serum	[36]
Mouse tandem IRGs	954/1[a] C15A[d]	Irgb1 C-terminal peptide CLSDLPEYWETGMEL	Rabbit serum	[13]
Phosphorylated mouse Irga6	87,558/4[a]	T108 phosphorylated Irga6	Rabbit serum	[37]
Mouse Irgm1	L115[e]	Mouse Irgm1 peptides QTGSSRLPEVSRSTE, NESLKNSLGVRDDD	Rabbit serum	[9]
Mouse Irgm1	1B2[e]	Mouse Irgm1 N-terminal peptide of long isoform CEAAPLLPNMAETHY	Mouse monoclonal	[38]
Mouse Irgm1	rbMAE15[e]	Mouse Irgm1 N-terminal peptide of short isoform MAETHYAPLSSAFPC	Rabbit serum	[39]
Mouse Irgm1	chMAE15A[e]	Mouse Irgm1 N-terminal peptide of short isoform MAETHYAPLSSAFPC	Chicken polyclonal IgY	[39]
Mouse Irgm2	H53/3[a,f]	Mouse Irgm2 N-terminal peptide MEEAVESPEVKEFEY	Rabbit serum	[9]
Mouse Irgc	39/3[a,g]	Mouse Irgc C-terminal peptides NGVEKGGSGEGGGEE KYILDSWKKHDSEEK	Rabbit serum	*Unpublished*
GRA7	2.1.2	*T. gondii* GRA7	Rat monoclonal	[40]

[a]Rabbit serum references followed by slash-number indicate the number of the rabbit bleed
[b]Both 10D7 and 10E7 antibodies recognize active Irga6 at the parasitophorous vacuolar membrane. However, 10E7 also recognizes IFNγ-induced inactive Irga6 expressed elsewhere in the cytoplasm, whereas 10D7 does not. 10D7 specifically detects both GTP-bound and denatured Irga6 [21]

^cThis antiserum may cross-react with other IRG proteins (*Lilue J, personal communication*)

^dThe 954/1 antibody recognizes the C-terminus of all IRG tandem proteins from laboratory mice and from several wild-derived mice. The peptide against which this antibody was raised is common to many of these proteins [13]

^eL115, 1B2, rbMAE15A, and chMAE15A antibodies recognize mouse Irgm1, but display differences in the recognition of the short and long isoforms [39]. 1B2 shows affinity for the long Irgm1 isoform. L115 was raised against peptides shared by the long and short isoforms of Irgm1, and recognizes both proteins. This study also produced two new antibodies raised against an N-terminal peptide of the short isoform—rbMAE15A and chMAE15A—which recognize the short isoform, but will also detect the long isoform of Irgm1, depending on the degree of expression of each protein. It's important to note that Springer et al. [39] showed that the commercially available antibodies ab69464 and ab69465 (Abcam) are not specific for mouse Irgm1, and cross-react with GST-Irgm2 and GST-Irgm3. These reagents are therefore not suitable to detect mouse Irgm1

^fH53 will detect Irgm2 from the C57BL/6J, C57BL/10J and C58/J laboratory strains and from a limited number of *Mus musculus castaneus* and *Mus musculus musculus* strains. Other strains carry an amino acid exchange in the Irgm2 N-terminus—V10D—rendering the protein unrecognizable by the H53 serum

^gDoes not recognize human IRGC (*Rohde C, personal communication*)

Table 2
Commercially available primary immunoreagents

Name	Recognized antigen	Type	Reference	Source
TP3	*T. gondii* P30 protein/ SAG1	Mouse monoclonal	sc-52,255	Santa Cruz
Anti-*Toxoplasma gondii*	*Toxoplasma gondii* lysates	Rabbit polyclonal	PU125-UP	Biogenex
Anti-*GFP*	Recombinant GFP	Goat polyclonal	AB0020	Sicgen
Anti-*Vinculin*	Synthetic peptide with partial Human Vinculin	Rabbit monoclonal	ab129002	AbCam
Anti-*HMGB1*	Synthetic peptide with partial Human HMGB1	Rabbit polyclonal	ab18256	AbCam

low toxicity. Additionally, transfected cell viability with Screen-Fect®A does not depend on serum-free medium [18].

2. DDCs are adherent cells; during the transfection it is necessary to first remove and discard the medium in each well (right after the complex formation step). Add fresh growth medium to the transfection complexes, mix with pipette (growth medium turns momentarily yellow) and immediately apply to cells [14].

3. Stock solutions of both interferons are made in sterile water. Murine IFNγ stock = 200 μg/ml or 1000 U/μl (5000× concentrated). Human IFNγ stock = 250 μg/ml (5000×). Both solutions are kept in small aliquots at −20 °C to avoid repeated freeze thaw cycles.

4. We typically use an MOI of ~2–10. Transgenic parasites expressing fluorescent protein (PRU-YFP, PRU-tomato) can be used to facilitate observation of host cell invasion in real-time.

5. We use a Zeiss Axio Observer Z1 fluorescence microscope located within our BSL-2 facility, equipped with an AxioCam MRm camera and Zen 2011 software (all ZEISS, Oberkochen, Germany). Because our microscope setup is not equipped with a CO_2 source, we include HEPES buffer to maintain pH levels during the acquisition time of <6 h. Imaging can be initiated shortly after infection or later. Longer acquisition times are possible with a proper CO_2 source associated to the microscope setup.

6. We plate 7.5×10^4 primary C57BL/6J MEFs/ well, 5×10^4 immortalized C57BL/6J DDCs/well, 2.5×10^5 L929 P2 cells/well, 2.8×10^5 RAW 264.7 macrophages/well or 1.2×10^5 Hs27 HFFs/well of a 12-well plate 2 days before infection.

7. Some suppliers provide IFNγ measured in international units (IU), others by mass. Typically, 1 mg purified IFNγ is equivalent to approximately 5×10^6 IU.

8. We collect adherent host cells using Accutase treatment; trypsin–EDTA can also be used but may result in higher autofluorescence in the green channel.

9. Thermo Fisher Scientific provides various LIVE/DEAD® solutions that allow for various experimental designs. The cytometers available in house favor the use of the LIVE/ DEAD® versions in Far Red for 633 or 635 nm excitation (Cat No. L10120) or Violet for 405 nm excitation (Cat No. L34958), with which we obtain comparable results (data not shown).

10. Following staining with the LIVE/DEAD® solution, washing and addition of 4% PFA, cells can be left in 4% PFA in the dark for up to 10 days prior to further processing or flow cytometry analysis without a discernible loss of LIVE/DEAD signal.

11. The BD Biosciences flow cytometry permeabilization/wash (P/W) buffer can be replaced by the following P/W buffer recipe: 1% fetal calf serum, 0.1% sodium azide, and 0.1% saponin. Simply filter-sterilize using a 0.2 μm filter and adjust pH to 7.4–7.6 with sodium hydroxide.

12. We use the goat anti-mouse IgG (H + L) secondary antibody, Alexa Fluor 488 conjugate, from Invitrogen (Cat No. A-11029) to detect the mouse TP3 anti-SAG1 antibody in cells previously stained with the Far Red LIVE/DEAD® dye for analysis with a FACSCalibur cytometer. We use the goat anti-mouse IgG secondary antibody, Alexa Fluor AF647 conjugate, from Abcam (Cat No. ab150115) to detect the mouse TP3 anti-SAG1 antibody in cells previously stained with Violet LIVE/DEAD® dye for analysis with a FORTESSA cytometer. Note the importance of using both primary and secondary

antibody reagents at saturation to maximize the resolution between infected and noninfected cells.

13. Generate ecotropic pseudotyped virus, which can only infect mouse or rat cells, or amphotropic pseudotyped virus, which can infect most mammalian cells (including human cells), by cotransfecting HEK 293T cells with either pCL-Eco or pCl-10A1, respectively [40].

Acknowledgments

The authors record their thanks to previous members of the laboratory who contributed to the development of the study of early postinfection events in *T. gondii* immunity and pioneered the application of several of these techniques. The present work would also not have been possible without the contributions of the service facilities of the IGC, in particular the Animal Facility, supported by the research infrastructure Congento, project LISBOA-01-0145-FEDER-022170, the Transgenics Facility, and the Antibody facility, both supported by Fundação Calouste Gulenkian, the Advanced Imaging Unit, supported by the project PPBI-POCI-01-0145-FEDER-022122 and the Flow Cytometry Unit, supported by the project LISBOA-01-0145-FEDER-007654.

This work was supported by central funds of the Instituto Gulbenkian de Ciência, by the Sonderforschungsbereiche 670 and 680 and Schwerpunkt 1399 of the Deutsche Forschungsgemeinde. Joana Loureiro received funding from the European Union's Horizon 2020 research and innovation program under the Marie Sklodowska-Curie Grant Agreement number 708694 entitled "*Toxoplasma* Sensing."

Author contributions: Subheading 1, Jonathan Howard; Subheading 2, Catalina Alvarez and Ben Mueller; Subheadings 3 and 4, Ana Lina Rodrigues and Joana Loureiro; Subheading 5, Joana Loureiro; Subheading 6, Claudia Campos. All authors contributed to the preparation and editing of the entire manuscript.

Appendix 1: Generating Mammalian Cell Lines Expressing an HMGB1-GFP Necrosis Reporter (Joana Loureiro)

Generation of the Mouse HMGB1-GFP Construct

A murine HMGB1 cDNA (mHMGB1) with an in-frame C-terminal eGFP moiety (mHMGB1-GFP) was shown to be functionally similar to untagged, endogenous HMGB1 [24]. Murine messenger RNA (mRNA) obtained using the Qiagen RNeasy Kit (Cat No. 74104) from C57BL/6J MEFs induced for 24 h with murine IFNγ. RNA was DNase-treated (Thermo Fisher Scientific

TURBO™ DNase, Cat No. AM2238) prior to cDNA synthesis (Invitrogen SuperScript III First-Strand Synthesis System, Cat No. 18080051). The 647 bp coding sequence of HMGB1 (Gene ID: 15289) was amplified from this cDNA (Herculase II Fusion DNA Polymerase, Agilent Technologies (Cat No. 600675) with primers JL1 and JL2 (see Table 3, below). After purification from an agarose gel (High Pure PCR Product Purification kit, Roche Cat. No. 11732668001), the amplicon was digested with EcoRI and SacII and cloned into EcoRI/SacII-digested Clontech's pEGFP-N3 plasmid (now discontinued), ligated using Gibson Assembly® Master Mix (New England Biolabs, Cat. No. E2611S) and transformed into One Shot® Mach1™-T1R Chemically Competent E. coli. Positive colonies were identified by colony PCR and the sequence of the fusion gene in the pEGFP-N3 expression vector confirmed using Primer S1.

A functional HMGB1-GFP fusion protein should display a mostly nuclear localization in living mammalian cells, consistent with the nucleus-cytoplasm shuttling dynamics of endogenous untagged HMGB1 [22]. Indeed, cells with green-fluorescent nuclei were readily visualized and a protein of the expected size (~50–60 kDa)—GFP protein (238 aa) ~27 kDa; mHMGB1 (215 aa) ~20–30 kDa—was detected by western blot after transfection of pEGFP-N3 expressing the mHMGB1-GFP fusion construct into HEK293T cells (ATCC® CRL-3216™) (data not shown).

Table 3
Primers used in generation of murine HMGB1-GFP constructs

Primer code	Primer name	Sequence (5′ → 3′)
JL1	mHMGB1EcoRI_fwd	CGAGCTCAAGCTTCGAATTCATGGGCAAAGGAGATCCTAAAAAGC
JL2	mHMGB1SacII_rev	GGATCCCGGGCCCGCGGATTCATCATCATCATCTTCTTCTTC
JL3	M6p_NcoI_HMGB1_Fwd	CTATAGAAGCTTGCCACCATGGATGGGCAAAGGAGATCCTAAAAAGC
JL4	M6p_NotI_GFP_Rev	GAGGGAGAGGGGCGGCCGCTTACTTGTACAGCTCGTCCATG
S1	pEGFP-N3_rev	TTTATGTTTCAGGTTCAGGGG
S2	pM6pSeq_fwd	CCGACCCCGGGGGTGGAC
S3	pM6Pseq_rev	CGTTCGGCCAGTAACGTTAG

**Generating
the Retroviral
mHGMB1-GFP
Expression Construct**

Because transfection efficiencies are often low in primary cells, we made a high-titer helper-free retroviral vector based on the pM6pBLAST system [25]: we used primers JL3 and JL4 (Table 3) to subclone the pEGFP-N3 mHMGB1-GFP cassette into pM6pBLAST. The ~1400 bp was digested with NcoI and NotI and cloned into Ncol/Notl pM6pBLAST. A clone confirmed to contain the correct sequence (primers S2 and S3) showed the expected protein behavior both by microscopy and western blot following transfection of the viral plasmid DNA into HEK 293Tcells (data not shown).

The pM6pBLAST-based viral plasmid was used to produce high-titer retroviruses expressing the mHMGB1-GFP gene through cotransfection with a packaging plasmid into HEK 293Tcells, and the retroviral supernatants of HEK 293T cultures were used to transduce mouse or human fibroblasts. Both procedures are described in detail below.

**Generation
of Mammalian Cell
Lines Expressing
the HMGB1-GFP
Reporter**

In our experience, retrovirus-mediated transduction of mouse and human fibroblasts is desirable for several reasons. It is highly efficient: we typically obtain >70% of cells displaying green nuclei within 1 day of HMGB1-GFP-retrovirus-mediated transduction. Moreover, retroviral transduction results in stable integration of the HMGB1-GFP cassette into the genome, leading to long-term expression. Additionally, the Blasticidin-S resistance gene present in pM6pBLAST allows enrichment for HMGB1-GFP expression in cells in culture by means of antibiotic (blasticidin) selection.

HEK293T cells used for virus packaging must be of low passage and must be very carefully maintained such that they never reach confluence; the viruses must be packaged with a viral envelope appropriately pseudotyped to ensure mouse or human cell tropism (*see* **Note 1**, below); the efficiency of virus transduction goes down *exponentially* with freeze-thawing of the virus-containing HEK293T cell culture supernatant, and therefore it is preferable to coordinate packaging and transduction so as to use freshly packaged virus.

*Protocol for HMGB1-GFP
Virus Production
in HEK293T Cells*

Material

1. DMEM supplemented with 10% heat-inactivated FCS, 1× NEAA, 1× penicillin–streptomycin, 1 mM sodium pyruvate, and 2 mM L-glutamine.

2. Cell culture incubator maintained at 37 °C with 10% CO_2.

3. Sterile Flat bottom 6-well plates (Tissue culture-treated).

4. Pipette filter tips (20, 200, and 1000 μl).

5. Serological Pipettes (5 and 10 ml).

6. 1.5 ml sterile microcentrifuge tubes.

7. ScreenFect®A plasmid transfection reagent and buffer (Incella Cat No. S-3001).

8. Retroviral DNA plasmid expressing murine HMGB1-GFP (fusion construct in pM6p.BLAST).

9. Packaging plasmid: pCL-Eco (mouse-pseudotyped envelope) plasmid or pCl-10A1 (human-pseudotyped envelope) [42].

10. 15 ml Falcon tubes.

11. 5 ml Plastic syringes.

12. Syringe Filters (Acrodisc® 25 mm Syringe filters with 0.45 μm Supor® Membrane).

Methods

Day −1: (Day before transfection) Plate cells at 750,000 cells/well in 6-well plates.

Day 0: (Day of transfection) Perform a visual assessment of confluence state of the cells. If cells are 65–75% confluent, you may proceed with the transfection procedure.

1. Replace medium on HEK293T cells—add 2 ml fresh FCS-containing DMEM (add medium VERY SLOWLY and CAREFULLY to the side walls of the wells, not directly to cells, or the cells will detach from the plate).

2. Make ScreenFect®A transfection mix and incubate for 20 min at RT as per the manufacturer's instructions. Transfection mix: dilute SFA reagent in SFA dilution buffer in tube A and dilute DNA in SFA dilution buffer in tube B. DNA dilution in Tube B: For each well of a 6 well plate, dilute 2.5 μg of retroviral plasmid DNA + 1.25 μg of pCL-Eco (encoding mouse-pseudotyped viral envelope) or pCl-10A1 (encoding human-pseudotyped viral envelope) in 240 μl of ScreenFect®A dilution buffer.

3. After 20 min of RT incubation, add the SFA-DNA mix dropwise and very carefully to HEK293T cells. Return cells to the incubator.

Day +1: Change medium—Replace medium (very carefully) on HEK293T cells.

Day +2: Collect 48 h virus supernatants.

1. Collect 48 h virus supernatants (sups) into 15 ml Falcon tubes and place sups at 4 °C Overnight.

2. Add 2 ml fresh serum-containing DMEM to each well and return HEK 293T cells to the incubator.

3. Optional: Plate target cells for infection after 18–24 h (Appendix 1.1.1.3).

Day +3: Collect 72 h virus supernatants.

1. Collect 72 h sups. Pool with 48 h virus supernatants.

2. Add polybrene to the (48 + 72) h supernatants to a final concentration of 8 μg/ml.

3. Filter through a 0.45 μm filter. Use supernatants immediately for infection of target cells (Appendix 1.1.1.3) or freeze aliquots at −20 °C. Note that the efficiency of virus transduction goes down exponentially with freeze-thawing.

Transduction of Target Cells with HMGB1-GFP-Expressing Retrovirus

Virus-mediated infection (transduction) by pCL-Eco or pCl-10A1-pseudotyped retrovirus has allowed us to generate HMGB1-GFP-expressing MEFs, DDCs, HFFs, and HeLa cells using the following protocol.

Material

1. DMEM supplemented with 10% heat-inactivated FCS, 1× NEAA, 1× penicillin–streptomycin, 1 mM sodium pyruvate, and 2 mM L-glutamine.

2. Cell culture incubator maintained at 37 °C with 10% CO_2.

3. Sterile flat bottom 12-well plates (Tissue culture-treated).

4. Pipette filter tips (20, 200, and 1000 μl).

5. Serological Pipettes (5 and 10 ml).

6. Mouse- or human-pseudotyped virus supernatants (filtered and polybrene-supplemented).

7. Target cells plated the day prior to retroviral transduction on 12-well plates.

8. Tabletop centrifuge equipped with a high-capacity microplate rotor and plate holders (preferably one that is capable of maintaining cells at 37 °C during spin infection).

9. Blasticidin-S hydrochloride (CAS 3513-03-9).

Methods

Day −1: Plate murine/human target cells∗ such that target cells are no more than 50–60% confluent at the time of transduction (there must be room on the plate for cells to divide, since it is during cell division that the retrovirus can access the cell nucleus and integrate into the host DNA).

   ∗MEFs and DDCs are plated at 20000 or 15,000 cells/well, respectively, HFFs are plated at 32000 cells/well of a 12-well plate.

   Day 0: Virus-mediated transduction of target cells.

1. Apply 37 °C-warm supernatants (filtered + supplemented with polybrene to 8 μg/ml) to target cells (typically 2 ml of virus supernatant/well of a 12-well plate).

2. Perform a spin-infection at 2200 rpm (~900 × g), at 37 °C, for 90 min. We use an Eppendorf centrifuge model 5810 R equipped with the A-4-81-MTP/Flex high-capacity microplate rotor (16.3 cm radius) with four plate holders.

3. After 90 min spin-infection, return cells to the 37 °C incubator.

Day +2 (48 h after target cell transduction): detach cells from plate and passage into 6-well plates and, if desired to increase the frequency of transduced cells, initiate selection with blasticidin-S HCl-containing DMEM. For antibiotic selection of pM6pBLAST-transduced MEFs we use 10 μg/ml of blasticidin; murine DDCs, human Hs27 fibroblasts and HeLa cells require higher blasticidin concentrations (15–20 μg/ml).

As early as 48 h after retrovirus transduction, expression of the mHGMB1-GFP fusion protein in mouse or human cells can be assessed. The predominantly nuclear localization and the electrophoretic mobility pattern of the mHGMB1-GFP reporter in C57BL/6J MEFs are shown in Fig. 9 (Table 3).

Appendix 2

See Fig. 10.

Appendix 3: Macro

```
/*    IJ macro to create ROIs for parasite, PV etc...
    by GabyGMartins @Instituto Gulbenkian Ciencia, Advanced
Imaging Facility - v0.2 2019-01-02
    macro assumes images are loaded with bioformats in imageJ/
FIJI as a composite hyperstack and reading of metadata
    expects pixel sizes to be properly scaled, as measurements
are performed in microns
    and that chromatic shift has been corrected - if there is
pixel-shift then measurements might not be accurate */
roiManager("reset");
run("Select None");
run("Make Composite");
run("Channels Tool..."); //activates channel tool and gives
user a chance to turn off unwanted channels (eg bright field)
waitForUser("turn off unwanted channels then OK");
//asks user to switch to PV channel and store in variable
PVchannel
PVchannel = getNumber("Which channel do you use to detect the
PV?", 3);
Stack.setChannel(PVchannel);
/*    Proceed to identifying semi-automatically the PV:
activates wand tool so user can click on parasite
```

```
       adjusting the "tolerance" of the wand the ROI matches the
shape of the PV
       a default tolerance value of 4500 work with our images; a
different default can be inserted below to accelerate to
process
       if magic wand fails user can also change ROI selection tool
manually and draw the parasite */

setTool("zoom"); //activates zoom function so user can zoom in
on parasite
waitForUser("Click on parasite to zoom in then click OK");
setTool("wand");
run("Wand Tool...", "tolerance=4500 mode=4-connected");
 // user can change the default tolerance here
waitForUser("Click inside the parasite to select and double
click on wand tool to adjust tolerance");
run("Enlarge...", "enlarge=0.1");
 //user here can change the area of the ring around PV
// stores the ROIcontaining the PV to ROImanager
roiManager("Add");
roiManager("Select", 0);
roiManager("rename", "PV")
//create band of cytoplasm outside of parasite and stores it as
cytosol in ROI manager
run("Make Band...", "band=1");
 //change thickness of band here
roiManager("Add");
roiManager("Select", 1);
roiManager("rename", "cytosol")
// create band of 0.8 µm representing the parasite's cortex and
call it "PVM"
roiManager("Select", 0);
run("Enlarge...", "enlarge=-0.8");
run("Make Band...", "band=0.8");
roiManager("Add");
roiManager("Select", 2);
roiManager("rename", "PVM")
// prepare ROImanager for measurements
roiManager("Select", newArray(0,1,2));
roiManager("Show All");
//activates several measurements and then stores measurements
into a results table
run("Set Measurements...", "area mean standard modal min shape
feret's integrated stack display redirect=None decimal=3");
roiManager("multi-measure measure_all");
```

References

1. Müller UB, Howard JC (2016) The impact of *Toxoplasma gondii* on the mammalian genome. Curr Opin Microbiol 32:19–25
2. Carruthers V, Boothroyd JC (2007) Pulling together: an integrated model of *Toxoplasma* cell invasion. Curr Opin Microbiol 10:83–89
3. Besteiro S, Dubremetz JF, Lebrun M (2011) The moving junction of apicomplexan parasites: a key structure for invasion. Cell Microbiol 13:797–805
4. Dubremetz JF (2007) Rhoptries are major players in *Toxoplasma gondii* invasion and host cell interaction. Cell Microbiol 9:841–848
5. Boothroyd JC, Dubremetz J-F (2008) Kiss and spit: the dual roles of *Toxoplasma* rhoptries. Nat Rev Microbiol 6:79
6. Martens S et al (2005) Disruption of *Toxoplasma gondii* parasitophorous vacuoles by the mouse p47-resistance GTPases. PLoS Pathog 1:0187–0201
7. Zhao YO, Khaminets A, Hunn JP, Howard JC (2009) Disruption of the *Toxoplasma gondii* parasitophorous vacuole by IFNg-inducible immunity-related GTPases (IRG proteins) triggers necrotic cell death. PLoS Pathog 5: e1000288
8. Fentress SJ et al (2011) Phosphorylation of immunity-related GTPases by a *Toxoplasma gondii* secreted kinase promotes macrophage survival and virulence. Cell Host Microbe 8:484–495
9. Khaminets A et al (2010) Coordinated loading of IRG resistance GTPases on to the *Toxoplasma gondii* parasitophorous vacuole. Cell Microbiol 12:939–961
10. Weiss LM, Kim K (2013) *Toxoplasma gondii*: the model apicomplexan – perspectives and methods: second edition. Elsevier, Amsterdam
11. Allen I (2013) Mouse models of innate immunity: methods and protocols, vol 1031. Humana Press, New York, NY
12. Antony VB, Owen CL, Hadley KJ (1989) Pleural mesothelial cells stimulated by asbestos release chemotactic activity for neutrophils in vitro. Am Rev Respir Dis 139:199–206
13. Lilue J, Müller UB, Steinfeldt T, Howard JC (2013) Reciprocal virulence and resistance polymorphism in the relationship between *Toxoplasma gondii* and the house mouse. elife 2013:1–21
14. Incella (2016) ScreenFect®A transfection reagent protocol. Incella, Baden-Württemberg, pp 1–5
15. Southern PJ, Berg P (1982) Transformation of mammalian cells to antibiotic resistance with a bacterial gene under control of the SV40 early region promoter. J Mol Appl Genet 1 (4):327–341
16. Chang PL et al (1986) Transformation of human cultured fibroblasts with plasmids carrying dominant selection markers and immortalizing potential. Exp Cell Res 167:407–416
17. Li LM et al (2015) ScreenFect A: an efficient and low toxic liposome for gene delivery to mesenchymal stem cells. Int J Pharm 488:1–11
18. Li L et al (2012) A biomimetic lipid library for gene delivery through thiol-yne click chemistry. Biomaterials 33:8160–8166
19. Fisch DH et al (2018) An artificial intelligence workflow for defining host-pathogen interactions. bioRxiv 408450. https://doi.org/10.1101/408450
20. Schindelin J et al (2012) Fiji – an open source platform for biological image analysis. Nat Methods 9:676–682
21. Papic N, Hunn JP, Pawlowski N, Zerrahn J, Howard JC (2008) Inactive and active states of the interferon-inducible resistance GTPase, Irga6, in vivo. J Biol Chem 283:32143–32151
22. Lotze MT, Tracey KJ (2005) High-mobility group box 1 protein (HMGB1): nuclear weapon in the immune arsenal. Nat Rev Immunol 5:331
23. Zhao YO et al (2009) *Toxoplasma gondii* and the immunity-related GTPase (IRG) resistance system in mice – a review. Mem Inst Oswaldo Cruz 104:234–240
24. Scaffidi P, Misteli T, Bianchi ME (2002) Release of chromatin protein HMGB1 by necrotic cells triggers inflammation. Nature 418:191–195
25. Bonaldi T et al (2003) Monocytic cells hyperacetylate chromatin protein HMGB1 to redirect it towards secretion. EMBO 22:5551–5560
26. Andersson U et al (2000) High mobility group 1 protein (Hmg-1) stimulates proinflammatory cytokine synthesis in human monocytes. J Exp Med 192:565–570
27. Tang D et al (2010) Endogenous HMGB1 regulates autophagy. J Cell Biol 190:881–892
28. Vanden Berghe T et al (2010) Necroptosis, necrosis and secondary necrosis converge on similar cellular disintegration features. Cell Death Differ 17:922–930

29. Bertho ÁL, Santiago MA, Coutinho SG (2000) Flow cytometry in the study of cell death. Mem Inst Oswaldo Cruz 95:429–433

30. Holmes KL et al (2014) International society for the advancement of cytometry cell sorter biosafety standards. Citometry A 85:434–453

31. Könen-Waisman S, Howard JC (2007) Cell-autonomous immunity to *Toxoplasma gondii* in mouse and man. Microbes Infect 9:1652–1661

32. Martens S et al (2004) Mechanisms regulating the positioning of mouse p47 resistance GTPases LRG-47 and IIGP1 on cellular membranes: retargeting to plasma membrane induced by phagocytosis. J Immunol 173:2594–2606

33. Zerrahn J, Schaible UE, Brinkmann V, Guhlich U, Kaufmann SHE (2002) The IFN-inducible Golgi- and endoplasmic reticulum-associated 47-kDa GTPase IIGP is transiently expressed during listeriosis. J Immunol 168:3428–3436

34. Carlow DA et al (1998) Specific antiviral activity demonstrated by TGTP, a member of a new family of interferon-induced GTPases. J Immunol 161:2348–2355

35. Maric-Biresev J et al (2016) Loss of the interferon-γ-inducible regulatory immunity-related GTPase (IRG), Irgm1, causes activation of effector IRG proteins on lysosomes, damaging lysosomal function and predicting the dramatic susceptibility of Irgm1-deficient mice to infection. BMC Biol 14:1–20

36. Pawlowski N et al (2011) The activation mechanism of Irga6, an interferon-inducible GTPase contributing to mouse resistance against *Toxoplasma gondii*. BMC Biol 9:7

37. Steinfeldt T et al (2010) Phosphorylation of mouse immunity-related gtpase (IRG) resistance proteins is an evasion strategy for virulent *Toxoplasma gondii*. PLoS Biol 8:e1000576

38. Butcher BA et al (2005) p47 GTPases regulate *Toxoplasma gondii* survival in sctivated macrophages. Infect Immun 73:3278–3286

39. Springer HM, Schramm M, Taylor G a, Howard JC (2013) Irgm1 (LRG-47), a regulator of cell-autonomous immunity, does not localize to mycobacterial or listerial phagosomes in IFN-γ-induced mouse cells. J Immunol 191:1765–1774

40. Fleckenstein MC et al (2012) A *Toxoplasma gondii* pseudokinase inhibits host irg resistance proteins. PLoS Biol 10:14

41. Naviaux RK, Costanzi E, Haas M, Verma IM (1996) The pCL vector system: rapid production of helper-free, high-titer, recombinant retroviruses. J Virol 70:5701–5705

42. Christova Y, Adrain C, Bambrough P, Ibrahim A, Freeman M (2013) Mammalian iRhoms have distinct physiological functions including an essential role in TACE regulation. EMBO Rep 14:884–890

Chapter 21

Image-Based Quantitation of Host Cell–*Toxoplasma gondii* Interplay Using HRMAn: A Host Response to Microbe Analysis Pipeline

Daniel Fisch, Artur Yakimovich, Barbara Clough, Jason Mercer, and Eva-Maria Frickel

Abstract

Research on *Toxoplasma gondii* and its interplay with the host is often performed using fluorescence microscopy-based imaging experiments combined with manual quantification of acquired images. We present here an accurate and unbiased quantification method for host–pathogen interactions. We describe how to plan experiments and prepare, stain and image infected specimens and analyze them with the program HRMAn (Host Response to Microbe Analysis). HRMAn is a high-content image analysis method based on KNIME Analytics Platform. Users of this guide will be able to perform infection studies in high-throughput volume and to a greater level of detail. Relying on cutting edge machine learning algorithms, HRMAn can be trained and tailored to many experimental settings and questions.

Key words *Toxoplasma gondii*, Host–pathogen interaction, High-content image analysis, Artificial intelligence, Machine learning, HRMAn, KNIME Analytics platform

---

1 Introduction

Toxoplasma gondii (*Tg*) is an obligate intracellular, eukaryotic parasite that can infect any nucleated cell of a warm-blooded animal [1]. Belonging to the family of apicomplexan parasites, it has adapted to an intricate life cycle centered on its feline definitive host [2]. *Tg* commonly infects humans through food contamination or contact with cats, albeit infection does not endanger healthy individuals, and will persist latently for the lifetime of the infected human host (Global seroprevalence estimated around 30%) [3]. However, infection in immunocompromised humans or primary infection during pregnancy, can cause severe disease called *toxoplasmosis* or cause congenital birth defects [4, 5].

Tg parasites can take different forms during the lifecycle, with tachyzoites being the highly replicative and infectious form present

Christopher J. Tonkin (ed.), *Toxoplasma gondii: Methods and Protocols*, Methods in Molecular Biology, vol. 2071,
https://doi.org/10.1007/978-1-4939-9857-9_21, © Springer Science+Business Media, LLC, part of Springer Nature 2020

during primary infection. Tachyzoites can be propagated easily and indefinitely in tissue culture, making them perfect for studying infection processes with *Tg* in vitro. To do so, infection experiments are performed by infecting host cells with freshly prepared tachyzoites. During infection, *Tg* rapidly invades host cells and establishes its own replicative niche within the cytosol, called the parasitophorous vacuole (PV) [6, 7]. *Tg* injects a plethora of effector proteins upon invasion and exports further proteins once residing within the PV in its new host cell, modulating the cell's response by, for example, suppressing cell-intrinsic immune responses or by blocking certain types of cell death [8, 9]. Within the PV *Tg* continues to grow and replicate and duplicates every 6–10 h [10]. Once *Tg* has replicated to a sufficient number or if the host cell cannot sustain more parasites, *Tg* egresses from the host cell, thereby rupturing the PV and the cell, and spreads to infect neighboring cells.

The PV is a highly modified compartment that was thought to be nonfusogenic with lysosomes and comprises a safe haven in which the parasite can grow [11–13]. However, more recently, it has become clear that PVs can be recognized by host factors within immune-stimulated murine [14–16] and human cells [17–19]. Consequently, this triggers cell-intrinsic immune responses, either slowing the growth of or killing the parasites.

To study infection processes, parasites or host cells are often manipulated, and infection is simply a readout for the effect of the manipulation. These can include genetic modification (deletion of certain genes or overexpression), silencing of genes with RNAi, or blocking specific enzymes with inhibitors. Whether the focus of the experiment is on the host cell or on the parasite itself will dictate the readout of the experiment.

As infection is a highly dynamic process, so is the readout chosen for quantification. Researchers often tend to score certain parameters by manual enumeration of immunofluorescence images. These parameters include the number of cells and parasites, replication of the parasite or deposition of host/parasite protein on the PV. However, manual counting limits the number of quantified parameters and valuable information may be lost, or interesting phenotypes missed. Furthermore, the process of manual counting is flawed, as human error is likely to be introduced. Thus, we identified the necessity to automate the process of image-based infection quantification.

We recently published an automated image analysis pipeline called HRMAn for quantification of host response to *Tg* infection [20]. As described above, it is imperative for infection biology to be able to quantify infection dynamics reliably and consistently. Here, we describe how to prepare samples for microscopy that give reproducible results and provide details on how to image them. We also briefly describe how to use the HRMAn analysis pipeline, but we

Table 1
Measurements and readouts provided by the HRMAn analysis pipeline

Readout	Explanation	Interpretation example	
		Host response	Parasite biology
% Infected cells	Proportion of infected cells	Infected cells	Infection efficiency
Vacuole to cell ratio	Number of detected PVs normalized to the cell number	Killing of parasites	Invasion efficiency
Pathogen load	Overall number of individual parasites normalized to the cell number	Killing and replication restriction	Invasion efficiency and growth rate
Infection levels	Distribution of cells containing a specified number of vacuoles (uninfected, 1 PV/cell, 2PVs/cell, ...)	Killing of parasites	Invasion efficiency
Mean pathogen size	Mean size of the PVs	Growth restriction	Growth rate
Vacuole position	Mean Euclidian distance of the PVs to the nucleus of the cell they are contained in	Transport of the PV	Parasite about to egress?
Inter vacuole distance	Mean Euclidian distance of different PVs within one cell	Transport of the PV	Clustering of PVs
Inter cell distance	Mean Euclidian distance between the nuclei of all cells	Clustering of cells	Modulation of cell motility
Fluorescence cytosol	Sum of the fluorescence signal in the cytosol of the cells	Defense protein production	Amount of secreted effector
Fluorescence nucleus	Sum of the fluorescence signal in the nucleus of the cells	Transcription factor activation	Amount of secreted effector
Ratio fluorescence nucleus/ cytosol	Ratio between the fluorescence signal in the cell's nucleus and cytosol	Transcription factor activation	Transport of effectors to the nucleus
Pathogen features	Pathogen size, shape, fluorescence	Effect on growth	Growth parameters
% Replicating pathogens	Proportion of parasites that have replicated (i.e., more than one parasite per vacuole)	Growth restriction	Growth rate
Replication distribution	Distribution of vacuoles based on how many parasites they contain, e.g., 1, 2, 4, or more than 4	Growth restriction	Growth rate
%Recruiting cells*	Proportion of infected cells that deposit defense proteins on at least one PV that they contain	Population response	Efficiency of *Tg* protein localization

(continued)

Table 1
(continued)

Readout	Explanation	Interpretation example	
		Host response	Parasite biology
Recruited vacuoles per cell*	Mean proportion of PVs that each cell marks with defense proteins	Individual response	Efficiency of *Tg* protein localization
Protein recruitment levels*	Overall proportion of marked vacuoles for individual channels of corecruitment of two proteins	Overall response levels	Display of *Tg* protein on PV, interaction of two *Tg* proteins
Vacuole coat distance*	Mean radial distance of the proteins on the PVM to the centroid of the PV	Recruitment sequence (temporal)	Exact localization of proteins (PVM, *Tg* membrane vs. IMC)
Vacuole coat thickness*	Thickness/fluorescence signal strength of the proteins on the PVM	Amount of recruited protein	Amount of *Tg* protein displayed
% Replicating pathogens (recruited)*	Proportion of parasites that have replicated (i.e., more than one parasite per vacuole) of only PVs that have been marked	Effect of recruitment on growth	Effect of *Tg* protein display on growth
Replication distribution (recruited)*	Distribution of vacuoles based on how many parasites they contain, of only PVs that have been marked	Effect of recruitment on growth	Effect of *Tg* protein display on growth

Overview and explanation of all readouts that are computed by HRMAn. All readouts can be used to either study the host response to infection with *Toxoplasma gondii* (*Tg*) or to study the parasite biology. All readouts can be obtained using the infection analysis, with the exception of those marked with an asterisk which are additionally obtained in the recruitment analysis. Examples for either application are provided
PV parasitophorous vacuole, *PVM* parasitophorous vacuole membrane, *IMC* inner membrane complex

want to note that for a more detailed instruction, we recommend visiting the homepage (https://hrman.org/) and use the provided tutorials. To learn more about the information that is extracted from the immunofluorescence images of infected cells, we provide an explanation of their meaning and how they can be interpreted from the host side "host response" or the parasite side "parasite biology" (Table 1).

To compute the readouts, HRMAn uses well-established image analysis and segmentation algorithms to detect cells and pathogens and combines this information with classical machine learning and cutting-edge artificial intelligence algorithms in the form of deep convolutional neural networks. This is wrapped into a user-friendly environment based on KNIME Analytics platform [21]. KNIME provides an intuitive graphical user interface and a modular architecture that will allow more experienced users to adapt and modify the analysis pipeline and tailor it to their needs. HRMAn can be used without any coding experience, but we recommend watching the tutorial videos and gaining some hands-on experience by using the example datasets provided on the homepage and on Dryad (*see* Subheading 2.6). Once comfortable with the analysis pipeline, users are enabled to perform infection experiment on a different scale, with virtually no limitation to the number of samples or replicates within each experiment.

2 Materials

2.1 General

- Micropipettes.
- Pipette controller.
- 15 mL and 50 mL conical tubes
- Microcentrifuge tubes.
- Serological pipettes.
- ddH$_2$O.
- Phosphate buffered saline (PBS), sterile filtered, suitable for cell culture.

2.2 Cell/Parasite Culture and Infection

- Tissue culture plates: 24-well or black-wall 96-well plates (Optional with coverslips glass-bottom, e.g., MACS Miltenyi, Imaging Plate CG 1.0 (96 well), # 130-098-264).
- Cell culture benchtop centrifuge with adaptors for multiwell plates.
- Appropriate cell culture medium with supplements for the used cell line.
- Optional: Trypsin–EDTA, for dislodging adherent cells.
- Human foreskin fibroblasts (HFFs), grown confluent in T25 flasks for propagation of *Tg* tachyzoites.
- DMEM with added 10% FCS, for propagation of HFFs and *Tg*-infected HFFs.
- Cell scrapers, 25 G needles and 10 mL syringes, for syringe-lysing *Tg* cultures.
- Trypan blue and hemocytometer (e.g., Immune Systems, Fast-read disposable counting slides #BVS100), for counting cells and parasite numbers.
- Gelatin; porcine skin gelatin (Sigma #G1890) made to 1% in ddH$_2$O.
- Ethanol, for disinfection.
- Coverslips; #1.5 thickness, 9–12 mm diameter.
- Optional: Phorbol 12-myristate 13-acetate (PMA) for differentiation of THP-1 cells into macrophages.

2.3 Specimen Preparation and Staining

- Formaldehyde; methanol-free formaldehyde 16% (e.g., Pierce #28908) diluted to give a final concentration of 4%.

- Optional: Ammonium chloride (NH_4Cl) solution, 50 mM dissolved in ddH_2O, sterile filtered.

- Permeabilization buffer; Prepare 10× stock in 50 mL volume. 2% (w/v) Bovine serum albumin Fraction V, 0.2% (w/v) saponin (e.g., Merck #47036) make to 50 mL in 10× PBS. Dispense 5 mL aliquots in 50 mL Falcon tubes, store −20 °C and make up to 50 mL with ddH_2O when required.

- Nuclear stain (e.g., Hoechst 33342 or DAPI).

- CellMask, plasma membrane stains for high-content screening (Thermo Fisher Scientific; HCS cell mask red #H32712, HCS cell mask green #H32714).

- Antibodies for staining and appropriate fluorescently labeled secondary antibodies for visualization (e.g., Alexa Fluor secondary antibodies by Molecular Probes, ThermoFisher).

- Mounting medium, a hardening mounting medium is required, for example Mowiol 4-88 (Sigma #81381) or ProLong Gold (ThermoFisher #P10144), when working with cells on coverslips.

- Microscope slides.

- Nontransparent plate seal, for sealing multiwell plates.

2.4 Imaging

- Fluorescence microscope or high-content imager equipped with CCD high-resolution, digital camera with ideally >12-bit dynamic range.

2.5 Image Analysis

- Computer capable of running KNIME Analytics platform version 3.4.2 or newer.

2.6 Online Resources

- The HRMAn analysis pipeline can be downloaded from: https://github.com/HRMAn-Org/HRMAn.

- More information and tutorial videos can be found here: https://hrman.org.

- Four different sample datasets for testing HRMAn can be downloaded from Dryad: https://doi.org/10.5061/dryad.6vq2mp0.

3 Methods

Quantification of the host cell response to *Tg* infection by imaging can be performed on different scales: small pilot experiments can be performed using manual image acquisition and specimens prepared on coverslips (*A*), whereas experiments that require testing of many different conditions can be performed in a high-throughput manner and are usually performed using multiwell plates (96-well or more, *B*). In steps where the sample preparation and analysis differ, we will refer to them as *A* or *B*, as indicated above. Furthermore, two types of analyses are possible using HRMAn, an "infection analysis" which quantifies infection dynamics as well as host cell responses and a "recruitment analysis" which additionally quantifies protein recruitment parameters at the PV.

3.1 Preparation of Host Cells for Infection

In general, cells need to be seeded in defined numbers at the start of an experiment. It is important to first determine the optimal seeding conditions and cell number for the experiment. If the cellular response is the target of the analysis, cells should be seeded as densely as feasible (to get as many of them imaged as possible) but they should not touch each other or grow fully confluent, otherwise image segmentation of the cells will be difficult and might result in inaccurate results (some example seeding densities and timelines of commonly used cell lines are provided in Table 2). For some cells it is advisable to coat plates in order for the cells to adhere better. We can recommend using gelatin as a substrate (*see* Box 1), but other substrates may be used if they work well for a particular cell type.

Box 1 Gelatin Coating

We find that gelatin-coating of plates significantly improves the attachment of cells during infection processes, which maintains equal numbers per well for imaging experiments. Perform the following steps to make up gelatin and coat plates:

– *Prepare gelatin*:

Add 1%(w/v) gelatin powder (e.g., Sigma #G1890 porcine skin gelatin) to ddH$_2$O and dissolve at 60 °C with stirring for 30 min. While liquid, filter through a bottle top filtration system (0.22 μm; e.g., StarLab CytoOne C6032-8233). Aliquot (10–50 mL) and store at 4 °C.

– *Coating plates*:

Before using, melt gelatin at 37 °C for 20–30 min until fully liquid. Add enough gelatin to cover bottom of the well(s) and incubate at 37 °C for 20 min or longer.

– *Seed cells*:

Aspirate excess gelatin from the well(s) and plate cells on top immediately.

Table 2
Example seeding densities and timelines of frequently used human cell lines

Cell line	Substrate	#/Well (A) (24-well)	#/Well (B) (96-well)	Seeding time point, comments
HFF	–	50,000	20,000	Seed 1 day before the experiment for individual cells or several days before if confluent monolayers are needed
HeLa	–	50,000	10,000	Seed 1 day before the experiment. This allows for cells to adhere and reach near confluence with the ability to segment the cells in image analysis. This also allows time for additional cell treatments
A549	–	50,000	10,000	
HUVEC	Gelatin	100,000	15,000	
THP-1	Gelatin	250,000	30,000	Seed 5 days prior to experiment in complete RPMI + 50 ng/mL PMA for differentiation. Replace medium after three days with complete RPMI to rest the cells

Cell numbers, growth substrate, and timeline for seeding five different human cell lines for *Toxoplasma gondii* infection experiments

In general, cells on coverslips are seeded in 24-well plates (*A*, *see* **Note 1**) whereas for high-throughput experiments they are seeded in 96-well plates (or other multiwell plates, *B*, *see* **Notes 1–3**). It is advisable to omit wells on the outer edge of a plate because they show more evaporation which can skew results. Instead fill them with sterile PBS or culture medium (whatever is available) to prevent evaporation from the cell-containing wells in the centre of the plate. Another consideration during the planning of experiments is the position of different treatment conditions on a plate. Make sure to change them during repeats of experiments to exclude any positional effects that may distort the data. When planning an experiment, it should also be considered to have some wells as uninfected controls, which can be used to track the effect of infection on the number of cells. We also recommend creating a plate map before starting the experiment to keep track of experiment conditions (for an example *see* Fig. 1a).

In some experimental settings the cells can be transfected with DNA or RNA before the infection. Additionally, cells can be pretreated with cytokines the evening before infection to induce responses or treated with inhibitors to manipulate their response. This depends on the type of experiment that is being performed (*see* **Note 4**).

3.2 Infection Procedure and Fixation of Samples

1. The day before infection, split *Tg* tachyzoites from freshly syringe-lysed HFFs onto new HFFs cells and let them grow to sufficient numbers overnight. Usually 1:5 splitting from a T25 flask into a new T25 flask with confluent HFFs gives

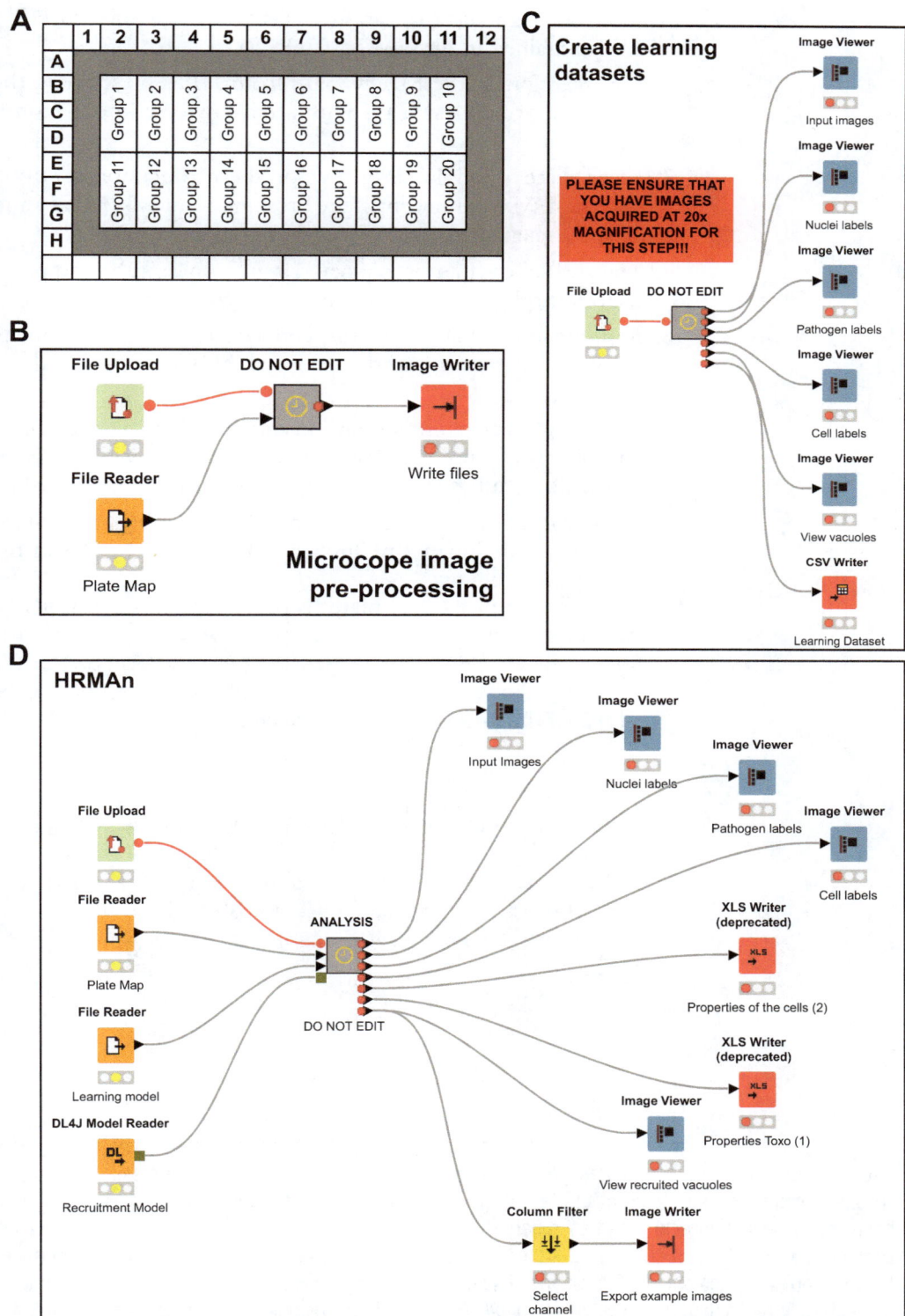

Fig. 1 Example plate layout and overview of the KNIME analysis pipelines used for HRMAn. (**a**) Example plate map of a 96-well plate, wells on the edge of the plate were omitted (gray) and individual sample groups are

sufficient high viability parasites (HFFs and *Tg*-infected HFFs are maintained in DMEM + 10% FCS).

2. For infection, harvest tachyzoites from HFFs by scraping the cells and syringe lysing through a 25 G needle into a 15 mL conical tube.

3. Clear lysate of cell debris by low speed centrifugation at $50 \times g$ for 5 min. Maximum centrifuge breaking is suitable for this and all subsequent steps.

4. Transfer supernatant into a new 15 mL conical tube and pellet tachyzoites by centrifugation at $600 \times g$ for 7 min.

5. Remove supernatant and resuspend *Tg* tachyzoites in complete medium, that is appropriate for the host cell line used for infection.

6. Take 10 μL tachyzoite suspension and mix 1:1 with trypan blue and fill 10 μL into a hemocytometer. Count viable parasites (unstained) and calculate their concentration.

7. Prepare dilutions of tachyzoites to have the appropriate number for the designated multiplicity of infection (MOI) in the appropriate volume:

   Infection in 24-well plates is performed using 450 μL *Tg* suspension per well (*A*), infection in 96-well plates is performed using 150 μL *Tg* suspension per well (*B*) (*see* Box 2). During infection, fresh cytokines and/or inhibitors can be added (if the inhibitors do not affect *Tg* itself, *see* **Note 4**).

Box 2 Example: Infection of THP-1 Cells in 60 Wells of a 96-Well Plate

THP-1 s were seeded as described above with 30,000 cells per well in the centre 60 wells of a 96-well plate. They all will be infected with *Tg* using a MOI = 3 in 150 μL per well.

Calculation:

– *Total Tg suspension needed*:

(continued)

Fig. 1 (continued) performed in triplicate wells (= technical replicates). We recommend making plate maps like the one depicted to keep track of the layout. (**b**) Overview of the "Microscope image pre-processing" pipeline (depicts user interface), used to rename and format images from any imaging platform before analyzing them with HRMAn. (**c**) Overview of the "Create learning datasets" pipeline (depicts user interface), used to create an annotated dataset for training of a decision-tree machine learning algorithm implemented in HRMAn to classify replication of *Toxoplasma gondii* (*Tg*) inside of its vacuole. (**d**) Overview of the "HRMAn" analysis pipeline (depicts user interface), used to perform high-content/ -throughput image analysis to study host-pathogen interaction of *Tg*

> **Box 2** (continued)
>
> 60 wells × 150 µL/well = 9 mL medium, make 10 mL to have some additional volume.
>
> – *Number of tachyzoites needed*:
>
> 30,000 host cells/well × 3 (MOI) = 90,000 *Tg*/well.
>
> – *Dilution*:
>
> (90,000 *Tg*/well)/(150 µL/well) = 600,000 *Tg*/mL.
>
> – *Result*:
>
> 10 mL × 600,000 *Tg*/mL = 6,000,000 *Tg* = 6×10^{6} *Tg*.
>
> → Prepare 10 mL medium with 6×10^{6} *Tg* tachyzoites and add 150 µL per well.

8. Once the *Tg* dilution for infection is prepared, add the appropriate volume per well and spin the plates at $500 \times g$ for 5 min (this helps to synchronize the infection). Place back in the tissue culture incubator at 37 °C, 5% CO_2.

9. 2 h post infection, any uninvaded/nonviable parasites are removed from the wells by aspirating the medium and carefully washing the infected cells three times with prewarmed PBS (*see* **Notes 5** and **6**). This prevents uninvaded parasites being included in the final analysis. The wells are then replenished with prewarmed complete medium. At this stage, cytokines and/or inhibitors can be added to the wells as appropriate (*see* **Note 4**).

10. After the required time of infection (2–24 h or more, depending on the experiment), wash cells twice with prewarmed PBS (*see* **Note 5**) and afterward add 450 µL PBS per well of a 24-well plate (*A*) or 150 µL per well of a 96-well plate (*B*).

11. To fix the cells add methanol-free 16% PFA to the samples, 150 µL per well of a 24-well plate (*A*) or 50 µL per well of a 96-well plate (*B*). This achieves 4% PFA final concentration.

12. Move samples to a light protected place (or cover with foil) and incubate for 15 min at room temperature.

13. Following incubation with 4% PFA, aspirate and discard the PFA into the appropriate waste and wash the cells three times with PBS (*see* **Notes 5** and **6**). Then fill all wells with PBS to cover the cells and leave at 4 °C overnight to quench residual PFA.

14. OPTIONAL: If specimen needs to be processed immediately, wash with 50 mM NH_4Cl to quench residual PFA and then wash again twice with PBS.

3.3 Staining of Fixed Specimens for Immunofluorescence Microscopy

1. Permeabilize the cells: Remove PBS from the samples and add 300 μL of permeabilization buffer per well of a 24-well plate (*A*) or 100 μL per well of a 96-well plate (*B*) and incubate 30 min at room temperature in the dark.

2. (*A*) Aspirate permeabilization buffer from the coverslips and proceed with staining. For coverslips, it is efficient to carefully pick them from the plate using fine point forceps and incubate inverted on a drop of staining solution on Parafilm (10–30 μL solution per 9–12 mm coverslip, respectively, is sufficient). In this instance, it is advisable to have the parafilm overlaying a sheet of prewet filter paper in a square petri dish to maintain a humid environment during incubation. (*B*) Remove permeabilization buffer from the 96-well plate (*see* **Note 7**) and proceed with adding staining solution (*see* below). For 96-well plates the minimum volume to add to cover all cells is 70 μL per well!

    Depending on the analysis you want to perform later on, decide on the staining procedure. Continue with **step 3** if you simply want to analyze the infection process or continue with **step 4** if you additionally want to analyze protein recruitment to the *Tg* vacuoles.

3. Staining for infection analysis:

    For simple infection analysis it is sufficient to have stained nuclei, cytosol and parasites. If nonfluorescent *Tg* lines were used for infection, perform antibody (Ab) staining as described below for host/parasite proteins (*see* **Note 8**).

    (a) Prepare staining solution: Permeabilization buffer + 1:2500 CellMask far red (for green parasites, use different color if the parasites express a different fluorophore) and 1:5000 Hoechst 33342 (or other nuclear stain).

    (b) Replace permeabilization buffer with 70 μL staining solution per well and incubate for 1 h at room temperature in the dark.

    (c) Continue with final wash steps.

4. Antibody-staining for protein recruitment analysis:

    For protein recruitment to *Tg* vacuoles analysis the cells have to be stained with an Ab against the protein of interest, if the protein is not tagged with a fluorescent protein. Furthermore, if nonfluorescent *Tg* lines were used for infection, perform Ab staining of them as well (*see* **Note 8**) (*see* Box 3).

    (a) Prepare first staining solution: Permeabilization buffer with added dilution of primary antibodies, add to the samples and incubate for 1 h at room temperature in the dark (*see* **Note 9**).

    (b) Wash three times with PBS.

(c) Prepare second staining solution: Permeabilization buffer with added dilution of appropriate secondary antibodies (coupled to fluorophores of choice) and 1:5000 Hoechst 33342, add to the samples and incubate for 1 h at room temperature in the dark (*see* **Note 9**).

(d) Continue with final wash steps.

5. Following staining wash all specimens at least five times with PBS to remove as much secondary antibody or unused stain as possible. This will result in less background during image acquisition. Coverslips need to be washed in ddH₂O and then mounted using Mowiol (or other mounting medium) onto glass microscope slides (*A*) or fill wells of the 96-well plates with 200 μL PBS per well and seal the plate using nontransparent plate seal (*B*).

At this point samples can be stored at 4 °C for more than a month, albeit some signal loss has to be expected.

Box 3 Example: Staining of HeLa Cells Infected with Colorless *Tg*

HeLa cells were infected with colorless *Tg* at a MOI = 3 for 6 h and we wanted to visualize ubiquitin and p62 decoration of vacuoles. To do this, we needed to stain the parasites and host cell proteins with antibodies:

– *First stain*:

Prepare permeabilization buffer with added rabbit anti-ubiquitin, goat anti-p62 and mouse anti-*Tg*SAG1*, add to samples and incubate for 1 h. Then perform wash steps.

– Second stain:

Prepare permeabilization buffer with added Hoechst 33342, anti-mouse-Alexa 488, anti-rabbit-Alexa 568, and anti-goat-Alexa 647*, add to samples and incubate for 1 h. Then perform final wash steps.

This will result in specimen that have blue nuclei, green *Tg*, red ubiquitin, and far-red p62. These samples can then be used to analyze (co)recruitment of the two proteins to the PV using HRMAn (*see* below).

*Example Abs! Use as appropriate and optimize for your own experiment.

3.4 Image Acquisition and Data Preparation

For image acquisition make sure to use the same standards as are applicable in general when using fluorescence microscopes:

1. Images should not only look "pretty" but represent quantifiable data.

2. Settings should be adjusted using a real sample and kept the same for an entire image acquisition dataset (i.e., several 96-well plates or coverslips) in order to be able to compare the different conditions later on.

3. Because images are obtained for quantitative analysis ensure that gain and offset are set to use the entire dynamic range of the detector, this prevents clipping of the dataset at either end.

4. Use of higher bit cameras (e.g.,12-bit) is advisable as they offer a higher dynamic range.

5. Data should be saved in a raw, uncompressed format such as .tiff.

In general, the use of high-content imaging systems, which were developed for automated image acquisition will solve many of these problems.

When imaging coverslips ensure that you acquire enough non-overlapping and randomly chosen fields of view (even if this means you image an empty spot on your coverslip)! Only like this can you ensure to get real insight into what was happening on your coverslip/in your well during infection (Loss of many cells or clumping of them in certain spots might actually represent an interesting phenotype!). To obtain an appropriately sized dataset, you should aim to image at least 1000 cells per condition which at a MOI of 1 should approximately result in a similar number of *Tg* vacuoles (this number may be smaller if cells were treated to become parasiticidal). The number of images required to reach these amount of cells depends on the magnification and camera detector size used for imaging. For example, collecting a grid of 5-by-5 adjacent fields of view containing approximately 50 cells each (at a magnification of 20× and when cells have been seeded according to the recommendations in Table 2) would give a suitable sample size for analysis.

As *Tg* is a reasonably large object, 20× magnification is sufficient for infection analysis and 40× magnification for protein recruitment analysis. Use of confocal imaging systems is not necessary at this point. If confocal images were acquired use the appropriate option in the image preprocessing step to create z-projections (*see* below).

1. Once the images are acquired and saved as single channel files they need to be prepared for analysis using HRMAn. Use the **"Microscope image pre-processing"** KNIME pipeline (Fig. 1b) from the HRMAn GitHub repository to prepare your dataset.

Table 3
Spreadsheet layout of the plate map used in the HRMAn analysis pipeline

Well	Sample group	Infected?
A01	1	0
A02	2	1
A03	2	1
A04	1	0
A05	3	1
. . .	. . .	. . .

Overview of the table layout of the plate map spreadsheet file used in the HRMAn analysis pipeline. Users can assign wells to defined sample groups by adding numbers into the respective column and indicate if the cells in the well were infected with *Toxoplasma gondii* in the last column. In the example, sample group 1 in wells A01 and A04 were uninfected, thus the 0. Following analysis, HRMAn will calculate the means and errors from the wells indicated in this table for the different sample groups. In the example above, the values of wells A02 and A03 would be used to create the mean value for sample group 2

2. Load the images into the program by specifying the location in the "**File upload**" node.

3. Load your plate map for the experiment (*see* below) into the program by specifying the .csv file in the "**Table reader**" node (Table 3).

4. Select the "**Image writer**" node on the right-hand side and start the pipeline by executing the node. (Right click and click execute in the menu that opens.)

5. The program will ask for the following:
   (a) The number of samples.
   (b) The number of fields per sample.
   (c) The number of channels.
   (d) The number of planes per field.

   Enter the values and confirm by clicking ok. Once all parameters are entered the program will display a summary and ask if they are correct.

6. The program will then automatically rename all images and write them into the same folder as your input images. If several planes were acquired, a z-projection is performed to reduce the amount of data (subject to future 3D-analysis update).

7. The files are now named according to the following scheme:
   A01f00d00∗, with A01 specifying the first well of the plate or representing the first sample/coverslip, f00 being the first field and d00 being the first channel.

It is important that all input images are named exactly according to this format!

As HRMAn was developed to work with images acquired in a plate format, this step ensures that data that did not originate from automated imaging of 96-well plates, or was named differently, will be analyzed and clustered correctly using similar plate maps (*see* below).

3.5 High-Content Image Analysis Using HRMAn

Once images are acquired and have been preprocessed (renamed), they are ready to be analyzed using HRMAn. The analysis runs in two stages: Stage 1 simply analyses common infection parameters and uses a decision tree machine learning algorithm to classify replication of the *Tg* parasites. This stage is based on well-established image analysis methods. Stage 2 uses a deep convolutional neural network (CNN) to classify recruitment of proteins to the PV. Before they can be used, the machine learning algorithms need to be trained:

3.5.1 Creating a Dataset for the Decision Tree Machine Learner

For this step you can use the **"Create learning datasets"** KNIME pipeline (Fig. 1c) that can be found in the HRMAn GitHub repository. It will help you to annotate individual *Tg* vacuoles based on how many parasites they contain. To run the pipeline, open it in KNIME and perform the following steps (to learn how to set up KNIME and the individual analysis pipelines, you can find video tutorials on https://hrman.org/):

(a) Use the **"File Upload"** node to load your images into the pipeline. It is important to have images acquired at a magnification of $20\times$ to have the right scaling! Make sure you have renamed your images according to the format described above (File name A01f00d01, A01f00d02, etc.).

(b) Select the **"Image Viewer"**-**Input images** node and execute it. This will start the analysis.

(c) The program will ask you for some information:

- The channel number and their order.

- The magnification you used to image.

- The pathogen type (enter a 1 for *Tg*).

(d) The program will then perform the first steps of the image analysis up to the segmentation. Once finished, the little traffic light underneath the node **"Image Viewer"**-**Input images** turns green. You can use this node to view the images that you have provided.

(e) Next use the **"Image Viewer"**-**Nuclei labels**, -**Pathogen labels** or -**Cell labels** to see the segmentation the program has performed and make sure they are good (*see* **Note 10**).

(f) Then select the **"Image Viewer"-View Vacuoles** node and the **"CSV Writer"-Learning dataset** node execute them. The csv writer node will write a table with the attributes of the *Tg* vacuoles to the defined output location. The last column in this document "Parasites/vacuole" will be empty.

(g) Then use the **"Image Viewer"-View Vacuoles** node to look at the individual cropped vacuoles. On the bottom you will see the vacuole ID, which will match the rows in the csv file. Determine the number of parasites (1, 2, 4, 4 or more) and type the value into the empty column of the csv file. As it becomes very difficult to determine the exact number of parasites if more than four parasites are contained within the same vacuole, we decided to pool them. If you encounter vacuoles like that, simply type in an eight and the machine learner will know what to do. Once you have finished annotating the vacuoles and every row in the csv file is filled in with the number of contained parasites, you can use this file for all future experiments using HRMAn analysis. Simply read it into the pipeline as described below.

3.5.2 Creating a Dataset for Training the CNN and Training

For creating datasets and training the deep neural network implemented in HRMAn ("HRMAlexNet"), we recommend watching the tutorial videos on hrman.org and following the detailed instructions provided there. Already trained models can be obtained from the GitHub repository (https://github.com/HRMAn-Org/HRMAn) or the homepage (https://hrman.org/).

Now the HRMAn analysis itself can be run. Please follow the instructions provided there to set up the program properly; Fig. 1d):

1. Use the **"File upload"** node to specify where HRMAn can find your images.

2. Using the **"File Reader"** node provide the plate map:
The template for a plate map can be found in the HRMAn repository (*see* Table 3 for the layout of the spreadsheet).

It is important that the file is saved as .csv and that the structure of the table (i.e., the index and the name of the columns) is not changed, as this could lead to errors in the program. In the plate map define which wells represent repeats of the same conditions by using continuous numbering of the different conditions on your plate. The program also needs to know if the cells in the sample were infected or if they represent uninfected, cells-only conditions. If they were infected this has to be represented with a 1, otherwise fill the cell with a 0.

3. Using the **"File Reader"** node to provide a learning model for the decision tree (*see* above for instructions on how to create this file).

4. Using the **"DL4J Model Reader"** node read in the file for the trained CNN (even if you are not performing recruitment analysis, provide a model here, as otherwise the program might crash. You can use the trained HRMAlexNet-Ubiquitin that can be downloaded from the GitHub repository).

5. Select the **"Image Viewer"**-**Input images** node and execute it. This will start the analysis.

6. HRMAn will ask you for some information:
   (a) The magnification that was used to image the cells: Simply enter the magnification as a number.
   (b) The pathogen you want to analyze: For *Tg* type a 1 and confirm by clicking ok.
   (c) The type of analysis you want to perform:
       For infection analysis (stage 1 only) type a 1.
       For recruitment analysis (stage 1 + 2) type a 2.
       Confirm by clicking ok (*see* Box 4).
   (d) The number of channels you used to image your cells (the default for infection analysis is three channels).
   (e) The order of your channels.

7. HRMAn will then perform the first steps of the analysis up to the segmentation. Once this is done, the traffic light indicator underneath the node **"Image Viewer"**-**Input images** turns green. You can use this node to view the images that you have provided.

8. Next use the **"Image Viewer"**-**Nuclei labels, -Pathogen labels** or **-Cell labels** to see the segmentation HRMAn has performed and make sure they are good (*see* **Note 10**).

9. If you are happy with the segmentation you can select and execute the **"XLS Writer"** -**Properties of the cells** and -**Properties Pathogens** nodes. This will start the rest of the analysis and write an .xlsx into your selected working directory. HRMAn indicates when the analysis is complete and following this the results file will open.

10. Save the file in a different location, for later analysis. (IMPORTANT: File will be overwritten once the analysis pipeline is executed again!).

Box 4 Example: Recruitment Analysis Using HRMAn

HeLa cells were infected with *Tg* for 6 h and stained for ubiquitin. The images were renamed and are ready for analysis.

- *Load the images, the plate map, learning models and start the analysis.*
- *Type in the information:*

  Cells were imaged at a magnification of 40× (type in 40), the pathogen was *Tg* (type in 1), HRMAn shall perform recruitment analysis (type in 2). Then double check the summary and confirm if correct (type in 1). Next, HRMAn wants to know the channel number, you have 3 channels (type in 3) and their order (type in as they come up). Then HRMAn wants to make sure that you have provided the correct plate map (type in 1). Then the analysis and segmentation will be performed.

- *Check the input images:*

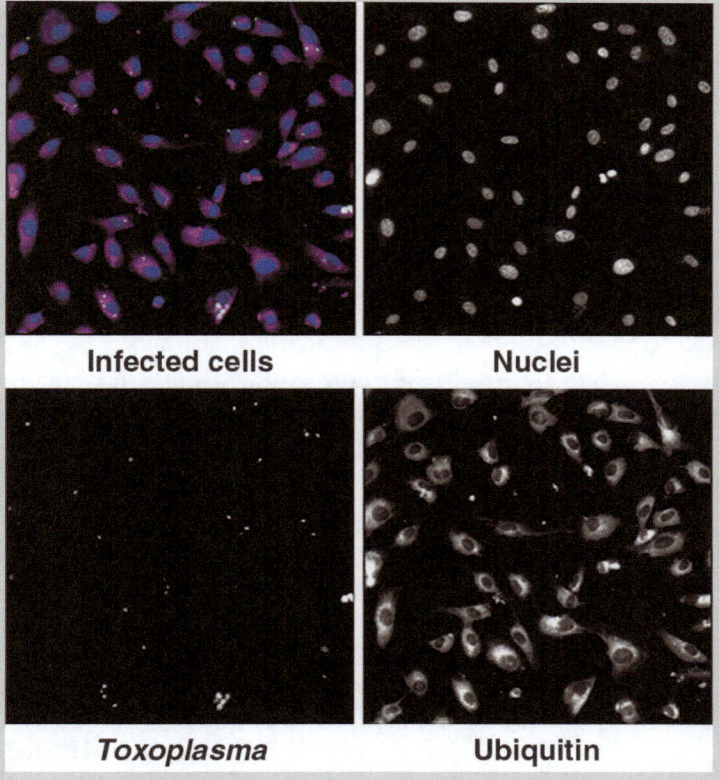

(continued)

Box 4 (continued)

All images loaded? Yes!

– *Check the nuclei/Tg/cell segmentation*:

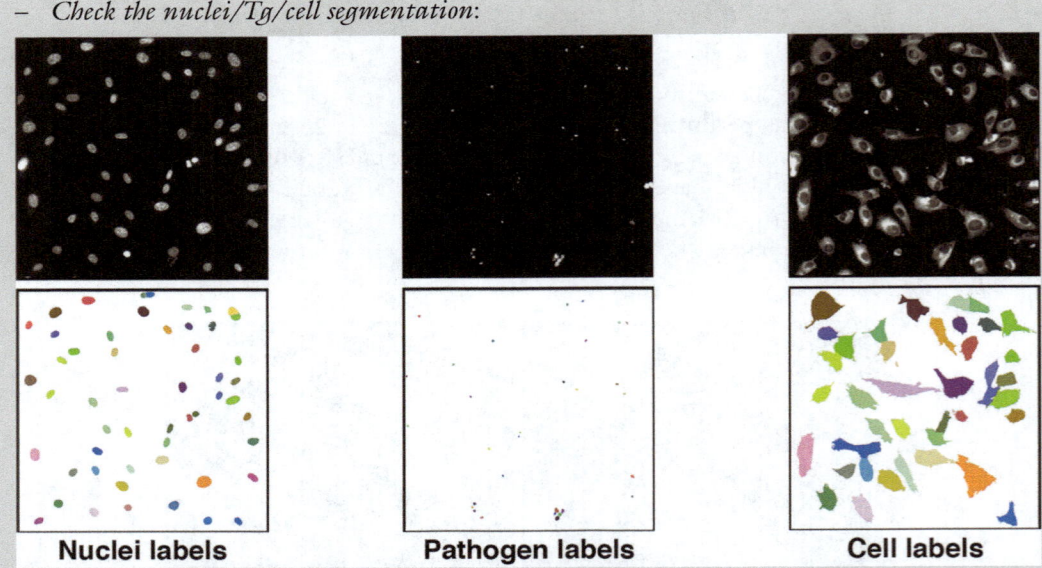

Segmentation ok? Yes!

– *Finish the analysis*:
   If all segmentations are good, select the output nodes and execute them. This will start
   the rest of the analysis and write the output file to your computer.

When the HRMAn analysis of the images is finished, the user is provided with a spreadsheet file that contains all computed results. This data can then be visualized using graph plotting programs. Here users need to ensure that all segmentation steps of the analysis have performed well and that the data is of the expected quality. Further, it is the user's responsibility to ensure data integrity and perform the appropriate statistical analysis.

Once familiar with HRMAn and KNIME analytics platform, it is easy to adapt the analysis pipeline exactly to the needs of the researcher using it, or extend it to measure more parameters. This allows study of the parasite biology, the host response to infection and the interplay of both sides. Importantly, HRMAn is open-source and employs neural network precision for the analysis of host protein recruitment to the pathogen. HRMAn has the potential to be tailored for the analysis of other intracellular pathogens (e.g., *Salmonella*, *Plasmodium*).

4   Notes

1. Use tissue culture treated plates.

2. Use black-wall plates to reduce scattered light. If higher magnification imaging is required ($>20\times$) it is advisable to use plates with a coverslip-thickness glass bottom. Handle glass-bottom plates with extra care, they are extremely fragile! We find that taping cardboard to the bottom helps prevent the glass from breaking. To reduce costs, higher magnification imaging can also be performed in plastic-bottom plates, depending on the microscope used for image acquisition, though this might increase background noise and negatively affect image quality.

3. Omit wells on the edge of the plate and fill them with sterile PBS to prevent evaporation and edge effects.

4. When using cell treatments such as cytokines or inhibitors, it is important to include appropriate no treatment and vehicle-only controls. Some inhibitors will need to be washed off the cells prior to infection as they may affect the invasion or growth of the parasite directly. We suggest washing twice with warmed medium or PBS.

5. When performing wash steps of cells, be very gentle to not wash away the cells. For cells that do not adhere well, we recommend using a wire manifold (e.g., Drummond Scientific Co., Straight, 8 places for 96-well plate, # 3-000-093) which is gentler and set to leave a residual amount of medium/PBS behind on washing. This not only minimizes damage to the cell layer by tips but also prevents poorly adherent cells from being drawn up with the medium/PBS on aspiration.

6. All solutions used during cell culture and staining should be filter-sterilized through a 0.22 μm filter to prevent microbe and dust contamination of samples.

7. We find that following fixation, inverting the plates and drying them by banging on a stack of paper is efficient and does not result in cell loss.

8. We find that anti-SAG1 (*Tg* surface antigen 1) is a well-performing stain for *Tg*. This antibody is available commercially (e.g., GeneTex mouse monoclonal, clone B754M #GTX38936).

9. Staining with antibodies needs to be optimized first! As antibodies are highly variable, we recommend using antibodies that have been used for immunofluorescence experiments before. Some companies validate their primary antibodies using siRNA negative controls and provide staining images for endogenous levels of protein, which can be helpful when selecting reliable

and specific antibodies. These steps can also be performed by the user. Initially it will be important to include primary only and secondary only antibody controls and where costaining is required to incorporate single stain controls. Make sure to use enough antibody to get a good signal without overstaining the sample which will create nonspecific background.

10. The HRMAn analysis pipeline has been designed to perform segmentation of nuclei, cells and *Tg* automatically using different automated normalization, thresholding and connected component analysis strategies combined with filtering. If the segmentation does not perform to the satisfaction of the user, it is possible to manually adjust the threshold used for segmentation. This can be achieved by opening the "Segmentation" node contained within the "Analysis" metanode and altering the threshold within the "Global Thresholder" used for the respective segmentation. However, the most common reasons for a failed segmentation is poor image acquisition/quality or a too high cell density. In these cases, we recommend preparing new samples.

Acknowledgments

We thank all members of the Frickel lab for productive discussion. This work was supported by the Francis Crick Institute, which receives its core funding from Cancer Research UK (FC001076), the UK Medical Research Council (FC001076), and the Wellcome Trust (FC001076). E.M.F. was supported by a Wellcome Trust Career Development Fellowship (091664/B/10/Z). D.F. was supported by a Boehringer Ingelheim Fonds Ph.D. fellowship. A.Y. and J.M. were supported by core funding to the MRC Laboratory for Molecular Cell Biology at University College London (J.M.), the European Research Council (649101-UbiProPox), the UK Medical Research Council (MC_UU12018/7).

Author Contribution: D.F., B.C., and E.M.F. wrote the manuscript. All authors contributed to revising the manuscript.

References

1. Sabin AB, Olitsky PK (1937) *Toxoplasma* and obligate intracellular parasitism. Science 85 (2205):336–338

2. Dubey JP, Miller NL, Frenkel JK (1970) The *Toxoplasma gondii* oocyst from cat feces. J Exp Med 132(4):636–662

3. Pappas G, Roussos N, Falagas ME (2009) Toxoplasmosis snapshots: global status of *Toxoplasma gondii* seroprevalence and implications

for pregnancy and congenital toxoplasmosis. Int J Parasitol 39(12):1385–1394

4. Beverley JK (1973) Toxoplasmosis. Br Med J 2 (5864):475–478

5. Luft BJ, Remington JS (1992) Toxoplasmic encephalitis in AIDS. Clin Infect Dis 15 (2):211–222

6. Morisaki JH, Heuser JE, Sibley LD (1995) Invasion of *Toxoplasma gondii* occurs by active

penetration of the host cell. J Cell Sci 108 (6):2457–2464

7. Suss-Toby E, Zimmerberg J, Ward GE (1996) *Toxoplasma* invasion: the parasitophorous vacuole is formed from host cell plasma membrane and pinches off via a fission pore. Proc Natl Acad Sci U S A 93(16):8413–8418

8. Besteiro S (2015) *Toxoplasma* control of host apoptosis: the art of not biting too hard the hand that feeds you. Microb Cell 2 (6):178–181

9. Krishnamurthy S, Konstantinou EK, Young LH, Gold DA, Saeij JPJ, Roth M (2017) The human immune response to *Toxoplasma*: autophagy versus cell death. PLoS Pathog 13 (3):e1006176

10. Goldman M, Carver RK, Sulzer AJ (1958) Reproduction of *Toxoplasma gondii* by internal budding. J Parasitol 44(2):161–171

11. Jones TC, Hirsch JG (1972) The interaction between *Toxoplasma gondii* and mammalian cells. II. The absence of lysosomal fusion with phagocytic vacuoles containing living parasites. J Exp Med 136(5):1173–1194

12. Mordue DG, Desai N, Dustin M, Sibley LD (1999) Invasion by *Toxoplasma gondii* establishes a moving junction that selectively excludes host cell plasma membrane proteins on the basis of their membrane anchoring. J Exp Med 190(12):1783–1792

13. Charron AJ, Sibley LD (2004) Molecular partitioning during host cell penetration by *Toxoplasma gondii*. Traffic 5(11):855–867

14. Virreira Winter S, Niedelman W, Jensen KD, Rosowski EE, Julien L, Spooner E et al (2011) Determinants of GBP recruitment to *Toxoplasma gondii* vacuoles and the parasitic factors that control it. PLoS ONE 6(9):e24434

15. Degrandi D, Kravets E, Konermann C, Beuter-Gunia C, Klümpers V, Lahme S et al (2013) Murine guanylate binding protein 2 (mGBP2) controls *Toxoplasma gondii* replication. Proc Natl Acad Sci U S A 110(1):294–299

16. Foltz C, Napolitano A, Khan R, Clough B, Hirst EM, Frickel E-M (2017) TRIM21 is critical for survival of *Toxoplasma gondii* infection and localises to GBP-positive parasite vacuoles. Sci Rep 7(1):5209

17. Selleck EM, Orchard RC, Lassen KG, Beatty WL, Xavier RJ, Levine B et al (2015) A noncanonical autophagy pathway restricts *Toxoplasma gondii* growth in a strain-specific manner in IFN-γ-activated human cells. MBio 6(5):e01157–e01115

18. Clough B, Wright JD, Pereira PM, Hirst EM, Johnston AC, Henriques R et al (2016) K63-linked ubiquitination targets *Toxoplasma gondii* for endo-lysosomal destruction in IFN-γ-stimulated human cells. PLoS Pathog 12 (11):e1006027

19. Clough B, Frickel E-M (2017) The *Toxoplasma* parasitophorous vacuole: an evolving host-parasite frontier. Trends Parasitol 33 (6):473–488

20. Fisch D, Yakimovich A, Clough B, Wright J, Bunyan M, Howell M et al (2019) Defining host–pathogen interactions employing an artificial intelligence workflow. elife 8:pii:e40560

21. Berthold MR, Cebron N, Dill F, Gabriel TR, Kötter T, Meinl T et al (2008) In: KNIME: the konstanz information miner (ed) Data analysis, machine learning and applications studies in classification, data analysis, and knowledge organization. Springer, Berlin, pp 319–326

Chapter 22

Metabolomic Analysis of *Toxoplasma gondii* Tachyzoites

Elizabeth F. B. King, Simon A. Cobbold, Alessandro D. Uboldi, Christopher J. Tonkin, and Malcolm J. McConville

Abstract

This protocol describes the use of ^{13}C-stable isotope labeling, combined with metabolite profiling, to investigate the metabolism of the tachyzoite stage of the protozoan parasite *Toxoplasma gondii*. *T. gondii* tachyzoites can infect any nucleated cell in their vertebrate (including human) hosts, and utilize a range of carbon sources that freely permeate across the limiting membrane of the specialized vacuole within which they proliferate. Methods for cultivating tachyzoites in human foreskin fibroblasts and metabolically labeling intracellular and naturally egressed tachyzoites with a range of ^{13}C-labeled carbon sources are described. Parasites are harvested and purified from host metabolites, with rapid metabolic quenching and ^{13}C-enrichment in intracellular polar metabolites quantified by gas chromatography–mass spectrometry (GC-MS) and liquid chromatography–mass spectrometry (LC-MS). The mass isotopomer distribution of key metabolites is determined using DExSI software. This method can be used to measure perturbations in parasite metabolism induced by drug inhibition or genetic manipulation of enzyme levels and is broadly applicable to other cultured or intracellular parasite stages.

Key words Metabolomics, ^{13}C-flux analysis, Intracellular pathogen, Toxoplasmosis, Mass spectrometry

---

1 Introduction

Parasitic protozoa belonging to the Phylum Apicomplexa are the cause of important and highly prevalent diseases in humans, including malaria (*Plasmodium falciparum*), cryptosporidiosis (*Cryptosporidium parvum*), and toxoplasmosis (*Toxoplasma gondii*). Current drug therapies for all of these diseases are limited and, in many cases, severely undermined by the emergence of drug resistance in clinical isolates [1–3]. As metabolic enzymes represent a major class of targets for antiparasitic drugs, new methods for quantitative analysis of parasite metabolism are needed. While genome-based annotations can provide a global view of the metabolic potential of these pathogens, a significant fraction of protein-encoding genes cannot be assigned a function based on homology. Moreover, existing genomic, transcriptomic, and proteomic

Christopher J. Tonkin (ed.), *Toxoplasma gondii: Methods and Protocols*, Methods in Molecular Biology, vol. 2071, https://doi.org/10.1007/978-1-4939-9857-9_22, © Springer Science+Business Media, LLC, part of Springer Nature 2020

approaches provide limited information on the precise structure of metabolic networks, metabolic fluxes, and the extent to which different metabolites are synthesized versus salvaged from the host. Metabolomic approaches are increasingly being used to fill some of these gaps and to complement other -omic approaches [4–6]. In particular, metabolite profiling, combined with stable isotope labeling experiments, has the potential to (a) determine whether annotated pathways are active in intracellular stages, (b) identify novel or unanticipated metabolic pathways that have not yet been annotated, (c) differentiate the role of parasite salvage versus de novo biosynthesis pathways, (d) functionally characterize the metabolic phenotype of parasite mutants, and (e) measure the mode of action of existing or new antiparasite drugs, as well as potential resistance mechanisms.

Detailed information on the metabolism of both the tachyzoite and bradyzoite lifecycle stages of *T. gondii* is crucial for understanding how these parasites survive and proliferate within different tissues and host cell types; identifying host factors that trigger differentiation of tachyzoites to bradyzoites (and vice versa) and in ultimately identifying potential new drug targets common to both major stages. Genome-scale stoichiometric models of *T. gondii* metabolism have been constructed, but suffer from a number of limitations, including the large number of genes of unknown function; the limited transcriptional flexibility of these parasites; and evidence that several highly conserved enzymes have been repurposed to have alternative functions in metabolism [8]. These limitations have provided an impetus for detailed metabolite profiling and ^{13}C-labeling studies to determine which pathways are active in vivo and to define the metabolic flexibility and major carbon sources used by intracellular tachyzoite stages. Initial ^{13}C-glucose/^{13}C-glutamine labeling studies with *T. gondii* infected human foreskin fibroblasts (HFFs) or naturally egressed tachyzoites showed that these stages co-utilized both carbon sources under physiological conditions and derived most of their ATP from mitochondrial respiration [7]. This result was unexpected, as previous studies had shown that the single pyruvate dehydrogenase complex was targeted to the apicoplast (a relic plastid) rather than to the mitochondrion, suggesting that a key step in the canonical mitochondrial TCA cycle was missing in these parasites. However, subsequent genetic and metabolomic studies showed that the function of mitochondrial PDH was performed by the branched chain α-amino acid dehydrogenase (BCKDH), which functioned exclusively as a PDH [8]. These initial profiling and ^{13}C-labeling studies also revealed the presence of an active γ-amino butyric acid (GABA) shunt in tachyzoites, which led to the annotation of three genes (previously of unknown function) that catalyzed the steps required for motility under nutrient-limited conditions [7]. Subsequent ^{13}C-labeling studies have further highlighted the metabolic flexibility of *T. gondii* tachyzoites and their capacity to switch between carbon sources following genetic ablation of key pathways or nutrient limitation. They have also provided insight into the role of metabolic futile cycles in regulating major fluxes in tachyzoite central carbon metabolism [9].

Here, we describe a method for mapping metabolic pathways in intracellular and extracellular stages of *T. gondii* tachyzoites using metabolite profiling and ^{13}C-labeling approaches. In this method, *T. gondii*-infected HFFs or egressed "extracellular" tachyzoites are metabolically labeled with ^{13}C-labeled carbon sources (i.e., ^{13}C-U-glucose, ^{13}C$_1$-glucose, ^{13}C$_{1,2}$-glucose ^{13}C-U-glutamate, ^{13}C-U-aspartate) under standard (non-perturbed) growth conditions. While the labeling studies described here are carried out over a single time point (4 h; corresponding to steady state equilibrium), cells can also be sampled at multiple time points to accurately measure labeling kinetics and metabolic flux. Care must be taken to ensure that parasites are harvested and separated from host cells/debris under conditions that effectively quench cell metabolism to prevent post-harvest changes in metabolite levels or labeling. Following metabolite extraction, the incorporation of ^{13}C-label into intracellular metabolite pools is quantified using either gas chromatography (GC) or liquid chromatography (LC)-mass spectrometry (MS) and the level of ^{13}C-enrichment in key metabolites across multiple metabolic pathways calculated after correcting for natural ^{13}C-abundance.

2 Materials

2.1 HFF and T. gondii Cultivation

1. Tissue culture hood.

2. D10 medium: Low glucose (1 g/L; 5.55 mM) DMEM media (sigma 5523) supplemented with 3.7 g/L sodium hydrogen carbonate, 1× GlutaMAX, 1× penicillin/streptomycin and 10% (*v/v*) cosmic calf serum.

3. D1 medium: Low glucose (1 g/L; 5.55 mM) DMEM media (sigma 5523) supplemented with 3.7 g/L sodium hydrogen carbonate, 1× GlutaMAX, 1× penicillin/streptomycin and 1% (*v/v*) foetal calf serum.

4. Phosphate-buffered saline (PBS).

5. 0.25% Trypsin/EDTA in DME (Sigma).

6. 80% ethanol (*v/v*) spray.

7. 25 cm^2 or 175 cm^2 filter-cap culture flasks (Falcon).

8. Incubator at 37 °C with 10% CO_2 atmosphere.

9. Autopipette, sterile plastic pipettes (10 and 50 mL).

2.2 Preparation of Extracellular Tachyzoites

1. Tissue culture hood.
2. 175 cm^2 flask of confluent HFFs—2× per replicate.
3. D1 medium (*see* Subheading 2.1).
4. Large ice bucket.
5. Smaller container appropriate for cold temperature and large enough to fit the bottom of a 175 cm^2 flask standing.
6. Ethanol, both absolute and 80% (*v/v*).
7. Dry ice pellets (solid CO_2).
8. Thermometer, with method to clean quickly in between quenches. For example, a falcon tube filled with 80% (*v/v*) ethanol to hold thermometer in between samples and paper towel to wipe it with.
9. Haemocytometer.

The following items should be cooled to 0–4 °C either on ice or in a fridge:

10. 50 mL falcon tube (2× per replicate), sterile.
11. PBS, sterile.
12. 26 G needle with Luer lock (1× per replicate), sterile.
13. 5 μm Minisart® NML Syringe Filter (Sartorius: 17594), or other appropriate 5 μm syringe filter (1× per replicate).
14. 5–10 mL plastic Luer lock syringe (2× per replicate).
15. Benchtop centrifuge with refrigeration.
16. Microfuge with refrigeration, or at 4 °C.
17. 4% (*w/v*) paraformaldehyde in PBS.
18. 1.5 mL Eppendorf tubes.

2.3 Preparation of Intracellular Tachyzoites

1. Tissue culture hood.
2. 175 cm^2 flask of confluent HFFs—2× per replicate.
3. D1 medium (*see* Subheading 2.1).
4. Haemocytometer.

The following items should be cooled to 0–4 °C either on ice or in a fridge:

5. Cell scrapers.
6. 50 mL falcon tube (2× per replicate), sterile.
7. PBS, sterile.
8. 26 G needle with Luer lock (1× per replicate), sterile.
9. 5 μm Minisart® NML Syringe Filter (Sartorius: 17594), or other appropriate 5 μm syringe filter (1× per replicate).
10. 5–10 mL plastic Luer lock syringe (2× per replicate).

11. Benchtop centrifuge with refrigeration.

12. Microfuge with refrigeration, or at 4 °C.

13. 4% (w/v) paraformaldehyde in PBS.

14. 1.5 mL Eppendorf tubes.

2.4 ^{13}C-U-Glucose Labeling

1. D1 medium with ^{13}C-U-glucose: DMEM medium basic formulation (Sigma 5030) supplemented with 1.032 g/L (5.55 mM) ^{13}C-U-glucose, 0.583 g/L L-glutamine, 0.11 g/L sodium pyruvate, 3.7 g/L sodium hydrogen carbonate, 1× GlutaMAX, and 1× penicillin/streptomycin and 1% (v/v) fetal calf serum.

2. PBS.

3. 175 cm^2 flask (or 50 mL falcon tube) for extracellular labeling.

4. 1.5 mL microfuge tube (for extracellular labeling).

2.5 Metabolite Extraction and Analysis by GC-MS

1. Chloroform (99.8% purity, GC-MS grade, *see* **Note 1**).

2. Methanol (99.9% purity, GC-MS grade).

3. Ultrapure water (18 MΩ, such as MilliQ).

4. 3:1 Methanol/ultrapure water—we routinely make up 15 mL methanol, 5 mL water and 5 μL 10 mM *scyllo*-inositol (so 400 μL will contain 1 nmol *scyllo*-inositol) but this will depend on the number of replicates being processed.

5. Microfuge at 4 °C and room temperature.

6. Methoxyamine hydrochloride made up in pyridine (20 mg/mL) immediately prior to use. Make up in a clean GC-MS vial and use a positive displacement pipette to add the pyridine. Cap vial swiftly and vortex to ensure no crystals remain.

7. *N,O*-bis(trimethylsilyl)trifluoroacetamide (BSTFA) +1% trimethylchlorosilane (TMCS) under argon atmosphere (preferably in 1 mL vials).

8. 1.5 mL tubes (safe-lock) (*see* **Note 1**).

9. Tweezers (*see* **Note 1**).

10. GC-MS vials (screw-cap, clear), vial inserts (250 μL pulled point glass) and screw caps (*see* **Note 1**).

11. Glass positive displacement pipettes.

12. Centrifugal evaporator for 1.5 mL microtubes (e.g., Christ RVC vacuum concentrator).

13. GC-MS system—such as an Agilent 6890 Series GC couples with a 5973 mass selective detector, and a 7683 series automatic liquid sampler. GC is performed with a 30 m DB-5 ms capillary column (J&W scientific; 250 μm i.d., 0.25 μm film thickness), incorporating a 10 m inert duraguard section. MS is

performed using electron impact (EI) or chemical ionisation (CI).

14. MSD Chemstation (ChemStation D.01.02.16, Agilent Technologies) is used for instrument control, editing/running the sample sequence and for data analysis.

15. DExSI is used for automated data analysis. [10].

2.6 Metabolite Extraction and Analysis by LC-MS

1. 80% acetonitrile (99.9% hyper grade (Merck) and MilliQ water) + 1 μM $^{13}C^{15}N$-aspartate (Cambridge Isotopes).

2. Ice-cold 1× PBS (approximately 50 mL).

3. Cold room or refrigerated microcentrifuge.

4. LC-MS vials (screw cap, clear glass, Agilent), vial inserts (250 μL pulled point glass, Agilent), and screw caps (Agilent).

5. SeQuant ZIC-pHILIC 5 μm polymeric column (150 × 4.6 mm; Merck) with guard column (ZIC-pHILIC 20 × 2.1 mm; Merck).

6. Hyper-grade acetonitrile (Merck).

7. 20 mM ammonium carbonate (HPLC grade; Fluka) made up in milli-Q water.

8. LC-MS system: we use an Agilent 1260 binary pump coupled to an Agilent 6545 Q-TOF but any high mass-accuracy full-scan MS would be suitable.

3 Methods

3.1 Host Cell Cultivation

1. *T. gondii* tachyzoites are typically cultivated in human foreskin fibroblasts (HFFs). The rate of growth and physiological state of intracellular tachyzoites is influenced by the host cell, so it is important to monitor the number of times HFF lines have been subcultured and overall health (*see* **Note 2**).

2. HFFs (obtained from ATCC) for passaging are maintained in 175 cm^2 filter-capped tissue culture flasks containing D10 medium at 37 °C in a humidified atmosphere of 10% CO_2.

3. When fully confluent and ready for passaging, the monolayer is washed with PBS before 5 mL of 0.25% Trypsin/EDTA in DME is added to the flask. The liquid is spread across the surface of the flask and incubated at 37 °C in 10% CO_2 for 1–5 min, or until the cells detach from the flask following percussive force.

4. D10 medium is added, to a final volume of 300 mL, and the HFFs are aliquoted into either 6 × 175 cm^2 flasks (50 mL each) used for experiments or 30 × 25 cm^2 flasks (10 mL each) used for passaging parasites.

5. HFFs are grown until fully confluent before infection with *T. gondii* tachyzoites.

6. To prepare host cells for infection, the medium is removed and replaced with D1 medium: 10 mL in 25 cm^2 flasks and 50 mL in 175 cm^2 flasks. Parasites are then added at an MOI appropriate for the strain and length of infection required (*see* **Note 3**).

3.2 Preparation of Extracellular Tachyzoites

1. At least three technical replicates of each parasite strain or condition are recommended for each experiment. For each technical replicate of extracellular tachyzoites, infect 2 × 175 cm^2 flasks of confluent HFFs with *T. gondii*. An MOI of 1:5 can be used for infection, although this is largely dependent on the parasite strain, the preferred length of time of parasite growth and the media components (*see* **Note 3**). A workflow for the following procedure is shown in Fig. 1a.

2. A dry ice/ethanol slurry is created by filling a large ice bucket with ice and placing a smaller container in the middle. Fill 2/3 with ethanol and add a handful of dry ice pellets. Add more as the pellets boil off during quenching.

3. Metabolite extraction is very time-sensitive; it is critical to ensure that all steps are done as quickly and consistently as possible to achieve good reproducibility. It is generally recommended to process a maximum of four flasks (two replicates) at a time.

4. Parasites are harvested when 70–90% of the parasites have egressed from the host cells. Cells are quenched by immersing the bottom of the flask in the dry ice/ethanol slurry. A clean thermometer is placed in the medium and the flask is agitated continuously. When the thermometer reaches 10 °C, remove the flask from the slurry and place on ice. There is a lag in the thermometer reading, so the culture will reach ~4 °C when put on ice. The cultures must not be allowed to freeze, as this results in parasite lysis. Parasites can also be quenched in a 50 mL falcon tube, although the rate of quenching is slower than in the large surface area flask.

5. All subsequent steps are performed at 0–4 °C, preferably in a cold room. The cultures are transferred to a 50 mL falcon tube and centrifuged at 1000 × g for 5 min at 0 °C. The supernatant (~1 mL) can be set aside for metabolite "footprinting" (*see* **Note 4**) analysis. The rest of the supernatant is removed and the pellet is resuspended in ice-cold PBS and the pellets of both flasks are combined.

6. Each replicate is passed through a 26 G syringe needle, followed by passage through a 5 μm filter. The resulting filtrate contains parasites free of host debris (*see* **Note 5**). These steps

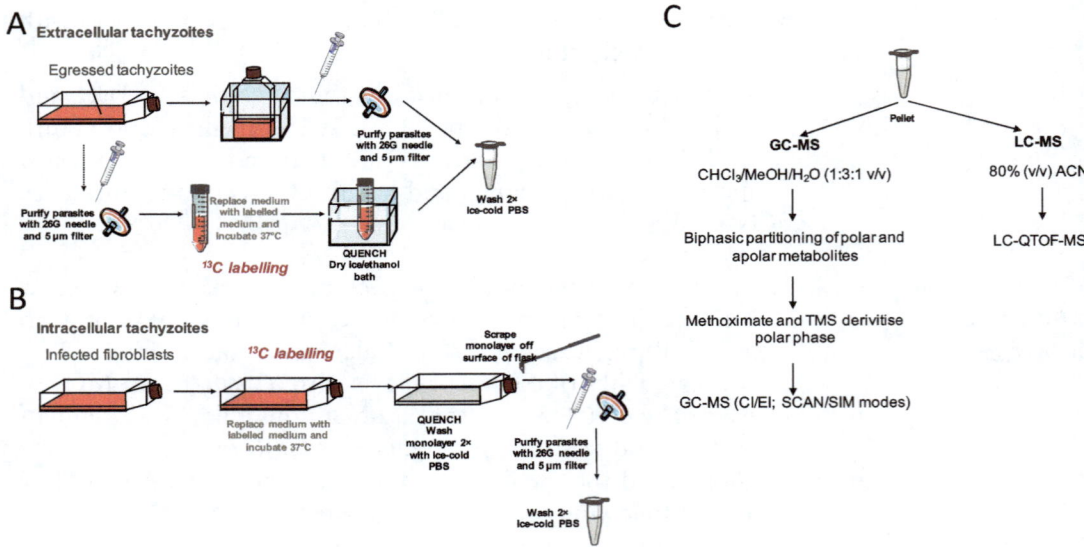

Fig. 1 Workflow for metabolite extraction of *T. gondii* tachyzoites. (**a**) Tachyzoites are allowed to egress from infected HFF and metabolically quenched and then separated from any host debris (by syringing and filtration) and medium metabolites (by washing in PBS) prior to extraction and metabolite profiling studies. Alternatively, egressed tachyzoites are separated from host debris without quenching and labeled with ^{13}C-labeled carbon sources, prior to metabolic quenching and metabolite extraction. (**b**) For ^{13}C-labeling of intracellular tachyzoites, adherent infected HFF monolayers are washed in labeling medium and then cultivated in medium containing the relevant ^{13}C-labeled carbon source. The monolayers are subsequently metabolically quenched, and parasites released and purified from host cells/debris (by syringing and filtration) and media components (by washing in PBS). (**c**) Parasite cell pellets are extracted in $CHCl_3/MeOH/H_2O$ (1:3:1 v/v) with subsequent biphasic partitioning to generate a polar and apolar metabolite fraction for GC-MS. Polar metabolites are derivatized by methoximation and TMS prior to GC-MS analysis. For LC-MS, metabolites are extracted in 80% (v/v) acetonitrile (ACN) prior to analysis

should be processed as quickly as possible, with due attention to safety. As syringe passage of large volumes of cells can lead to high back-pressure and longer processing time, it is recommended to syringe lyse less than 20 mL at a time.

7. Purified parasites are centrifuged at $1000 \times g$ for 5 min at 0–4 °C in a benchtop centrifuge. The supernatant is removed and the pellet resuspended with 1 mL ice-cold PBS and transferred to a 1.5 mL Eppendorf tube. Parasites are pelleted once again and resuspended in 1 mL ice-cold PBS.

8. An aliquot of the suspension (10 μL) is fixed in 90 μL 4% PFA for cell counting (*see* **Note 6**). The rest of the suspension is centrifuged at $14,000 \times g$ for 30 s at 4 °C, and the supernatant and pellet kept on ice, ready for extraction.

9. Fixed parasites are counted using a haemocytometer (in duplicate), while cell pellets are kept on ice There should be between 5×10^7 and 2×10^8 cells in each tube, depending

on the yield of purified parasites. Lower parasite numbers will result in decreased sensitivity. All samples in the experiment should have approximately the same cell count prior to extraction.

3.3 Preparation of Intracellular Tachyzoites

1. For analysis of intracellular tachyzoites, four 175 cm^2 flasks of confluent HFFs per replicate are infected with parasites. The MOI is dependent on the strains used, the preferred length of time of parasite growth and the media components (*see* **Note 3**). The workflow for this procedure is shown in Fig. 1b.

2. Parasites are harvested when >90% of the host cells contain >32 tachyzoites, prior to initiation of parasite egress and host cell lysis. Medium is removed and metabolism quenched by washing the host cell monolayer twice with ice-cold PBS (pH 7.4) and cells subsequently suspended by scraping cells into 5 mL ice cold PBS. All subsequent steps are undertaken at 4 °C in a cold room.

3. As metabolite extraction needs to be done quickly, it is advisable to process a maximum of four flasks at a time. Suspensions of metabolically quenched host cells are passed through a 26 G needle, and the lysate subsequently filtered through a 5 μm filter (*see* **Note 7**). The filtrate primarily contains live parasites free of host cell debris (*see* **Note 3**). As syringe passage of large volumes of cells can lead to high back-pressure and longer processing time, it is recommended to syringe lyze less than 20 mL at a time.

4. Purified parasites are centrifuged at 1000 × *g* for 5 min at 0–4 °C in a benchtop centrifuge. The supernatant is removed and the pellet resuspended in 1 mL ice-cold PBS, transferred to a 1.5 mL Eppendorf tube and washed with a further 1 mL of ice-cold PBS.

5. An aliquot (10 μL) of the penultimate cell suspension is taken and fixed in 90 μL 4% PFA to determine parasite numbers (*see* **Note 6**). The rest of the suspension (1 mL) is spun at 14,000 × *g*, 30 s at 4 °C.

6. PFA-fixed parasites are counted on a haemocytometer.

3.4 ^{13}C Labeling of Metabolites

1. ^{13}C-labeling studies can be used to identify metabolic pathways that are active in vivo and distinguish between de novo versus salvage pathways. A selection of ^{13}C-labeled precursors are commercially available, which can be used individually or in parallel to monitor the activity of pathways of central carbon metabolism. In this protocol we describe the use of ^{13}C-U-glucose to label multiple pathways in tachyzoite central carbon metabolism, including glycolysis, the pentose phosphate pathway, the TCA cycle and glycosylation pathways.

2. D1 medium lacking glucose is prepared from powder (sigma 5030) to which is added ^{13}C-U-glucose (*see* **Note 8**). The latter is added at the same molar concentration as unlabeled glucose in standard medium (i.e., 1.032 g/L ^{13}C-glucose instead of 1.00 g/L ^{12}C-glucose).

3. The protocols shown below (Subheadings 3.4.1 and 3.4.2) are for metabolite labeling of parasites from Subheadings 3.2 and 3.3, respectively (Fig. 1a, b).

3.4.1 Labeling Extracellular Tachyzoites

1. Extracellular tachyzoites are prepared as described in Subheading 3.2 (Fig. 1a). Unquenched cultures are transferred to a 50 mL falcon tube and centrifuged at $1000 \times g$ for 5 min. The supernatant is removed and the pellet resuspended in PBS. Experimental groups are pooled and passed through a 26 G needle, followed by passage through a 5 μm filter (*see* **Note 5**).

2. The parasite suspension are transferred to a 1.5 mL microfuge tube, and washed in PBS (1 mL) by centrifugation in a microfuge at $14,000 \times g$ for 30 s.

3. Washed parasite pellets are suspended in 1 mL D1 labeling medium and added to a 175 cm^2 flask containing 49 mL of labeling medium. Labeling can also be performed in a 50 mL falcon tube.

4. Parasites are incubated at 37 °C in 10% CO_2. Aliquots can be removed and cold quenched at regular intervals (i.e., every hour for 4 h) to monitor changes in ^{13}C-incoporation into different metabolites, or replicate samples can be harvested at a single time point (such as after 4 h, when steady-state equilibrium in high turnover intermediates has been achieved).

5. Quenching is carried out as previously described using a dry ice/ethanol bath. As parasites have been purified from host cells already, **step 6** from Subheading 3.2 can be omitted. After centrifugation (**step 7**), 1 mL of supernatant can be set aside for metabolite "foot-printing" analysis. Follow Subheading 3.2 from this stage onward.

3.4.2 Labeling of Intracellular Tachyzoites

1. HFF cells are infected with *T. gondii* tachyzoites as described in Subheading 3.3 (Fig. 1b). When the parasites are 6+ hours away from egressing (*see* **Note 9**), medium is removed and the monolayer is washed $2\times$ with PBS and replaced with labeling medium. Labeling is carried out at 37 °C in 10% CO_2. Either a time course can be carried out with samples quenched every hour for 4 h, or multiple replicates can be generated at a single time point (such as 4 h).

2. Parasites are quenched and purified from host cells as described in Subheading 3.3 from **step 2**.

3.5 Metabolite Extraction for Polar Metabolites to Analyze by GC-MS

1. Cell pellets from Subheadings 3.2 and 3.3 are used here (Fig. 1c).

2. Chloroform (100 µL) is added to the chilled cell pellets. The tube is capped and scraped across the rack to rapidly suspend the pellet in solvent.

3. Methanol/water (3:1 v/v; 400 µL) containing 1 nmol *scyllo*-inositol is added to generate a monophasic solution (final ratio chloroform/methanol/water, 1:3:1 v/v) and the tube scraped across a rack and vortexed rigorously to facilitate extraction. The suspension is sonicated briefly in a sonicating bath to further aid dispersal and then centrifuged at 14,000 × *g*, 10 min at 4 °C (*see* **Note 10**).

4. The supernatant is transferred to a fresh tube containing 200 µL water at room temperature, (final ratio chloroform/methanol/water, 1:3:3 v/v) and samples centrifuged at 14,000 × *g* for 10 min at room temperature. The upper aqueous phase is carefully transferred to a fresh 1.5 mL tube, ensuring the interface is not disturbed. At this stage, both the upper aqueous phase (containing polar metabolites) and lower organic phase (containing apolar metabolites) can be stored at −80 °C.

5. For analysis of polar metabolites, the aqueous phase is transferred to GC-MS inserts 75–100 µL at a time and dried in vacuo using a Christ RVC vacuum concentrator (room temperature). In parallel, metabolite mix and appropriate standards are dried under the same conditions. Samples are washed in 2 × 50 µL methanol and the inserts carefully transferred to GC-MS vials using clean tweezers. It is imperative that the samples are completely dry.

6. Freshly prepared methoxyamine chloride solution (20 µL, 20 mg/mL in pyridine) is added using a positive displacement glass pipette. Vials are immediately capped, vortexed and incubated overnight with gentle agitation on an orbital shaker or plate rocker at room temperature.

7. BSTFA +1% TMCS (20 µL) is added to each vial 1 h prior to GC-MS analysis. Samples are vortex mixed and incubated at room temperature. Derivatisation time should be kept constant across samples.

8. GC is performed using a DB5ms capillary column incorporating a fused 10 m inert duraguard using the parameters shown in Table 1 and retention time locking. MS can either be performed in electron ionisation (EI) or chemical ionization (CI) mode. Metabolite identification is based on GC retention times and the highly reproducible mass spectra generated during GC-EI-MS, compared to authentic standards that are run in parallel with the samples (custom-made metabolite mix)

Table 1
GC-MS settings

	Electron impact (EI)	Chemical ionization (CI)
Ionization source	Inert EI ion source, 250 °C *Agilent part number G3170-65760*	CI ion source complete, 300 °C *Agilent part number G3170-65403* CI reagent gas, methane 14%
Detector	Full scan, 50–500 *m/z* range SIM can also be performed	Full scan, 50–700 *m/z* range. SIM can also be performed
Injection	1× wash of syringe with hexane (discarded) 4× wash with sample (not discarded) 1 μL injection of sample (no pre- or post-injection delay) 3× wash with methanol (discarded) 5× wash with hexane (discarded)	
Inlet	General purpose split/splitless liner with glass wool tapered and deactivated, held at 270 °C *E.g., Agilent part number 5183-4711*	
Carrier gas	Helium—ultra high purity Constant column flow rate of 1.4 mL/min Inlet purged at 50 mL/min for 60 s, gas saver at 15 mL/min after 60 s	
Capillary column	A multipurpose, low bleed column suitable for GC-MS *E.g., Agilent part number J&W 122-5532G. Length: 40 m (10 m DuraGuard + 30 m 08% column); Internal diameter: 0.25 mm, film thickness: 0.25 μm; Phase: 08–5 ms* *Other suitable columns include Agilent J&W VF-5ms EZ Guard, 30 m/10 m, 0.25 mm, 0.25*	
Oven program	70 °C, 2 min hold Ramp from 70 to 294 °C at 12.5 °C/min Ramp from 295 to 320 °C at 25°C/mm 320 °C, 3 min hold *Total run time: 24 min*	
Transfer line	250 °C	

and/or vendor-based EI mass spectra. GC-CI-MS provides a complementary analytical mode to GC-EI-MS, and the generation of mass spectra in which the molecular ion can dominate. GC-CI-MS is particularly well suited for quantitating the relative abundance of different metabolite isotopomers generated during ^{13}C-labeling experiments as the molecular ions cover all possible isotopomers, while diagnostic fragment ions created during CI (or EI) MS can provide information on the position of labeled carbons.

3.6   GC-MS Data Analysis

GC-MS chromatograms are processed using ChemStation software (Agilent Technologies) while the automated identification annotation and quantitation of stable-isotope labeled metabolites is performed using the DExSI software package [10]. ChemStation

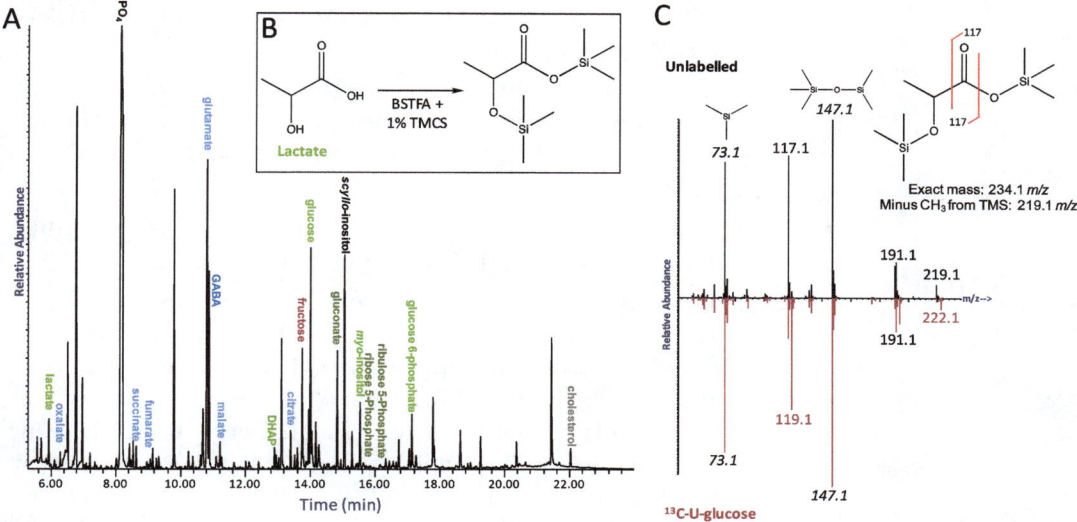

Fig. 2 GC-MS analysis of *T. gondii* metabolites. (**a**) GC-MS chromatogram of *T. gondii* PruΔ*hxgrt* tachyzoite polar metabolites (key intermediates in central carbon metabolism glycolysis (light green), the pentose phosphate pathway (dark green), neutral sugars (red), the TCA cycle (light blue) and select host-derived metabolites (in black). The chromatograms also contain TMS derivative of phosphate, derived from the PBS wash and the *scyllo*-inositol internal standard. (**b**) Structure of L-lactate before and after derivatization with BSTFA +1% TMCS. (**c**) Mass spectra of lactate from unlabeled compared to ^{13}C-U-glucose labeled PruΔ*hxgrt* tachyzoites

allows detection of metabolites based on retention time and mass spectra/diagnostic ions relative to authentic standards or vendor-provided mass spectral libraries (Fig. Fig. 2a). Retention time locking is performed following column cutting or replacement using the metabolite mix.

The DExSI software is an open source application that can be used to quantitate the relative or absolute abundance of metabolite isotopomers in a fully automated fashion [10]. The software implements commonly used calculations in metabolite/isotopomer quantification, such as natural isotope abundance correction and fractional labeling. DExSI contains functions for visualizing data (heatmaps, changes in fractional labeling over time, etc.) and for exporting processed data to Microsoft Excel or to metabolite pathway mapping software packages, such as VANTED [11]. DExSI and ChemStation are used in tandem to ensure correct identification of metabolites in DExSI.

3.7 Metabolite Extraction and Analysis by LC-MS

1. Parasite pellets are generated as outlined in Subheadings 3.2 and 3.3 (Fig. 1c).

2. 80% acetonitrile (200 μL containing 1 μM ^{13}C^{15}N-asparate as the internal standard) is added to each sample and the cell pellet

rapidly resuspended and drawn across a microcentrifuge rack to ensure thorough mixing.

3. Cell extracts are immediately centrifuged ($14,000 \times g$, 5 min) and the supernatant, containing polar metabolites, collected and transferred directly to 250 μL glass inserts in 1.5 mL LC-MS vials.

4. Samples are stored at 4 °C if LC-MS analysis is performed within 18 h, or at −80 °C if longer storage is required.

5. Samples are loaded into an autosampler maintained at 4 °C and 5–10 μL of the extracts are injected onto a SeQuant ZIC-pHILIC column (5 μM, 150 × 4.6 mm, Millipore) coupled to a 1200 series HPLC system (Agilent). Polar metabolites (including major intermediates in central carbon metabolism) are detected using the gradient described in Table 2 and a flow rate of 0.3 mL/min. Solvent A (20 mM ammonium carbonate in water) and B (100% acetonitrile) are prepared fresh before each LC-MS run.

6. MS detection is performed using an Agilent Q-TOF mass spectrometer 6545 operating in negative ESI mode, with the MS tuned to low mass range and optimized for labile ions. Mass spectra are collected (85–1200 *m/z*) between 2 and 28 min at 0.9 spectra/second in centroid mode. The gas temperature is set to 150 °C, drying gas 10 L/min, nebulizer 20 psig, sheath gas temperature 300 °C, sheath gas flow 10 L/min, capillary voltage 2500 V and the nozzle voltage 200 V. The MS threshold is set between 100 and 500 to ensure manageable file size. An internal reference ion solution is continually run throughout the chromatographic separation and the 119.03632 (purine) and 981.99509 (hexakis adduct) *m/z* ions used to maintain mass accuracy.

7. Metabolite identification is achieved using a collection of 150 pure metabolite standards grouped into five samples. Each standard sample is sequentially injected onto the LC-MS instrument and metabolite identification based on the retention time and exact mass.

8. Each sample and standard LC-MS .d file is converted to .the mzXML format using MS convert and uploaded into the MAVEN software package [12, 13]. Alignment of samples is performed using a polynomial degree of 5 with 1000 iterations. Moreover, the alignment is limited to 1000 groups (with each group containing at least three good peaks) and the minimum ion intensity threshold set to 30,000.

9. *m/z* feature extraction is performed using the following settings: mass domain resolution = 10 ppm, time domain resolution = 10 scans, minimum number of good peaks = 6, minimum signal/baseline ratio = 5, minimum peak width = 5

Table 2
LC-MS gradient settings

Time (min)	Flow rate (mL/min)	Solvent A (20 mM Ammonium Carbonate)	Solvent B (acetonitrile)
0	0.3	20	80
0.5	0.3	20	80
15.5	0.3	50	50
17.5	0.3	70	30
18.5	0.3	95	5
21	0.3	95	5
23	0.3	20	80
29.5	0.3	20	80

scans, and the minimum peak intensity $= 3000$. This typically results in 5000–12,000 individual m/z groups.

10. A targeted metabolite analysis is performed by searching a predefined metabolite library containing approximately 150 metabolites with specific retention times which correspond to the same set of metabolites run in **step** 7. A 10 ppm mass window and 0.5 min retention time window are used for metabolite identification. The integrated area top for each positively assigned metabolite is then exported, along with any isotopolog data that is extracted from a ^{13}C-labeling experiment.

11. For untargeted analyses, pairwise comparisons (untreated vs treated) are performed in the MAVEN software package from the total list of extracted m/z features with a minimum fold-difference of 1.5, missing values set to 300 and significance determined using an adjusted P value <0.01 using the Benjamini post hoc test for multiple hypothesis testing. Each statistically significant feature is then visually inspected and any co-eluting adducts, in-source fragments and isotopolog m/z features removed. The observed mass of each m/z feature is then searched against the METLIN database [14, 15] using M-H and M + Cl adducts. Plausible metabolite assignments are then confirmed with pure standards where possible or MS-MS spectra acquisition. Briefly MS-MS spectra for m/z features of interest are collected using the preferred auto MS-MS method using collision voltages of 10, 20 and 40 V. MS-MS spectra are searched against the METLIN database within the Agilent Qualitative Workstation software package.

12. Isotopolog data is corrected for the natural abundance of carbon using established procedures [16] with the following formulas:

$$M^0_{real} = \frac{M^0_{measured}}{0.989^N}$$

$$M^{+1}_{real} = \frac{M^{+1}_{measured}}{0.989^{N-1}} - 0.011\,N \times M^0_{real}$$

$$M^{+2}_{real} = \frac{M^{+2}_{measured}}{0.989^{N-2}} - 0.011^2 \times \frac{N}{2(N-1)} \times M^0_{real} - 0.011 \times (N-1) \times M^{+1}_{real}$$

where M^0 is the amount of the monoisotopic compound, M^{+1} is the amount of the compound with one ^{13}C atom, M^{+2} is the amount of the compound with two ^{13}C atoms. N is the number of carbon atoms in the molecule, "real" refers to values corrected natural isotope abundance and "measured" refers to raw values determined by LC-MS.

4   Notes

1. All solvents used for samples should be the highest quality and purity. All water used should be ultrapure (18.1 MΩ—MilliQ water is considered ultrapure). All tubes, vials, tweezers, etc. should be free of contaminants and stored under dust-free conditions. Work areas should be kept clean and gloves should always be worn while handling tubes, solvents, vials, etc. We have found that the use of Eppendorf-branded tips and tubes minimizes the level of plasticizers detected by GC-MS.

2. Metabolomics experiments should be carried out using healthy host cells. It is recommended to use HFFs that have been passaged less than ten times (1:4 split each time) and to initiate infection when the HFF have reached confluency. If HFF cultures are visibly more spread out and are growing slower, a fresh stock should be thawed.

3. We have found that 5×10^7 tachyzoites cell equivalents are required for robust GC-MS analysis and 5×10^6 tachyzoite cell equivalents for LC-MS analysis of polar metabolites. The number of parasites used for infection depends on the experiment being performed. The type II strain PruΔ*hxgprt* requires 3 days to fully egress when an MOI of 2 was used. As each strain and growth conditions will influence the time of parasite egress, it may be necessary to adjust the timings or MOIs outlined in this protocol. For example, if infected HFF are being cultivated under glucose depleted conditions, the MOI of a slow-growing

strain may need to be increased to ensure parasites egress within 3–4 days, and prevent host cell death from glucose deprivation.

4. Metabolite "foot-printing" refers to the analysis of the culture supernatant to determine metabolites which have been consumed or excreted by the parasite/host cells [17]. Metabolite levels in the culture supernatant can be determined by GC-MS, LC-MS, or NMR. Samples for this can be stored at −20 °C prior to analysis.

5. These steps are important in the liberation and purification of parasites from host cells. While filtration is the most effective and efficient method of purification, it is known to result in a low yield of parasites [18]. Filtration with a 5 μm filter can result in a loss of ~75% of parasites, though this will vary between different filter material. It is important to carefully check the resultant parasite preparations by microscopy for any host cells or debris. Needle passage alone does not entirely disrupt all the host cells. Trypan blue staining of preparations following needle passage typically shows both stained (dead) and unstained (live) host cells, while staining of preparations after filtration should contain no detectable host cells. Uninfected host cells can be used as a control for level of host cell metabolite cross contamination, although *see* [19] for caveats.

6. This protocol ensures normalization by cell count is as accurate as possible by taking a sample at the last step before extraction.

7. As the purification of intracellular parasites from HFF can be time-consuming, it may be necessary to perform extraction on smaller batches and subsequently pool samples to make individual replicate samples. Note that the metabolic quenching protocol used here is robust and produces highly reproducible results for most metabolites. However, the levels of some high turnover metabolites (i.e., ATP) can change during post-quenching steps and this needs to be assessed empirically.

8. The 1% FCS used in labeling medium, contains ~ 6 mM glucose which needs to be factored in when calculating the specific activity of the ^{13}C-glucose in labeling experiments. The amount of $^{12}C/^{13}C$-glucose (or other ^{13}C-labeled metabolites) in the medium can be measured directly by GC-MS or LC-MS by sampling an aliquot of the culture medium at the beginning and end of the labeling period.

9. The labeling can be initiated at earlier time points if the *T. gondii* strain has a fast doubling time (>6 h). As labeling often takes up to 4 h, parasites may egress before quenching, decreasing the yield of parasites.

10. Previous studies have included an extraction step at 60 °C for 15 min [7]. While this may enhance extraction of metabolites, heat can cause significant degradation of metabolites and should be avoided where possible [20].

References

1. Alday PH, Doggett JS (2017) Drugs in development for toxoplasmosis: advances, challenges, and current status. Drug Des Devel Ther 11:273–293

2. Gamo F-J (2014) Antimalarial drug resistance: new treatments options for plasmodium. Drug Discov Today Technol 11:81–88

3. Miyamoto Y, Eckmann L (2015) Drug development against the major diarrhea-causing parasites of the small intestine, cryptosporidium and giardia. Front Microbiol 6:1208

4. Jang C, Chen L, Rabinowitz JD (2018) Metabolomics and isotope tracing. Cell 173:822–837

5. Dumas M-E (2012) Metabolome 2.0: quantitative genetics and network biology of metabolic phenotypes. Mol Biosyst 8:2494

6. Kloehn J, Blume M, Cobbold S et al (2016) Using metabolomics to dissect host–parasite interactions. Curr Opin Microbiol 32:59–65

7. MacRae JI, Sheiner L, Nahid A et al (2012) Mitochondrial metabolism of glucose and glutamine is required for intracellular growth of *Toxoplasma gondii*. Cell Host Microbe 12:682–692

8. Oppenheim RD, Creek DJ, Macrae JI et al (2014) BCKDH: the missing link in apicomplexan mitochondrial metabolism is required for full virulence of *Toxoplasma gondii* and plasmodium berghei. PLoS Pathog 10: e1004263

9. Blume M, Nitzsche R, Sternberg U et al (2015) A *Toxoplasma gondii* gluconeogenic enzyme contributes to robust central carbon metabolism and is essential for replication and virulence. Cell Host Microbe 18:210–220

10. Dagley MJ, McConville MJ, Wren J (2018) DExSI: a new tool for the rapid quantitation of 13C-labelled metabolites detected by GC-MS. 34:1957–1958

11. Junker BH, Klukas C, Schreiber F VANTED: a system for advanced data analysis and visualization in the context of biological networks. BMC Bioinformatics 7:109

12. Clasquin MF, Melamud E, Rabinowitz JD (2012) LC-MS data processing with MAVEN: a metabolomic analysis and visualization engine. Curr Protoc Bioinforma:1–23

13. Melamud E, Vastag L, Rabinowitz JD (2010) Metabolomic analysis and visualization engine for LC-MS data. Anal Chem 82:9818–9826

14. Smith CA, O'Maille G, Want EJ et al (2005) METLIN: a metabolite mass spectral database. Ther Drug Monit 27:747–751

15. Zhu Z-J, Schultz AW, Wang J et al (2013) Liquid chromatography quadrupole time-of-flight mass spectrometry characterization of metabolites guided by the METLIN database. Nat Protoc 8:451–460

16. Yuan J, Bennett BD, Rabinowitz JD (2008) Kinetic flux profiling for quantitation of cellular metabolic fluxes. Nat Protoc 3:1328–1340

17. Kell DB, Brown M, Davey HM et al (2005) Metabolic footprinting and systems biology: the medium is the message. Nat Rev Microbiol 3:557–565

18. Wu L, Chen S x, Jiang X g et al (2012) Separation and purification of *Toxoplasma gondii* tachyzoites from in vitro and in vivo culture systems. Exp Parasitol 130:91–94

19. Carey MA, Covelli V, Brown A et al (2018) Influential parameters for the analysis of intracellular parasite metabolomics. 3(2):e00097-18

20. Fang M, Ivanisevic J, Benton HP et al (2015) Thermal degradation of small molecules: a global metabolomic investigation. Anal Chem 87:10935–10941

Chapter 23

Label-Based Mass Spectrometry Approaches for Robust Quantification of the Phosphoproteome and Total Proteome in *Toxoplasma gondii*

Malgorzata Broncel and Moritz Treeck

Abstract

Protein phosphorylation plays a key role in regulating biological processes. Over 30% of the proteome is phosphorylated in most organisms and unraveling the function of the kinases that mediate these phosphorylation events requires the technology to reliably measure phosphorylation on proteins under various conditions. Advances in mass-spectrometry instrumentation, sample preparation, and labeling technologies now offer a range of quantification methods, each with their advantages and disadvantages. Here we describe in detail two different quantification methods, that is, stable isotope labeling by amino acids in cell culture and tandem mass tagging, combined with phosphopeptide enrichment strategies to measure the phosphoproteome of *Toxoplasma* parasites.

Key words SILAC, TMT, LC-MS/MS, Phosphoproteome, Proteome, TiO_2, IMAC, High pH reverse phase fractionation, *Toxoplasma gondii*

---

1 Introduction

Phosphorylation is one of the most prevalent posttranslational modifications in *Toxoplasma* affecting >30% of the predicted proteome [1]. It regulates numerous cellular processes throughout the life cycle of this apicomplexan parasite. Moreover, phosphorylation appears to be a regulatory mechanism also outside the parasite boundaries [1] as it plays roles in the interaction of *Toxoplasma* with the host cell. Although several proteome-wide phosphoproteomic studies have been performed in *Toxoplasma* [1–5], robust and reliable quantification of phosphorylation sites within an intracellular parasite is not trivial.

Mass spectrometry (MS)-based proteomics provides a powerful approach for analysing the phosphorylation state of cell. This technique allows not only proteome wide phosphopeptide identification but also robust quantification of thousands of individual phosphorylation sites. Importantly, quantitative information

Christopher J. Tonkin (ed.), *Toxoplasma gondii: Methods and Protocols*, Methods in Molecular Biology, vol. 2071, https://doi.org/10.1007/978-1-4939-9857-9_23, © Springer Science+Business Media, LLC, part of Springer Nature 2020

about the total proteome, that is, all nonphosphorylated peptides, can be obtained within the same workflow to ensure that differential phosphorylation is not due to changes in protein level. Quantitation of phosphorylation can be accomplished by employing either label-free or label-based approaches, each having their particular pros and cons [6]. Label-free workflows are straightforward, flexible in terms of experimental design and cost effective, however they suffer from reproducibility issues as each sample is processed separately and variability can be introduced during each of the many steps in the phosphoproteomic workflow. Moreover, as each sample is analyzed individually during LC-MS/MS, data acquisition times are high and reliable quantification depends heavily on the reproducibility of chromatographic separations. Label-based techniques on the other hand take advantage of metabolic (e.g., stable isotope labeling by amino acids in cell culture, SILAC) or isobaric (e.g., tandem mass tags, TMT) tagging of proteins or peptides, respectively [7, 8]. Each sample/replicate is labeled with a different reagent with a specific mass and mixed (multiplexed) early in the proteomic workflow. The multiplexed sample is then processed and LC-MS/MS analyzed as one entity thus bypassing problems with variability and reproducibility of label-free approaches. As the mass difference between the labeled peptides derived from each sample/ replicate is known, the multiplexed sample can be deconvoluted and individual quantifications extracted (Fig. 1). Although the number of samples/replicates to be directly compared in label-based experiments is limited (currently 10 for TMT) and the associated sample preparation cost is much higher than in label-free workflows, both SILAC and TMT-based quantitative phosphoproteome profiling gained wide popularity due to generally more confident quantifications and multiplexed data acquisition. It is worth emphasizing that SILAC and TMT strategies can, in principle, be used interchangeably (even as orthogonal validation) in addressing biological phenomena, the only limitation being the multiplexing capability of each approach (3-plex and 10-plex, respectively).

In this chapter, we present detailed protocols for SILAC and TMT-based quantitative proteomics (phospho and proteome) of intracellular *Toxoplasma gondii*. Our protocol describes metabolic as well as TMT sample labeling strategies, two-step sequential phosphopeptide enrichment and fractionation for improved phosphosite coverage. In addition, we present details of our routine MS acquisition methods, including the recently developed MultiNotch MS3 strategy for TMT [9]. Finally, we provide examples of SILAC and TMT data processing/analysis by the freely available MaxQuant/Perseus software platforms [10, 11]. In our SILAC-based quantitative proteomic workflow (Fig. 1a) parasites are cultured in media containing unlabeled arginine or lysine (henceforth referred to as "light") or media containing 13C15N arginine and 13C15N

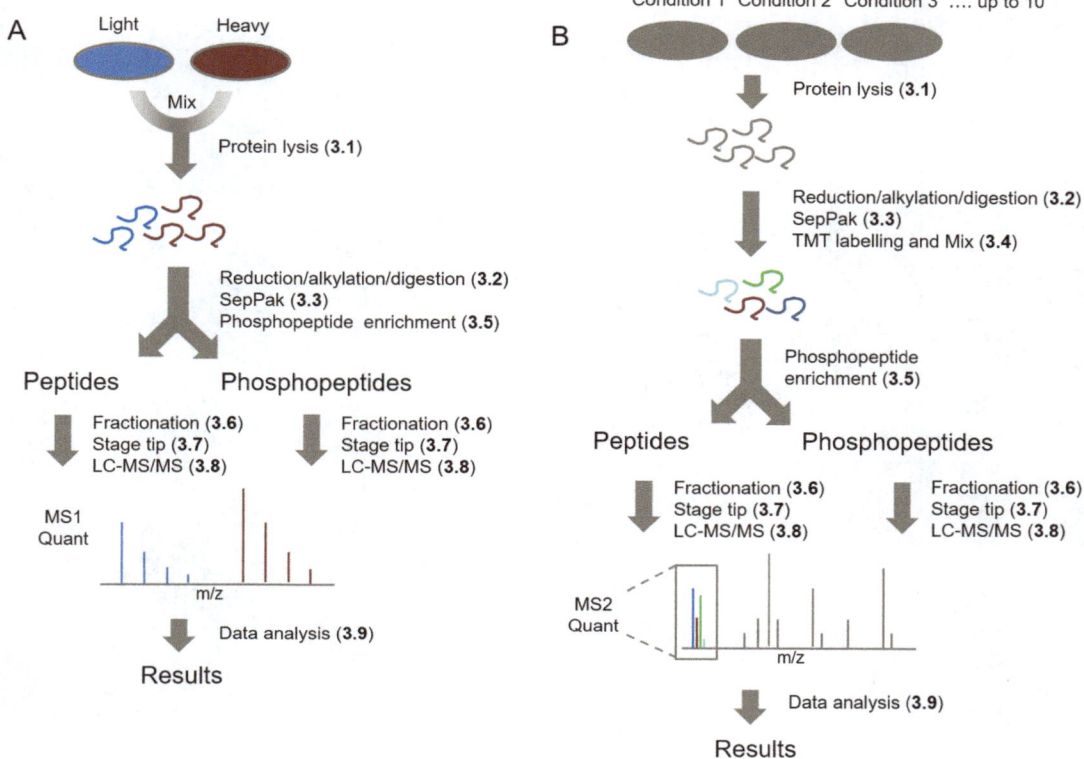

Fig. 1 Schematic representation of phosphoproteomic workflows for **(a)** SILAC and **(b)** TMT labeled samples

lysine (henceforth referred to as "heavy") and after protein extraction with urea-based buffers the samples are mixed in 1:1 ratio. Following cysteine reduction and alkylation, proteins are digested to peptides and after purification on SepPak phosphopeptides are extracted by two consecutive metal-based affinity enrichments, namely titanium dioxide (TiO_2) and immobilized metal affinity chromatography (IMAC). Enriched phosphopeptides as well as a fraction of the flowthrough that contains all nonphosphorylated peptides (i.e., total proteome) are fractionated and subjected to a final desalting step before LC-MS/MS analysis on a Q-Exactive mass spectrometer. In our TMT-based quantitative proteomic workflow (Fig. 1b) parasites are cultured in standard media. Each sample/replicate is then lysed and its protein content quantified. Equivalent amounts of each sample are then reduced, alkylated, digested, and SepPak purified. Next the samples are separately TMT labeled and then combined. Salts and unreacted TMT reagents are then removed via SepPak. Phosphopeptides are isolated from the total proteome by the two-step sequential enrichment followed by sample fractionation (as above) before LC-MS/MS analysis on a Fusion Lumos mass spectrometer. Generated raw data is then analyzed with MaxQuant/Perseus. Application of the

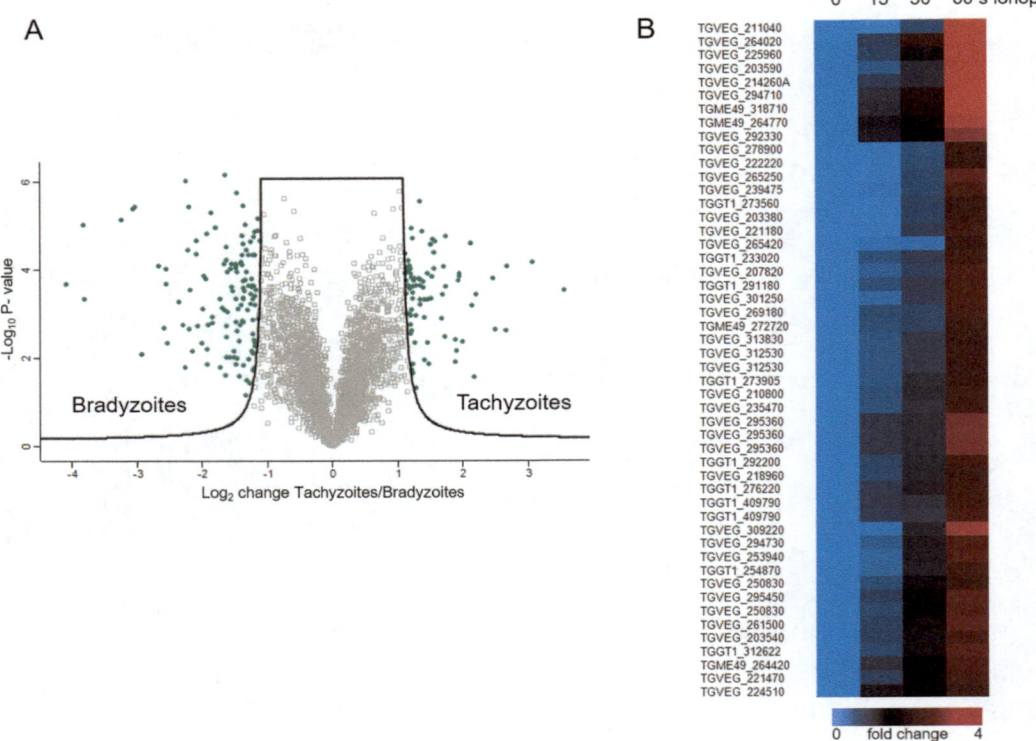

Fig. 2 Examples of quantification of changes in phosphorylation (**a**) during stage conversion from tachyzoites to bradyzoites using SILAC and (**b**) during time course of ionophore treatment of intracellular *Toxoplasma gondii* using TMT labeling; color coding in the heat map (scale at the bottom) represents fold change (log2 treated/untreated) in phosphorylation level between conditions

abovementioned quantitative workflows allowed us to profile phosphorylation changes during stage conversion in *Toxoplasma gondii* in case of SILAC (Fig. 2a) as well as during time course of ionophore treatment in case of TMT labeling (Fig. 2b). Despite the fact that host background constituted up to 70% of our samples we were able to robustly identify and quantify thousands of phosphorylation sites in *Toxoplasma gondii*.

2   Materials

Prepare all buffers and solutions using LC-MS grade solvents (water, acetonitrile and methanol) and use low protein-binding microcentrifuge tubes for sample handling.

2.1   Cell Culture, Lysis, and Protein Concentration Determination

1. *Toxoplasma* strain RH and Prugniaud (Pru).

2. Culture media:
   (a) TMT experiments: DMEM GlutaMAX supplemented with 10% FBS.

(b) SILAC experiments: DMEM containing 13C15N arginine and 13C15N lysine (R10K8) heavy media and DMEM containing unlabeled arginine and lysine (R0K0) light media supplemented with 10% dialyzed FBS; stage conversion media: RPMI pH 8.1 supplemented with 1% dialyzed FBS.

3. 8 μM calcium ionophore A23187 in Ringer's buffer.

4. Lysis buffer: 8 M urea with protease and phosphatase inhibitors, prepare fresh and place on ice before cell lysis.

5. PBS.

6. Pierce bicinchoninic acid (BCA) assay kit.

2.2 Protein Reduction, Alkylation, and Digestion

1. 50 mM ammonium bicarbonate.

2. 0.5 M dithiothreitol (DTT) in 50 mM ammonium bicarbonate. Prepare fresh just before use.

3. 1 M iodoacetamide (IAA) in 50 mM ammonium bicarbonate. Prepare fresh, protect from light.

4. MS grade LysC and Trypsin.

5. Trifluoroacetic acid.

2.3 Peptide Desalting on SepPak

1. C18 SepPak Light cartridges 100 mg.

2. Vacuum manifold.

3. Acetonitrile.

4. 50% acetonitrile/0.5% acetic acid.

5. 0.1% trifluoroacetic acid.

6. 0.5% acetic acid.

7. Vacuum centrifuge.

2.4 TMT Labeling

1. TMT 10-plex kit.

2. 50 mM Na-Hepes pH 8.5.

3. Dry acetonitrile.

4. 5% hydroxylamine in 50 mM Na-Hepes pH 8.5.

5. Formic acid.

6. Vacuum centrifuge.

7. Ultrasonic bath.

2.5 Phosphopeptide Enrichment

1. Titanium dioxide:
   (a) Titansphere beads.
   (b) Loading buffer: 80% acetonitrile/5% trifluoroacetic acid/1 M glycolic acid.
   (c) Wash buffer 1: 80% acetonitrile/1% trifluoroacetic acid.

(d) Wash buffer 2: 10% acetonitrile/0.2% trifluoroacetic acid.

(e) Elution buffer 1: 1% ammonium hydroxide.

(f) Elution buffer 2: 5% ammonium hydroxide.

(g) Vacuum centrifuge.

(h) Ultrasonic bath.

2. IMAC:

(a) High-Select™ Fe-NTA Phosphopeptide Enrichment Kit (product no. A32992).

(b) Water.

(c) pH paper.

(d) Vacuum centrifuge.

(e) Ultrasonic bath.

2.6 High pH Reverse-Phase Fractionation

1. Pierce High pH Peptide Fractionation Kit (product no. 84868).

2. Water.

3. Acetonitrile.

4. 0.1% trifluoroacetic acid.

5. 2% trifluoroacetic acid.

6. Vacuum centrifuge.

7. Ultrasonic bath.

2.7 Stage Tip

1. 3M Empore™ Solid Phase Extraction Disks C18.

2. 200 μL pipette tips.

3. Methanol.

4. 1% trifluoroacetic acid.

5. 50% acetonitrile/5% trifluoroacetic acid.

6. Vacuum centrifuge.

7. Ultrasonic bath.

2.8 LC-MS/MS

1. 50-cm Easy Spray PepMap column (75 μm inner diameter, 2 μm particle size).

2. Dionex Ultimate 3000 RSLC nano.

3. HPLC solvent A: 0.1% formic acid/5% DMSO.

4. HPLC solvent B: 80% acetonitrile/0.1% formic acid/5% DMSO.

5. QExactive mass spectrometer.

6. Fusion Lumos mass spectrometer.

2.9   Data Analysis

1. MaxQuant http://coxdocs.org/doku.php?id=maxquant:start
2. Perseus http://coxdocs.org/doku.php?id=perseus:start

---

3   Methods

3.1   Cell Culture, Lysis, and Protein Concentration Determination

Cell culture conditions and parasite lines used will vary depending on the user defined biological question under investigation.

1. For TMT-based experiments grow RH parasites in DMEM Glutamax supplemented with 10% FBS. Infect one T150 flask of confluent human foreskin fibroblasts (HFFs) per condition with fivefold excess of *Toxoplasma*, that is, at MOI = 5. After 24 h wash with 10 mL of PBS and treat intracellular parasites with 8 μM calcium ionophore on a heated plate at 37 °C for 0, 15, 30, and 60 s.

2. For SILAC-based experiments grow Pru parasites in heavy/light media for at least 6–7 lytic cycles to ensure efficient (>90%) heavy label incorporation (*see* **Note 1**). To induce stage conversion, change light media to the stage conversion media and culture for 3 days at 37 °C and ambient CO_2 level. Use at least one infected T150 flask of HFFs per heavy/light condition, wash with PBS (2×) before lysis.

3. Lyse intracellular parasites on ice with 3 mL of ice-cold lysis buffer, scrape vigorously and collect into 15 mL Falcon tubes.

4. Sonicate lysates on ice (3 × 30 s at 30% duty cycle) and spin at 3200 × *g* for 20 min to remove insoluble material.

5. Remove a 100 μL aliquot and determine protein concentration (*see* **Note 2**).

3.2   Protein Reduction, Alkylation, and Digestion

1. For TMT experiments take equivalent amounts of protein for each sample/replicate (*see* **Note 3**).

2. For SILAC experiments mix heavy and light lysate in 1:1 ratio (*see* **Note 4**).

3. Place protein lysates in 15 mL Falcon tubes and add freshly prepared 0.5 M DTT solution to obtain a final concentration of 5 mM. Vortex samples and incubate at 56 °C for 30 min.

4. Allow samples to cool down to room temperature and add fresh solution of 1 M IAA to obtain a final concentration of 14 mM. Briefly vortex and incubate in the dark for 30 min.

5. Quench the reaction with DTT (add equal volume as above) and incubate 15 min in the dark.

6. Dilute samples 2× with 50 mM ammonium bicarbonate to reduce the concentration of urea to <4 M, add LysC and incubate at least 2 h at 37 °C (*see* **Note 5**).

7. Dilute samples 2× with 50 mM ammonium bicarbonate to reduce the concentration of urea to <2 M and add trypsin at a ratio of 1:50 (enzyme to protein). Incubate overnight at 37 °C.

8. Place on ice for 10 min and quench trypsin with trifluoroacetic acid (4 μL/1 mL of lysate), then leave on ice for 10 additional min.

9. Spin at full speed for 20 min and recover the supernatant.

3.3 Peptide Purification on SepPak

1. Use C18 SepPak Lite, 100 mg bed volume (maximum sample load 5 mg per column) in conjunction with a vacuum manifold to desalt the samples.

2. Wash SepPak with 3 mL of acetonitrile.

3. Condition SepPak with 1 mL 50% acetonitrile/0.5% acetic acid.

4. Equilibrate SepPak with 3 mL 0.1% trifluoroacetic acid.

5. Load sample (acidified supernatant from Subheading 3.2).

6. Desalt sample with 3 mL of 0.1% trifluoroacetic acid.

7. Wash with 1 mL of 0.5% acetic acid.

8. Elute peptides with 1.2 mL of 50% acetonitrile/0.5% acetic acid.

9. Dry eluates by vacuum centrifugation.

3.4 TMT Labeling

1. Dissolve samples at 1 mg/mL in 50 mM Na-Hepes pH 8.5 then add acetonitrile to a final concentration of 30% (v/v).

2. TMT reagents are prepared fresh. Equilibrate frozen TMT reagents at RT for 15 min and spin quickly to collect at the bottom of the tube. Dissolve TMT reagents with acetonitrile (41 μL per 0.8 mg of reagent), incubate for 5 min, mix occasionally and spin down before adding reagents to samples (*see* **Note 6**).

3. Mix gently and incubate for 1 h at RT.

4. Quench unreacted TMT reagents with 5% hydroxylamine/50 mM Na-Hepes pH 8.5 to get a final concentration of 0.3% (v/v) and incubate for 15 min at RT.

5. Acidify with formic acid to pH~2 (check on pH paper).

6. Mix 2 μL of each labeling reaction and dilute to 300 μL with 1% formic acid. Stage tip (*see* Subheading 3.7) and run test LC-MS/MS (*see* Subheading 3.8 and Table 1, section 3.8.2) to check equal protein labeling (reporter intensity) between conditions. If no ratio variation >1.5 is observed, mix all at 1:1 ratio and speedvac to dryness (*see* **Note 7**).

7. Purify via SepPak (*see* **Note 8** and proceed as in Subheading 3.3) and speedvac to dryness.

3.5 Phosphopeptide Enrichment

3.5.1 Titanium Dioxide

All centrifugation steps are performed for 1 min at $2000 \times g$

1. Weigh out 5 mg of titanium dioxide beads per 1–2 mg of sample (*see* **Note 9**).

2. Add 1 mL of loading buffer to each sample and sonicate for 20 min.

3. Add the fully solubilized sample to the beads and vortex the suspension for 10 min.

4. Spin the samples down, remove most of the supernatant (do not disturb the beads) and store it at $-80\ ^\circ$C for the subsequent IMAC enrichment (*see* Subheading 3.5.2).

5. Add 150 µL of loading buffer to the beads for the first wash step, agitate for 10 min, spin down then remove the supernatant and discard.

6. Add 150 µL of 80% acetonitrile/1% trifluoroacetic acid to the beads for the second wash step, agitate for 10 min, spin down then remove the supernatant and discard.

7. Add 150 µL of 10% acetonitrile/0.2% trifluoroacetic acid to the beads for the third wash step, agitate for 10 min, spin down then remove the supernatant and discard.

8. The beads and bound phosphopeptides have now been washed. Dry the beads in a vacuum centrifuge for 30 min.

9. Phosphopeptides must now be eluted from the beads using successive high pH solutions. Add 100 µL of 1% ammonium hydroxide to the beads for the first elution step, agitate for 10 min, spin down then collect the supernatant.

10. Add 100 µL of 5% ammonium hydroxide to the beads for the second elution step, agitate for 10 min, spin down then collect the supernatant and combine with the first elution.

11. Dry eluates by vacuum centrifugation immediately and store at $-80\ ^\circ$C (*see* **Note 10**).

3.5.2 IMAC

IMAC enrichment is performed according to the manufacturer's instructions. All centrifugation steps are performed for 30 s at $1000 \times g$.

1. SepPak purify the titanium dioxide supernatant from Subheading 3.5.1 point 4 above (*see* **Note 11** and Subheading 3.3).

2. Solubilize desalted samples in 200–500 µL of Binding/Wash Buffer in an ultrasonic bath for 20 min. Use pH paper to verify that sample pH is <3.

3. Remove the bottom closure of the spin column and loosen the screw cap. Place column in a 2 mL microcentrifuge collection tube and spin down to remove storage buffer.

4. Add 200 µL of Binding/Wash Buffer, spin down and discard the flowthrough. Repeat this step once.

5. Cap the bottom of the column with a white Luer plug. Place the column with the plug into the empty microcentrifuge tube.

6. To bind phosphopeptides add the suspended peptide sample to the equilibrated spin column. Mix by pipetting up and down once and incubate for 30 min.

7. Carefully remove the bottom plug and loosen the screw cap. Place the column into the microcentrifuge tube, spin down, retain the flowthrough and store at −80 °C (*see* **Note 12**).

8. Wash column by adding 200 µL of Binding/Wash Buffer. Spin down, discard the flowthrough and repeat this step two additional times for a total of three washes.

9. Wash column by adding 200 µL of LC-MS grade water, spin down and discard the flowthrough.

10. To elute phosphopeptides place column in a new microcentrifuge tube and add 100 µL of Elution Buffer. Spin down and retain the eluate. Repeat this step once.

11. Dry the combined eluates immediately in a vacuum concentrator (*see* **Note 10**). Store at −80 °C.

3.6 High pH Reverse-Phase Fractionation

Fractionation is performed according to the manufacturer's instructions.

1. Remove the protective white tip from the bottom of the column and place the column into a 2 mL sample tube. Centrifuge at $5000 \times g$ for 2 min to remove the solution and pack the resin material. Discard the liquid.

2. To condition the column load 300 µL of acetonitrile, place the spin column back into a 2 mL sample tube and centrifuge at $5000 \times g$ for 2 min. Discard acetonitrile and repeat once.

3. Wash the spin column twice with 0.1% trifluoroacetic acid solution as above. The column is now ready for use.

4. Dissolve up to 100 µg of sample (*see* **Note 13**) in 300 µL of 2% trifluoroacetic acid solution using a sonicating bath.

5. Place the spin column into a new 2 mL sample tube. Load 300 µL of the sample solution onto the column and centrifuge at $3000 \times g$ for 2 min. Discard the flowthrough.

6. Place the column into a new 2 mL sample tube. Load 300 µL of water onto the column and centrifuge again. Discard the flowthrough.

7. Place the column into a new 2 mL sample tube. Load 300 μL of the appropriate elution solution prepared depending on the sample type:

    (a) For the phosphoproteome prepare eight solutions with increasing concentration of acetonitrile (5%, 7.5%, 10%, 12.5%, 15%, 17.5%, 20%, and 50%) in 0.1% triethylamine,

    (b) for the TMT labeled proteome prepare nine solutions with increasing concentration of acetonitrile (5%, 10%, 12.5%, 15%, 17.5%, 20%, 22.5%, 25%, and 50%) in 0.1% triethylamine,

    centrifuge at $3000 \times g$ for 2 min to collect the eluates (*see* **Note 14**).

8. Evaporate the liquid contents of each fraction to dryness using vacuum centrifugation (*see* **Note 10**).

3.7 Stage Tip

1. Prepare stage tips with Empore C18 membrane and pack into a 200 μL pipette tips (*see* **Note 15**).

2. Resuspend peptides in 100 μL of 1% trifluoroacetic acid using a sonicating bath for 20 min.

3. Wash each tip with 100 μL methanol using centrifugation ($1000 \times g$, 2 min).

4. Equilibrate each tip with 200 μL of 1% trifluoroacetic acid using centrifugation ($1000 \times g$, 3 min).

5. Load and bind the samples using centrifugation ($250 \times g$, 3 min).

6. Wash each tip with 300 μL of 1% trifluoroacetic acid using centrifugation ($1000 \times g$, 3 min). Repeat for a total of two washes (*see* **Note 16**).

7. Elute peptides with 50 μL of 50% acetonitrile/5% trifluoroacetic acid by centrifugation ($250 \times g$, 2 min).

8. Take to dryness by vacuum centrifugation and store at $-80\,°C$.

3.8 LC-MS/MS

Dissolve samples in LC-MS grade 0.1% trifluoroacetic acid, sonicate for 20 min and spin down ($21,000 \times g$, 20 min) to remove any insoluble material. Transfer to autosampler vials and load on a 50 cm Easy Spray PepMap column equipped with an integrated electrospray emitter. Perform reverse phase chromatography using the RSLC nano with a binary buffer system (solvent A: 0.1% formic acid/5% DMSO; solvent B: 80% acetonitrile/0.1% formic acid/5% DMSO) at a flow rate of 250 nL/min. Run SILAC samples on a linear gradient of 2–35% B in 90 min with a total run time of 120 min, including column conditioning. Run TMT labeled samples on a linear gradient of 5–35% B in 140 min followed by 35–60% B in 10 min with a total run time of 180 min including column conditioning (*see* **Note 17**). Specific MS and MS/MS scan

Table 1
Mass spectrometry acquisition parameters for SILAC (3.8.1) and TMT (3.8.2, 3.8.3) labeled samples

	SILAC (3.8.1)	TMT (MS2) (3.8.2)	TMT (MS3) (3.8.3)
Instrument	QExactive	Fusion Lumos	Fusion Lumos
Run time	120 min	180 min	180 min
Detector	Orbitrap	Orbitrap	Orbitrap
Full MS scan	300–1800 *m/z*	400–1400 *m/z*	400–1500 *m/z*
Resolution	70,000	120,000	120,000
AGC target	1e6	4e5	4e5
Max IT	250 ms	100 ms	50 ms
Exclusion	20 s	60 s	60 s
MS2 scan	from 100 *m/z*	from 100 *m/z*	400–1200 *m/z*
Resolution	17,500	50,000	30,000
AGC target	5e4	2e5	5e4
Max IT	120 ms	86 ms	80 ms
Loop	10 most abundant	3 s	3 s
Isolation window	2 *m/z*	0.7 *m/z*	0.7 *m/z*
Collision energy	28	38	35
Activation type	HCD	HCD	CID
Multistage activation	No	No	Yes
MS3 scan	NA	NA	100–500 *m/z*
SPS precursors			5
Resolution			60,000
AGC target			1e5
Max IT			105
Isolation window			2 *m/z*
Collision energy			65
Activation type			HCD

parameters for SILAC and TMT acquisition are summarized in Table 1 (*see* **Note 18**).

3.9 Data Analysis

3.9.1 MaxQuant

Load raw data files to MaxQuant (*see* **Note 19**). Use *Toxoplasma gondii* (ToxoDB [12]) and *Homo sapiens* (UniProt [13]) proteome fasta files (*see* **Note 20**) to enable peptide identification from the acquired MS/MS spectra. Select cysteine carbamidomethylation as a fixed modification whereas methionine oxidation, acetylation of protein N-terminus, and phosphorylation as variable modifications. Set the enzyme specificity to trypsin with maximum of two missed cleavages. The following parameters are preset in the software: precursor mass tolerance for the first search (20 ppm) and for the main search (4.5 ppm), false discovery rate on protein, peptide, and site level (1%). Enable "Unique and razor peptides" mode to allow identification and quantification of proteins in groups (razor peptides are uniquely assigned to protein groups and not to individual proteins) and "Match between runs" option for fractionated samples (time window 0.7 min). For SILAC: set experiment type as standard and multiplicity to 2 (for double SILAC). Specify heavy labels used (e.g., Arg10 and Lys8) and enable "Re-quantify" feature. For TMT: set experiment type as reporter ion MS2 or MS3 (depending on the used LC-MS/MS method) and specify the isobaric labels (e.g., 10-plex TMT, *see* **Note 21**) as well as the reporter mass tolerance (we use 0.003 Da).

3.9.2   Perseus

Process MaxQuant search results further using Perseus (*see* **Note 22**). For phosphosite quantification analysis load Phospho(STY)sites.txt (*see* **Note 23**) whereas for total proteome quantification analysis load ProteinGroups.txt. Filter data to remove contaminants and IDs originating from reverse decoy sequences. For total proteome analysis remove also entries only identified by site. Log2 transform H/L ratios (SILAC) or reporter intensities (TMT) and log10 transform intensities (total, H, L). Check sample distribution (histogram) and normalize by median subtraction to remove systematic bias. Filter data for at least one valid value to remove nonquantified entries. Perform statistical analysis (*see* **Note 24**) to identify significantly changing phosphosites or protein levels. Correlate phosphosite quantification with protein abundance derived from the acquired experimental data to ensure that differential phosphorylation is not due to change in protein level. To ensure high confidence in peptide/protein IDs monitor such parameters as PEP, peptide score, razor and unique peptides and sequence coverage (*see* **Note 25**). For confident phosphosite assignment apply localization probability and localization score difference cut offs of $\geq 90\%$ and ≥ 10, respectively. For quantification control, verify raw MS1 (SILAC) and MS2/MS3 (TMT) scans to ensure correct assignment of labeling pairs and reporter ions, respectively.

4   Notes

1. We routinely confirm heavy label incorporation via MS whereby 20 µg of heavy lysate is processed (reduced, alkylated, and digested) and an aliquot equivalent to 500 ng of protein injected onto LC-MS/MS (*see* Subheading 3.8 and Table 1, section 3.8.1). In addition, sample labeling should be performed in forward as well as reversed manner. Reverse labeled samples serve as quantification controls as well as biological replicates. Finally, once heavy labeled parasites have been obtained they can be frozen down and stored for subsequent experiments.

2. We use the Pierce BCA assay for quantifying protein concentration, however any available method that is compatible with urea should suffice. The BCA kit allows up to 3 M urea therefore samples need to be diluted accordingly (1:3 in our case).

3. We usually take between 0.5 and 1 mg of protein per condition.

4. We usually work with 1 mg of protein per condition.

5. In order to decrease the number of trypsin missed cleavages we pretreat our samples with LysC. We generally use 30 μg of enzyme per TMT 10-plex and 5 μg per SILAC sample. Incubate lysates with LysC for 2–5 h at 37 °C.

6. We use the medium size TMT 10-plex kit (product no. 90111) which contains 3×0.8 mg per TMT label. According to the manufacturer instructions 0.8 mg of reagent can label 25–100 μg of digested proteins. We and others however found that 0.8 mg of reagent is sufficient to label 300–350 μg. For labeling of 1 mg of digested proteins we pool all three vials together (2.4 mg reagent total).

7. In addition to mixing checks we also verify individual label incorporation (routinely >98%). For this we take 5 μL aliquot of each labeling reaction, dilute in 100 μL of 1% formic acid and stage tip before LC-MS/MS (we use a 65 min method on QExactive, MS1 scan as in 3.8.1, MS2 scan parameters: Resolution 35,000, AGC target 1e5, max IT 60 ms). Freeze the lysates at −80 °C while performing MS verification.

8. For TMT 10-plex with 1 mg protein per condition we divide the sample in two equal parts to ensure that protein load is <5 mg per SepPak (max. loading capacity is 5 mg for a 100 mg SepPak).

9. In case of TMT labeled samples we use 1 mL of loading buffer per 2 mg protein and then divide the sample to get 2 mg protein per 5 mg of titanium dioxide beads. For example, in case of TMT 10-plex experiment with 1 mg protein per condition (10 mg total), we dissolve in 5 mL of loading buffer and divide in five samples (2 mg each per 5 mg of beads).

10. Phosphopeptides are not stable under basic conditions and cannot be stored in elution buffer. In case when immediate sample drying is not possible, acidify the elution with formic acid (to a final concentration of 3%).

11. For TMT labeled samples we combine the titanium dioxide supernatants. In case the total protein amount is >5 mg divide this pooled sample between two SepPaks. After desalting we again divide the sample to get ca. 2 mg per IMAC column.

12. Be careful as the manufacturer's instruction says discard the flowthrough at this point. The flowthrough contains all unbound peptides, that is, the total proteome necessary to validate that any quantified changes in phosphorylation are not due to the altered protein level. Therefore we need to *retain* the flowthrough.

13. In case of the phosphoproteome we pool samples from both enrichment steps (TiO_2 and IMAC). We estimate phosphopeptide content to be ca. 3% of the total protein, so in case of a TMT 10-plex experiment with 1 mg protein per label (10 mg total) this would be roughly 300 µg and would require three fractionation columns (100 µg capacity each). In case of the total proteome we remove an aliquot equivalent to a 100 µg of protein (from Subheading 3.5.2, **step 7**), speedvac to dryness and dissolve in 300 µL of 2% trifluoroacetic acid.

14. TMT-labeled proteome samples require an additional column wash with 300 µL of 5% acetonitrile/0.1% triethylamine to remove unreacted TMT reagent. Discard this first wash fraction.

15. Prepare stage tips (one per sample) by cutting a little disc of the membrane with a blunt needle (18 Gauge) and pack with a capillary. Ensure that the disc is tightly packed in the tip to prevent sample loss during loading.

16. For TMT labeled proteome samples (e.g., the mixing check or individual label incorporation check), add a third wash step with 200 µL of 5% acetonitrile/1% trifluoroacetic acid to remove unreacted TMT labels.

17. We use longer LC methods with extended gradient for TMT labeled samples due to larger initial sample size and increased hydrophobicity of TMT labeled peptides, respectively, compared to SILAC experiments.

18. For total proteome analysis: in case of SILAC we use acquisition parameters listed in Table 1, section 3.8.1 with the following modifications in MS2 scan parameters: max IT 50 ms; for TMT we use acquisition parameters listed in Table 1, section 3.8.2 with the following modifications in MS2 scan parameters: AGC target 5e4, max IT 54 ms.

19. For introduction to MaxQuant *see* [10].

20. Generate fasta files (we use ToxoDB and UniProt) and add to Andromeda (search engine integrated into MaxQuant) sequence databases using the following parsing rules >([^]*) for *T. gondii* and >.*\|(.*)\| for human.

21. Update correction factors (specification sheet is provided with the TMT kit) for each TMT label in Andromeda modifications list.

22. For introduction to Perseus *see* [11].

23. It is important to also check phosphoenrichment efficiency, for this load Modification specific peptides.txt and calculate percentage of phosphorylated vs all quantified peptides.

24. After verifying normal sample distribution we usually apply t-test based statistics. To ensure enough statistical power we

most frequently perform our experiments in biological triplicates. When correcting for multiple hypothesis testing, we use
Benjamini–Hochberg FDR.

25. In general PEP should be small (< 0.01) as this is the probability that a given PSM is incorrect, peptide score should be
high (for modified peptides >40), number of razor and unique
peptides per protein should be >2, and the higher the
sequence coverage the better.

Acknowledgments

This work was supported by funding to M.T. from the Francis
Crick Institute (https://www.crick.ac.uk/), which receives its core
funding from Cancer Research UK (FC001189; https://www.can
cerresearchuk.org), the UK Medical Research Council (FC001189;
https://www.mrc.ac.uk/), and the Wellcome Trust (FC001189;
https://wellcome.ac.uk/). M.B. and M.T. are also supported by a
grant from the NIH (R01AI123457).

References

1. Treeck M, Sanders JL, Elias JE, Boothroyd JC
(2011) The phosphoproteomes of plasmodium
falciparum and *Toxoplasma gondii* reveal
unusual adaptations within and beyond the
parasites' boundaries. Cell Host Microbe
10:410–419

2. Treeck M, Sanders JL, Gaji RY et al (2014) The
calcium-dependent protein kinase 3 of *Toxoplasma* influences basal calcium levels and functions beyond egress as revealed by quantitative
phosphoproteome analysis. PLoS Pathog 10:
e1004197

3. McCoy JM, Stewart RJ, Uboldi AD et al (2017)
A forward genetic screen identifies a negative
regulator of rapid Ca^{2+}–dependent cell egress
(MS1) in the intracellular parasite *Toxoplasma
gondii*. J Biol Chem 292:7662–7674

4. Nebl T, Prieto JH, Kapp E et al (2011) Quantitative in vivo analyses reveal calcium-
dependent phosphorylation sites and identifies
a novel component of the *Toxoplasma* invasion
motor complex. PLoS Pathog 7:e1002222

5. Jia Y, Marq JB, Bisio H et al (2017) Crosstalk
between PKA and PKG controls
pH-dependent host cell egress of *Toxoplasma
gondii*. EMBO J 36:3250–3267

6. Riley NM, Coon JJ (2016) Phosphoproteomics in the age of rapid and deep proteome
profiling. Anal Chem 88:74–94

7. Ong SE, Blagoev B, Kratchmarova I et al
(2002) Stable isotope labeling by amino acids
in cell culture, SILAC, as a simple and accurate
approach to expression proteomics. Mol Cell
Proteomics 1:376–386

8. Thompson A, Schäfer J, Kuhn K et al (2003)
Tandem mass tags: a novel quantification strategy for comparative analysis of complex protein
mixtures by MS/MS. Anal Chem
75:1895–1904

9. McAlister GC, Nusinow DP, Jedrychowski
MP et al (2014) MultiNotch MS3 enables
accurate, sensitive, and multiplexed detection of differential expression across cancer
cell line proteomes. Anal Chem
86:7150–7158

10. Tyanova S, Temu T, Cox J (2016) The Max-
Quant computational platform for mass
spectrometry-based shotgun proteomics. Nat
Protoc 11:2301–2319

11. Tyanova S, Temu T, Sinitcyn P et al (2016) The
Perseus computational platform for compre-
hensive analysis of (prote)omics data. Nat
Methods 13:731–740

12. http://toxodb.org/toxo/

13. UniProt C (2015) UniProt: a hub for protein
information. Nucleic Acids Res 43:
D204–D212

INDEX

Christopher J. Tonkin (ed.), *Toxoplasma gondii: Methods and Protocols*, Methods in Molecular Biology, vol. 2071,
https://doi.org/10.1007/978-1-4939-9857-9, © Springer Science+Business Media, LLC, part of Springer Nature 2020